W9-BKU-391

REVIEW COPY

Please submit two tear sheets of review.

U.S. list price: $159.00

Monophasic Action Potentials

Bridging Cell and Bedside

Edited by

Michael R. Franz, MD, PhD

Professor of Medicine and Pharmacology
Georgetown University Medical Center
Director of Cardiac Electrophysiology
Division of Cardiology
Veterans Affairs Medical Center
Washington, DC

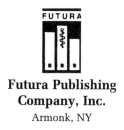

Futura Publishing Company, Inc.
Armonk, NY

Library of Congress Cataloging-in-Publication Data

Monophasic action potentials : bridging cell and bedside / edited by
   Michael R. Franz.
      p.   cm.
   Includes bibliographical references ad index.
   ISBN 0-87993-430-1 (alk. paper)
   1. Electrocardiography.   2. Heart—Electric properties.
3. Arrhythmias.   I. Franz, M. R. (Michael R.), 1949–   .
   [DNLM: 1. Action Potentials—physiology.   2. Arrhythmia—
physiopathology.   3. Anti-Arrhythmia Agents.
4. Electrocardiography.   5. Heart Conduction System—
physiopathology.   WG 330 M7512 1999]
   RC683.5.E5M65   1999
   616.1'207547—dc21
   DNLM/DLC
   for Library of Congress   99–25522
                                                                              CIP

Copyright © 2000
Futura Publishing Company, Inc.

Published by
Futura Publishing Company
135 Bedford Road
Armonk, New York 10504

LC#: 99-25522
ISBN#: 0-87993-430-1

Printed in the United States on acid-free paper.

Foreword from the Basic Scientist's View

I am pleased and honored by Dr. Franz's request that I write a foreword for his book *Monophasic Action Potentials: Bridging Cell and Bedside.* I have not used the technique of recording monophasic action potentials for some time, but I welcome an opportunity to review some early studies made with Paul Cranefield and to summarize the conclusions we reached about the utility of the method.

Burdon-Sanderson and Page published what probably are the earliest records of monophasic "injury" potentials in 1883. Subsequently there were many recordings of the activity-dependent changes in potential differences between injured and normal cardiac muscle for which a variety of means were used to induce the injury. A problem with these studies was the tendency for the local injury to "heal" rather promptly with a consequent return of biphasic deflections. Scheutz used a combination of pressure and maintained suction to create long-lasting injury, and reviewed his own work and that of others in 1936. Subsequently, in 1938, Eyster showed that maintained suction provided stable records for reasonably long intervals, and Cranefield used this method in 1951 to study certain electrical characteristics of ventricular muscle during activity. In 1958 we joined Surawicz in an experiment that directly compared monophasic potentials and transmembrane action potentials recorded simultaneously from the isolated, perfused rabbit heart using the suction technique for one and a floating microelectrode for the other. We reevaluated these comparisons in 1960 in *Electrophysiology of the Heart.* We concluded that although there were some quantitative differences between monophasic records and records of transmembrane potential (ie, the value of the injury potential differed from that of the resting potential; in the monophasic record the relative value of the overshoot was exaggerated and the upstroke was slower and often distorted by fast deflections), the monophasic record provided an adequate representation of the voltage-time course of the plateau and phase 3 of repolarization.

In 1968 Surawicz and associates used suction electrode catheters to record monophasic potentials from human right atrium and right and left ventricular endocardium. They were discouraged from continuing this type of study because of evidence that the suction caused some degree of histologically demonstrable tissue damage. Most recently, in 1986, Franz demonstrated that stable and reliable monophasic tracings could be recorded from the human heart through the use of a catheter electrode and maintained pressure. Since then, this method has been used widely for studies on the in situ hearts of human and experimental animals and has provided a great deal of useful information on alterations in action potential duration, the time course of repolarization, and the occurrence of afterdepolarizations as a result of disease, drugs, and physiologic modulators. This is information about the electrical activity of the in situ heart that cannot be obtained by other means.

On final comment probably is worth while. It was recognized at the outset that the monophasic record reflected the potential difference between injured (depolarized) and normal myocardium and, thus, early records often were termed *injury potentials*. Regardless of the method used, injury always is present. There is no evidence, however, that this type of injury causes any adverse outcomes that might limit the use of this technique.

Brian F. Hoffman, MD
David Hosack
Professor of Pharmacology
Department of Pharmacology
Associate Dean
Columbia University
College of Physicians and
    Surgeons
New York, NY

Foreword from the Clinical Electrophysiologist's View

Potential Future Uses of Monophasic Action Potential Recordings

I am delighted to participate in some small way to this magnum opus on monophasic action potential (MAP) recordings. We are all deeply indebted to Dr. Michael Franz for making available to basic and clinical electrophysiologists a unique tool that allows for measurements of the "electrical soul" of cardiac cell. This volume aptly summarizes the incredible breadth of utilization of this tool in terms of adding to our understanding of basic electrophysiologic phenomena. Much of this is due to the ready availability of a tool that allows for faithful reproduction of cellular action potentials.

From the point of view of the clinician, I can see much wider use of the MAP recordings in clinical medicine. First, the recording of MAP at multiple cardiac sites gives the clinician important insights into the presence of inhomogeneities of repolarization. The hope remains that MAP recordings will help explain known electrocardiographic precursors that are associated with increased risk of sudden death. These include marked lengthening of the T wave and presence of abnormal U wave, as well as T wave alternans. Further explanation of the underlying mechanisms of these abnormalities may hopefully improve the clinician's ability to better define a population at high risk for sudden cardiac death. Recent exciting work has focused on the primacy of repolarization abnormalities in the genesis of ventricular fibrillation. The same arguments can be applied to the clinical situations of explaining how rapid atrial arrhythmias deteriorate into atrial fibrillation.

In addition, I would imagine that with further refinements (elimination of motion artifacts), MAP recordings might eventually be used for intracardiac mapping. The limitations of both unipolar and bipolar electrode recordings as mapping tools are well appreciated. In contrast, the very sharp upstroke of the MAP recording allows for precise delineation of cellular activation, better lending itself to automated analyses of complex rhythms.

One additional clinical use of MAP recordings is in the assessment of antiarrhythmic drugs. The MAP recording allows for precise delineation of changes in refractoriness, and allows for the elucidation of use dependency effects of drugs. In addition, multiple recordings allow for assessment of drug-induced effects on the homogeneity of changes in cellular refractoriness in response to drugs' effects.

Finally, in this era of clinical electrophysiology so dominated by both catheter ablation and device therapy, it is indeed important, in terms of future advances, to possess a tool which allows for bright minds to better explore and understand mechanisms of arrhythmias. We are indeed greatly indebted to Dr. Michael Franz and to those who contributed to this unique work, for giving us the tools to ask more probing questions to advance our knowledge—all in terms of the betterment of patient care.

Melvin M. Scheinman, MD
Professor of Medicine
Division of Cardiology
University of California
    of San Francisco
San Francisco, CA

Preface

I can't overstate my gratitude to the outstanding scientists who contributed to this book and provided their latest data on myocardial repolarization. I am deeply honored by their work that made this book a true encyclopedia of what is new and important in the use of monophasic action potentials (MAPs) and myocardial repolarization.

This book was designed to be the first comprehensive account of the nature and use of MAPs and of how they can help in our understanding of repolarization-related electrophysiology and its abnormalities that lead to arrhythmias. MAPs have undergone a fascinating history and a remarkable renaissance that lives today in many areas of electrophysiologic research, both basic and clinical. Undoubtedly, this is in large part due to the fact that MAP recordings allow one to gain insight, in an intact isolated or in situ heart, into the processes surrounding myocardial repolarization. This is an area that has received growing attention during the last decade.

Initially, I had planned to divide this volume into two major sections: an experimental research section and a clinical use section of the MAP recording technique. After surveying the material, I realized that many topics in either sections have direct counterparts in the other. The MAP recording technique is being used by both experimental and clinical researchers for the same reason: to establish knowledge of repolarization and the many factors that modulate normal and abnormal repolarization, and do so in the intact heart. Therefore, in this book, both experimental and clinical electrophysiologic studies are combined under related subject headings. This also underscores the primary purpose of the MAP technique, and the title of this book, which is to bridge "cell and bedside."

In closing, I would like to thank Jacques Strauss and Steven Korn at Futura Publishing Company for their openness and encouragement for this book. A special thanks is also awarded to Joanna Levine, who as production editor was extremely meticulous and helpful during every stage of the book's preparation.

Michael R. Franz

Contributing Authors

J. A. Abildskov, MD   Professor of Medicine, Nora Eccles Harrison Cardiovascular Research and Training Institute and the Division of Cardiology, University of Utah, Salt Lake City, UT

Michèle Adam, MD   Electrophysiologist, Department of Cardiology, University Hospital Santa Maria of Terni, Terni, Italy

Matthias Antz, MD   Division of Cardiovascular Surgery, University KIEL, KIEL, Germany

Charles Antzelevitch, PhD   Research Scientist, Masonic Medical Research Laboratory, Utica, NY

Evan Atkinson, BS   Graduate Student, Department of Biomedical Engineering, Tulane University, New Orleans, LA

Vincenzo Barbaro, PhD   Biomedical Engineering Laboratory, Instituto Superiore di Sanitá, Rome, Italy

Klaus Bargheer, MD   Kurklinik Fallingbostel, Fallinbostel, Germany

Pietro Bartolini, PhD   Biomedical Engineering Laboratory, Instituto Superiore di Sanitá, Rome, Italy

Steffen Behrens, MD   Medizinische Klinik II, Kardiologie and Pulmologie, Universitaetsklinikum Benjamin Franklin, Free University Berlin, Berlin, Germany

Fulvio Bellocci, MD   Associated Professor of Cardiology, Institute of Cardiology, Catholic University of the Sacred Heart, Rome, Italy

Shlomo A. Ben-Haim, MD, DSc   Cardiovascular Laboratory, The Bruce Rappaport Faculty of Medicine, Technion-Israel Institute of Technology, Haifa, Israel

†Deceased

Martin Borggrefe, MD, FESC   Hospital of the Westfälische Wilhelms-Universität Münster; Department of Cardiology and Angiology and Institute of Arteriosclerosis Research, Münster, Germany

Günter Breithardt, MD, FESC, FACC   Hospital of the Westfälische Wilhelms-Universität Münster; Department of Cardiology and Angiology and Institute of Arteriosclerosis Research, Münster, Germany

Giovanni Calcagnini, PhD   Biomedical Engineering Laboratory, Instituto Superiore di Sanitá, Rome, Italy

Ronald W. F. Campbell, MB, ChB, FRCP, FESC[†]   Professor of Academic Cardiology, Department of Academic Cardiology, Freeman Hospital, Newcastle upon Tyne, England

Edward B. Caref, PhD   Cardiology Division, Department of Medicine, State University of New York Health Science Center and Veterans Affairs Medical Center, Brooklyn, NY

Mary E. Chavez, CVT   VA Medical Center, Washington, DC

Peng-Sheng Chen, MD   Pauline and Harold Price Chair in Cardiac Electrophysiology Research, Professor of Medicine, University of California, Los Angeles; Division of Cardiology, Department of Medicine, Cedars-Sinai Medical Center and UCLA School of Medicine, Los Angeles, CA

William T. Clusin, MD, PhD   Associate Professor, Cardiology Division, Stanford University School of Medicine, Stanford, CA

Ruben Coronel, MD, PhD   Experimental Cardiologist, Department of Experimental Cardiology, Cardiac Research Center, Academic Medical Center, Amsterdam, The Netherlands

Angelika Costard-Jaeckle, MD   Division of Cardiovascular Surgery, University KIEL, KIEL, Germany

Marieke de Groot, MD, PhD   Fellow, Department of Cardiology, Cardiovascular Research Institute Maastricht, University of Maastricht, Maastricht, The Netherlands

Paul Dorian, MD, MSc   Arrhythmia Service, St. Michael's Hospital, University of Toronto, Toronto, Canada

Steven N. Ebert, PhD   Assistant Professor, Department of Pharmacology, Georgetown University Medical Center, Washington, DC

Lars Eckardt, MD   Hospital of the Westfälische Wilhelms-Universität Münster; Department of Cardiology and Angiology and Institute of Arteriosclerosis Research, Münster, Germany

Geoffrey Eddlestone, PhD   Research Scientist, Masonic Medical Research Laboratory, Utica, NY

Steward Edwards   Chief Executive Officer, Conway-Stewart Medical, Sunnyvale, CA

Kenneth A. Ellenbogen, MD   Professor of Medicine, Director of Cardiac Electrophysiology, Medical College of Virginia and Hunter Holmes McGuire Veterans Affairs Medical Center, Richmond, VA

Nabil El-Sherif, MD   Professor of Medicine and Physiology, Director of Electrophysiology, Department of Medicine, State University of New York Health Science Center at Brooklyn; Chief, Cardiology Division, The Veterans Affairs Medical Center, Brooklyn, NY

Erica D. Engelstein, MD   Assistant Professor of Medicine, Indiana University School of Medicine, Indianapolis, IN

C. Larissa Fabritz, MD   Assistentin und Wissenschaftliche Mitarbeiterin der Klinik und Poliklinik für Kinderheilkunde, Allgemeine Kinderheilkunde, Westfälische Wilhelms-Universität Münster, Münster, Germany

Guilherme Fenelon, MD   Federal University of Sao Paulo, Paulista School of Medicine; Department of Clinical Electrophysiology, Sao Paulo Hospital, Sao Paulo, Brazil

Peter Fenici, MD   Fellow in Internal Medicine, Clinical Physiology–Biomagnetism Research Center, Catholic University of Sacred Heart, Rome, Italy

Riccardo Fenici, MD   Professor of Cardiology, Director, Clinical Physiology–Biomagnetism Research Center, Catholic University of Sacred Heart, Rome, Italy

Ross D. Fletcher, MD   Chief of Staff, VA Medical Center; Professor of Medicine, Georgetown University Medical Center, Washington, DC

Parwis C. Fotuhi, MD   Postdoctoral Fellow, Department of Medicine, the University of Alabama at Birmingham, Birmingham, AL; Recipient of a "Habitationsstipendium der Deutschen Forschungsgmeinschaft"

Michael R. Franz, MD, PhD, FACC   Professor of Medicine and Pharmacology, Georgetown University Medical Center; Director of Cardiac Electrophysiology, Division of Cardiology, Veterans Affairs Medical Center, Washington, DC

Lior Gepstein, MD   Lecturer, Cardiovascular Laboratory, The Bruce Rappaport Faculty of Medicine, Technion-Israel Institute of Technology, Haifa, Israel

Rajiva Goyal, MD   Director of Electrophysiology, Bay Medical Center, Bay City, MI

Axel Haverich, MD   Hannover Medical School, Hannover, Germany

Wilhelm Haverkamp, MD   Hospital of the Westfälische Wilhelms-Universität Münster; Department of Cardiology and Angiology and Institute of Arteriosclerosis Research, Münster, Germany

Gal Hayam, BSc   Cardiovascular Laboratory, The Bruce Rappaport Faculty of Medicine, Technion-Israel Institute of Technology, Haifa, Israel

Daniel P. Higham, MBBS, MRCP   Consultant Physician/Cardiologist, Department of Cardiology, Wansbeck General Hospital, Northumberland, England

Stefan H. Hohnloser, MD   Director of Electrophysiology, Department of Medicine, Division of Cardiology, J. W. Goethe University, Frankfurt, Germany

Luc Hondeghem, MD, PhD   Professor of Pharmacology, KU Leuven; President of HPC n.v., Oostende, Belgium

Raymond E. Ideker, MD, PhD   Professor of Medicine, Department of Medicine, Professor of Physiology, Department of Physiology, Professor of Biomedical Engineering, Department of Biomedical Engineering, the University of Alabama at Birmingham, Birmingham, AL

Warren M. Jackman, MD, FACC   Professor of Medicine (Cardiology), George Lynn Cross Research Professor, Director of Clinical Electrophysiology, University of Oklahoma Health Sciences Center, Oklahoma City, OK

Michiel Janse, MD   Professor of Experimental Cardiology, Head of the Department of Experimental Cardiology, Cardiac Research Center, Academic Medical Center, Amsterdam, The Netherlands

Robert Johna, MD   Hospital of the Westfälische Wilhelms-Universität Münster; Department of Cardiology and Angiology and Institute of Arteriosclerosis Research, Münster, Germany

Janice L. Jones, PhD   Professor, Department of Physiology and Biophysics, Georgetown University and Cardiac Research Laboratory, Department of Veterans Affairs Medical Center, Washington, DC

Hrayr S. Karagueuzian, PhD   Director, Basic Cardiac Electrophysiology, Professor of Medicine, University of California, Los Angeles; Division of Cardiology, Department of Medicine, Cedars-Sinai Medical Center and UCLA School of Medicine, Los Angeles, CA

Pamela E. Karasik, MD   Assistant Professor of Medicine, Department of Cardiology, Department of Veterans Affairs and Georgetown University Medical Centers, Washington, DC

Young-Hoon Kim, MD   Associate Professor, Division of Cardiology, Department of Medicine, Korea University, Seoul, Korea

Paulus F. Kirchhof, MD   Assistent und Wissenschaftlicher Mitarbeiter der Medizinischen Klinik und Poliklinik, Innere Medizin C–Kardiologie und Angiologie, Westfälische Wilhelms-Universität Münster, Münster, Germany

Stephen B. Knisley, PhD   Associate Professor of Biomedical Engineering, Department of Biomedical Engineering, the University of Alabama at Birmingham, Birmingham, AL

Bjoern C. Knollmann, MD   Research Fellow, Department of Pharmacology and Institute for Cardiovascular Sciences, Georgetown University, Washington, DC

Ryszard B. Krol, MD, PhD   Clinical Assistant Professor of Medicine, UMDNJ-New Jersey Medical School, Newark, NJ; Attending Physician, Arrhythmia & Pacemaker Service, Eastern Heart Institute-Atlantic Health System, General Hospital Center at Passaic, Passaic, NJ; Electrophysiology Research Foundation, Millburn, NJ

Robert W. Kurz, MD   Specialist for Internal Medicine and Intensive Care Medicine, First Medical Department, Donauspital, Vienna, Austria

Kenneth R. Laurita, PhD   Assistant Professor of Medicine and Biomedical Engineering, Case Western Reserve University, Cleveland, OH

Ralph Lazzara, MD, FACC   Natalie O. Warren Professor of Medicine, George Lynn Cross Research Professor, Director Cardiac Arrhythmia Research Institute, University of Oklahoma Health Sciences Center, Oklahoma City, OK

S. Douglas Lee, MD   St. Michael's Hospital, University of Toronto, Toronto, Canada

Bruce B. Lerman, MD   H. Altschul Master Professor of Medicine, Cornell University Medical College; Chief, Division of Cardiology, Director, Cardiac Electrophysiology Laboratory, New York Hospital–Cornell Medical Center, New York, NY

Imad Libbus, MS   Research Scientist, Case Western Reserve University, Cleveland, OH

Paul R. Lichtlen, MD   Hannover Medical School, Hannover, Germany

Xiao-Ke Liu, MD   Graduate Student, Department of Pharmacology, Georgetown University Medical Center, Washington, DC

Robert L. Lux, PhD   Professor of Medicine, Nora Eccles Harrison Cardiovascular Research and Training Institute and the Division of Cardiology, University of Utah, Salt Lake City, UT

Lisa Malden, PhD   Associate Clinical Engineer, St. Jude Medical, CRMD, Sunnyvale, CA

Toshihisa Miyazaki, MD   Assistant Professor, Cardiopulmonary Division, Department of Internal Medicine, Keio University School of Medicine, Tokyo, Japan

Annibale Sandro Montenero, MD   Chief of Cardiology Department, University Hospital Santa Maria of Terni, Terni, Italy

Fred Morady, MD   Professor of Internal Medicine, Division of Cardiology, Department of Internal Medicine, The University of Michigan Medical Center, Ann Arbor, MI

Sandra Morelli, PhD   Biomedical Engineering Laboratory, Instituto Superiore di Sanità, Rome, Italy

Bruce D. Nearing, PhD   Assistant Professor, Division of Cardiology, Institute for Prevention of Cardiovascular Disease, Beth Israel Deaconess Medical Center, Boston, MA

David M. Newman, MD, FACC Arrhythmia Service, St. Michael's Hospital, University of Toronto, Toronto, Canada

Satoshi Ogawa, MD Professor, Cardiopulmonary Division, Department of Internal Medicine, Keio University School of Medicine, Tokyo, Japan

Tohru Ohe, MD National Cardiovascular Center, Osaka, Japan; Professor of Medicine, Okayama University Medical School, Okayama, Japan

S. Bertil Olsson, MD, PhD Professor, Department of Cardiology, University Hospital, Lund, Sweden

Tobias Opthof, PhD Electrophysiologist, Experimental Cardiology, Cardiac Research Center, Academic Medical Center, Amsterdam, The Netherlands

Claudio Pandozi, MD Chief, Electrophysiology Laboratory, Department of Heart Diseases, San Filippo Neri Hospital, Rome, Italy

Atul Prakash, MD, MRCP Clinical Assistant Professor of Medicine, UMDNJ-Robert Wood Johnson School of Medicine, New Brunswick, NJ; Attending Physician, Arrhythmia & Pacemaker Service, Eastern Heart Institute-Atlantic Health System, General Hospital Center at Passaic, Passaic, NJ; Electrophysiology Research Foundation, Millburn, NJ

Michael J. Reiter, MD, PhD Professor of Medicine (Cardiology), Director, Cardiac Arrhythmia Service, University of Colorado Health Sciences Center, Denver, CO

David S. Rosenbaum, MD Associate Professor of Medicine, Biomedical Engineering, Physiology, and Biophysics, Case Western Reserve University; Chief, Cardiac Arrhythmia Service, Cleveland Veterans Affairs Medical Center, Cleveland, OH

Fred Sachs, PhD Professor of Physiology and Biophysics, Department of Physiology and Biophysics, State University of New York at Buffalo, Buffalo, NY

Philip T. Sager, MD Associate Professor of Medicine, UCLA School of Medicine; Director of Cardiac Electrophysiology, West Los Angeles Veterans Affairs Medical Center, Los Angeles, CA

Sanjeev Saksena, MD, FACC, FESC Clinical Professor of Medicine, UMDNJ-Robert Wood Johnson School of Medicine, New Brunswick, NJ; Director Arrhythmia & Pacemaker Service, Eastern Heart Institute-Atlantic Health System, General Hospital Center at Passaic, Passaic, NJ; Electrophysiology Research Foundation, Millburn, NJ

Massimo Santini, MD, FACC, FESC   Professor, Chief of the Department of Heart Diseases, San Filippo Neri Hospital, Rome, Italy

Tadashi Satoh, MD   Research Associate in Cardiology, First Department of Internal Medicine, Tokyo Medical and Dental University School of Medicine, Tokyo, Japan; Codirector, Clinical Electrophysiology Laboratory, Department of Cardiology, Sohka City Hospital, Saitama, Japan

Melvin M. Scheinman, MD   Professor of Medicine, Division of Cardiology, University of California at San Francisco, San Francisco, CA

Claus Schmitt, MD   Elektrophysiologische Abteilung, Klinik für Herz- und Kreislauferkrankungen, Deutsches Herzzentrum München an der Technischen Universität München, München, Germany

Juergen Schreieck, MD   Elektrophysiologische Abteilung, Klinik für Herz- und Kreislauferkrankungen, Deutsches Herzzentrum München an der Technischen Universität München, München, Germany

Alaa Eldin Shalaby, MD   Fellow in Cardiac Electrophysiology, University of California Los Angeles School of Medicine; West Los Angeles Veterans Affairs Medical Center, Los Angeles, CA

Hugh Sharkey, RN   Executive Vice President and Chief Technology Officer, Oratec Interventions Inc., Menlo Park, CA

Wataru Shimizu, MD, PhD   Research Scientist, Masonic Medical Research Laboratory, Utica, NY; Codirector, Clinical Cardiac Electrophysiology Laboratory, National Cardiovascular Center, Osaka, Japan

Serge Sicouri, MD   Research Scientist, Masonic Medical Research Laboratory, Utica, NY

Bruce S. Stambler, MD   Director, Clinical Electrophysiology and Pacing, Associate Professor of Medicine, University Hospitals of Cleveland, Cleveland, OH

Bela Szabo, MD, PhD   Associate Professor of Research, Department of Medicine, University of Oklahoma Health Sciences Center, Veterans Administration Medical Center of Oklahoma, Oklahoma City, OK

Oscar H. Tovar, MD   Associate Professor, Department of Physiology and Biophysics, Georgetown University and Cardiac Research Laboratory, Department of Veterans Affairs Medical Center, Washington, DC

Natalia Trayanova, PhD   Associate Professor, Department of Biomedical Engineering, Tulane University, New Orleans, LA

S. Cora Verduyn, PhD Postdoc, Netherlands Heart Foundation, Department of Experimental Cardiology, Cardiovascular Research Institute Maastricht, Maastricht, The Netherlands

Richard L. Verrier, PhD, FACC Associate Professor of Medicine, Harvard Medical School; Institute for Prevention of Cardiovascular Disease, Beth Israel Medical Center, Boston, MA

Mauro Villani, MD Assistant in the Electrophysiology Laboratory, Department of Heart Diseases, San Filippo Neri Hospital, Rome, Italy

Marc A. Vos, PhD Associate Professor of Experimental Cardiology, Department of Cardiology, Cardiovascular Research Institute Maastricht, University of Maastricht, Maastricht, The Netherlands

Hein J. J. Wellens, MD, PhD Chairman of Cardiology, Department of Cardiology, Academic Hospital Maastricht, Maastricht, The Netherlands.

Mark A. Wood, MD Associate Professor of Medicine, Assistant Director of Cardiac Electrophysiology, Medical College of Virginia and Hunter Homes McGuire Veterans Administration Medical Center, Richmond, VA

Raymond L. Woosley, MD, PhD Professor and Chairman, Department of Pharmacology, Georgetown University Medical Center, Washington, DC

Tsu-Juey Wu, MD Attending Physician, Staff Electrophysiologist, Division of Cardiology/Internal Medicine, Taichung Veterans General Hospital, Taichung, Taiwan

Gan-Xin Yan, MD, PhD Research Scientist, Masonic Medical Research Laboratory, Utica, NY

Masaaki Yashima, MD Instructor, Department of First Internal Medicine, Nippon Medical School, Tokyo, Japan

Shiwen Yuan, MD, PhD Department of Cardiology, University Hospital, Lund, Sweden

Markus Zabel, MD Fellow in Electrophysiology, Department of Medicine, Division of Cardiology, Klinikum Benjamin Franklin, Free University, Berlin, Germany

Paolo Zecchi, MD Chief, Department of Cardiology, Institute of Cardiology, Catholic University of the Sacred Heart, Rome, Italy

Xiaohong Zhou, MD Assistant Professor of Medicine, Department of Medicine, the University of Alabama at Birmingham, Birmingham, AL

Douglas P. Zipes, MD Distinguished Professor of Medicine, Pharmacology, and Toxicology, Director, Division of Cardiology, Krannert Institute of Cardiology, Indiana University School of Medicine, Indianapolis, IN

Bernhard Zrenner, MD Elektrophysiologische Abteilung, Klinik für Herz- und Kreislauferkrankungen, Deutsches Herzzentrum München an der Technischen Universität München, München, Germany

Andrew C. Zygmunt, PhD Research Scientist, Masonic Medical Research Laboratory, Utica, NY

Contents

**Section V.
Torsades de Pointes and Other
Triggered Ventricular Arrhythmias**

**Section VIII.
Antiarrhythmic Device-Related Uses of
Monophasic Action Potential Recording**

Section I

Monophasic Action Potential Methodology:
Introduction

Monophasic action potential (MAP) recordings have stood at the cradle of cardiac electrophysiology, having been used long before the microelectrode technique was invented. The first MAP recordings date back to the last century (soon to be 2 centuries ago), when only primitive methods were available. Over the last 30 years, the MAP method has seen a remarkable comeback. It is now being recognized that action potential recordings from the intact or in vivo heart are essential for the understanding of many electrophysiologic and arrhythmia problems that cannot be explored sufficiently in dissected heart tissue or single-cell preparations. Isolation of tissue or cells from the context of the whole organ often removes the very object of investigation, such as reentry mechanisms, whole-heart dispersion of repolarization, mechanoelectrical feedback, and "real life" ischemia, just to name a few.

Meanwhile, the methodology of MAP recording has been refined to become more safe and simple, so that it would prove acceptable for the clinical electrophysiologic laboratory, where its use is helpful to discern arrhythmia mechanisms and teach interested fellows about basic electrophysiology in the human heart. New techniques have evolved, such as single-catheter MAP recording pacing catheters and multiple-site MAP recording mapping from endocardium and epicardium. Lately, attempts have even been made to obtain intramural MAP recordings; however their validity has not yet been proven.

Despite the relative simplicity of obtaining MAP recordings, the exact mechanism of the MAP genesis is still not understood. Even the simple question: "which of the two electrodes necessary to record the MAP is the one which records the local electrophysiologic information?" has puzzled the minds of great electrophysiologists in the past and still does today.

1

In this opening section, the above topics are all reviewed by experts in the field. This section concludes with practical advice on how to obtain and ascertain quality MAP recordings in patients.

1

Theory Underlying the Suction Electrode Method and Early Use in Clinical Research

S. Bertil Olsson, MD, PhD and Shiwen Yuan, MD, PhD

Initial Background

The obvious event of breakthrough concerning the knowledge of the electrophysiology of individual cardiac cells was the construction of the microelectrode,[1] allowing recording of the true electrical gradient over the cellular membrane. The electrical recordings meant to illustrate transmembranal electrical events that were performed prior to this technique were, of course, not possible to evaluate in a truly reliable way until the microelectrode technique was available. The similarities and differences between the true myocardial transmembrane action potential recorded with microelectrode and the monophasic action potential (MAP) recorded with the earlier available technique were not explored in detail until 10 years after the introduction of the microelectrode,[2] presumably because the new technique rapidly replaced the old one.

The MAP technique had been developed and used in animal experiments, using a bipolar recording technique and a suction device applied to the epicardial surface of exposed hearts.[3,4] It was, however, well known that different types of reversible or nonreversible localized myocardial

From Franz MR (ed): *Monophasic Action Potentials: Bridging Cell and Bedside.*
©Futura Publishing Company, Inc., Armonk, NY, 2000.

injuries were the prerequisites for the recording of the electrical signals, which were named MAPs.[5-7]

The fact that the different recording techniques resulted in a monophasic electrical myocardial signal later prompted a clear definition of MAP. Today, *"the MAP is defined as the electrical event of a cardiac cycle, recorded with a differential DC* [direct current] *recording technique between an exploring electrode terminal in direct contact with or in the immediate vicinity of an area of depolarized myocardium and an indifferent electrode terminal in close proximity to the exploring one."*[8] A unipolar electrogram from the indifferent electrode terminal must, however, not record any current of injury.[9] This definition restricts the recording so that it must be done with bipolar technique, and underlines the control of signal quality, allowing exclusion of bipolar "injury-to-injury" phenomena. Nowadays, the bipolar technique is unanimously accepted, although signal quality identification by following the unipolar indifferent terminal lead is seldom reported. It should be mentioned, however, that unipolar signals from depolarized myocardial areas may yield important information concerning myocardial repolarization.[10] Since these signals contain major far-field electric components,[11] it may be appropriate to name them current-of-injury potentials in order to distinguish them from true MAPs.

Based on an idea of recording cellular atrial myocardial events from a transseptal puncture needle,[8] and on the experience gained from adopting the original suction electrode principle in the study of transmembranal ionic turnover during the cardiac cycle in frogs,[12] a recording device meant for recording of MAPs from the intact heart via a cardiac catheter was developed and applied in humans[13] and animals.[14] This device was constructed in a way which allowed bipolar recording technique across the boundaries of a reversible localized myocardial depolarization, induced by the combination of catheter suction against the endocardial wall and potassium perfusion within the area of recording. Furthermore, the signal quality was controlled by continuously recording the unipolar electrogram from the indifferent electrode terminal, thus fulfilling the demands of today's definition of MAPs.

The technical limitations of this recording device were, however, obvious, especially for recording in humans. A further development of the technique was therefore made, resulting in a bipolar suction electrode catheter that was easier to use.[11] Although the technique was based on the suction electrode principle, it was observed that the mere pressure of the catheter tip against the endocardial wall resulted in a MAP which improved in quality and rose in amplitude with increasing pressure.[9,11] Figure 1 illustrates the principle of the suction electrode catheter device and the design of the catheter. For safety reasons, this catheter was exclusively used in right-sided cardiac catheterizations.

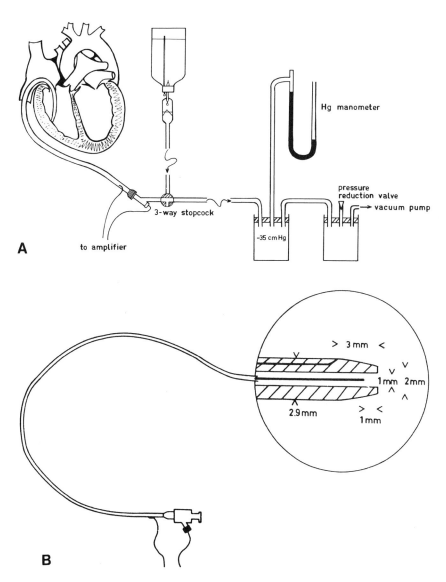

Figure 1. Schematic illustration of the first suction electrode catheter device that allowed recording of monophasic action potentials of the intact human heart with acceptable precision (**A**). Note the position of the two electrode terminals at the tip of the catheter (**B**). After the catheter tip was pressed against the endocardial wall, a monophasic signal appeared. The signal quality improved after the application of suction within the catheter. Reproduced from Reference 10, with permission.

First Recordings in Humans

The initial recordings in humans with the improved device were done almost exclusively in patients undergoing diagnostic cardiac catheterizations, mostly due to valvular heart diseases.[9,15-17] In addition, atrial MAPs were recorded in a series of patients undergoing DC conversion of long-lasting atrial fibrillation, immediately before and after reestablishment of sinus rhythm.[18] The content of the first 5 publications was also published as a PhD thesis, in which an extended analysis of the material was made, including validation of method precision.[9] Figure 2 presents representative MAP recordings from the right atrium and ventricle.

Although unpublished, the initial validation included an attempt to estimate the total duration of a MAP. Since this measure had a poor reproducibility and since publications on action potential durations at that time used several different repolarization levels, investigators decided to give a measure of duration of good reproducibility that was as close as possible to the total duration.[9] Publications involving measurements of duration of MAPs have thereafter almost always used the same repolarization level, 90%, although a level closer to the refractory period, for instance 75%, perhaps would be more appropriate.

In addition to the MAP duration, amplitude and amplitude-normalized repolarization rate, as well as time relation to electrocardiographic evidence of excitation, were studied. None of these measurements have attracted so much interest, however, as the duration.

Atrial Recordings

Atrial repolarization in humans was only observed in selected cases as a Ta wave, and thus was almost entirely unexplored until the initial studies with the MAP method were published. Atrial MAPs recorded during sinus rhythm using the improved suction electrode device[11] had an amplitude between 3.1 and 17.7 mV.[9,15] The duration at 90% repolarization varied in these recordings between 216 and 421 milliseconds. The obvious need for normal values concerning atrial MAP in humans prompted an extended study, including validation of effects of pacing and physical training.[19]

A completely new and challenging observation was the association between short atrial MAP duration and propensity for arrhythmia relapse when the recordings were done immediately following DC conversion of long-lasting atrial fibrillation.[18] Atrial myocardial repolarization was also studied during atrial fibrillation and flutter.[15] In no case was it possible to observe a signal level that corresponded with the resting membrane potential. Instead, atrial fibrillation was characterized by different fibrillatory cycle durations starting at different levels of repolarization of the preceding

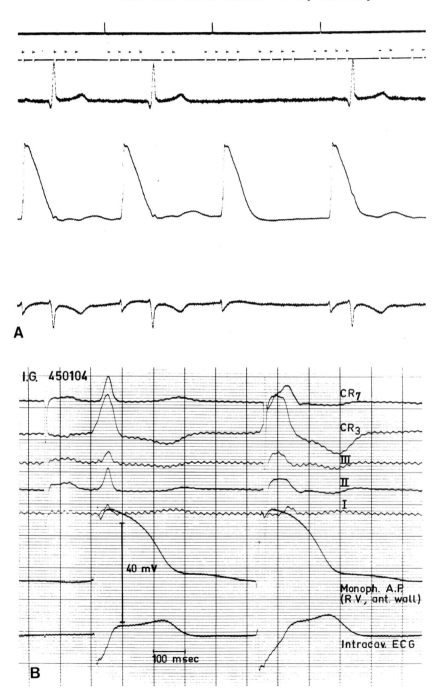

Figure 2. Representative recordings of right atrial (**A**) and right ventricular (**B**) MAPs from initial studies using the suction electrode catheter.

cycle, while atrial flutter evidenced a more extended but always incomplete repolarization. Later, a mathematical extrapolation technique allowed calculations of a theoretical MAP duration as well as a theoretical "resting potential" in atrial fibrillatory MAP recordings.[20] Interestingly, suction electrode recording attempts during intermittent atrial standstill in two patients failed to illustrate any voltage drop, thus suggesting a depolarized atrial myocardium.[9]

Ventricular Recordings

With use of the suction electrode method, the amplitude of ventricular MAP recordings were higher than at the atrial level and ranged between 13.1 and 47.8 mV.[16] When it was possible to obtain recordings from more than one position within the right ventricle, at least one had a MAP amplitude exceeding 20 mV. Although little attention has been paid to the MAP amplitude, MAP recordings from selected patients with constrictive cardiac disease illustrated that a 20-mV right ventricular MAP amplitude discriminated between constrictions of pericardial and myocardial origins, the latter never exceeding this amplitude (S.B. Olsson, unpublished observations, 1980).

The relation between the right ventricular MAP duration and the QT interval was evaluated early and, although the MAP duration varies spatially, a close correlation was found.[16] Interestingly, there was no relation between the duration of the right atrial MAP and the right ventricular MAP, when these recordings could be performed at almost identical heart rates.[9]

Later, a series of right ventricular MAP recordings from healthy individuals was reported, also illustrating in greater detail the relationship between MAP, ventricular effective refractory period (VERP), and QT time, measured in different ways.[21] The MAP duration is correlated to the VERP; however, their relation is not always linear, especially under the effect of antiarrhythmic drugs that have disparate effects on MAP duration and VERP. At fluoroscopically identical sites, the ratio between VERP and MAP duration was 0.96 ± 0.05 in a group of 48 healthy men.[21]

Genesis of the MAP: Result from a Computer Modeling Study

To study the electric origin of the MAP, Hirsch et al[22] established a computer model that relates the MAP recorded by use of the suction electrode technique to the intracellular action potential. In this model, the tissue under the exploring electrode is divided into 50,000 elements, with fast propagation in the intact part and different extents of slow conduction in the "injured" part of the tissue. The MAPs generated from this model were consistent with those recorded using the suction electrode technique, supposing the total area of "injury" was not more extensive than the size of the electrode (Fig. 3). The result of this modeling study supports the commonly accepted hypothesis that the MAPs are recorded between an area of reversible injury, or local depolarization, and an indifferent electrode. The injured or depolarized area, which is the prerequisite for the MAP recording, can be produced by applying a suction, mechanical pressure, or even thermal and chemical factors onto the endocardium or the epicardium.[9,11,23] Thus, the cells immediately subjacent to the tip electrode are depolarized and electrically inactivated, while the adjacent cells surrounding these depolarized cells are unaffected. An electrical gradient then develops between the unexcitable cells and adjacent normal cells. The MAPs reflect the voltage time course of the normal cells surrounding the injured cells. Both the injured and the normal cells contribute equally to the genesis of the boundary current, which produces the MAP field potential. In this sense, the MAP recorded using the suction electrode technique does not differ from that recorded using the currently used contact electrode technique.

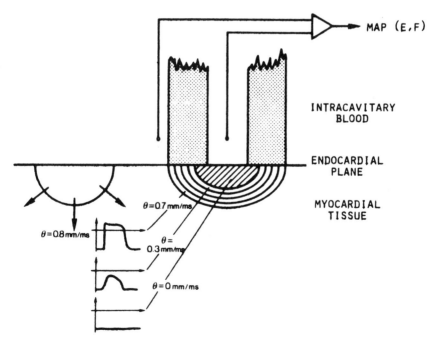

Figure 3. Schematic illustration of the genesis of MAP tested in a computer modeling study by Hirsch et al. It is assumed that there is a gradual depolarization of the cells immediately beneath the MAP electrode. Reproduced from Reference 22, with permission.

Studies of the Effects of Antiarrhythmic Drugs

Since prolongation of the action potential duration is a property of many antiarrhythmic drugs and is considered a prerequisite for their efficacy, the evaluation of the drug effects on MAP duration became one of the main foci in the early applications of the suction electrode technique. In 1973, Olsson et al[24] recorded MAPs from the right atrium in 9 patients with paroxysmal atrial fibrillation before and after 4 or more weeks of oral administration of amiodarone, and found that the atrial MAP duration was prolonged in all of the patients by an average of 30%.[24] The effect of amiodarone shown in laboratory animals[25] was thus verified in the clinical setting.[24] A significant prolongation of both MAP duration and VERP after intravenous injection of amiodarone was later verified.[26] Based on MAP recording using the suction electrode technique, the effects of many other antiarrhythmic drugs, such as mexiletine, flecainide, melperone, sotalol, metoprolol, lignocaine, procainamide, metoprolol, verapamil, and even digoxin and atropine were evaluated by the same group.[27-36]

With the spread of the suction electrode technique, evaluations of antiarrhythmic drugs were also conducted in other centers. Gavrilescu et al[37] found that quinidine prolonged both right atrial and right ventricular MAP duration and, more interestingly, it prolonged the right atrial MAP duration to a greater degree for atrial premature beats than for sinus beats, which may explain why quinidine can prevent atrial arrhythmias in doses that do not influence sinus rhythm.[37,38] Endresen et al[39,40] documented that disopyramide prolonged MAP duration and VERP with an increased VERP-MAP duration ratio, while lidocaine shortened both MAP duration and VERP without clear change of their ratio. Duff et al[41] and Endresen et al[42] studied the effect of propranolol on repolarization in patients and found a shortening of MAP duration while VERP remained unchanged. Echt et al[43] demonstrated that sotalol prolonged the MAP duration and the effective refractory period at both the atrial and the ventricular level. A similar class III action of bunaphtine has also been documented in human subjects.[44,45] Amlie et al[46,47] administered digoxin under autonomic blockade in dogs and found shortening of both VERP and MAP duration with an increased VERP-MAP duration ratio.

Among the early applications of the suction electrode technique was Harper and Olsson's[34] use of the sharp upstroke of the MAPs to measure the local activation time for studying the influence of antiarrhythmic drugs on intraventricular conduction velocity. They demonstrated subnormal and supernormal conduction of premature beats and found an increased period of subnormal conduction with the abolition of the supernormal conduction period following the administration of mexiletine (Fig. 4).

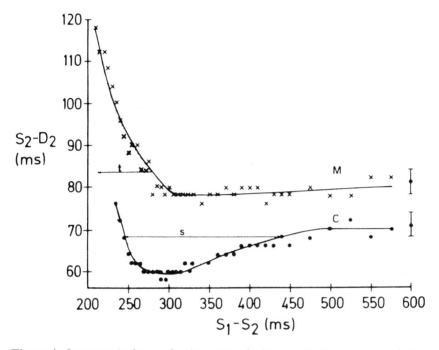

Figure 4. Intraventricular conduction curves during ventricular programmed stimulation, analyzed by measuring the distance from the stimulus artifact (S2) to the onset of the MAP upstroke (D2) in the extra beats. In the control recording (C), a phase of supernormal conduction (s) is clearly visible. After the administration of mexiletine (M) there is no obvious supernormal conduction phase but there is a substantial delay of the conduction in the earliest extra beats, ie, a phase of subnormal conduction (t). Reproduced from Reference 34, with permission.

Thus, the use of MAP recording in antiarrhythmic drug study allowed the findings of the cellular electropharmacology in vitro to be verified in a clinical setting in vivo.

Rate Adaptation and Spatial Dispersion of the MAP Duration

Rate Adaptation of the MAP Duration

It is well known that the MAP duration is influenced by the change of heart rate and/or rhythm, the electrical restitution, which has been extensively studied and is now verified as an intrinsic electrophysiologic feature of the myocardium.[9,17,48–52] Characterization of the rate-dependent changes of MAP duration in patients with arrhythmias may give insight into the contribution of cellular mechanisms to the arrhythmogenic substrate.[53-56]

The earliest observation of the rate adaptation of the MAP duration in humans was conducted using the suction electrode technique. In 1971, Olsson[9,17,57] observed that during sinus or junctional rhythm and pacing, a rapid heart rate was associated with a shorter atrial and ventricular MAP duration and a slow heart rate with a relatively longer MAP duration. Similarly, during programmed stimulation and atrial fibrillation, a short cycle length was associated with a MAP of short duration and vice versa (Fig. 5). It is interesting that the rate-related changes of MAP duration were different for atrial and ventricular MAPs. The shortening of atrial MAP was caused by a relatively steeper final repolarization, while that of the right ventricular MAP was not only during phase 3 but also during the plateau phase. On the other hand, pacing-induced heart rate increase shortened the MAP merely during the plateau phase. This was also the case when the stimulation cycle was abruptly shortened, while a sudden

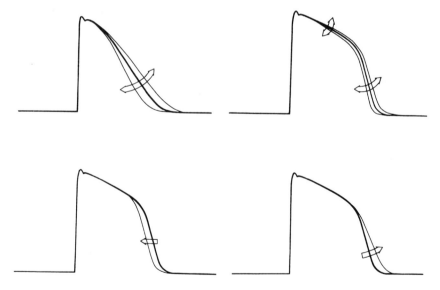

Figure 5. Schematic illustration of the rate-related changes of the MAP duration and contour in a group of patients. Upper left: the atrial MAP was shortened at faster heart rate and prolonged at slower heart rate, with the changes mainly during phase 3. Upper right: the changes of the ventricular MAP duration was not only during phase 3, but also during the plateau phase. The ventricular MAP duration changed similarly following short and long intervals during atrial fibrillation. Lower left: pacing-induced heart rate increase or abrupt shortening of the cycle length shortened merely the plateau phase of the ventricular MAP. Lower right: an abrupt prolongation of the cycle length prolonged phase 3 of the ventricular MAP with a decreased repolarization rate. Reproduced from References 14 and 17, with permission.

prolongation of the cycle length resulted in a MAP prolongation due to a relative slowing of phase 3.[17] Similarly, a rate adaptation was noted when the ventricular MAP was studied during atrial fibrillation[17] (ie, there was a direct relation between the duration of the MAP, both phase 2 and phase 3, and the preceding cycle length [Fig. 5]). The different changes of the contour of the MAP may suggest variable uses of different ionic channels of the cellular membrane, although cellular myocardial electrophysiology was inadequately explored at the time of the recordings in order to allow such speculations.

Intra-Atrial and Intraventricular Differences of MAP Duration

Increased dispersion of repolarization is now considered an important mechanism linked to the development of tachyarrhythmias. The dispersion of repolarization can be evaluated by recording MAPs from multiple sites in the atrium and/or ventricle. In one of the earliest of such observations, Olsson studied the intra-atrial and intraventricular difference of the MAP duration by recording MAPs sequentially and correlating the local MAP duration to the P or Q wave onset. He found that in the atrium, the site activated earlier associated with a MAP of shorter duration and vice versa, while the opposite relation was found in the ventricle.[9] This may represent the very first observation of dispersion of repolarization in humans.

Limitations of the Suction Electrode Technique

For proper MAP recordings, the tip of the suction electrode catheter should be kept in close adherence to the endocardium by the application of a negative pressure of as much as -350 mm Hg. Thus, a certain volume of tissue is sucked into the lumen of the catheter and there is a risk of injury to the tissue, although the injury caused by the suction of less than 2 minutes is reversible. To avoid permanent injury, the continuous suction time (ie, the recording time) cannot exceed 2 minutes. This limits the technique to the observations of short-term phenomena; the effects of interventions or the long-lasting effects cannot be evaluated with reliability, even though careful replacement of the catheter to the previous site was used before and after intervention and during observation of long-lasting effects.

The suction electrode technique requires suction pump, three-way stop cocks, air-bubble filter, and other precautions. Comparing with the currently used contact electrode technique, the suction electrode technique is more cumbersome and more complicated. Furthermore, due to the potential risk for arterial air emboli, the suction electrode technique is not suitable for left-sided MAP recording.

References

1. Ling G, Gerard RW. The normal membrane potential of frog sartorius fibers. *J Cell Comp Physiol* 1949;34:383.
2. Hoffman BF, Cranefield PF, Lepeschkin E, et al. Comparison of cardiac monophasic action potentials recorded by intracellular and suction electrodes. *Am J Physiol* 1959;196:1297-1301.
3. Schütz E. Monophasische Actionsströme vom in Situ durchbluteten Säugetierherzen. *Klin Wschr* 1931;10(31):1454-1456.
4. Schütz E. Elektrophysiologie des Herzens bei einphasischer Ableitung. *Ergebnisse der Physiologie* 1936;38:493-523.
5. Wilson FN, MacLeod AG, Barker PS. *The Distribution of the Currents of Action and of Injury Displayed by Heart Muscle and Other Excitable Tissues.* Ann Arbor: University of Michigan Press; 1933.
6. Eyster JAE, Meek WJ, Goldberg H, Gilson WE. Potential changes in an injured region of cardiac muscle. *Am J Physiol* 1938;124:717.
7. Eyster JAE, Gilson WE. The development and contour of cardiac injury potentials. *Am J Physiol* 1945/46;145:507.
8. Olsson B, Yuan S. Historical development of the monophasic action potential recording technique. In Franz MR, Schmitt C, Zrenner B (eds): *Monophasic Action Potentials.* Heidelberg: Springer-Verlag; 1997:3-21.
9. Olsson SB. *Monophasic Action Potentials of Right Heart. Suction Electrode Method in Clinical Investigations* [PhD dissertation]. Göteborg: University of Göteborg, Elanders Boktryckeri AB; 1971.
10. Shabetai R, Surawicz B, Hammill W. Monophasic action potentials in man. *Circulation* 1968;38:341-352.
11. Olsson SB, Varnauskas E, Korsgren M. Further improved method for measuring monophasic action potentials of the intact human heart. *J Electrocardiol* 1971;4:19-23.
12. Sjöstrand U. *Analysis of Ionic Tracer Movements During Single Heart Cycles* [PhD dissertation]. Uppsala, Sweden: Uppsala University; 1964.
13. Korsgren M, Leskinen E, Sjöstrand U, Varnauskas E. Intracardiac recording of monophasic action potentials in the human heart. *Scand J Clin Lab Invest* 1966;18:561-564.
14. Sjöstrand U. A method for intracardiac recording of monophasic action potentials in the dog heart in situ. *Acta Physiol Scand* 1966;68:58.
15. Olsson SB. Monophasic action potentials from right atrial muscle recorded during heart catheterization. *Acta Med Scand* 1971;190:369-379.
16. Olsson SB. Right ventricular monophasic action potentials during regular rhythm. A heart catheterization study in man. *Acta Med Scand* 1972; 191(3):145-157.
17. Olsson SB, Varnauskas E. Right ventricular monophasic action potentials in man. Effect of abrupt changes of cycle length and of atrial fibrillation. *Acta Med Scand* 1972;191(3):159-166.

18. Olsson SB, Cotoi S, Varnauskas E. Monophasic action potential and sinus rhythm stability after conversion of atrial fibrillation. *Acta Med Scand* 1971;190(5):381-387.

19. Brorson L. *Electrophysiological properties of right atrium. Studies in Healthy Males and in Patients with Supraventricular Tachyarrhythmias* [PhD dissertation]. Göteborg: University of Göteborg; 1975.

20. Olsson SB, Cai N, Edvardsson N, Talwar KK. Prediction of terminal atrial myocardial repolarisation from incomplete phase 3 data. *Cardiovasc Res* 1989;23(1):53-59.

21. Edvardsson N. *Cellular Effects of Antiarrhythmic Agents* [PhD dissertation]. Göteborg: Göteborg University; 1983.

22. Hirsch I, Edvardsson N, Olsson SB, Broman H. Cardiac monophasic action potentials related to intracellular action potentials. A modeling study. In Hirsch I (ed): *On the Generation, Analysis and Clinical Use of Cardiac Monophasic Action Potentials. Thesis.* Göteborg: Vasastadens Bokbinderi; 1984:(I)1-58.

23. Olsson SB, Brorson L, Edvardsson N, Varnauskas E. Estimation of ventricular repolarization in man by monophasic action potential recording technique. *Eur Heart J* 1985;6(suppl D):71-79.

24. Olsson SB, Brorson L, Varnauskas E. Class 3 antiarrhythmic action in man. Observations from monophasic action potential recordings and amiodarone treatment. *Br Heart J* 1973;35(12):1255-1259.

25. Singh BN, Vaughan Williams EM. The effect of amiodarone, a new anti-anginal drug, on cardiac muscle. *Br J Pharmacol* 1970;39:657-668.

26. Blomström P, Bodnar J, Edvardsson N, et al. Acute effect of intravenous amiodarone on ventricular refractoriness and repolarization. *PACE* 1987;10(4 part II):1004. Abstract.

27. Edvardsson N, Hirsch I, Emanuelsson H, et al. Sotalol-induced delayed ventricular repolarization in man. *Eur Heart J* 1980;1:335-343.

28. Edvardsson N, Olsson SB. Effect of intravenous melperone on atrial repolarization in man. *Scand J Clin Lab Invest* 1981;41(1):87-90.

29. Edvardsson N, Olsson SB. Effects of acute and chronic beta-receptor blockade on ventricular repolarisation in man. *Br Heart J* 1981;45(6):628-636.

30. Edvardsson N, Hirsch I, Olsson SB. Right ventricular monophasic action potentials in healthy young men. *PACE* 1984;7(5):813-821.

31. Edvardsson N, Hirsch I, Olsson SB. Acute effects of lignocaine, procainamide, metoprolol, digoxin and atropine on human myocardial refractoriness. *Cardiovasc Res* 1984;18(8):463-470.

32. Edvardsson N, Olsson SB. Induction of delayed repolarization during chronic beta-receptor blockade. *Eur Heart J* 1985;6(suppl D):163-169.

33. Harper RW, Olsson SB, Varnauskas E. Effect of mexiletine on monophasic action potentials recorded from the right ventricle in man. *Cardiovasc Res* 1979;13(6):303-310.

34. Harper RW, Olsson SB. Effect of mexiletine on conduction of premature ventricular beats in man: A study using monophasic action potential recordings from the right ventricle. *Cardiovasc Res* 1979;13(6):311-319.

35. Olsson SB, Harper RW. Mexiletine effect on monophasic action potential (MAP) of right ventricle in man. *Acta Med Scand Suppl* 1978;615(93):93-98.

36. Olsson SB, Edvardsson N. Clinical electrophysiologic study of antiarrhythmic properties of flecainide: Acute intraventricular delayed conduction and prolonged repolarization in regular paced and premature beats using intracardiac

monophasic action potentials with programmed stimulation. *Am Heart J* 1981;102(5):864-871.

37. Gavrilescu S, Dragulescu SI, Luca C, et al. The effects of quinidine on the monophasic action potential of the right atrium in patients with atrial fibrillation. *Agressologie* 1976;17(2):11-18.

38. Gavrilescu S, Luca C. Right ventricular monophasic action potentials in patients with long QT syndrome. *Br Heart J* 1978;40(9):1014-1018.

39. Endresen K, Amlie JP, Forfang K. Effects of disopyramide on repolarisation and intraventricular conduction in man. *Eur J Clin Pharmacol* 1988;35(5):467-474.

40. Endresen K, Amlie JP. Acute effects of lidocaine on repolarization and conduction in patients with coronary artery disease. *Clin Pharmacol Ther* 1989;45(4):387-395.

41. Duff HJ, Roden DM, Brorson L, et al. Electrophysiologic actions of high plasma concentrations of propranolol in human subjects. *J Am Coll Cardiol* 1983;2(6):1134-1140.

42. Endresen K, Amlie JP. Effects of propranolol on ventricular repolarization in man. *Eur J Clin Pharmacol* 1990;39(2):123-125.

43. Echt DS, Berte LE, Clusin WT, et al. Prolongation of the human cardiac monophasic action potential by sotalol. *Am J Cardiol* 1982;50(5):1082-1086.

44. Bonatti V, Finardi A, Cabasson J, Botti G. Effects of Bunaphtine on right atrial and ventricular monophasic action potentials in man. Preliminary note. *G Ital Cardiol* 1976;6(3):440-449.

45. Bonatti V, Finardi A, Cabasson J, Botti G. A study of the mechanism of the action of Bunaphtine recording the myocardial monophasic action potentials in man. Conclusive report. *G Ital Cardiol* 1976;6(8):1378-1383.

46. Amlie JP, Refsum H. Vagus-induced changes in ventricular electrophysiology of the dog heart with and without beta-blockade. *J Cardiovasc Pharmacol* 1981;3(6):1203-1210.

47. Amlie JP, Storstein L, Watanabe H. Digoxin- and digitoxin-induced changes in monophasic action potential of the right ventricle of the dog heart. *Cardiovasc Res* 1980;14(3):130-136.

48. Franz MR, Schaefer J, Schoettler M, et al. Electrical and mechanical restitution of the human heart at different rates of stimulation. *Circ Res* 1983;53:815-822.

49. Seed WA, Noble MI, Oldershaw P, et al. Relation of human cardiac action potential duration to the interval between beats: Implications for the validity of rate corrected QT interval (QTc). *Br Heart J* 1987;57(1):32-37.

50. Endresen K, Amlie JP. Electrical restitution and conduction intervals of ventricular premature beats in man: Influence of heart rate. *PACE* 1989;12(8):1347-1354.

51. Morgan JM, Cunningham D, Rowland E. Electrical restitution in the endocardium of the intact human right ventricle. *Br Heart J* 1992;67(1):42-46.

52. Morgan JM, Cunningham AD, Rowland E. Relationship of the effective refractory period and monophasic action potential duration after a step increase in pacing frequency. *PACE* 1990;13(8):1002-1008.

53. Morgan JM, Cunningham D, Rowland E. Dispersion of monophasic action potential duration: Demonstrable in humans after premature ventricular extrastimulation but not in steady state. *J Am Coll Cardiol* 1992;19(6):1244-1253.

54. Yuan S, Wohlfart B, Olsson SB, Blomström-Lundqvist C. The dispersion of repolarization in patients with ventricular tachycardia. A study using simultaneous monophasic action potential recordings from two sites in the right ventricle. *Eur Heart J* 1995;16(1):68-76.

55. Yuan S, Blomström-Lundqvist C, Pehrson S, et al. Dispersion of repolarization following double and triple programmed stimulation: A clinical study using the monophasic action potential recording technique. *Eur Heart J* 1996;17:1080-1091.

56. Yuan S, Blomström-Lundqvist C, Pripp C-M, et al. Signed value of monophasic action potential duration difference. A useful measure in evaluation of dispersion of repolarization in patients with ventricular arrhythmias. *Eur Heart J* 1996;17(8 suppl):275.

57. Olsson SB. Recording of monophasic action potentials in the study of atrial dysrhythmias. *G Ital Cardiol* 1972;2(4):536-541.

2

Monophasic Action Potentials Recorded by Contact Electrode Method:

Genesis, Measurements, and Interpretations

Michael R. Franz, MD, PhD

Introduction

Monophasic action potentials (MAPs) are extracellularly recorded waveforms that under optimal conditions can reproduce the repolarization time course of transmembrane action potentials (TAPs) with high fidelity.[1-3] While TAP recordings require the impalement of an individual cardiac cell by a glass microelectrode and therefore generally are limited to in vitro preparations, MAPs can be recorded from the endocardium and epicardium of the in situ beating heart, including that of a human subject. MAP recordings therefore are suitable for studying characteristics of local myocardial electrophysiology—especially of repolarization—in the whole-heart and clinical settings (Table 1). However, despite the growing use of the MAP recording method, there still are surprisingly little hard data on the exact mechanism by which MAPs are created and recorded. New methods for recording MAPs recently have been proposed, and new theories and models have been suggested to explain the mechanisms that underlie the genesis of the MAP signal. This chapter reviews old and new information

From Franz MR (ed): *Monophasic Action Potentials: Bridging Cell and Bedside.*
©Futura Publishing Company, Inc., Armonk, NY, 2000.

Table 1
Advantages and Disadvantages of MAP Recordings Compared to
Intracellular Recordings

Disadvantages of MAP Recordings:

1. No information on <u>absolute</u> voltage of resting and action potential amplitude.
2. No reliable information on <u>absolute</u> upstroke velocity.
3. Multicellular recording (averaging) may mask distinct features of individual myocardial cells.

Advantages of MAP Recordings:

1. Allows recordings from the intact, in situ, human heart.
2. Identification of the effects on repolarization of heart mechanics, antiarrhythmic drugs, ischemia, rate and rhythm, afterdepolarizations, in normal and diseased human myocardium.
3. Multicellular recording: averages electrophysiologic properties over many cells, making recordings more representative.

on the MAP genesis and its particular recording modes. It also highlights some important MAP quality criteria and guidelines for correct interpretation of MAPs and how to avoid artifacts.

Brief History of MAP Recording Techniques

The "Injury" Method

The first MAP was recorded in 1882 by Burdon-Sanderson and Page,[4] who placed one electrode on the intact epicardial surface and the other on an injured site of a frog heart, and thereby captured the phasic electrical changes of the cardiac cycle on a charcoal-covered recording drum. Burdon-Sanderson and Page produced this injury by cutting into the myocardium, and termed these recordings *monophasic action currents* (later to be replaced by monophasic action *potentials*). Until then, electrodes placed on intact heart tissue had been recording *multiphasic* deflections, similar to those recorded today in the human electrophysiology laboratory by conventional electrode catheters; so the term *monophasic* was a logical choice. It was believed for several decades that such monophasic action potentials could only be produced by traumatic tissue injury or cellular disruption. Methods such as cutting, stabbing, or burning of a myocardial site were invented to produce monophasic "injury" currents.[5] In 1934 Schuetz[6] introduced the suction electrode for experimental MAP recording. In 1966, Korsgren and coworkers[7] used a suction electrode catheter in a patient and recorded, for the first time, MAPs from the in situ ventricular endocardium. This pioneering step subsequently was amplified by the work of Olsson and coworkers,[8-10] who refined the suction electrode technique and demonstrated the value of MAP recording in exploring human cardiac electrophysiology, mainly of the right atrium. Injury was still deemed necessary, and to do this "cautiously" in the human heart by suction technique required the use of three-way stop cocks, bubble filters to prevent air emboli, and other precautions.[8] Because this technique was cumbersome and raised patient safety concerns, the suction electrode technique never gained wide acceptance in the clinical electrophysiologic laboratory.

The "Contact" Electrode Method

The first nontraumatic method for recording MAPs was published in 1935 by Jochim et al.[11] These authors demonstrated that MAPs can be obtained by simply pressing an electrode against the epicardium of the toad ventricle while merely touching another electrode to the nearby epicardium (Fig. 1). They also showed that the MAP is positive with respect to zero if the pressure electrode is the active electrode (connected to the positive amplifier input). This important observation went largely unnoticed for many years. However, their observation was, in both methodology and

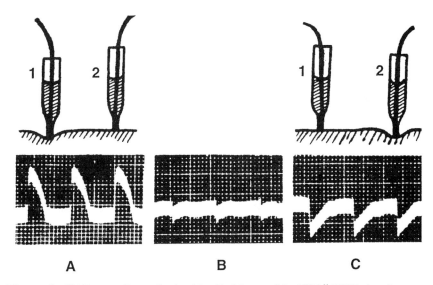

A   B   C

Figure 1. MAP recordings obtained by Jochim et al in 1935.[11] MAP signals were generated by pressing an electrode against the epicardium of a toad heart. When the positive electrode (labeled 1) was pressed against the epicardium, a positive MAP was obtained (**A**). A biphasic electrogram was obtained when both electrodes merely touched the epicardium (**B**). When the negative electrode (labeled 2) was pressed against the epicardium, a negative MAP was obtained (**C**).

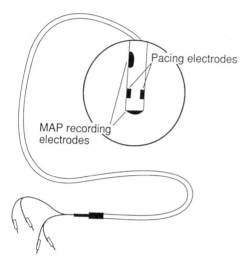

Figure 2. Sketch of contact electrode catheter design for recording MAPs from endocardium in patients or large animals. Shown is the most widely used version (the MAP-pacing combination catheter), which includes small-surface pacing electrodes located 2 mm proximal to the catheter tip in an orthogonal position. MAP electrodes are made of high-grade silver-silver chloride powder suspended in special polymeric matrix. Pacing electrodes are made of platinum-iridium. This catheter also incorporates a bidirectional steering feature (not shown). Additional designs are described in previous publications by Franz.[26,56]

interpretation, surprisingly similar to the current principle of recording MAPs by contact electrode.

The contact electrode technique for clinical use was developed between 1980 and 1983 by Franz et al,[12,13] and was later expanded to allow simultaneous electrical stimulation with the same catheter without excessive pacing artifacts[14] (Fig. 2). Catheters and probes for endocardial and epicardial MAP recording were developed for clinical studies and for experimental studies.[15-17] The contact electrode technique allows one to record MAPs without suction but rather by pressing a nonpolarizable electrode gently against the endocardium or epicardium. The ability to record MAPs by the nontraumatic contact electrode technique refuted the previous contention that myocardial injury (or suction) is a prerequisite for MAP recording. Besides being more simple and clinically safe, the contact electrode method provides MAP recordings that, due to lack of myocardial injury, are stable over time. This allows the clinical electrophysiologist to monitor MAPs over periods of several hours from the same endocardial site to assess, for instance, the effects of antiarrhythmic drugs or cycle length changes on local myocardial repolarization.[13,18]

Genesis of the MAP: Old and New Theories

The MAP is measured with an extracellular electrode which has a diameter of 1 to 2 mm and therefore cannot enter a single cardiac cell. This has given rise to much debate about the genesis of the MAP. The early literature on MAP measurements focused on the central issue of whether the MAP signal is recorded with the electrode in contact with *injured* (depolarized) myocardium or with the electrode in contact with *uninjured* (intact) myocardium. Hans Schaefer,[19,20] a vehement protagonist of the former assumption, argued that MAPs can only be obtained when injury is present and therefore the electrode in contact with injured muscle must be the different electrode. Others countered that injured cells are electrically inactive and therefore the electromotive force producing the MAP must originate from the uninjured cells.[21-23] As will be explained later, the truth appears to lie in the middle.

The "Schuetz-Hypothesis" on Injury Potentials

Based on experiments in frog hearts, from 1934 to 1936 Schuetz[6,24] promoted the theory that the MAP is the voltage drop that is recorded between the different electrode (in contact with injured myocardium) and the indifferent electrode (in contact with uninjured myocardium). He assumed leak current flow between the injured cells and the uninjured myocardium and explained the MAP by the following simple equation:

$$E_{inj} = E_m \times (R_e + R_i) / R_i \qquad (1)$$

where E_{inj} is the MAP voltage, E_m is the transmembrane voltage, R_e is the extracellular resistance, and R_i is the intercellular resistance. This hypothesis assumes that the MAP is the result of a voltage source, with all electromotive generators in parallel. An increase in extracellular resistance (for instance by drying the heart's surface) would result in a greater MAP amplitude (which in fact occurred), and a decrease in extracellular resistance by wetting the heart's surface with electrolyte solution would decrease the MAP amplitude (which also is true for injury potentials in this setting). This hypothesis also assumes that short circuiting between the injured cells and the extracellular space is minimized by using a tight electrical seal between the MAP recording electrode and the surrounding tissue. The suction electrode method was promoted to some extent because it was believed to provide such a seal. This theory has some semblance to the sucrose-gap technique which is used to record the TAP in vitro without transmembrane impalement.[25]

The "Volume Conductor" Hypothesis

Based on the following observations, Franz[26] concluded that the Schuetz hypothesis does not apply to the contact electrode method but that the contact electrode MAP results from a *current* source and is governed by

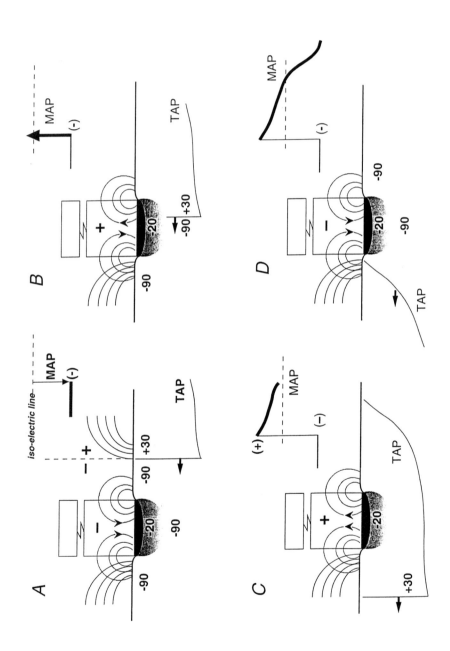

Figure 3. Diagram illustrating the genesis of MAP recording by contact electrode. **A.** Late electrical diastole. The myocardial cells are -90 mV negative inside with respect to outside. Pressure of the tip electrode (black ellipsoid) against the myocardium results in constant depolarization of the subjacent cell volume (shaded hemisphere). A fixed depolarization to –20 mV is assumed but could be slightly larger or smaller. The potential gradient across the boundary between the normal diastolic potential and the fixed depolarization underneath the contact electrode creates current flow (circular lines) which, in the extracellular space, flows from normal to depolarized tissue. Under the present volume conductor conditions, this creates a current sink and a corresponding sink potential at the contact electrode site. The MAP recording (inside in upper right) shows a steady potential negative to zero. An arriving action potential wave, which carries an inside potential of +30 mV near the upstroke, is shown to the right of the contact electrode site. **B.** Early electrical systole. The action potential wave arrives at the contact electrode site. The cell volume depolarized by the contact pressure is unexcitable and maintains its potential at –20 mV. Its initial +30 mV inside brings to the contact site a relative positive inside charge and a relative negative outside charge. This leads to a reversal of the boundary current and field potential polarity. The MAP now moves in a positive direction and inscribes an upstroke and early phase 1. **C.** Midelectrical systole. The propagating action potential wave has completely encompassed the MAP recording site. As the TAP wave gradually repolarizes, the boundary gradients gradually diminish. The MAP undergoes slow repolarization which nears the isoelectric line as the TAP potential approaches the potential in the pressure-depolarized cell volume. **D.** End-electrical diastole. The propagating TAP wave recedes from the MAP electrode contact site. Voltage gradients return to their preexisting (diastolic) state. The cycle is completed and results in a MAP recording that faithfully resembles the original TAP recording. MAP = monophasic action potential recorded from extracellular space. TAP = transmembrane action potential recorded from intracellular space.

volume conductor theory. 1) The contact electrode obtains MAPs from the endocardium while surrounded by the blood pool in the ventricular or atrial cavity and has no surrounding seal, suggesting that the extracellular resistance has no influence on the amplitude of the MAP. This was confirmed by experimental studies in small animal hearts.[26] 2) The number of cells (single electromotive generators) contributing to the MAP seems important because greater contact pressure between the tip electrode and myocardium increases the MAP amplitude.[16] Furthermore, MAPs of greater amplitude are recorded from ventricular myocardium than from atrial myocardium or from larger hearts (eg, canine and human hearts) as compared to small hearts (eg, those of rabbits), suggesting that wall thickness beneath the MAP tip electrode plays a role in determining the MAP amplitude.[26] This suggests that the MAP amplitude is related to the volume of cells that contribute to the MAP genesis, and that the MAP signal results from a current source, with individual electromotive generators more or less in series.

Figure 3 schematically depicts the hypothesis by which the contact electrode method produces and records MAPs. Pressure exerted focally against the myocardium depolarizes the group of cells subjacent to the electrode to a level estimated at −30 to −20 mV with respect to the diastolic extracellular reference potential. Because sodium channels remain inactivated at these voltage levels, these cells are unexcitable and thus unable to participate in the periodic depolarizations and repolarizations that occur in the adjacent (normal) myocardium. The group of cells depolarized by the contact electrode provide a "frozen" potential that contrasts with the time-varying potential in the unaffected adjacent cells. Assuming preserved electrical coupling, this causes a time-varying electrical gradient between the depolarized (unexcitable) cells subjacent to the electrode and the adjacent (excitable) cells. This electrical gradient produces current flow across the boundary between these two states. During electrical *diastole*, this gradient results in a *source* current emerging from the normal cells and a *sink* current descending into the depolarized cells subjacent to the MAP electrode. The *sink* current produces a *negative* electrical field that is proportional to the strength of current flow, which depends on the potential gradient and the number of cells that contribute to the interface between the subjacent depolarized and the adjacent nondepolarized cells. During electrical *systole*, the normal cells adjacent to the MAP electrode undergo complete depolarization which overshoots the zero potential by some 30 mV, whereas the already depolarized and therefore refractory cells subjacent to the MAP electrode cannot further depolarize and maintain their potential at the former reference level. As a result, the former current *sink* reverses to a current *source*, producing an electrical field of opposite polarity. According to this hypothesis, the MAP recording reflects the voltage time course of the normal cells that bound the surface of the volume of cells depolarized by the contact pressure. Thus, both the depolarized ("electrically frozen") cells and the active cells of the neighboring myocardium contribute to the genesis of the boundary current that produces the MAP field potential; one cannot exist without the other.

How Accurate are MAP Recordings?

The accuracy with which MAP recordings reflect the local cellular depolarization and repolarization was examined in several studies which compared the MAP with the simultaneously recorded TAP.[1-3] These studies have pointed out a number of similarities and dissimilarities between the MAP and TAP.

MAP Amplitude and Resting Potential

Both the diastolic and action potential amplitude are markedly less in the MAP as compared to the TAP. The amplitude of the contact electrode MAP typically ranges between 5 and 50 mV, although values as high as 81 mV have been reported.[26] Despite this variability, which depends on the contact pressure and tissue type (see above), *relative* changes in the MAP resting and action potential amplitude can be interpreted as long as a stable baseline recording is obtained before and after the intervention.[15,27]

Repolarization Time Course

The MAP faithfully reflects the duration as well as the configuration of the repolarization phases 1 through 3 of the TAP.[2,28] Figure 4 shows TAP and MAP recordings obtained simultaneously from closely adjacent sites in an isolated, perfused rabbit septum preparation during interventions which influence the action potential duration (APD) and configuration.[28] Each panel shows TAP and MAP signals superimposed onto each other after they have been rescaled to match in amplitude. With each of the interventions shown, changes in the shape and duration are nearly identical in the TAP and MAP recordings.

Upstroke Velocity

The maximum upstroke velocity (V_{max}) of the MAP is much smaller than that measured with an intracellular electrode. In the canine heart, V_{max} of the ventricular MAP averages 7 V/s[15] as compared to 200 to 300 V/s in

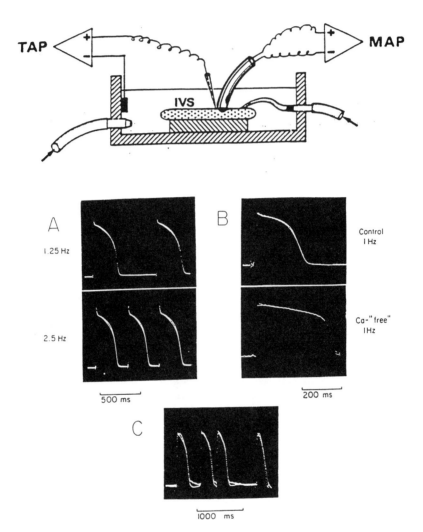

Figure 4. Comparison of monophasic (MAP) and transmembrane (TAP) action potential recorded simultaneously from closely adjacent sites in a rabbit isolated, perfused intraventricular septum (IVS) preparation. In A, the rate of pacing was increased from 1.25 Hz to 2.5 Hz, resulting in significant shortening of the action potential duration. The recordings in B show the effect of replacing the normal perfusing and bathing solution with a calcium-free solution. With the pacing rate maintained at 1 Hz, the action potential greatly increases in plateau duration, resulting in a more rectangular configuration. The effects of an extrasystole and a subsequent pause on action potential duration are shown in C. With all of these interventions, changes in the shape and duration are nearly identical in the TAP and MAP recordings. From Reference 28.

the transmembrane record.[29] The smaller rise velocity of the MAP is due in part to its smaller amplitude and in part to the fact that the MAP electrode records the electrical activity from a group of cells whose depolarizations occur sequentially with time. Despite the marked difference in absolute magnitude of V_{max} between TAP and MAP recordings, relative changes in V_{max} may provide important information. Franz et al[15] demonstrated during acute ischemia that V_{max} of the MAP decreased by 95% at only 5 minutes of coronary artery occlusion. This makes the MAP upstroke velocity a highly sensitive marker of myocardial ischemia. Under stable recording conditions, MAPs also provide reliable measures of drug-induced changes in V_{max} that can help classify use-dependent properties of sodium channel blocking drugs.[27]

Upstroke and Phase 1 Morphology

Using high band-width amplification, the upstroke of the MAP contains a rapid deflection, appearing as a biphasic notch within the MAP upstroke or as a spike overshooting or undershooting it.[2,13] This notch is the remnant of the "intrinsic deflection" seen in the myocardial surface electrogram prior to applying contact pressure and the development of the MAP. This intrinsic deflection may appear as a positive spike immediately preceding the MAP plateau phase, mimicking an "overshoot potential" or "phase 1 repolarization." This, however, should not be taken as evidence that the MAP reflects recordings from specialized conductive tissue or that the spike-and-dome morphology reflects the transient outward current (I_{to}) channel activity of epicardial myocardium as suggested by some investigators.[30] As Figure 5 shows, during excitations originating from different ectopic ventricular sites with their attending alterations in activation sequence, the upstroke phase alters it shape and overshoot potential despite the fact that the MAP electrode remains at a constant location. There currently is no reliable method to eliminate the intrinsic deflection which, in contrast to the remote QRS, originates from myocardium very near the exploring MAP tip electrode. For this reason, we define the MAP amplitude as the distance from the baseline to the crest of its plateau phase, and not to the peak of the upstroke. It also underscores why the rise velocity of the MAP upstroke cannot be equated with that of the TAP.

Afterdepolarizations

Basic electrophysiologic studies have provided strong evidence that afterdepolarizations play a significant role in the genesis of triggered arrhythmias such as torsades de pointes. These afterdepolarizations,

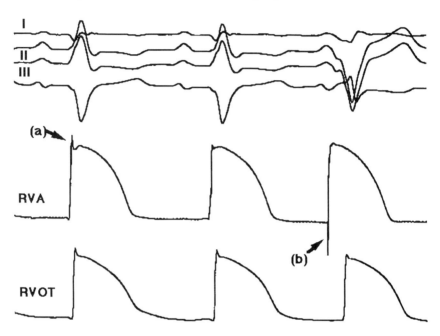

Figure 5. Demonstration that the upstroke of the MAP is not a reliable rendition of the cellular action potential's phase 1 and 2. Variation in the ventricular activation sequence, as visible by surface electrocardiogram (ECG) changes can cause changes in the upstroke phase, mimicking "spike and dome" configuration (a) or absence of it with clipped upstrokes and negative spike. These changes can occur despite otherwise stable and accurate repolarization features of the MAP and should not be interpreted as features characteristic of special cell groups I, II and III designate ECG leads and RVA and RVOT MAP recordings from the right ventricular apex and outflow tract, respectively.

which can be distinguished between early (EAD) and delayed (DAD) afterdepolarizations, cannot be detected by conventional intracardiac recordings. MAP recordings have been used to detect EADs or DADs during experimental[31-36] and clinical[37-41] electrophysiologic studies and to relate them to triggered arrhythmias. However, it is extremely important that stringent quality criteria are applied to the MAP recording before abnormalities are interpreted in the final repolarization time course as EADs or DADs. "Humps" and "wobbles" in the MAP recording may simply be the result of unstable electrode contact (see below: movement artifacts). The following criteria may be helpful in distinguishing true EADs or DADs from movement artifacts: 1) experimental conditions usually allow the investigator to obtain baseline recordings before beginning interventions. These baseline recordings should be stable with a smooth phase 3 and a horizontal phase 4 without appreciable deviations. 2) EADs, when they occur in response to interventions such as application of catecholamines or APD-prolonging drugs, or short-long pacing sequences, should be critically evaluated to determine if they bear sufficient morphologic resemblance to, and behavior compliant with, data known from transmembrane recordings. 3) Washout of the inducing agent or cessation of the interventional pacing protocol should result in disappearance of EADs and return to baseline MAP tracings. Even then, no absolute proof of the validity of the EADs or DADs is obtained. There will always be a degree of uncertainty that diminishes proportionally with the experience of the investigator and his/her ability to suppress bias. This author believes, after careful inspection of the experimental protocols and figures, that the work presented in References 34 to 44 is convincing and supports the usefulness of MAP recordings for the purpose of identifying EADs or DADs under the given experimental conditions.

Movement Artifacts

One of the most important limitations of MAP recordings is that they may be distorted by motion artifacts caused by the beating heart. The MAP amplitude is (within limits) proportional to the contact pressure exerted by the electrode against the myocardium. Unless correct positioning of the catheter tip electrode permits precise tracking of the wall motion, the rhythmic dilatation and contraction of the ventricle will alternatingly lessen and increase the contact pressure. This may result in transient amplitude changes of the MAP signal. These transient potential changes take a positive or negative direction depending on the time of pressure change with respect to the phase of the MAP signal. Diastolic dilatation of the ventricle may cause a decrease in contact pressure, resulting in a decrease in diastolic MAP amplitude. Because the diastolic phase of the MAP is negative with respect to zero potential, a decrease in diastolic MAP amplitude may be misinterpreted as "spontaneous diastolic depolarization" or "DADs." Conversely, systolic contraction of the ventricle may increase the contact pressure between the catheter tip and the endocardium, resulting in a transient increase in MAP amplitude. Because the systolic phase of the MAP is positive with respect to zero potential, an increase in systolic MAP amplitude may cause an elevation of the later part of the MAP or produce false "EADs." An example of an MAP tracing presumably distorted by the above described contact pressure changes is shown in Figure 6. Compared with the correct waveform (broken line), the MAP shows a rapidly upward sloping potential during diastole. This is most likely due to loss of endocardial electrode contact during diastolic relaxation (outward motion) of the ventricular wall. These movement artifacts can be minimized by using highly elastic catheters and careful positioning which allows the distal

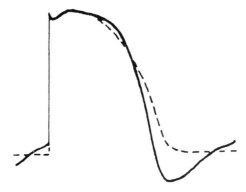

Figure 6. Artifacts in the MAP recording (solid line) due to unstable contact between the catheter tip electrode and the endocardium. Dotted line shows stable recording. See text for discussion.

catheter shaft to flex back and forth during the ventricular contraction and relaxation process, thereby maintaining steady contact pressure.

Mechanoelectrical Feedback

The issue of motion artifacts is further complicated by the fact that nonuniform ventricular contraction and relaxation can produce true electrophysiologic changes. A yet little understood phenomenon known as contraction-excitation coupling[42] or mechanoelectrical feedback[43] can lead to changes in APD,[44,45] afterdepolarizations,[46,47] and even arrhythmias.[48] The mechanism underlying these electrophysiologic effects is believed to be myocardial stretch. Nonuniformity of ventricular contraction and relaxation[49] creates conditions under which some wall segments undergo excessive lengthening during diastole or even late systole, causing regional heterogeneity of load-induced electrophysiologic changes. Some investigators have discarded afterdepolarizations in MAP recordings categorically as movement artifacts because they did not observe the same afterdepolarizations in intracellular microelectrode recordings.[50] However, to ensure stable microelectrode impalements, intracellular recordings are usually obtained from excised, mechanically relatively quiescent preparations which do not experience physiologic load or length changes. Thus, validation of the MAP by comparing it against the "gold standard" of the TAP must fail in this respect. This makes the reliable distinction between "true" and "false" motion-induced MAP changes one of the greatest challenges of the MAP method.

Determining the MAP Duration

Because the asymptotic end of repolarization makes precise measurement of total MAP duration difficult, the MAP duration is usually deter-

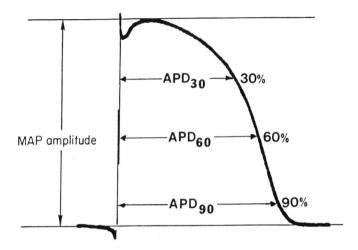

Figure 7. Method of analysis of the MAP signal. The amplitude of the MAP is measured as the distance from the diastolic baseline to the crest of the MAP plateau phase, not the peak of the upstroke. The duration of the MAP signal is measured as the interval, along a line horizontal to the diastolic baseline, from the fasted part of the MAP upstroke (or the intrinsic deflection, if discernible) to the desired repolarization level. The example shows evaluation of MAP duration at 30%, 60%, and 90% repolarization. From Reference 13.

mined at a repolarization level of 90% (or another fraction) with respect to the MAP amplitude. The MAP amplitude is defined here as the distance from the baseline to the crest of the MAP plateau, not its upstroke peak (Fig. 7).[13] Others have suggested the use of the intersection between the diastolic baseline and a tangent placed on phase 3 repolarization,[51] although this may produce more arbitrary results depending on the slope of final repolarization. We define the beginning of the MAP as the instance of fasted rise time of the MAP upstroke or, if detectable, the notch of the intrinsic deflection that is superimposed onto the MAP upstroke.[13]

Are Chronic MAP Recordings Possible?

Permanent monitoring of local activation and repolarization characteristics would be very desirable. This, if combined with an implantable telemetry device, could be used to monitor the effects of antiarrhythmic drugs on myocardial repolarization at specific intervals, or in relation to the onset of proarrhythmic events. Progression of cardiomyopathy and heart transplant rejection are other fields that would benefit from continuously available MAP interrogation. As understanding of the cellular basis of arrhythmias grows, abnormal changes of MAP signals recorded by permanent electrodes and transmitted by telemetry may become predictors and warning signals of life-threatening arrhythmic events.

Unfortunately, this does not seem possible with currently available MAP methods. MAPs have a tendency to decrease their amplitude and change their morphology over time. The MAP signal deterioration is much more rapid (minutes) with techniques that create MAPs by frank cellular injury, such as suction or stabbing the tissue with a needle or plunge electrode. MAP signal deterioration is gradual (several hours) with the contact electrode, especially when only moderate contact pressure is applied. The loss in MAP amplitude over time is associated with two important features. One is that as the MAP amplitude decreases, the initial spike becomes more prominent. This spike is the remnant of the intrinsic deflection (which becomes unmasked as the MAP plateau amplitude decreases) and should not be confused with a spike-and-dome configuration of TAPs as was done by Tande et al.[30] The second feature that accompanies the decrease in the MAP amplitude is that the loss in total (plateau) amplitude is primarily due to a decrease in the diastolic voltage of the MAP. The mechanisms underlying the amplitude decrease of injury potentials was studied extensively by De Mello et al,[52] who concluded that it is promoted by cellular uncoupling between the injured and normal cells. Several experiments led De Mello to believe that this electrical uncoupling takes place at the site of gap junctions and that calcium and proton ion accumulation at these sites plays a pivotal role.[53-55]

How *Local* Are MAP Recordings?

Because any type of MAP electrode is too large to enter a single cardiac cell, it is obvious that the MAP does not reflect single-cell action potentials by either transmembrane voltage or individual-cell repolarization characteristics. Instead, it has long been recognized that the MAP reflects a summation potential derived from a multitude of cells in close vicinity of the exploring MAP electrode.[1] While there appears to be general consensus that the MAP is created by local depolarization, the exact "field of view" of the MAP (both in the lateral and vertical direction from the MAP electrode) is uncertain. Obviously, the diameter of the exploring MAP electrode will to some extent determine the area from which the electrical activity of individual cells are sampled. However, an even greater influence on the spatial resolution of the MAP, or how stringently and accurately the MAP reflects local electrical activity and not also far-field potentials, appears to be determined by the position of the MAP *reference* electrode.

Different versus *Indifferent* Electrode: Which One Records the Map?

Based on experimental observations and theoretical deductions (see earlier in this chapter), it is evident that the MAP originates from cells in the immediate vicinity of the electrode that causes persistent depolarization. It is also evident that to obtain an upright MAP signal, the MAP exploring electrode must be connected to the positive input of the amplifier, and the reference electrode to the negative input. The frequently used MAP contact electrode design[13,14] has a tip electrode (the *exploring* MAP electrode) and a *reference* electrode 5 mm proximal to the tip. Thus, it appears that the MAP is recorded in bipolar fashion and therefore is a "bipolar" signal. This, however, is not the case. It seems helpful to first define the nature of unipolar versus bipolar recordings with regard to the MAP genesis.

Unipolar Recordings

A unipolar recording is defined as a set up in which one electrode (the exploring electrode) is in close contact with the tissue of interest and the other (the reference electrode) is situated elsewhere, at a distance from the site of interest. In experimental animal studies and in human electrophysiologic studies, the reference electrode often is placed remote from the heart (eg, the catheter insertion site) or the Wilson central terminal is used. Because most electrophysiologic recording circuits use differential amplification, the advantage of unipolar recording is that the information obtained at the site of interest is not canceled out by similar information from a site in its immediate vicinity. The disadvantage is that the large distance between the exploring electrode and the reference electrode includes electrical potentials that originate outside the area of interest. The extent by which such far-field potentials may contaminate the local information depends on, among other factors, the geometry between the axis formed by the exploring and reference electrodes and the spread of electromotive fields generated elsewhere in the heart.

Bipolar Recordings

A bipolar recording is defined as a set up in which both electrodes (which are fed into a differential amplifier) are located close to each other (usually not more than 10 mm apart in clinical electrophysiologic studies and often much closer in experimental studies). The advantage of such close bipolar recording is that far-field potentials are effectively cancelled out, leaving only information that originates within the perimeter of the bipolar electrode axis. This is the method of choice in clinical electrophysiologic studies where the emphasis lies on discerning local electrical activation (wave fronts). Activation wave fronts occupy very small distances due to their rapid onset. The disadvantage of this bipolar arrangement is that it cancels out information on the local *repolarization* process which, due to its longer duration, has a much larger spread. Adjacent T waves of similar duration and magnitude will be reduced to very small and sometimes unrecognizable potentials.

Monophasic versus Biphasic Electrograms

Monophasic electrograms are defined as those which deflect in only one dominant direction. The MAP is, by definition, a monophasic electrogram. In fact, the term *monophasic action potential* or *monophasic action current* was already used in 1882 by Burdon-Sanderson and Page who recorded the first (unipolar) MAP from the frog epicardium.[4] Previously, electrograms obtained from heart tissue were biphasic or multiphasic signals. At first sight, the monophasicity of the MAP suggests that it is recorded by a unipolar recording set up. This, however, is not necessarily true. Depending on the method of analysis, the monophasic portion of the electrogram is as local and as distant as is the ST elevation in a precordial lead in a patient having an acute myocardial infarction: both may be prominent and both may lack spatial specificity.

Unipolar MAP Recordings

By coupling the active MAP-exploring electrode with a remote electrode, such as a Wilson central terminal, a monophasic potential is still obtained, but it will also contain far-field potentials.[13] The extent by which these far-field potentials contribute to the local MAP signal is often unpredictable. If an area of myocardial depolarization caused by ischemia or other causes exists remote from the MAP recording site, the field potential created across its boundaries may contaminate the local MAP signal to a greater or lesser extent, depending on the particular geometry of the current sources with respect to the position of the two MAP electrodes. This problem is reminiscent of difficulties encountered in interpreting precordial ST segment elevations or depressions when more than one ventricular wall segment is injured by ischemia.[57] Reciprocal changes, cancellations, and expansions all may occur, making the precise localization of the primary injury difficult.

"Close-Bipolar" MAP Recordings

The problem of MAP contamination by far-field potentials was recognized by Olsson,[8] who advocated a "close-bipolar" MAP recording approach. The electrical field potential, which is caused by applying suction or contact pressure to the myocardium and which creates the MAP, seems to be confined to a finite region not extending much beyond the area of depolarization. An electrode placed 5 mm proximal to the depolarizing tip electrode usually is far enough away from the MAP generating current and therefore can be used as a reference electrode that is indifferent to the monophasic field. This close-bipolar electrode arrangement provides a very small solid angle toward more remote electrical forces and, by using differential amplification, greatly reduces far-field potentials. It is the close-bipolar technique that makes the MAP recording truly *local* as the following two examples illustrate.

1. Figure 8 compares 2 recordings, one unipolar and one close-bipolar, with the exploring MAP electrode position unchanged, during normal and ectopic ventricular activation. The unipolar MAP shows major differences in morphology during ectopic activation while the close-bipolar MAP does not. This underscores the fact that, using the close-bipolar technique, the MAP measures only *local* depolarization and repolarization events.
2. Figure 9 shows 3 types of recordings obtained simultaneously from the anterior left ventricular epicardium of the in situ canine heart: 1) the close-bipolar MAP; 2) the unipolar MAP; and 3) the unipolar electrogram. These 3 signals were recorded by 3 independent, high-impedance, differential amplifiers. Any 2 of the 3 recordings are the sum of the third (similar to the 3 Einthoven leads). (See details in figure legend.) Occlusion of the left anterior descending coronary artery resulted in a decrease in the amplitude of the close-bipolar MAP and a concomitant increase in the ST segment of the unipolar electrogram, with both changes being nearly reciprocal to each other. The unipolar MAP, however, remained almost unchanged. At a later stage, with the ischemic region having progressed to complete injury, the close-bipolar MAP has become an isoelectric potential, indicating absence of local electrical activity. The unipolar electrogram has become monophasic, showing remnants of the QRS complex. The unipolar MAP is still monophasic with little change from its baseline state. Therefore, it must be concluded that unipolar MAP recordings are not a reliable measure of local electrophysiologic activity but are sensitive to influences originating from potential gradients at distant sites. Only close-bipolar MAP recordings reflect the local electrophysiologic changes during regional ischemia.

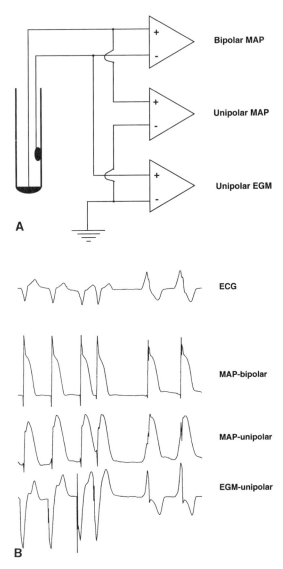

Figure 8. **A.** Diagram of 3-channel recording of close-bipolar MAP, unipolar MAP, and unipolar electrogram (EGM). **B.** Comparison of unipolar and close-bipolar MAP recording during beats of varying ventricular activation sequence. The unipolar MAP shows significant distortions in its waveform and duration, while the close-bipolar MAP retains essentially the same morphology with changes in duration due to cycle length changes. The lowest tracing shows the unipolar EGM, which was recorded from the proximal MAP electrode against the remote reference. It appears that the unipolar MAP is a hybrid between the close-bipolar MAP and the unipolar EGM. All three recordings were obtained from the same catheter located at the right ventricular outflow tract.

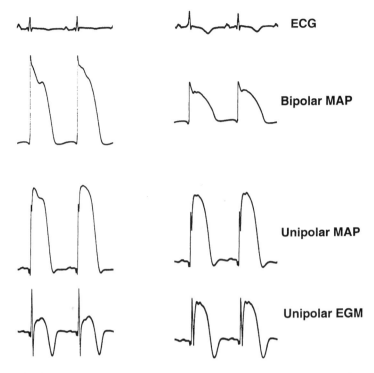

ECG

Bipolar MAP

Unipolar MAP

Unipolar EGM

Figure 9. Comparison of the effects of regional myocardial ischemia (produced by occlusion of the left anterior descending coronary artery [LAD]) on the close-bipolar and unipolar MAP and unipolar electrogram (EGM). The three recordings were obtained simultaneously from the epicardium of the LAD region using the circuit arrangement shown in Figure 8A. Acute ischemia resulted in substantial decrease in the amplitude of the close-bipolar MAP recording. The unipolar EGM showed prominent ST segment elevation. The unipolar MAP recording, in contrast to the close-bipolar MAP recording, showed little change.

"Field of View" of MAP Recordings

Even with the close-bipolar MAP recording technique, the actual spatial resolution of the MAP has not been determined with accuracy. Levine et al[58] addressed this issue by analyzing the "foot" of MAP signals recorded from slices of canine myocardium, and found that approaching electrical activity may be seen from areas as far as 10 mm from the MAP tip electrode. However, these recordings were obtained from a slice of canine myocardium that was not perfused but only superfused and, therefore, were based on a thin superficial layer of surviving myocardium. Furthermore, only a unipolar recording technique was applied. The "foot" of the MAP therefore overestimated far-field electrical activity and underestimated electromotive forces originating from deeper, yet local, cells.

One obvious determinant for the field of view is the size of the MAP tip electrode that produces and explores the boundary currents between the depolarized cells and adjacent normal cells (see above). The spatial resolution cannot be less than the tip electrode diameter (typically 1 to 2 mm). Another determinant is the distance and the solid angle between the tip electrode and the reference electrode with respect to the MAP voltage field source. The "Franz electrode" technique uses an interelectrode distance of 5 mm or less. When the tip electrode is kept in an ideal position perpendicular to the myocardial surface, the solid angle with respect to areas lateral to the tip electrode is very small, resulting in effective cancellation of remote electromotive sources if differential amplification is used. Franz et al[2] impaled with microelectrodes myocardial cells in the immediate vicinity of the contact site of the MAP electrode and measured *normal* transmembrane resting and action potentials as close as 0.1 mm to the MAP tip electrode circumference, suggesting that the area of depolarized tissue which constitutes the MAP boundary is confined to the MAP electrode size. These authors also recorded MAPs across a sharp transmural infarct border and noted an abrupt transition from normal to ischemic MAP signals within less than 5 mm of the ischemic border.[15] This further supports the view that the MAP signal reflects electrical activity from a very small area, not less than the electrode size and probably not more than 5 mm in diameter.

"Depth of View" of MAP Recordings

The "depth of view" with which the MAP electrode senses the electrical activity of myocardial tissue beneath the MAP contact electrode has not yet been determined. The fact that MAP recordings from thicker wall segments (left ventricle, large animals) have substantially greater amplitudes than recordings from thin-walled tissue (right atrium, small animals)[26] suggests that tissue at some considerable depth beneath the exploring electrode contributes to the genesis of the MAP signal. In another validation study, Ino et al[3] compared simultaneous MAP and TAP recordings from canine endocardium, epicardium, and isolated Purkinje strands. In endocardial preparations composed of superficial (1 to 2 cell layers) Purkinje fibers with deeper ventricular muscle cells, the action potential at 50% and 90% repolarization (APD_{50} and APD_{90}, respectively) of MAPs more closely reflected the underlying deeper ventricular muscle cells rather than the superficial Purkinje fibers. Tetrodotoxin shortened Purkinje fiber APD and slightly lengthened that of ventricular muscle. Simultaneously recorded MAP showed an intermediate change in APD. These data support the assumption that the depth of field reaches into deeper myocardial layers; however, how deep exactly is not known.

Are Intramural MAP Recordings Possible?

The impetus for intramural MAP recordings comes from the desire to record disparities of APDs across the myocardial wall of the intact heart, because it has been shown by microelectrode techniques that such disparity exists and that midmyocardial cells (M cells) have longer APDs and are more prone to exhibit EADs at slow rates than are epicardial or endocardial cells.[59,60] Thus, the recording of truly local intramyocardial MAP recordings would advance the understanding of the mechanism of many arrhythmias, most notably of the torsades de pointes variety. Attempts have been made to obtain MAPs intramyocardially by inserting a multipolar plunge electrode into the myocardial wall and coupling it with a reference electrode placed on a remote (epicardial) site of the ventricle.[61] The initial injury (monophasic) potential resulting from inserting the plunge electrodes into the myocardial wall was allowed to subside until a normal electrogram was recorded. The remote electrode site was then depolarized with KCl. This led to a new monophasic recording. This MAP was of reversed polarity when connected to the amplifier in conventional manner (see above). To make this MAP upright, the exploring (intramural) electrode was coupled to the negative amplifier input and the KCl electrode to the positive amplifier input. As discussed earlier, this suggests that the monophasic portion of the recording derives from the remote (KCl) electrode and not from the intramural plunge electrodes.

Because of the wide spacing between the intramyocardial electrode and the remote KCl electrode, these "intramural MAP recordings," by definition, represent largely unipolar MAP recordings which are subject to contamination by far-field potentials in much the same way as unipolar electrograms. Superimposition of disparate T wave durations on these MAPs may give the impression that MAPs of different duration are recorded from different intramural sites. Such recordings, while to some degree reflecting intramural differences, are not truly local as obtained by the close-bipolar technique but are hybrids of local and far-field potentials.

It appears from the above discussion that the MAP itself is a unipolar recording, despite the fact that the MAP reference electrode is positioned nearby. Unlike conventional bipolar recordings, however, the reference electrode is located proximal to the site of MAP genesis (ie, perpendicularly away from the field that is measured as the MAP). It is, however, the proximal, closely adjacent reference electrode which makes the MAP truly local.

Conclusion

MAP recordings have come a long way and are now an integral part of electrophysiologic studies that are concerned with understanding basic electrophysiology and arrhythmia mechanisms in the intact heart. MAP recordings in the clinical laboratory have confirmed many basic electrophysiologic principles, and observations from human heart MAP recordings have spawned experimental research not previously recognized as clinically important. However, while the methodology of MAP recording by contact electrode technique is relatively simple, the understanding of the abilities and limitations of the MAP and its proper interpretations are not. While falling short of intracellular recordings in several aspects, MAP recordings have the advantage of providing accurate reflections of the repolarization time course of a local multicellular sample in the intact, beating heart (Table 1). Future developments and refinements of the MAP recording technique will undoubtedly advance our possibilities further, including possibly longer term and simultaneous multiple-site MAP mapping.

References

1. Hoffman BF, Cranefield PF, Lepeschkin E, et al. Comparison of cardiac monophasic action potentials recorded by intracellular and suction electrodes. *Am J Physiol* 1959;196:1297-1301.
2. Franz MR, Burkhoff D, Spurgeon H, et al. In vitro validation of a new cardiac catheter technique for recording monophasic action potentials. *Eur Heart J* 1986;7:34-41.
3. Ino T, Karagueuzian HS, Hong K, et al. Relation of monophasic action potential recorded with contact electrode to underlying transmembrane action potential properties in isolated cardiac tissues: A systematic microelectrode validation study. *Cardiovasc Res* 1988;22:255-264.
4. Burdon-Sanderson J, Page FJM. On the time-relations of the excitatory process in the ventricle of the heart of the frog. *J Physiol* 1882;2:385-412.
5. Schuetz E. Einphasische Aktionsstroeme vom in situ durchbluteten Saeugetierherzen. *Z Biol* 1932;92:441-452.
6. Schuetz E. Weitere Versuche mit einphasischer Aufzeichnung des Warmblueter-Elektrokardiogramms. *Z Biol* 1934;95:78-90.
7. Korsgren M, Leskinen E, Sjöstrand U, Varnauskas E. Intracardiac recording of monophasic action potentials in the human heart. *Scand J Clin Lab Invest* 1966;18:561-564.
8. Olsson SB. Monophasic action potentials from right atrial muscle recorded during heart catheterization. *Acta Med Scand* 1971;190:369-379.
9. Olsson SB. Atrial repolarization in man. Effect of beta-receptor blockade. *Br Heart J* 1974;36:806-810.
10. Brorson L, Olsson SB. Atrial repolarization in healthy males. Studies with programmed stimulation and monophasic action potential recordings. *Acta Med Scand* 1976;199:447-454.

11. Jochim K, Katz LN, Mayne W. The monophasic electrogram obtained from the mammalian heart. *Am J Physiol* 1935;111:177-186.

12. Franz M, Schottler M, Schaefer J, Seed WA. Simultaneous recording of monophasic action potentials and contractile force from the human heart. *Klin Wochenschr* 1980;58:1357-1359.

13. Franz MR. Long-term recording of monophasic action potentials from human endocardium. *Am J Cardiol* 1983;51:1629-1634.

14. Franz MR, Chin MC, Sharkey HR, et al. A new single catheter technique for simultaneous measurement of action potential duration and refractory period in vivo. *J Am Coll Cardiol* 1990;16:878-886.

15. Franz MR, Flaherty JT, Platia EV, et al. Localization of regional myocardial ischemia by recording of monophasic action potentials. *Circulation* 1984;69:593-604.

16. Franz MR, Bargheer K, Rafflenbeul W, et al. Monophasic action potential mapping in human subjects with normal electrocardiograms: Direct evidence for the genesis of the T wave. *Circulation* 1987;75:379-386.

17. Franz MR, Costard A. Frequency-dependent effects of quinidine on the relationship between action potential duration and refractoriness in the canine heart in situ. *Circulation* 1988;77:1177-1184.

18. Franz MR, Swerdlow CD, Liem LB, Schaefer J. Cycle length dependence of human action potential duration in vivo. Effects of single extrastimuli, sudden sustained rate acceleration and deceleration, and different steady-state frequencies. *J Clin Invest* 1988;82:972-979.

19. Schaefer H. Theorie des Potentialabgriffs beim Elektrokardiogramm, auf der Grundlage der "Membrantheorie." *Pflüegers Arch* 1942;245:72-97.

20. Schaefer H, Peña A, Schölmerich P. Der monophasische Aktionsstrom von Spitze und Basis des Warmblüterherzens und die Theorie der T-Welle des EKG. *Pflügers Arch* 1943;246:728-745.

21. Sugarman H, Katz LN, Sanders A, Jochim K. Observations on the genesis of the electrical currents established by injury to the heart. *Am J Physiol* 1940;130:130-143.

22. Cranefield PF, Eyster JAE, Gilson WE. Electrical characteristics of injury potentials. *Am J Physiol* 1951;167:450-457.

23. Eyster JAE, Gilson WE. The development and contour of cardiac injury potential. *Am J Physiol* 1946;145:507-520.

24. Schuetz E. Elektrophysiologie des Herzens bei einphasischer Ableitung. *Ergebn Physiol Exper Pharmakol* 1936;38:493-620.

25. Antzelevitch C, Moe GK. Electrotonically mediated delayed conduction and reentry in relation to "slow responses" in mammalian ventricular conducting tissue. *Circ Res* 1981;49:1129-1139.

26. Franz MR. Method and theory of monophasic action potential recording. *Prog Cardiovasc Dis* 1991;33:347-368.

27. Koller B, Franz MR. New classification of moricizine and propafenone based on electrophysiologic and electrocardiographic data from isolated rabbit heart. *J Cardiovasc Pharmacol* 1994;24:753-760.

28. Franz MR, Burkhoff D, Lakatta EG, Weisfeldt ML. Monophasic action potential recording by contact electrode technique: In vitro validation and clinical applications. In Butrous GS, Schwartz PJ (eds): *Clinical Aspects of Ventricular Repolarization*. London: Farrand Press; 1989:81-92.

29. Draper MH, Weidmann S. Cardiac resting and action potentials recorded with an intracellular electrode. *J Physiol (Lond)* 1951;115:74-94.

30. Tande PM, Mortensen E, Refsum H. Rate-dependent differences in dog epi- and endocardial monophasic action potential configuration in vivo. *Am J Physiol* 1991;261:H1387-H1391.

31. Patterson E, Szabo B, Scherlag BJ, Lazzara R. Early and delayed afterdepolarizations associated with cesium chloride-induced arrhythmias in the dog. *J Cardiovasc Pharmacol* 1990;15:323-331.

32. Ben-David J, Zipes DP. Differential response to right and left ansae subclaviae stimulation of early afterdepolarizations and ventricular tachycardia induced by cesium in dogs. *Circulation* 1988;78:1241-1250.

33. Priori SG, Corr PB. Mechanisms underlying early and delayed afterdepolarizations induced by catecholamines. *Am J Physiol* 1990;258:H1796-H1805.

34. Vera Z, Pride HP, Zipes DP. Reperfusion arrhythmias: Role of early afterdepolarizations studied by monophasic action potential recordings in the intact canine heart during autonomically denervated and stimulated states. *J Cardiovasc Electrophysiol* 1995;6:532-543.

35. Vos MA, Verduyn SC, Gorgels AP, et al. Reproducible induction of early afterdepolarizations and torsade de pointes arrhythmias by d-sotalol and pacing in dogs with chronic atrioventricular block. *Circulation* 1995;91:864-872.

36. Zabel M, Hohnloser SH, Behrens S, et al. Electrophysiologic features of torsades de pointes: Insights from a new isolated rabbit heart model. *J Cardiovasc Electrophysiol* 1997;8:1148-1158.

37. Habbab MA, El-Sherif N. Drug-induced torsades de pointes: Role of early afterdepolarizations and dispersion of repolarization. *Am J Med* 1990;89:241-246.

38. Morgan JM, Lopes A, Rowland E. Sudden cardiac death while taking amiodarone therapy: The role of abnormal repolarization. *Eur Heart J* 1991;12:1144-1147.

39. El-Sherif N, Bekheit SS, Henkin R. Quinidine-induced long QTU interval and torsade de pointes: Role of bradycardia-dependent early afterdepolarizations. *J Am Coll Cardiol* 1989;14:252-257.

40. Shimizu W, Ohe T, Kurita T, et al. Epinephrine-induced ventricular premature complexes due to early afterdepolarizations and effects of verapamil and propranolol in a patient with congenital long QT syndrome. *J Cardiovasc Electrophysiol* 1994;5:438-444.

41. Shimizu W, Ohe T, Kurita T, et al. Effects of verapamil and propranolol on early afterdepolarizations and ventricular arrhythmias induced by epinephrine in congenital long QT syndrome. *J Am Coll Cardiol* 1995;26:1299-1309.

42. Lab MJ. Contraction-excitation feedback in myocardium. Physiological basis and clinical relevance. *Circ Res* 1982;50:757-766.

43. Lab MJ. Monophasic action potentials and the detection and significance of mechanoelectric feedback in vivo. *Prog Cardiovasc Dis* 1991;34:29-35.

44. Lerman BB, Burkhoff D, Yue DT, et al. Mechanoelectrical feedback: Independent role of preload and contractility in modulation of canine ventricular excitability [published erratum appears in *J Clin Invest* 1986;77:2053]. *J Clin Invest* 1985;76:1843-1850.

45. Franz MR, Burkhoff D, Yue DT, Sagawa K. Mechanically induced action potential changes and arrhythmia in isolated and in situ canine hearts. *Cardiovasc Res* 1989;23:213-223.

46. Franz MR, Cima R, Wang D, et al. Electrophysiological effects of myocardial stretch and mechanical determinants of stretch-activated arrhythmias [published erratum appears in *Circulation* 1992;86:1663]. *Circulation* 1992;86:968-978.

47. Zabel M, Koller BS, Sachs F, Franz MR. Stretch-induced voltage changes in the isolated beating heart: Importance of the timing of stretch and implications for stretch-activated ion channels. *Cardiovasc Res* 1996;32:120-130.
48. Franz MR. Mechano-electrical feedback in ventricular myocardium. *Cardiovasc Res* 1996;32:15-24.
49. Housmans PR, Chuck LH, Claes VA, Brutsaert DL. Nonuniformity of contraction and relaxation of mammalian cardiac muscle. *Adv Exp Med Biol* 1984; 170:837-840.
50. Olsson SB, Blomstrom P, Blomstrom-Lundqvist C, Wohlfart B. Endocardial monophasic action potentials. Correlations with intracellular electrical activity. *Ann N Y Acad Sci* 1990;601:119-127.
51. Olsson SB. Right ventricular monophasic action potentials during regular rhythm. A heart catheterization study in man. *Acta Med Scand* 1972;191:145-157.
52. De Mello WC, Motta GE, Chapeau M. A study on the healing-over of myocardial cells of toads. *Circ Res* 1969;24:475-487.
53. De Mello WC. Effect of intracellular injection of calcium and strontium on cell communication in heart. *J Physiol (Lond)* 1975;250:231-245.
54. De Mello WC. Influence of the sodium pump on intercellular communication in heart fibres: Effect of intracellular injection of sodium ion on electrical coupling. *J Physiol (Lond)* 1976;263:171-197.
55. De Mello WC. The role of cAMP and Ca on the modulation of junctional conductance: An integrated hypothesis. *Cell Biol Int* 1983;7:1033-1040.
56. Franz MR. Bridging the gap between basic and clinical electrophysiology: What can be learned from monophasic action potential recordings? *J Cardiovasc Electrophysiol* 1994;5:699-710.
57. Coronel R, Wilms-Schopman FJ, Opthof T, et al. Injury current and gradients of diastolic stimulation threshold, TQ potential, and extracellular potassium concentration during acute regional ischemia in the isolated perfused pig heart. *Circ Res* 1991;68:1241-1249.
58. Levine JH, Moore EN, Kadish AH, et al. The monophasic action potential upstroke: A means of characterizing local conduction. *Circulation* 1986; 74:1147-1155.
59. Sicouri S, Fish J, Antzelevitch C. Distribution of M cells in the canine ventricle. *J Cardiovasc Electrophysiol* 1994;5:824-837.
60. Sicouri S, Antzelevitch C. Drug-induced afterdepolarizations and triggered activity occur in a discrete subpopulation of ventricular muscle cells (M cells) in the canine heart: Quinidine and digitalis. *J Cardiovasc Electrophysiol* 1993;4:48-58.
61. Nesterenko VV, Weissenburger J. Experimental evidence for re-interpretation of basis for the monophasic action potential: A new technique with large amplitude and stable transmural signals. *Circulation* 1995;92(suppl I):I299. Abstract.

3

Computer Model of Monophasic Action Potential Genesis

Natalia Trayanova, PhD, Lisa Malden, PhD and Evan Atkinson, BS

Introduction

Monophasic action potentials (MAPs) are extracellularly recorded waveforms. Unlike conventional extracellular recordings (ie, electrograms), which are used widely to determine the pattern of activation in the heart, MAPs mimic the time course of local repolarization.[1] This remarkable feature makes MAPs an invaluable tool for studying cellular recovery processes not only in experimental but also in clinical settings.[2]

Despite the increased attention that MAPs have received over recent years in both experimental and clinical studies, the genesis of the MAP is not yet well understood. Current MAP recordings are obtained by pressing an electrode of relatively large diameter (about 1 mm or more[1]) against the myocardial surface (see Fig.1, panel A for schematic representation of the MAP electrode). The size of the electrode tip ensures that the recording is extracellular, as the tip is too large to penetrate a single myocyte. An understanding of why MAP signals closely follow the repolarization course of transmembrane action potentials (TAPs) could help improve their correlation with TAPs and could contribute to advancements in MAP recording techniques.

From Franz MR (ed): *Monophasic Action Potentials: Bridging Cell and Bedside.* ©Futura Publishing Company, Inc., Armonk, NY, 2000.

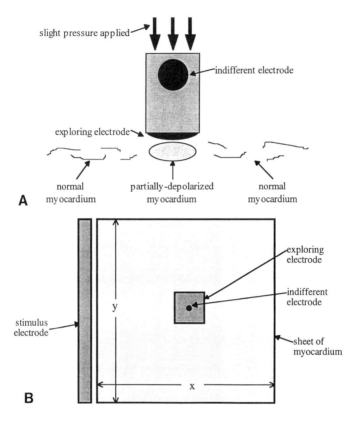

Figure 1. A. Schematic of the MAP electrode. The tip of the MAP electrode is pressed against the myocardial surface. The indifferent electrode must also have electrical continuity with the myocardium. The contact medium is either blood for endocardial readings or saline-soaked foam rubber, mounted on the electrode, for epicardial readings. **B.** Representation of the model geometry used to simulate MAPs on a sheet of myocardium.

Deducing from the available data regarding MAP signals, Franz[1] hypothesized that the mechanical pressure exerted on the myocardium subjacent to the recording electrode depolarizes and inactivates the cells in this region while leaving the adjacent cells largely unaffected. Thus, an electrical gradient is established between the depolarized cells and the normal cells. This gradient exists during both diastole, when the pressured cells are more depolarized than the rest of the myocardium, and systole, when the normal cells undergo complete depolarization and achieve values of transmembrane potential higher than those of the injured cells. Thus, cells on both sides of the injury boundary contribute to the generation of a boundary current that gives rise to the extracellular potential recorded by the MAP electrode.

The goal of the research discussed in this chapter is to conduct simulation experiments to test Franz's hypothesis. More specifically, the intent of the study is to model extracellular potentials generated by the passage of a propagating wave through a region of depolarized cells surrounded by normal myocardium. This investigation builds on the modeling studies of Hirsch,[3] Malden,[4] and Malden and Henriquez.[5] Using a cellular automata model, Hirsch[3] examined the extracellular potentials associated with a region of ischemic properties; the calculated potentials resembled MAP recordings. Malden, alone[4] and with Henriquez,[5] attempted to simulate MAPs by employing more realistic membrane kinetics and modeling the MAP electrode as a region of passive membrane properties. The present study extends the latter line of inquiry. We employ various electrical representations of the injured cells in the calculation of MAPs. The simulated MAPs are then compared to experimentally recorded signals, and conclusions regarding the level of depolarization of the injured cells are made. In this comparison, of particular significance is the fact that clinically recorded MAPs are characterized by a 1:2 ratio of systolic to diastolic potential magnitude (as measured from the zero reference line) regardless of the peak-to-peak magnitude of the MAP signal.[1]

Model Description

Geometry

To explore tissue behavior that can give rise to MAP signals, we used a 2-dimensional computer model of a square sheet of anisotropic myocardium. While the model allows for variable sheet dimensions, most of the simulations were performed using dimensions 1×1 cm, dictated by our intent to compare our simulation results with those of previous simulation studies.[4,5] In the tissue preparation, myocardial fibers were assumed to run parallel to the Cartesian x axis. The MAP electrode was modeled by a 1×1 mm exploring electrode located centrally on the tissue and a 0.1×0.1 mm indifferent electrode located centrally and 0.5 cm above the sheet (see Fig. 1, panel B). In addition to merely being in electrical contact with the tissue, the exploring electrode established a region of injury. Despite the simplified representation of the MAP electrode in the model, its dimensions correspond to those of MAP electrodes used in experimental and clinical recordings.[1,6]

The MAP electrode recorded electrical activity associated with a planar wave propagating across the tissue (referred to here as *systole*). The wave was elicited by line stimulation of the left tissue edge (shown in Fig.1, panel B), ie, the wave propagated along fibers from left to right. The membrane kinetics in our model were represented by the Luo-Rudy (phase

I) membrane equations.[7] The stimulus used to elicit the planar propagating wave was of strength -300 $\mu A/cm^2$ and duration 1 millisecond. The planar wave was launched 500 milliseconds after the application of the "pressure" (ie, after 500 milliseconds of *diastole*), thus allowing time for the potentials in the tissue to equilibrate.

Governing Equations

The transmembrane potential in the tissue was calculated using the following differential equation:

$$BI_m = C_m \frac{\partial V_m}{\partial t} + I_{stim} + \sum I_{ion} = \beta \left(\sigma_{ix} \frac{\partial^2 V_m}{\partial x^2} + \sigma_{iy} \frac{\partial^2 V_m}{\partial y^2} \right) \tag{1}$$

which assumes that the extracellular potentials in the tissue are much smaller than the intracellular potentials, ie, the tissue is represented by a monodomain approximation.[8] V_m denotes the transmembrane potential (mV); I_m is the transmembrane current density ($\mu A/cm^2$); C_m is the specific membrane capacitance ($\mu F/cm^2$); I_{stim} and I_{ion} are the stimulus and ionic currents densities ($\mu A/cm^2$); and σ_{ix} and σ_{iy} are the intracellular conductivities (mS/cm) along and across the fibers, respectively. The surface-to-volume ratio of the membrane, β (cm^{-1}), is equal to $2/a$ where a is the radius of a typical fiber in the tissue (or half of the tissue thickness in the z direction).

Boundary conditions were imposed on the transmembrane potential at the tissue borders. In this study we assumed that the myocardial sheet is insulated, thus no-flux boundary conditions applied. In terms of transmembrane potential, the no-flux boundary conditions on the tissue borders reduce to:

$$\frac{\partial V_m}{\partial n} = 0 \tag{2}$$

where n denotes the direction normal to the edges of the sheet.

The MAP electrode records the extracellular potentials of the tissue. To calculate the extracellular potential, Φ_e, the following expression was used[9]:

$$\Phi_e(x_0,y_0) = \frac{2a}{4\pi\sigma_e} \int_{y1}^{y2} \int_{x1}^{x2} \frac{I_v(x,y)}{R} dxdy \tag{3}$$

It represents the extracellular potential at a point with coordinates (x_0,y_0) in the tissue, as generated by sources distributed over the myocardial sheet. The volume density of the transmembrane current, I_v($\mu A/cm^3$), constitutes the source for the extracellular potential. It is related to the transmembrane current density, I_m, by the expression $I_v = \beta I_m = (2/a) I_m$. The limits of the integrals correspond with the boundaries of myocardium in x and y directions, and R represents the distance in cm between a source point of coordinates (x,y) and a field point of coordinates (x_0,y_0). The conductivity of the extracellular space is denoted as σ_e (mS/cm).

Representation of Tissue Behavior Under the MAP Electrode

For this research we used the following modeling strategies to represent altered electrical behavior of the cells in the pressure region:

- *Assume that the tissue under the MAP electrode tip has a fixed value of transmembrane potential higher than the normal resting potential.* In this case, all cells that belong to the injured region are assumed to have the same, constant transmembrane potential regardless of whether the remaining myocardium is in systole or in diastole. The injured cells are not electrically affected by the surrounding tissue because the transmembrane potential in the region of injury is "clamped" at a certain level. However, at rest, the fixed potential of the injured region does have an effect on the surrounding tissue—it contributes to elevated resting potentials of the cells surrounding the injured region. For sufficiently high values of the clamped potential, the current at the boundary between injured and normal cells is suprathreshold, thus generating a wave that propagates outwardly from the injury boundary. Based on Franz's[1] theory that cells under the MAP electrode are depolarized to potentials less than 0 mV, we clamped the transmembrane potential under the MAP electrode to levels in the range of –10 to –70 mV.* Mathematically, this was accomplished by forcing the transmembrane potential of the injured cells to a constant value rather than allowing it to be governed by the normal ventricular myocardial kinetics of the Luo-Rudy (phase I) model.
- *Assume that the tissue under the MAP electrode tip has an elevated resting potential.* In this case, the injured cells are assumed to have high values of resting potential and are thus inactivated by depolarization. The potential of the injured cells is not clamped. Thus, when an action potential propagates through the healthy tissue, current from surrounding healthy cells contributes to electrotonic changes in the transmembrane potential of the injured cells. In diastole, the high resting potential of the injured cells affects the normal tissue, somewhat elevating the resting potentials of cells surrounding the pressure region. Similar to the case of clamped transmembrane potential in the injured region (see above item),

---

* The values of clamped potential used here differ from the value of –75 mV used in a simulation by Malden included in Reference 4.

very high values of resting potential under the MAP electrode can lead to strong currents flowing off the injury line, exciting the normal myocardium. In this research, we raised the resting potential of the cells in the pressure region to values in the range of –40 to –10 mV. The choice of this range was dictated by our intent to inactivate the cells under the MAP electrode while keeping their resting potential below 0 mV. Mathematically, we achieved elevated values of resting potential by altering the extracellular potassium concentration in the pressure region and thus the Nernst potentials E_K and E_{K1} (= E_{Kp}) in the Luo-Rudy model. Table 1 presents the potassium concentrations and Nernst values associated with the values of resting potential used in this study. The extracellular potassium concentration and corresponding Nernst potentials were used as initial conditions in the pressure region (instead of the normal tissue initial conditions in the Luo-Rudy membrane model) when solving the differential equation for V_m (eq. 1). Figure 2 depicts the transmembrane potential of a membrane patch under normal conditions as well as in cases when the resting potential is raised in the manner discussed above. When the resting potential is elevated to –40 mV and beyond, the patch becomes inactivated as demonstrated by its passive response to current stimulation.

* *Assume that the tissue under the MAP electrode tip is inexcitable.* Such an assumption was made for the first time in the pilot MAP simulation studies of Malden alone[4] and Malden and Henriquez.[5] Under this condition, the membrane is modeled as a passive resistor-capacitor network. Mathematically, the term I_{ion} in equation 1 is replaced by $(V_m - V_{rest})/R_m$, where R_m (mS/cm^2) is the membrane-specific resistance at rest. From the Luo-Rudy membrane equations, one can calculate the value of R_m as 3.5 kΩcm^2.[4] In our simulations, we used this value of the membrane resistance to calculate the MAPs. (Additional simulations were carried out with decreased membrane resistance to represent pressure-induced increases in leakage current through the membrane and to assess how it is reflected in the MAP magnitude.) When the injured region of myocardium is considered passive, there is no potential difference across the injury boundary during diastole. Potential gradients arise only

---

Table 1
LR1 Model Parameters Altered in Order to Simulate
Elevated Resting Potential in the Injured Tissue

Targeted V_r (mV)	$[K]_e$ (mM)	E_K (mV)	$E_{Kl} = E_{Kp}$ (mV)	Actual V_r (mV)
–40	31	–39.21	–41.28	–40.13
–30	45	–29.88	–31.31	–30.01
–20	67.5	–19.52	–20.46	–20.01
–10	101.5	–8.94	–9.54	–10.01

LR1 = Luo-Rudy (phase I).

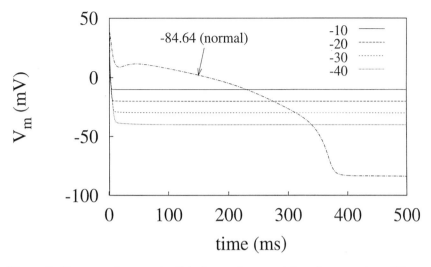

Figure 2. Transmembrane potential of a membrane patch under normal conditions and for elevated resting potential (in the range of –40 to –10 mV).

during systole. Current from normal cells undergoing an action potential in the vicinity of the MAP electrode "invades" the pressure region and changes the transmembrane potential of the cells subjacent to the MAP electrode. Despite its magnitude, this change is purely electrotonic since the cells cannot be excited. The difference between electrotonic transmembrane potential under the MAP electrode and the active behavior of the surrounding cells gives rise to border currents that are expected to contribute to extracellular potentials recorded by the MAP electrode. Although the MAPs simulated under the conditions of passive region of pressure have been, to a large extent, explored previously by Malden, alone[4] and with Henriquez,[5] we included them in this study for reasons of completeness and so that we could make comparisons with MAPs that were simulated using other representations of the injured region (see above items).

Numerical Considerations and Parameter Values

To calculate the transmembrane potential distribution throughout the myocardial sheet as well as under the MAP electrode tip, the finite difference forward Euler method was used. The sheet was discretized into nodes 0.01 cm apart. Thus, a 1-cm^2 sheet consists of 100×100 nodes. A time step of 0.01 millisecond was used in the calculations. The boundary conditions (eq. 2) were implemented, ensuring spatial second-order accuracy. Table 2 summarizes the numerical values of all parameters used in this study.

Table 2
Descriptions and Values of Tissue Material Constants
and LR1 Model Parameters

	Variable	Description	Value
Tissue	R_m	membrane resistance per unit area	3.54 kΩ/cm^2
	C_m	membrane capacitance per unit area	1.0 μF/cm^2
	σ_{ix}	intracellular conductance, longitudinal	3.333 mS/cm
	σ_{iy}	intracellular conductance, transverse	0.654 mS/cm
	σ_e	extracellular conductance, bath	10 mS/cm
	dx, dy	spatial increment (nodal dimensions)	0.01 cm
	a	fiber radius (half of tissue thickness)	0.0008 cm
	I_{stim}	extracellular stimulus current (for 1 msec)	−300 μA/cm^2
LR1 Model	V_m	transmembrane potential	−84.64 mV*
	PR_{NaK}	permeability ratio, sodium to potassium	0.01833
	$[Ca]_i$	intracellular concentration (initial), calcium	0.002 mM
	$[Na]_i$	intracellular concentration, sodium	18 mM
	$[Na]_e$	extracellular concentration, sodium	140 mM
	$[K]_i$	intracellular concentration, potassium	145 mM
	$[K]_e$	extracellular concentration, potassium	5.4 mM*
	E_{Na}	Nernst potential, sodium	54.4 mV
	E_K	Nernst potential, potassium	−77 mV*
	$E_{Kl} = E_{Kp}$	driving force, secondary potassium currents	−88 mV*

*Values for physiologically normal ventricular myocardium. These values were altered appropriately when simulating elevated resting potential.
LR1 = Luo-Rudy (phase I).

Results

As described in the *Methods* section, pressure is applied to the tissue at t = 0 milliseconds, and a propagating planar wave front is launched from the left tissue border at 500 milliseconds. The period after 500 milliseconds represents the "normal activation of the tissue." The wave front propagates through the sheet, and the centrally located electrode "records" an injury-induced extracellular potential (MAP). We used the three modeling strategies described to represent altered electrical behavior of the cells under the MAP electrode.

Clamped Transmembrane Potential in the Injured Region

Panel A of Figure 3 shows the extracellular potential (MAP) recorded in the center of the tissue. These MAPs are generated with the assumption that cells subjacent to the tip of the MAP electrode can be adequately represented as a region of fixed transmembrane potential, V_{clamp}, of a value

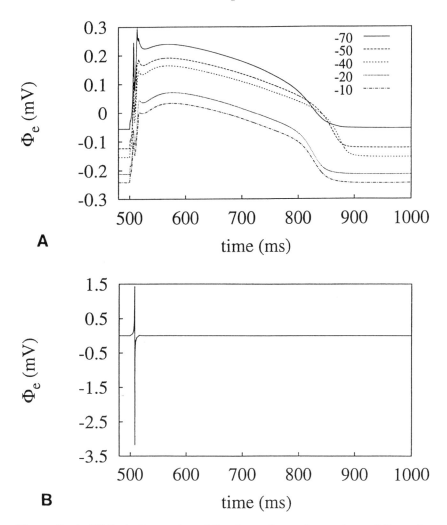

Figure 3. A. MAPs in the center of the tissue for various values of V_{clamp}, the transmembrane potential of the injured region. **B.** The normal extracellular potential at the same site.

higher than the resting potential of normal tissue* (see first item in preceding section). For purposes of comparison, the normal (ie, if V_m were not clamped) extracellular potential at the same location is shown in panel B of Figure 3. This figure demonstrates that in the examined range of V_{clamp} from –70 to –10 mV, the resulting MAPs have a shape similar to that of the TAP. They are characterized with a biphasic intrinsic deflection in the

---

*The resting potential of normal tissue is –84.64 mV, as calculated from the Luo-Rudy membrane model.

upstroke similar to that of the clinically recorded MAPs,[1] and they have a repolarization phase following a distinct plateau region. The biphasic intrinsic deflection takes the shape of a biphasic extracellular potential under normal conditions (similar to Fig. 3, panel B); it is a result of the propagation of the wave front past the point of recording. The similarity of MAP to the TAP is illustrated in Figure 4, in which the MAPs are displayed together with a normal TAP; their magnitudes are normalized with respect to the maximum plateau magnitude of the TAP. For all values of V_{clamp}, the duration of the MAP is somewhat shorter than the duration of the TAP, an observation consistent with in vitro and in vivo MAP recordings.[10] The MAP generated for $V_{clamp} = -40$ mV has a duration closest to the duration of the TAP.

To better understand the electrophysiologic phenomena that underlie the generation of MAP signals, it is necessary to examine the currents generated in the vicinity of the MAP electrode before and after the arrival of the "normal activation." Immediately after the application of pressure to the tissue by the MAP electrode (ie, while tissue is in diastole), a potential gradient is established across the border of the injured region. Panel A of Figure 5 illustrates the spatial distribution of transmembrane potential along the central fiber in the tissue 500 milliseconds after the application of pressure. For values of V_{clamp} between -70 and -40 mV, the potential difference established across the injury boundary is insufficient to produce a current capable of exciting the surrounding tissue. Thus, after the application of the pressure, some equilibration between the potentials of the "injured" cells and the surrounding normal cells takes place (Fig. 5, panel A), resulting in an elevated resting potential of the cells surrounding the

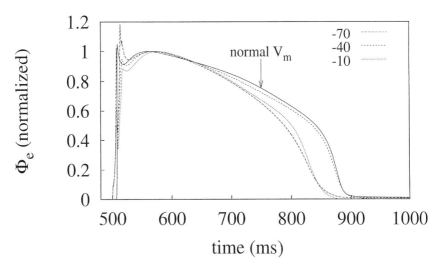

Figure 4. MAPs as in Figure 3, panel A, normalized with respect to the maximum plateau magnitude of the normal transmembrane action potential.

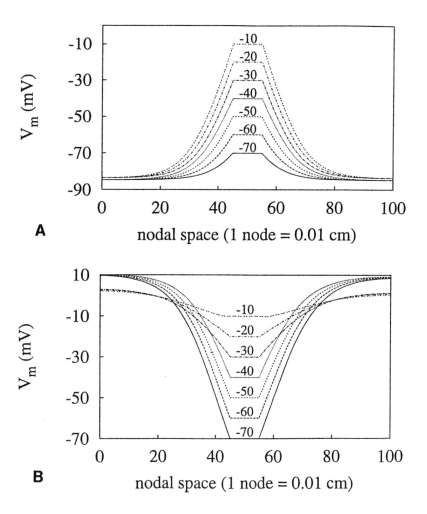

Figure 5. Spatial distribution of transmembrane potential along the central fiber in the tissue for various values of V_{clamp}: **A.** in diastole, 500 milliseconds after the application of pressure to the central region of the tissue; **B.** in systole, 50 milliseconds after the onset of "normal activation."

MAP electrode. As V_{clamp} is fixed at values above −40 mV, the boundary current becomes sufficient to excite the surrounding tissue. In this case, following the application of pressure to the tissue, a wave front propagates outwardly from the injured region (not shown here). The 500-millisecond interval from the application of the pressure to the launch of the "normal activation" propagating wave at the left tissue border allows the initial pressure-generated wave to pass completely through the sheet. Moments just before the arrival of the normal activation wave, as shown in panel

A of Figure 5, the spatial distribution of potential is unaffected by this initial outward wave front propagation. Overall, after application of pressure to the tissue (and the subsequent passage of an outward wave front, if any), current flows from the injured region toward the surrounding cells; the magnitude of this current is larger for higher values of V_{clamp}. This is demonstrated in panel A of Figure 6, which presents the spatial distribution of the transmembrane current volume density, I_v, along the central fiber in the sheet. Current density is localized around the borders of the pressure region; its absolute magnitude increases with the elevation of V_{clamp}. The

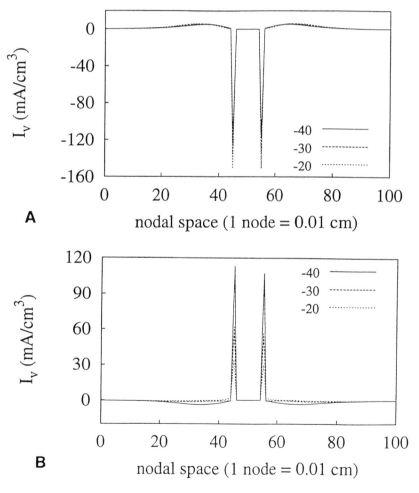

Figure 6. Spatial distribution of the transmembrane current volume density, I_v, along the central fiber in the tissue for various values of V_{clamp}: **A.** in diastole, 500 milliseconds after the application of pressure to the central region of the tissue; **B.** in systole, 50 milliseconds after the onset of "normal activation."

sign of the current density reflects the fact that it is directed from the injured tissue toward the normal cells.

The direction of this current is reversed during the normal activation of the sheet when the magnitude of the transmembrane potential of the surrounding cells is larger than V_{clamp}. Thus, during systole, a potential gradient is created, and current flows from the normal cells toward the injured region. Panel B of Figure 5 depicts the spatial distribution of transmembrane potential along the central fiber in the tissue 50 milliseconds after the onset of the normal activation wave. At this time, the sheet is at a plateau potential.* Panel B of Figure 6 illustrates the spatial distribution of transmembrane current volume density along the central fiber in the sheet 50 milliseconds after the onset of the normal activation wave (550 milliseconds after pressure applied). The two positive peaks correspond to the surge of current from normal tissues into injured tissue at the borders. The magnitude of the current decreases with the elevation of V_{clamp}. This systolic current lasts as long as the cells surrounding the MAP electrode region are at a potential larger than V_{clamp}, indicating that the duration of the MAP cannot be longer than the duration of the TAP. The latter observation is consistent with experimental evidence.[11] Figure 7 shows the transmembrane current volume density in time for 3 values of V_{clamp}. The current consists of diastolic and systolic phases and an overall shape that resembles the TAP.

When examining Figure 3, of particular interest is the fact that with the elevation of V_{clamp} in the pressure region, the take-off (baseline) level

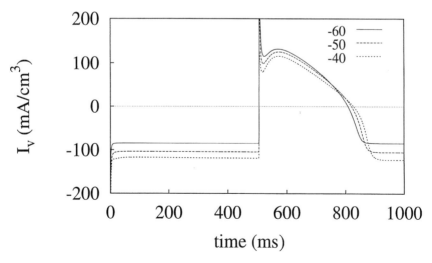

Figure 7. Time course of the transmembrane current volume density for 3 values of V_{clamp}. The node is located centrally on the left border of the pressure region.

*Note that normal plateau potential is approximately 10 mV, which decreases to 2 mV in cases when a pressure-generated wave precedes the normal activation.

of the MAP decreases, ie, the MAP shifts toward more negative values of extracellular potential. Such behavior is characteristic of the time course of I_v at the border as well (Fig. 7); the latter is the current source for the extracellular potential (MAP) as evident from equation 3. This behavior is consistent with the fact that for high values of V_{clamp} the diastolic current is larger than the systolic (compare Fig. 6, panels A and B, see also Fig. 7). The solid line in Figure 8 presents the ratio of systolic to diastolic magnitude of the MAP signal as a function of the clamp potential in the injured tissue. The horizontal dashed line corresponds to the experimentally observed ratio of 1:2.[1] Clearly, since the latter value of the ratio appears to be a consistent feature of the MAP signal that is independent of the peak-to-peak magnitude of the MAP,[1] this group of simulations indicates that the pressure exerted by the MAP electrode appears to depolarize the tissue to a value of approximately –27 mV.

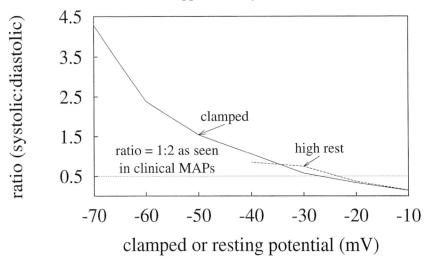

Figure 8. Ratio of systolic to diastolic MAP magnitude as a function of V_{clamp} (solid line) or V_r (dashed line) in the injured region. The dotted line corresponds to the experimentally observed ratio of 1:2.

Elevated Resting Potential in the Injured Region

The second group of simulation results in this study refers to MAPs calculated under the assumption that the region of injury has an elevated resting potential, V_r (see second item in *Representation of Tissue Behavior Under the MAP Electrode* section). Figure 9 shows the MAPs for different values of V_r, while Figure 10 shows the normal TAP together with some of the normalized MAPs. The MAPs corresponding to values of V_r in the range

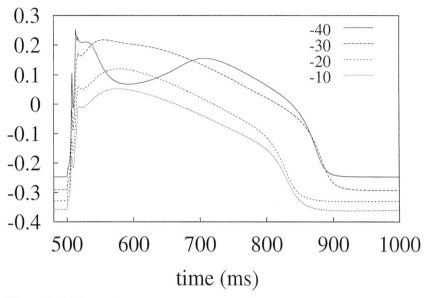

Figure 9. MAPs in the center of the tissue for 4 values of V_r, the resting potential of the injured region.

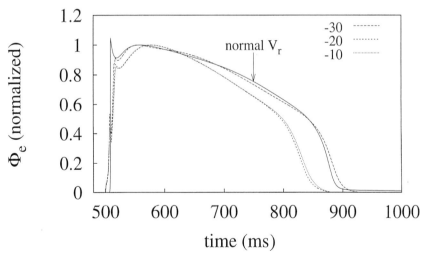

Figure 10. MAPs as in Figure 9, normalized with respect to the maximum plateau magnitude of the normal transmembrane action potential.

of −30 to −10 mV have shapes similar to the normal TAP and thus are consistent with experimental observations. The remaining MAP (V_r = −40 mV) has a different shape, characterized by a dip during the plateau phase; the shape of the MAPs for lower values of V_r (not shown here) is similar. The events underlying this phenomenon can be best understood by examining the current flow during diastole and systole. During diastole (after the application of pressure to the central portion of the sheet), a potential difference and current flow is established from injured cells toward healthy cells in a manner similar to the behavior shown in panel A of Figure 5. Unlike the clamped case, however, an action potential is not elicited from the pressure region until V_r reaches −30 mV (as opposed to −40 mV in the clamped case). The spatial characteristics of this current are similar to the ones shown in panel A of Figure 6. During systole, however, the potential of the injured region changes. Although the cells in that region are completely or partially inactivated (depending on the value of V_r) and may not be able to generate an action potential, the transmembrane potential in the region changes due to current contribution from surrounding cells that are undergoing a normal activation. Figure 11 presents the transmembrane potential in the center of the injured region during systole; the normal TAP is also included in the figure for comparison. The magnitude of the former decreases with increase in the deviation of V_r from the normal resting potential in the pressure region. For high values of V_r (ie, V_r > −20 mV), the transmembrane potential of the injured cells changes by only a few millivolts for the entire duration of the normal activation.

The transmembrane potential curve corresponding to V_r = −40 mV in Figure 11, however, exhibits a large change in magnitude, indicating the presence of an active component in membrane potential. Keeping in mind that a cell undergoing a normal action potential is adjacent to a cell undergoing the transmembrane potential corresponding to V_r = −40 mV, one can

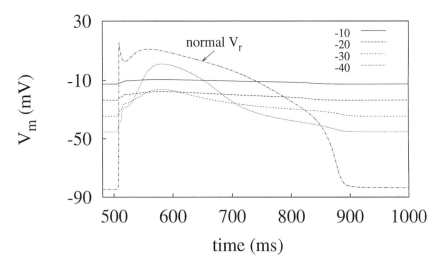

Figure 11. Transmembrane action potential (TAP) at the center of the injured region during systole for 4 values of V_r. The normal TAP is also shown for comparison.

appreciate the dynamics of the current flowing between the two regions. During and after the upstroke, there is a large amount of current flowing from the normal cells to the injured (compare the normal TAP with the curve for $V_r = -40$ mV). This current decreases dramatically as time progresses, due to increase in the transmembrane potential of the injured cells. During the repolarization of the adjacent normal cells, the border current increases again, as the transmembrane potential in the pressure region subsides. The dynamics of this current flow are evident in Figure 12, which illustrates the time course of I_v for a node located centrally on the left border of the pressure region. The solid curve corresponds to $V_r = -40$ mV; it is this transmembrane current behavior that is reflected in the MAP shown in Figure 9.

This second group of simulation results also demonstrates a shift in MAP potentials toward more negative values with the elevation of the resting potential in the injured region (Fig. 9). This behavior and the reasons for it are identical to the ones described in the first group of simulations above. The dashed line in Figure 8 presents the ratio of systolic to diastolic magnitude of the MAP signal as a function of the resting potential in the injured tissue (in the range of -40 to -10 mV). Under the assumption made here (elevated V_r in the injured region), the dashed line intersects the 1:2 level of systolic to diastolic magnitude at -24 mV (ie, the clinically observed ratio of systolic to diastolic magnitude of the MAP signal is achieved when the resting potential in the injured region assumes a value of -24 mV).

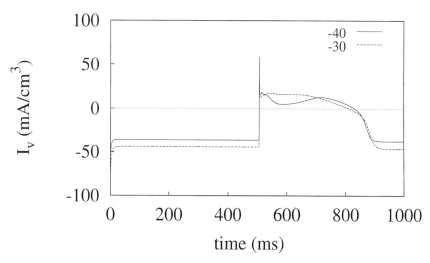

Figure 12. Time course of the transmembrane current volume density for two values of V_r. The node is located centrally on the left border of the pressure region.

Passive Membrane Properties of the Injured Region

We conducted further simulation experiments to examine whether representation of the injured region as passive tissue could result in a MAP that was consistent with experimental recordings. The calculated MAP is shown in Figure 13 together with two other MAPs for comparison: one corresponding to V_{clamp} = –20 mV, and another corresponding to V_r = –20 mV. The "passive" MAP is characterized by a zero take-off potential level. The reason for this behavior is that, at diastole, both normal and injured regions have the same resting potentials, and thus there is no diastolic border current. In the passive case, current flows from normal cells toward injured cells during systole only. This current causes a passive change in transmembrane potential in the pressure region, shown in Figure 14 together with the normal TAP. The potential difference between normal and passive transmembrane potentials generates a MAP during systole. Increasing the value of the specific membrane resistance R_m in a manner suggested by Malden,[4] thus making the passive region more 'leaky," alters only the absolute magnitude of the MAP and not its relation to the zero reference value (not shown here). Since the lack of diastolic phase of the MAP is a behavior that is not consistent with experimental and clinical recordings, the assumption that the MAP region can be considered passive tissue does not appear sustainable.

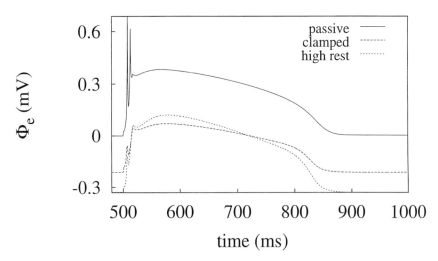

Figure 13. MAPs at the center of the tissue, assuming the MAP region is passive, has a fixed transmembrane potential of –20 mV, and has an elevated resting potential of –20 mV.

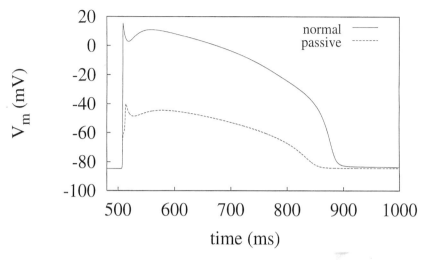

Figure 14. Transmembrane potential at the center of the tissue, assuming the MAP region is passive and is composed of normal, healthy cells.

Discussion

This simulation study explores the pressure-induced electrical behavior of the myocardium that results in the generation of extracellular signals (MAPs), the time course of which mimics the local repolarization in the tissue. The goal of the research is to unravel the genesis of the MAP signals. We test the hypothesis advanced by Franz[1] that postulates that MAPs are due to the depolarization of cells under the pressure electrode. This depolarization establishes potential gradients and thus induces current flow across the border between normal and injured tissue. This current flow exists in both systole and diastole; it flows from injured to normal cells at rest, and from normal to injured tissue during activation.

Our simulation results prove Franz's hypothesis. Assuming that the tissue under the MAP electrode is depolarized, we calculated the extracellular potential in the center of this injured region. The wave shapes obtained here very closely resemble experimentally and clinically recorded MAPs.[1] We were able to show that, indeed, pressure-generated depolarization results in systolic and diastolic currents localized around the border of the MAP region. These border currents serve as sources for the extracellular potential recorded by the MAP electrode.

We represented depolarization in the pressure region as 1) a fixed transmembrane potential of a value higher than the resting potential, and 2) an elevated resting potential. In the first case, the potentials of the injured cells are not affected by the neighboring activity of normal cells. In the second case, however, the transmembrane potential of the injured cells increases during systole due to current flow from adjacent healthy active cells. In both cases, we found that the 1:2 ratio of systolic to diastolic MAP signal amplitudes is achieved if the cell depolarization following the application of pressure is at a level of −20 to −30 mV. Our simulations indicate that, at this level of initial depolarization (ie, elevated resting potential), any change in transmembrane potential in the injured region during systole is of the order of a few millivolts. Thus, the transmembrane potential always remains below the level of the neighboring systolic potential. The latter condition ensures continuous current flow from normal to injured cells during systole. If the initial depolarization is at a level below −30 mV, the cells in the injured region are not completely inactivated. They generate an action potential which, although of magnitude significantly below normal, increases the transmembrane potential in the injured region to a level not far from the plateau potential of the surrounding normal cells, thus diminishing the current flow into the injured region. This decrease in the border current is reflected as a dip in the plateau of the MAP signal. Such a dip has not been observed experimentally, indicating that the level of depolarization of the pressured cells is above −30 mV. It is possible that in clinical MAP recordings the rhythmic contraction of the heart lessens the contact pressure of the MAP electrode. If pressure is decreased, then the level of depolarization under the MAP electrode might drop as well. This in turn could result in MAP signals that exhibit the plateau dip as shown in Figure 9 for $V_r = -40$ mV. As documented by Franz,[1] motion artifacts of this type have been in fact observed during clinical MAP recordings.

In this study we also conducted simulations in which we represented the injured region as passive tissue, ie, tissue of the same resting potential as normal cells but lacking excitability. The transmembrane potential of the injured region can increase only due to electrotonic contribution from neighboring active cells. This representation and its contribution to the formation of MAP was previously explored in detail by Malden, alone[4] and with Henriquez,[5] and it was included here only for the purpose of comparison. Using the passive representation, we found that the MAP signals are only positive, ie, they do not exhibit diastolic and systolic phases of reversed sign as observed in clinical MAPs.[1] The reason behind this behavior is that there is no potential difference between normal and injured cells in diastole. In addition, the calculated "passive" MAP has an intrinsic deflection in the upstroke, the shape of which is not consistent with experimental observations (Fig. 13). Thus, we concluded that representing the region under the MAP electrode as passive does not adequately reflect the underlying cellular behavior.

The simulation results also provide insight into the close relationship between the MAP signal and the repolarization phase of the TAP. Indeed, Franz et al[11] demonstrated that the mean absolute difference in duration

(APD_{90}) between simultaneous intracellular and MAP recordings was 5.4 milliseconds (11.3 milliseconds standard deviation). We found that a MAP mimics the local repolarization process because the duration of the *change* in current flow between normal and injured cells lasts as long as the activation of the healthy cells adjacent to the MAP electrode. In diastole, there is a constant current flow across the line of injury. During systole, this current decreases and subsequently reverses direction. The duration of this *change* in the border current is equal to the duration of the TAP in healthy cells (see Figs. 7 and 12), and the border current is the source for the MAP signal (see eq. 3). In equation 3, the MAP is shown to be a result of the convolution of the current density with a function representing the inverse distance between the point of recording and a location in the myocardium. Since the borders of the injured region are very close to the point of recording (here the center of the injured region), the current flow at the borders has the largest contribution to the MAP signal. Thus, inadvertently, the MAP signal reflects the repolarization of the healthy cells adjacent to the MAP electrode.

In contrast to the faithful representation of TAP repolarization time course by the MAP signal, the MAP magnitude differs greatly from the TAP magnitude. Experimental study[12] documents typical MAP amplitudes in the range of 10 to 50 mV, although values up to 81 mV have been measured. The current understanding of MAP signals relates the MAP amplitude to the amount of cells contributing to the genesis of the MAP signal; thus recordings from the left ventricle and those in large animals exhibit larger magnitudes.[1] In contrast, we use a model of a small 2-dimensional sheet of myocardium (1 cm^2) to calculate the MAPs. The magnitudes of the calculated signals are therefore very small and nowhere near clinically recorded MAP amplitudes. To verify that tissue size contributes to the magnitude of the recorded MAP signal, we conducted additional simulations with different tissue sizes. Figure 15 demonstrates that changing the tissue size alters the magnitude of the MAP signal without affecting the ratio of diastolic to systolic deflections. Thus, we expect that computer simulations will be able to truly reproduce the MAP amplitude only after the inclusion of the appropriate dimensions of the tissue preparation in the model.

We anticipate an extension of our research to incorporate representations of the 3-dimensional fibrous myocardial structure. The advantage of doing so will be not only the calculation of MAP signals of magnitude closer to those experimentally recorded but also a more faithful representation of tissue behavior after the application of the pressure electrode. In the present model, the diastolic border current established in the tissue after the contact with the MAP electrode is sufficient to excite neighboring cells for values of V_{clamp} or V_r above −30 mV. Thus, a wave front propagating outwardly from the injured region precedes the recording of the MAP. In

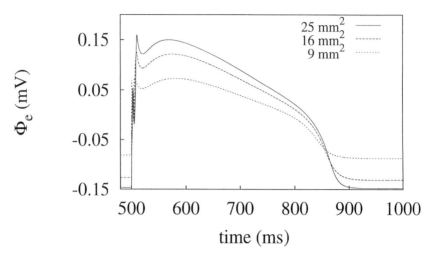

Figure 15. MAPs in the center of the tissue for various sizes of the myocardial sheet. The injured region is assumed to have a clamped potential of –40 mV.

3 dimensions, a much larger border current will be needed to achieve the same effect. Therefore, a propagating wave may not follow the application of pressure to the tissue in cases where the injured cells are depolarized to more than –30 mV. Thus, we anticipate that, using 3-dimensional tissue models, we will be able to better represent the events that lead to the genesis of the MAP signal.

Our study has other limitations as well. First, the model assumes the same level of initial depolarization throughout the MAP region. This corresponds to equally distributed pressure over the tip of the MAP electrode, which is not likely to be valid in reality. Nonetheless, we expect that, provided the variation in pressure does not result in large changes in the level of depolarization throughout the MAP region, the calculated MAPs will be very similar to the ones obtained in this study. Second, the MAPs calculated here correspond to a single point in the center of the tissue, while the real MAP is recorded from the entire hemispherical tip of the MAP electrode and thus represents the weighted average of the extracellular potentials at all points in the injured region. Taking such a weighted average will not only affect the MAP magnitude. Simulations by Malden, alone[4] and with Henriquez,[5] have shown that the pointwise extracellular potentials in the pressure region vary depending on the distance from the boundary to the injured region. Thus, the weighted-average MAP may differ slightly in shape from MAPs simulated at a single point. Despite its limitations, the present modeling study provides considerable insight into the genesis of MAP signals and will contribute to further advancements in MAP recording techniques and applications.

References

1. Franz MR. Method and theory of monophasic action potential recording. *Prog Cardiovasc Dis* 1991;33:347-368.
2. Franz MR. Bridging the gap between basic and clinical electrophysiology: What can be learned from monophasic action potential recording? *J Cardiovasc Electrophysiol* 1994;5:699-710.
3. Hirsch I. *On the Generation, Analysis and Clinical Use of Cardiac Monophasic Action Potentials.* Technical report 146. Göteborg, Sweden: Chalmers University of Technology; 1984.
4. Malden LJ. *Mechanisms Contributing to the Appearance of Monophasic Action Potentials* [Master's thesis]. Durham, NC: Duke University; 1994.
5. Malden LJ, Henriquez CS. A quantitative examination of the basis of monophasic action potentials. *PACE* 1994;17:822. Abstract.
6. Lang V, Ströbel J, Bolz A, Schaldach M. Field theoretical approach to the origin of the monophasic action potential for optimizing geometry of implantable leads. In *19th International Conference.* Chicago: IEEE/EMBS; 1997:185-187.
7. Luo C, Rudy Y. A model of the ventricular cardiac action potential. *Circ Res* 1991;68:1501-1526.
8. Henriquez CS. Simulating the electrical behavior of cardiac muscle using the bidomain model. *Crit Rev Biomed Eng* 1993;21:1-77.
9. Spach MS, Miller WT III, Miller-Jones E, et al. Extracellular potentials related to intracellular action potentials during impulse conduction in anisotropic canine cardiac muscle. *Circ Res* 1979;45:188-204
10. Franz MR, Cohen T, Lee R, et al. Correlation between action potential duration and effective refractory period in vivo: Results from 25 patients with normal right ventricular myocardium. *PACE* 1991;14:703. Abstract.
11. Franz MR, Burkhoff D, Spurgeon H, et al. In vitro validation of a new cardiac catheter technique for recording monophasic action potentials. *Eur Heart J* 1986;7:34-41.
12. Franz MR, Burkhoff D, Lakatta EG, et al. Monophasic action potential recording by contact electrode technique: In vitro validation and clinical applications. In Butrous GS, Schwartz PJ (eds): *Clinical Aspects of Ventricular Repolarization.* London: Farrand; 1989:81-92.

4

Multiple Monophasic Action Potential Recording with a Single Magnetocardiographically Localizable Amagnetic Catheter

Riccardo Fenici, MD
and Peter Fenici, MD

Introduction

The identification of the mechanisms of focal arrhythmias and the localization of their substrate is sometimes difficult with conventional electrophysiologic study. The introduction of monophasic action potential (MAP) recording with the suction catheter electrode technique[1,2] was the first attempt to improve the resolution of electrophysiologic study by filling the gap between experimental and clinical electrophysiology. Indeed this method was an interesting tool for clinical investigation of the dynamics of endocardial repolarization[3-7] and local conduction disturbances.[3,8] After-depolarization-like signals were also observed in patients and, as early as

This work was supported by the Italian National Research Council (CNR), owner of patents: Ital. Patent N. 1219855, May 24, 1990; US Patent N. 5 056 517, Oct.15, 1991; Eur. Patent N. 0428812, March 08, 1995.

From Franz MR (ed): *Monophasic Action Potentials: Bridging Cell and Bedside.*
©Futura Publishing Company, Inc., Armonk, NY, 2000.

1978, triggered automaticity was suggested as a possible mechanism for human arrhythmias.[9-11] However, as the suction technique is somewhat cumbersome, the method was used only in a limited number of electrophysiology laboratories,[3-11] and its safety was considered controversial. A significant step forward for MAP recording was the contact electrode technique,[12] which is easier and practically risk-free. Franz et al[12-14] systematically investigated this approach and developed the combination catheter, which triggered a widespread interest for the method and its clinical application for the study of repolarization[15-21] and afterdepolarizations.[22-27] Since the early 1970s it had been felt that multiple MAP recordings, either sequential[16] or simultaneous with more than one catheter,[17,20,21,26,27] were useful to quantify, in patients, the dispersion of repolarization and refractoriness on a beat-to-beat basis. The following, however, were major limitations for multiple recordings: 1) the need for multiple catheters; 2) the spatial resolution of local recordings, which cannot be precisely defined and kept stable during long-term studies; 3) the lack of electroanatomic integration of the electrophysiologic information obtained; and 4) the lack of preoperative knowledge of the 3-dimensional (3-D) coordinates of the arrhythmogenic substrate, where the MAP catheter would more easily detect electrophysiologic abnormalities. Recently novel catheter-based technologies have been developed for accurate single-catheter endocardial activation mapping and for nonfluoroscopic 3-D navigation of electrophysiologic catheters,[28-30] to speed up ablation procedures. None of these technologies can be used for preoperative noninvasive localization of the arrhythmogenic target and to combine such "a priori" knowledge with the navigation of MAP catheters in order to improve the diagnostic resolution of the electrophysiologic study.

This chapter describes a new method for multiple simultaneous MAP recording with a single amagnetic catheter[31] that can be localized with the magnetic source imaging (MSI) technique[32] into a 3-D model or magnetic resonance imaging (MRI) slices of the patient's heart, to integrate spatially the electrophysiologic information obtained with MAP recording. MSI is a contactless imaging technique that provides noninvasive localization of focal arrhythmias, based on the body surface mapping of cardiac magnetic fields.[33-39]

The Amagnetic Catheter

The multipurpose amagnetic catheter for magnetocardiographic (MCG)-guided multiple simultaneous MAP recording is patented by the Italian National Research Council.[40] The catheter, which is 6F or 7F, has several different configurations and features a variable number of nonpolarizable amagnetic electrodes at the tip, arranged in such a way that current dipoles of different geometry and strength can be generated in the patient's heart, without artifacts induced by ferromagnetic materials, or spurious magnetic fields. Modified versions also feature additional lumens for the purpose of fluid infusion, or to insert steerable wires and optic fibers that are suitable for laser ablation.[40] This amagnetic catheter was first used to test the accuracy of MCG localization both in phantoms and in patients.[41-43]

In the simplified configuration, shown in Figure 1, panel a, the amagnetic catheter is capable of recording 4 simultaneous MAPs, with a spatial resolution of 4 mm^2. Unlike the conventional 1-mm catheter tip electrode, the diameter of each tip electrode of the amagnetic catheter is only 0.2 to 0.3 mm. Therefore, as compared with standard MAP catheters, each terminal electrode of the amagnetic catheter is in contact with approximately one fifth the amount of myocardial cells. The proximal (reference) electrode is a 1-mm ring, placed at 5 mm from the tip. If used for pacing, the stimulation thresholds obtained with this catheter range between 0.1 and 0.5 mA, as a function of the geometry of the pacing dipole. The 3-D position of the catheter's tip can be automatically calculated using MSI, which is described later (Fig. 1, panels c and d).

Multiple MAP Recording

The amagnetic catheter is very reliable for multiple simultaneous MAP recording with a well defined and high spatial resolution.[43] For analog recording, all tip electrodes are connected to the positive input of high-impedance, DC-coupled, optically isolated differential preamplifiers. The reference electrode is connected to the negative input of the amplifier. With this recording set up, MAP signals are oriented upward. The recording bandwidth is from DC to 1 kHz. Analog signals are recorded with a Siemens Mingograph recorder (frequency response DC to 1 kHz), at the paper speed of 100 and 200 mm/s, and stored in magnetic tape.

For digital processing, although MAPs of apparently comparable morphology can be recorded with the new standard electrophysiologic multichannel digital recording equipment, which generally provides a band-pass filtering of 0.05 to 500 Hz and digitization at 1 kHz (Figs. 2 through 4), a proper bandwidth for MAP recording is DC to 1kHz, which is wide enough to cover the frequency content of the MAP signal (Fig. 5), and needs a sampling frequency of only 4 kHz (with at least 12-bit resolution). The wider recording bandwidths (DC to 3 or 5 kHz) proposed by Franz[14] and by Yuan[20] are surely ideal for analog recordings, but would theoretically imply a sampling frequency of 12 to 20 kHz for proper digitization.[44] This is not practical for multichannel long-term recordings, which require a large disk capacity to store the data. Indeed, at standard resolution the

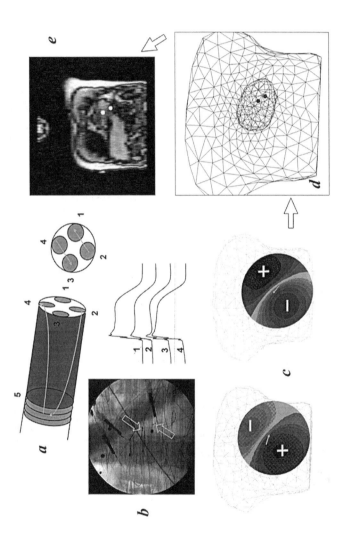

Figure 1. a. Schematic drawing of the magnetic source imaging (MSI) localizable anagmetic catheter for multiple MAP recording, and its multimedial imaging. **b.** Fluoroscopy (2 amagnetic catheters), frontal view. **c.** Isocontour plots of the magnetic field component perpendicular to the frontal surface of the sensors (positive [+] areas indicate magnetic flux toward the chest, while negative values [–] denote flux out of the chest). The field distributions generated by the 2 catheters are both dipolar but inverted according to the polarity of the current impressed to the catheters. **d.** MSI localizations of the 2 catheters in the 3-D model of a patient's heart. **e.** Transfer of localizations on magnetic resonance imaging slices.

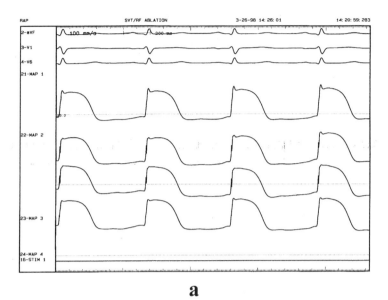

a

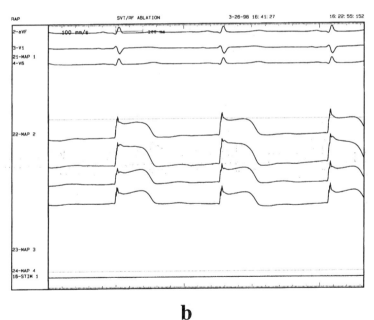

b

Figure 2. a. Example of single-catheter multiple MAP recording from the right ventricle. **b**. The quality of the MAP signals after 2 hours, during which the catheter tip electrodes were repetitively used to activate artificial dipoles for magnetic source imaging localization and imaging. (Prucka Eng. Inc recorder: bandwidth 0.05 to 500 Hz. Notch filter 50Hz. Sampling frequency 1 kHz.)

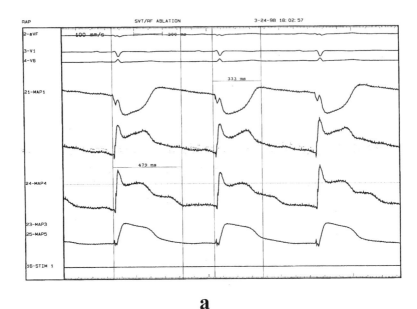

a

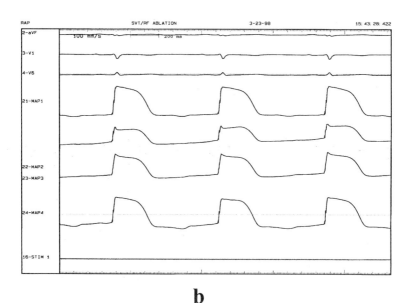

b

Figure 3. **a**. Example of bad endocardial contact of the catheter: MAP 1 is negative MAP 2 and MAP 3 feature a steplike prolongation of phase 3 mimicking early afterdepolarization (EAD). **b**. After better endocardial contact is achieved in the same area, all MAPs are positive and their duration is quite similar, without evidence of repolarization abnormalities or EADs.

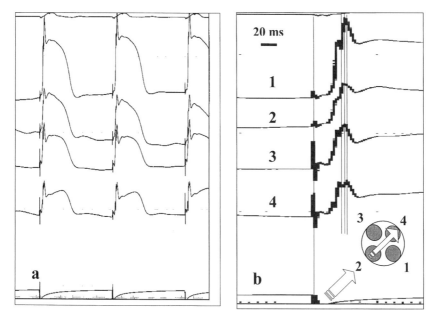

Figure 4. a. Four simultaneous MAP recordings from the right ventricular (RV) midseptum during pacing (with a second pacing catheter at the RV apex). All MAPs are positive, however the morphology of MAP 4 is evidently altered and the phase 0 is more notched, suggesting unfavorable contact of the fourth tip electrode. **b**. Due to the 1-kHz sampling frequency, high resolution of local activation sequence under the tip electrodes is not optimal. The timing is: first 2; second 1 and 3 simultaneously; last 4. This suggests the direction of the propagation wave front shown in the sketch (lower right corner).

signal restitution also seems good with a 1-kHz sampling frequency[20,44] (Figs. 2, 3, 4 and 6). Nevertheless, according to the sampling theorem,[45] the signal must be sampled at a rate that is at least twice the frequency of its highest Fourier component, to avoid the possibility that the higher frequency components of the signal will have an uncontrolled disturbing effect ("aliasing") on the computed Fourier coefficients. A sampling frequency of 4 kHz is also the minimum resolution time (0.25 milliseconds) required for precise evaluation of local activation time between electrodes located at a distance of 1.5 to 2.0 mm, assuming that the physiologic conduction velocity of endocardial Purkinje network is in the order of 2 m/s.

Custom software has been developed for automatic analysis of MAP signals, that is similar to that reported by others.[20,44] The program automatically detects the diastolic baseline, the upstroke, the crest, and the offset of the MAPs, although the operator can interactively adjust all parameters before starting the automatic computation, which provides automatic cal-

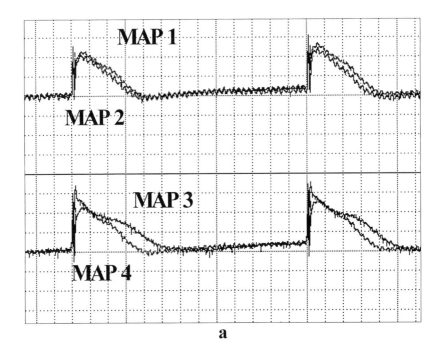

a

b   c

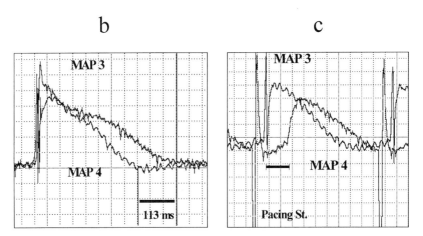

Figure 5. In a patient with lone atrial fibrillation, **a**. 4 right atrial MAPs from the interatrial septum (MAP 1-2 and MAP 3-4 are shown superimposed for comparison); **b**. in sinus rhythm, evident dispersion of local atrial repolarization between MAP 3 and MAP 4 (113 milliseconds), without significant difference of local activation time; **c**. during atrial pacing (with a second catheter) both MAPs shorten. MAP 4 changes from "fast" to "slow" morphology, with evident dispersion of local activation time (70 milliseconds). (Bandwidth: DC to 1 kHz. No notch filter. Sampling frequency 4 kHz.)

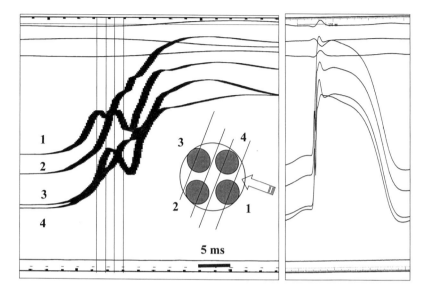

Figure 6. Four MAP recording from the right ventricular outflow tract. High-resolution analysis of the local activation sequence under the tip electrodes, in sinus rhythm. The MAP sequence (measured at first peak of each MAP) is: 1, 4, 2, 3. This gives the direction of the propagation wave front indicated by the open arrow on the sketch of the catheter tip (center). The time separation between the peaks is 1.2 milliseconds, the separation between two subsequent electrodes is about 1.1 mm. This gives a calculated propagation velocity of approximately 0.9 m/s.

culation of MAP duration at 50% (d50%) and 90% (d90%) of repolarization, and local activation time for each MAP. Once the length of the recording to be analyzed is defined, the program displays, beat by beat, the calculated values on the waveforms, and their average ± standard deviation at the end. As indexes of local dispersion of conduction and repolarization, the coefficient of variation of local activation time and of d50% and d90% can be also automatically calculated and displayed.

In a recent clinical study[43] the single-catheter multiple MAP recordings technique was used to monitor the stability of orthogonal endocardial contact during MSI localization of the amagnetic catheter in the right ventricle of patients without ventricular arrhythmias. The average amplitude of the right ventricular MAP was 23±9 mV. Local variation coefficients of right ventricular MAP d50% and d90% were 7.4% and 3.1%, respectively. After 2 hours, the signals were still very stable (Fig. 2, panel b), although the patients had been moved from one bed to another 4 times, and the recording electrodes had been alternatively used to induce different pacing dipoles for MSI localization of the catheter. The amplitude of the MAP signal decreased by about 50%. The coefficient of variation of local activation time was 1.1%.

The average amplitude of right atrial MAP was 5.9 ± 2 mV. In patients with lone atrial fibrillation, local abnormalities of repolarization and of conduction can be evidenced with single-catheter multiple MAP recording, as shown in Figure 5.

The Magnetic Source Imaging Method

MSI is the newest noninvasive method for functional electrophysiologic imaging, based on body surface mapping of the magnetic field generated by cardiac electrophysiologic phenomena (called *magnetocardiography* or *MCG*).[33-35] It provides quantitative 3-D localization and imaging of cardiac arrhythmias, which has been demonstrated in several clinical studies.[36-39] An example of MSI of the site of origin of a ventricular extrasystole is shown in Figure 7.

MCG is recorded with superconducting sensors called *SQUID* (Semi Quantum Interference Device).[33] The sensors are cooled in liquid helium

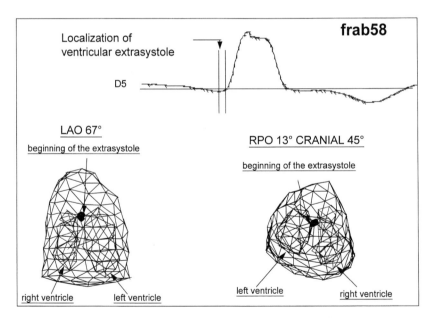

Figure 7. Example of magnetic source imaging localization and 3-D imaging of the site of onset of ventricular extrasystoles, originating in the interventricular septum. Two fluoroscopy-like projections (left anterior oblique [LAO], right posterior oblique [RPO]) of the 3-D model of the patient's heart have been selected, angled to show the septum between the endocardial surfaces of the right and left ventricles.

(–271°C) inside a cylindrical Dewar that is supported by a gantry system. Mapping can be done either sequentially with a single SQUID or simultaneously with multichannel instrumentation. The former method has been used since 1982 in the unshielded catheterization room of the Biomagnetism Center at the Catholic University of Rome,[34] where MCG was sequentially mapped from 36 chest points with a superconducting radiofrequency SQUID coupled to a second-order gradiometer (featuring a 1.5-cm pickup coil and 5-cm baseline) in order to reduce the influence of background electromagnetic noise. The sensors were immersed in liquid helium inside a cylindrical Dewar, supported by a gantry system. A COMB filter was used to reject power line interference (50 Hz) and harmonics. Final amplification, before analog-to-digital conversion (at 12-bit resolution and 1-kHz sampling rate), was provided by a conditioning unit, with a recursive high-pass filter of the first order, intermediate adjustable gain amplifiers, and a final Bessel low-pass filter of the eighth order (bandpass between 0.016 and 250 Hz). The overall sensitivity of the system was 50 fT/√Hz.

Presently multichannel MCG recording is done only in high-performance, shielded rooms, which provide state-of-the-art signal-to-noise ratio (SNR) during the recording, with a sensitivity of about 5 fT/√Hz, and allow quasi real-time localization of the sources of interest on a beat-to-beat basis.[46] Our multichannel MCG recordings were performed, both in patients and in phantoms, with a 67-channel cardiomagnetometer in the BioMag shielded room at the Helsinki University Central Hospital (HUCH). All MCG signals were bandpassed at 0.01 to 500 Hz and digitized with a sampling frequency of 2 kHz. Before MCG recordings, thorax coordinates were defined by digitizing a set of reference points, which were used to transfer MCG localization in MR images and for comparison with fluoroscopic images with the same coordinate system.

Mathematical Models

For the localization of the catheter, the so-called magnetic inverse solution must be solved.[47] A moving equivalent current dipole in a semi-infinite space or in a realistic torso model is used in the computation. Both volume conductors are assumed to be homogeneously conductive as the best compromise between reality of the model and time required for the calculation. The 3-D realistic, homogeneous torso model of the patient surface is tessellated with plane triangles[48] (Figs. 1, 7, and 8), using the boundary element calculations (BEM). In the BEM the electric potential is assumed to be linear in each triangle, and the discretized integral equations for the electric potential and the magnetic field can be manipulated into matrix equations which can be quickly solved.[47] The six parameters (position and moment) of a current dipole are estimated with nonlinear

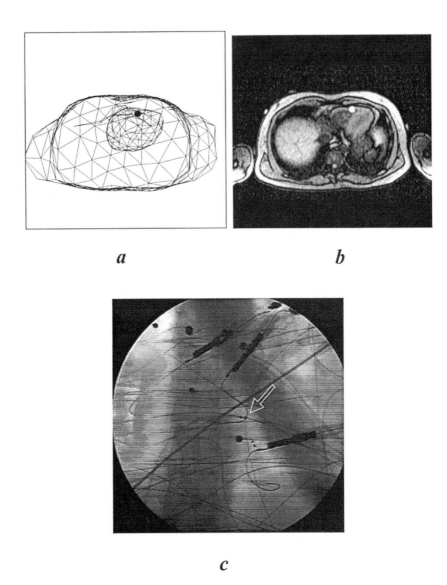

a

b

c

Figure 8. In the same patient as in Figure 1, transaxial views of the boundary element torso model (boundary element calculations) (**a**), and of magnetic resonance imaging (**b**), which shows proper localization of the catheter placed at the mid anterior wall of the right ventricle (white and black dots) **c**. Frontal fluoroscopic image is shown for comparison (the localized catheter is marked by the white open arrow).

least squares fitting.[49] For each patient, the BEM of the torso is calculated with use of his or her own MRI images.[50] The heart volume is placed inside the torso after the calculations are made, to improve the anatomic imaging of the localization figures. When the recordings are performed in the shielded room, the SNR is optimal and all inverse computations can be done beat to beat from raw MCG data. Without shielding, signal averaging and/or digital filtering are necessary to improve the SNR before the calculation of the inverse solution.

3-D Imaging of the MAP Catheter

The first validation study performed in patients was carried out at the Catholic University of Rome,[51,52] with single-channel instrumentation in an unshielded electrophysiology laboratory. In that noisy environment, the average 3-D localization error was 11.2 ± 5.6 mm.

More recently the accuracy of MSI for the imaging of the 3-D position of the tip of the new multipurpose amagnetic catheter for high-resolution multiple MAP recording was evaluated with the state-of-the-art multichannel instrumentation in the BioMag Center of the Helsinki University Central Hospital.

The intrinsic accuracy of the MSI system was preliminarily quantified with phantom measurements simulating both a semi-infinite homogeneous volume conductor[41] and a realistic torso model with homogeneous conductivity.[42] The reproducibility of the measurements was tested by repeating the same measurement 5 times and computing the coefficient of variation and the coefficient of reproducibility.[53] With this advanced experimental set up, the beat-to-beat localization accuracy of the catheter in a realistic torso phantom was as good as 2 mm. The reproducibility of the method, tested in repeated recording sessions, was demonstrated by the coefficient of variation of 3-D localization (1.37%) and by the coefficient of reproducibility of 2.6 mm.

In patient studies,[42,43] the 3-D localization of the tip of the catheter was calculated from stimulus peaks generated by 10 mA fed into the catheter's dipoles. The polarity of the magnetic field induced by the stimulus varied in the individual patients, depending on the direction of the artificial dipole (Fig. 1, panel c). The accuracy of the MSI localization was evaluated by: 1) mismatch with fluoroscopy, and 2) anatomic location of the equivalent current dipole (ECD) in MRI slices (Figs. 1 and 8). The position of the amagnetic MAP catheter is imaged into the 3-D model of the patient's heart with sufficient accuracy for electroanatomic integration of the MAP recordings. The 3-D images of the heart can be rotated by the operator in real time during the electrophysiologic study. The transfer of the localization figures on the MRI slices confirms the anatomic reliability of the model (Figs. 1 and 8).

New Information

Compared to conventional MAP recording, MSI-guided multiple close-bipolar MAP recording from the 4 tip electrodes provides much new information:

1. The 3-D position of the catheter can be localized without the use of fluoroscopy, and the local MAP recordings can be associated to a specified anatomic position.
2. The axial position of the catheter against the endocardium can be easily monitored. Indeed if all of the tip electrodes are equally in touch with the endocardium, the quality of all 4 MAP recordings is comparable (Fig. 2 and Fig. 3, panel b). If one electrode is not properly touching the endocardium, the corresponding MAP is distorted or even reversed in polarity (Fig. 3, panel a and Fig. 4).
3. The number of myocardiocytes in contact with each tip electrode is smaller, thus minimizing spatial averaging of the relative contribution to the MAP signal generated by different cells (Purkinje versus contractile myocytes). The upstroke (phase 0) is usually sharper.
4. As the interelectrode distance is fixed for each catheter configuration, the sequence of local endocardial depolarization, the direction of the propagating wave front, and the propagation velocity in respect to the geometry of the recording assembly can be precisely defined (Figs. 4 and 6).
5. The local propagation velocity at the site of MAP recording can be independently calculated from MSI localization data.[34,42]

Present Limitation and Future Developments

Preliminary observations[32] suggest that preoperative MSI study of the arrhythmia can be used to drive the MAP catheter as close as possible to the arrhythmogenic area, where multiple MAP recording can discover localized arrhythmogenic mechanisms such as dispersion of repolarization,[31] abnormal local conduction with microreentry,[8] or afterdepolarizations[32] (see also Figs. 4 and 5). The combined information of 3-D MSI localization of the catheter and of the detection of the local geometry of endocardial activation, inferred by the multiple MAP recording, can be useful to detect and localize microreentry circuits and multiple simultaneous activation wave fronts in patients with atrial fibrillation.[54]

In summary, single-catheter, MSI-guided multiple MAP recording is a new low-invasivity method for high-resolution electrophysiologic study from (or very close to) arrhythmogenic areas. Presently, the major limitation of the method is the lack of commercially available multichannel MSI mapping systems that work in electrophysiology laboratories with the same sensitivity achievable in a high-performance shielded room. Indeed an optimal SNR ratio during the recordings is still a critical requirement for MCG accuracy; in our unshielded electrophysiology laboratory the localization uncertainty was almost 4 times higher than in the shielded room used in Helsinki.[43,52] Furthermore, additional effort in mathematical modeling and software development are needed to integrate the electroanatomic information provided by MSI localization of arrhythmias with that inferred by multiple local MAP recording, and to improve the 3-D anatomic representation of the catheter.

In recent computer simulation work, a comparable 3-D localization accuracy was reported.[55] An obvious alternative to MSI may be the use of body surface potential mapping (BSPM)[56,57] to image and drive the MAP catheter. Recent experimental and clinical measurements, however, have shown that, with the presently used models, BSPM localization error is at least twice that obtained with MSI.[42,58] Thus, at the moment, BSPM functional imaging can be complementary but not alternative to MSI. Moreover, the contactless MSI method is much faster and more well accepted by the patient, as it avoids the placement of 60 to 123 electrodes. This implies that further investments are needed to construct a more compact multichannel MSI instrumentation that is reliable in unshielded electrophysiology laboratories. With fast developing technology, such instrumentation for electrophysiologic study could be available in the near future, with a significant drop in cost which would favor a wider clinical application of the method. Meanwhile, the amagnetic catheter for multiple MAP recording warrants further experimental and clinical investigation to evaluate whether its high spatial resolution can be useful to improve the accuracy and diagnostic power of clinical electrophysiology.

Acknowledgments: We are grateful to Professor Luigi Donato for providing the financial support, and to Mr. Luigi Venturelli for developing the prototypes of the amagnetic catheters. We are also indebted to Dr. Jukka Nenonen, Dr. Markku Mäkijärvi, Dr. Katja Pesola, Dr. Lauri Toivonen, Dr. Petri Koronen, and Professor Toivo Katila, for their invaluable contributions in retesting the catheter and method, and also in the BioMag Laboratory of the Helsinki University Central Hospital, within the EU HCM BIRCH Programme. The Neuromag Ltd. (Helsinki) is acknowledged for supporting this research with their advanced software for MSI. We warmly thank Dr. Donatella Brisinda, Dr. Andrea Giorgi, and Dr. Maria Pia Ruggieri, who sustained the burden of clinical work during the preparation of this manuscript.

References

1. Korsgren M, Leskinen E, Sjöstrand U, Varnauskas E. Intracardiac recording of monophasic action potentials of the human heart. *Scand J Lab Invest* 1966;18:561-564.

2. Olsson SB, Varnauskas E, Korsgren M. Further improved method for measuring monophasic action potentials of the intact human heart. *J Electrocardiol* 1971;4:19-23.

3. Olsson SB. *Monophasic Action Potentials of Right Heart. Suction Electrode Method in Clinical Investigations* [PhD dissertation]. Göteborg: University of Göteborg, Elanders Boktrykeri AB; 1971.

4. Gavrilescu S, Cotoi, Pop T. The monophasic action potential of right atrium. *Cardiology* 1972;57:200-207.

5. Fenici R, Bellocci F, Zecchi P, et al. Monophasic action potential of human heart. Preliminary results with a new technique. *Acta Med Rom* 1973;11:300-312.

6. Puech P, Cabasson J, Latour H, et al. Study of monophasic action potentials of the myocardium by endocavitary approach. *Arch Mal Coeur* 1974;64:1117-1122.

7. Fenici R, Marchei M, Bellocci F, Zecchi P. Effect of Bunaphtine on right atrial repolarization in man. *Br Heart J* 1977;39:787-794.

8. Fenici R, Masselli M, Zeppilli P, Pirrami MM. Clinical recordings of monophasic action potentials: Demonstration of intra-atrial conduction block in sinus node region and possible role in reentrant supraventricular tachycardia. *Am Heart J* 1981;102(1):124-128.

9. Fenici R, Marchei M, Colonna P, et al. Right ventricular monophasic action potential recording in man after suicidal digoxin ingestion. *VIII World Congress of Cardiology*. Abstr. no. 1480; Tokyo: 1978.

10. Fenici R, Colonna P, Marchei M, et al. Monophasic action potential recording and afterpotentials in one patient with paroxysmal atrial fibrillation. *VIII World Congress of Cardiology*. Abstr. no. 1459; Tokyo: 1978.

11. Fenici R. Right ventricular monophasic action potentials in patients with long Q-T syndrome. *Br Heart J* 1979;42:615-616.

12. Franz M. Long-term recording of monophasic action potentials from the human endocardium. *Am J Cardiol* 1983;51:1629-1634.

13. Franz MR, Burkhoff D, Spurgeon H, et al. In vitro validation of a new catheter technique for the recording the monophasic action potential. *Eur Heart J* 1986;7:34-41.

14. Franz MR. Method and theory of measuring monophasic action potential recording. *Prog Cardiovasc Dis* 1991;33:347-368.

15. Olsson SB. Estimation of ventricular repolarization in man by monophasic action potential recording technique. *Eur Heart J* 1985;6:71-79.

16. Franz MR, Bargheer K, Rafflenbeul W, et al. Monophasic action potential mapping in human subjects with normal electrocardiograms: Direct evidence for the genesis of the T wave. *Circulation* 1987;75:379-386.

17. Morgan JM, Cunningham D, Rowland E. Dispersion of monophasic action potential duration: Demonstrable in humans after premature ventricular extrastimulation but not in steady state. *J Am Coll Cardiol* 1992;19:1244-1253.

18. Franz MR. Bringing the gap between the basic and clinical electrophysiology. *J Cardiovasc Electrophysiol* 1994;5(8):699-710.

19. Yuan S, Blomstrom-Lundqvist C, Olsson SB. Monophasic action potentials: Concepts to practical clinical applications. *J Cardiovasc Electrophysiol* 1994;5:287-308.

20. Yuan S. *Dispersion of Ventricular Repolarisation. A Study in Patients with Ventricular Arrhythmias Using Monophasic Action Potential Recording Technique* [PhD dissertation]. Lund: University of Lund; Grahns Boktrykeri AB; 1995.

21. Yuan S, Wohlfart B, Olsson SB, Blomstrom-Lundqvist C. The dispersion of repolarization in patients with ventricular tachycardia. *Eur Heart J* 1995;16:68-76.

22. Levine JH, Spear JF, Guarnieri T, et al. Cesium-chloride-induced long QT syndrome: Demonstration of afterdepolarizations and triggered activity in vivo. *Circulation* 1985;72:1092-1103.

23. Vassallo JA, Kassidy DM, Kindwall KE, et al. Nonuniform recovery of excitability in the left ventricle. *Circulation* 1988;78:1365-1372.

24. Gough WB, Raphael H. The early afterdepolarization as recorded by monophasic action potential technique: Fact or artifact? *Circulation* 1989;80(suppl II):II130.

25. El-Sherif N, Bekheit SS, Henkin R. Quinidine-induced long QT interval and torsade de pointes: Role of bradycardia-dependent early after depolarizations. *J Am Coll Cardiol* 1989;14:252-257.

26. Habbab MA, El-Sherif N. Drug-induced torsade de pointes: Role of early afterdepolarizations and dispersion of repolarization. *Am J Med* 1990;89:241-246.

27. Shimizu W, Ohe T, Kurita T, et al. Early afterdepolarizations induced by isoproterenol in patients with long QT syndrome. *Circulation* 1991;84:1915-1923.

28. Peters SN, Jackman WN, Schilling RJ, et al. Human left ventricular endocardial activation mapping using a novel noncontact catheter. *Circulation* 1997;95:1658-1660.

29. Gepstein L, Hayam G, Ben-Haim S. A novel method for nonfluoroscopic catheter-based electroanatomical mapping of the heart. *Circulation* 1997;95:1611-1622.

30. Johnson SB, Packer DL. Intracardiac ultrasound guidance of multipolar atrial and ventricular mapping basket applications. *J Am Coll Cardiol* 1997;29:202A. Abstract.

31. Fenici P, Ruggieri MP, Fenici R. Multiple simultaneous monophasic action potential recordings with a single biomagnetically localizable amagnetic catheter. *Eur Heart J* 1996;17:282A.

32. Fenici R, Melillo G. Biomagnetically localizable multipurpose catheter and method for MCG guided intracardiac electrophysiology, biopsy and ablation of cardiac arrhythmias. *Int J Card Imaging* 1991;7:207-215.

33. Siltanen P. Magnetocardiography. In Macfarlane PW, Lawrie TDW (eds): *Comprehensive Electrocardiology*. London: Pergamon Press; 1989:1405-1434.

34. Fenici RR, Melillo G, Masselli M. Clinical magnetocardiography: Ten years experience at the Catholic University of Rome. *Int J Card Imaging* 1991;7:(3-4):151-167.

35. Nakaya Y. Magnetocardiography. *Clin Phys Physiol Meas* 1992;13:191-229.

36. Hombach V, Kochs M, Weissmuller P, et al. Localization of ectopic ventricular depolarization by ispect-radionuclide ventriculography and by magnetocardiography. *Int J Card Imaging* 1991;7(3-4):225-235.

37. Oeff M, Burghoff M. Magnetocardiographic localization of the origin of ventricular ectopic beats. *PACE* 1994;17:517-522.

38. Fenici R, Covino M, Cellerino C, et al. Magnetocardiographically guided catheter ablation. *J Interv Cardiol* 1995;8(suppl):825-836.

39. Moshage W, Achenbach S, Göhl K, Bachmann K. Evaluation of the non-invasive localization accuracy of cardiac arrhythmias attainable by multichannel magnetocardiography (MCG). *Int J Card Imaging* 1996;12:47-59.

40. Fenici R. Consiglio Nazionale delle Ricerche. Biomagnetically localizable multipurpose catheter and method for MCG guided intracardiac electrophysiology, biopsy and ablation of cardiac arrhythmias. United States Patent Documents [19], Patent N.5 056 517, Oct.15, 1991.

41. Fenici R, Fenici P, van Bosheide J. Amagnetic catheter for biomagnetically guided endocardial mapping and ablation of cardiac arrhythmias. In Reichl H, Heuberger A (eds): Micro System Technologies. Berlin: VDE-Verlag GmbH; 1996:711-716.

42. Fenici R, Pesola K, Mäkijärvi M, et al. Nonfluoroscopic localization of an amagnetic catheter in a realistic torso phantom by multichannel magnetocardiography and body surface potential mapping. *PACE* 1998;21(11 pt. 2):2485-2491.

43. Fenici RR, Pesola K, Korhonen P, et al. Magnetocardiographic pacemapping for non-fluoroscopic localization of intracardiac electrophysiology catheters. *PACE* 1998;21(11 pt. 2)2492-2499.

44. Franz MR, Kirchhof PF, Fabritz CL, Zabel M. Computer analysis of monophasic action potentials: Manual validation and clinically pertinent applications. *PACE* 1995;18(pt. I):1666-1678.

45. Lehmann H. Signal processing. In Williamson SJ, Romani GL, Kaufman L, Modena I (eds): *Biomagnetism: An Interdisciplinary Approach*. New York: Plenum Press; 1983:591-624.

46. Simelius K, Ahonen A, Huotilainen M, et al. BioMag: Functional brain and heart research in clinical environment. *Proc XVII Annu Int Conf IEEE Eng Med Biol Soc*. Montreal, Canada: September 1995: CD-ROM.

47. Nenonen J. Solving the inverse problem in magnetocardiography. *IEEE Eng Med Biol Mag* 1994;13:87-96.

48. Horacek M. Digital model for studies in magnetocardiography. *IEEE Trans Magn* 1973;9:440-444.

49. Marquardt DW. An algorithm for least-squares estimation of nonlinear parameters. J SIAM 1963;11: 431-441.

50. Lötjönen J, Sipilä O, Nenonen J, et al. Individual boundary element models for magnetocardiographic applications. *Proc 18th Annu Int Conf IEEE Eng Med Biol Soc*, 1996: CD-ROM.

51. Fenici R, Melillo G, Cappelli A, et al. Magnetocardiographic localization of a pacing catheter. In Williamson SJ, Hoke M, Stroink G, Kotani M (eds): *Advances in Biomagnetism*. New York: Plenum Press; 1989:361-364.

52. Fenici R, Melillo G. Magnetocardiography: Ventricular arrhythmias. *Eur Heart J* 1993;14(suppl. E):53-60.

53. Altman DG, Bland JM. Measurements in medicine: The analysis of method comparison studies. *Statisticians* 1983;32:307-317.

54. Holm M, Johansson R, Brandt J, et al. Epicardial right free wall mapping in chronic atrial fibrillation. *Eur Heart J* 1997;18:290-310.

55. Hren R, Zhang X, Stroink G. Comparison between electrocardiographic and magnetocardiographic inverse solutions using the boundary element method. *Med Biol Eng Comput* 1996;34:110-114.

56. Dubuc M, Nadeau R, Tremblay G, et al. Pacemapping using body surface potential maps to guide catheter ablation of accessory pathways in patients with Wolff-Parkinson-White syndrome. *Circulation* 1993;87:135-143.

57. Sippens-Groenewegen A, Spekhorst H, van Hemel H, et al. Localization of the site of origin of postinfarction ventricular tachycardia by endocardial pacemapping. *Circulation* 1993;88:2290-2306.

58. Pesola K, Fenici R, Mäkijärvi M, et al. Comparison of localisation accuracy of magnetocardiographic and body surface potential mapping using an amagnetic stimulation catheter. *11th International Conference on Biomagnetism, Biomag98*. Sendai, Japan: 1998.

5

The Monophasic Action Potential-Pacing Combination Catheter:

Assessing the Relationship Between Repolarization and Excitability In Vivo

Michael R. Franz, MD, PhD

Conventional electrode catheters used in electrophysiologic studies for the purpose of programmed electrical stimulation have several ring electrodes that are placed sequentially along the distal end of the catheter. In a typical quadripolar catheter, the two most distal electrodes are used for pacing, and the proximal electrode pair is used for recording the electrogram. The distance between the electrode rings varies but is commonly between 5 and 10 mm. Because of the rather large electrode spacing, it is often uncertain whether the recorded electrogram indicates the local evoked response or includes some conduction delay between local capture and activation at the recording electrodes. Furthermore, with such conventional electrode configuration, the stimulus artifact is very large and often overshadows the response electrogram evoked by the stimulus. This complicates interpretation of the response time to local capture.

The monophasic action potential (MAP)-pacing combination catheter differs from this conventional electrophysiologic catheter design in two important aspects: 1) the primary recording electrode is not proximally

From Franz MR (ed): *Monophasic Action Potentials: Bridging Cell and Bedside.* ©Futura Publishing Company, Inc., Armonk, NY, 2000.

located but forms the distal tip of the catheter, with the reference electrode only 5 mm proximal to the tip, and 2) the pacing electrodes are situated halfway between the tip and reference recording electrodes, in an orthogonal fashion (Fig. 1). This electrode configuration provides for extremely low capture thresholds (0.02 to 0.25 mA; mean 0.09 mA), reducing the interference between the pacing artifact and the recorded signal to a minimum.[1] Several factors likely account for the unusually low capture threshold and minimal stimulus artifacts. First, the pacing electrodes used in this catheter have a smaller surface area than conventional ring electrodes and therefore emit higher current densities. Second, the electrical field produced by the pacing current is positioned horizontally above the vertical field that produces the MAP, with subsequently less contamination of the latter. Third, the MAP catheter provides and ensures close and stable contact with the endocardium (unstable contact would result in no or unstable MAPs). Fourth, and perhaps most important, only the tip (MAP) electrode is in contact with depolarized myocardium, while the stimulus electrodes usually do not exert pressure against the endocardium. This prevents the pacing site from being depolarized and made relatively refractory, which would result in increased capture thresholds.

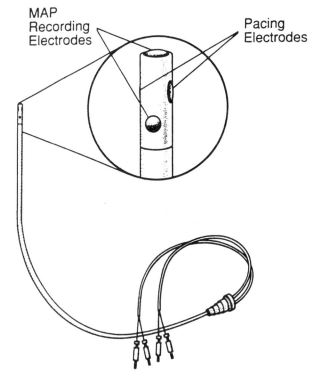

MAP
Recording
Electrodes

Pacing
Electrodes

Figure 1. Schematic of MAP-pacing combination catheter.

Relationship Between MAP Duration and Refractory Period Measured Simultaneously at the Same Site

Conventional electrophysiologic catheters allow determination of the effective refractory period (ERP) at a given endocardial site but cannot elucidate the relationship between the action potential duration (APD) and the ERP. The MAP-pacing combination catheter places electrical stimuli in the immediate vicinity of the MAP recording site. This allows the electrophysiologist to measure both the ERP and APD simultaneously and at nearly identical sites.[1]

Figure 2 shows two simultaneous MAP recordings obtained with two MAP-pacing combination catheters, one positioned in the right ventricular outflow tract and the other in the right ventricular apex. The first 3 beats shown are driven by stimuli from the catheter positioned in the outflow tract, and the last 2 beats from the catheter in the apex. During pacing, stimulus artifacts are seen immediately preceding the MAP upstroke in the record from the corresponding catheter (see arrows in Fig. 2). These stimulus artifacts are smaller than the MAP signal, in this example amounting to 8% and 75% of the MAP amplitude. On average, stimulus artifact amplitudes of twice diastolic threshold stimuli amount to $33 \pm 17\%$ of MAP amplitude, and often occur in a direction opposite to that of the MAP upstroke. Thus, there is seldom any obfuscation of even the initial phase of the MAP signal evoked by the closely adjacent stimulus.

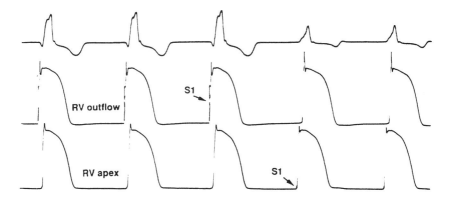

Figure 2. MAPs recorded simultaneously from right ventricular apex and outflow tract while pacing is performed first from one, then the other catheter. Note the small size of the stimulus artifacts (arrows) and the fact that MAP morphology remains essentially unchanged despite a change in ventricular activation sequence. From Reference 1, with permission.

Figure 2 also demonstrates that the MAP signal does not change appreciably in configuration or duration when the stimulation site is switched from the right ventricular outflow tract to the right ventricular apex. In contrast, the surface electrocardiogram (ECG) shows a marked change in morphology when the ventricular activation site is altered. Thus, neither the altered ventricular activation sequence nor the proximity of the electrical stimulus affected the repolarization time course of the local MAP recording.

Both APD and ERP are known to vary substantially from site to site in the ventricle.[2] A precise and reliable evaluation of the relationship between the ERP and the APD should therefore be carried out at the same myocardial site. Figure 3 demonstrates how the endocardial ERP is determined simultaneously with the concomitant MAP duration (APD) at nearly identical sites. The ability to assess the ERP/APD relationship or ERP/APD ratio is important because the normal relationship between myocardial repolarization and excitability can be altered by myocardial disease or antiarrhythmic drug treatment.

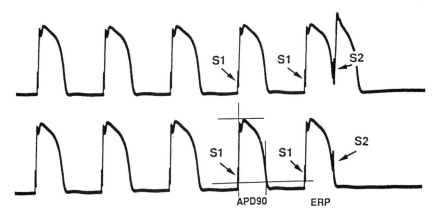

Figure 3. Determination of simultaneously measured effective refractory period (ERP) and MAP duration at 90% repolarization (APD$_{90}$). The premature stimulus (twice diastolic threshold strength) in the upper tracing still captures the myocardium. In the lower tracing, the stimulus interval is 5 milliseconds shorter and fails to capture. This interval equals the ERP and can be compared with the APD$_{90}$ of the same or immediately preceding response. From Reference 1, with permission.

The ERP/APD Relationship in Normal Myocardium

In normal ventricular myocardium and in the absence of sodium channel blocking drugs, the relationship between the MAP duration and the ERP in the canine[1,3] and human[4,5] heart has been shown to be constant and independent of heart rate. These studies showed (both in animal and human in situ hearts) that the ERP/APD ratio resides within a very small margin of 0.75 to 0.85 or, in terms of repolarization level, the ERP for twice diastolic threshold stimuli ends at repolarization levels between 75% and 85% (Fig. 4). This provides an important reference with which to compare the ERP/APD relationship under the influence of antiarrhythmic drugs or disease.

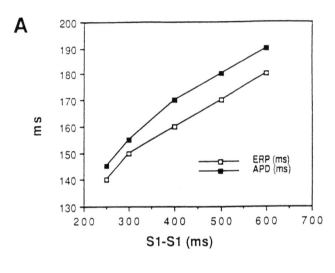

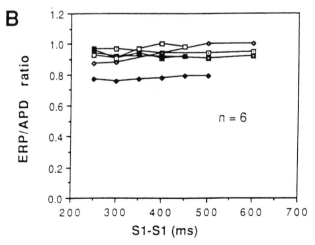

Figure 4. A. Parallelism of effective refractory period (ERP) and MAP duration at 90% repolarization (APD$_{90}$) measured at the same site at different cycle lengths. **B.** Constancy of ERP/APD$_{90}$ ratio at different sites over the same range of cycle lengths as in A. Different sites had slightly different ratios, but the site-specific ratio remained constant within a narrow range.

Modulation of the ERP/APD Relationship by Antiarrhythmic Drugs

Myocardial disease such as ischemia, or antiarrhythmic drug treatment, can alter the normal relationship between repolarization and refractoriness. Sodium channel blocking drugs tend to prolong the ERP even in the absence of APD prolongation or even if they shorten APD. Such a disproportionate increase in ERP relative to APD results in an increased ERP/APD ratio (or postrepolarization refractoriness [PRR]), and has been reported for lidocaine, procainamide, quinidine, mexiletine, and other class I antiarrhythmic agents.[3,4,6,7]

PRR caused by sodium channel blocking drugs may increase with increasing stimulation frequency.[6-8] Simultaneous determinations of MAP durations and ERP are therefore useful in verifying the use-dependent electrophysiologic profile of antiarrhythmic drugs predicted from in vitro studies and may aid in understanding the antiarrhythmic mechanisms of such drug effects in the human heart. (Chapters 25 and 26 provide greater detail on this area of research.)

An example of rate (use)-dependent increase in the ERP/APD ratio is given for an experimental MAP study in Figure 5, panel A and for a clinical MAP study in Figure 5, panel B. As the basic pacing cycle length is decreased from 600 to 250 milliseconds, the APD shortens successively but the ERP undergoes much less shortening and actually lengthens. This results in a marked increase in the ERP/APD ratio or PRR at short cycle lengths. It has been suggested that an increase in the ERP/APD ratio or creation of PRR produces a "window of refractoriness," which prevents premature stimuli from capturing the myocardium during the vulnerable period. Experimental studies have demonstrated that certain drug combinations that exhibit greater clinical efficacy and better tolerance than single drug treatment produce rate-dependent PRR in an additive fashion.[9,10]

Visualizing the Relationship Between Repolarization and Excitability During Routine Electrocardiographic Studies

Figure 6 shows MAP recordings along with 4 surface ECGs and a His bundle recording in a patient with inducible ventricular tachycardia. Programmed ventricular stimulation was performed with the MAP-pacing catheter positioned at the right ventricular outflow tract. The first 2 responses shown are sinus beats. When pacing through the MAP catheter begins, stimulus artifacts appear as sharp downward deflections immediately before the MAP upstroke but cause no further interference with the MAP signal. Following an 8-beat train at an S1-S1 cycle length of 600

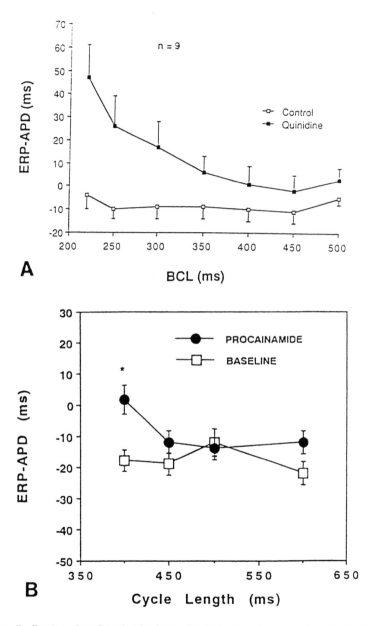

Figure 5. During class I antiarrhythmic drug treatment, successive shortening of the paced cycle length results in a progressive increase of the effective refractory period—action potential duration (ERP-APD) difference. **A.** Epicardial data from canine heart during quinidine treatment. From Reference 1, with permission. **B.** Endocardial data from human heart during procainamide treatment. From Reference 4, with permission.

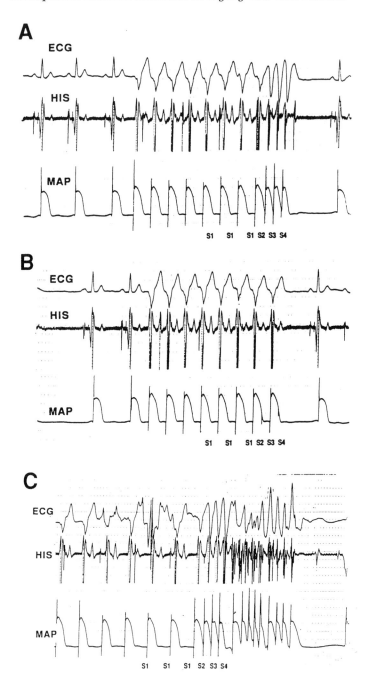

Figure 6. Programmed stimulation with the MAP-pacing catheter in a patient with inducible ventricular tachycardia. See text for details.

milliseconds, 3 extrastimuli (S2-S4) are administered at the shortest coupling intervals that elicit a propagated ventricular response. The upstroke of each extrastimulus response thus marks the end of the ERP of the previous response. Panel A shows that the first extrastimulus (S2) causes significant shortening of the subsequent APD (S2 response) relative to the regularly paced APD (S1 response). The concomitant decrease in S2 ERP allows S3 to capture at a shorter coupling interval than S2. S3, in turn, produces further shortening of APD and ERP, allowing S4 to capture the ventricle at a yet shorter interval.

Panel B shows that when the S2 coupling interval is decreased by 5 milliseconds, S2 fails to capture the ventricle and a relative pause occurs until the next extrastimulus (S3). This pause results in a longer APD as compared to the APD following a successful S2 capture. The S4 stimulus, although administered at the same coupling interval as in the previous train, now fails to capture the ventricle. The simultaneously recorded MAP allows us to appreciate that failure to capture is due to APD prolongation (resulting from the missing S2 response), which causes S4 to fall onto an earlier, refractory repolarization level.

Panel C shows the same drive and extrastimulus train as panel A, but in contrast to panel A, in this example extrastimulation induces nonsustained ventricular tachycardia of 9-beat duration. As appreciated by comparison with the surface ECG and conventional intracardiac tracings, the MAP recording provides clear definition of the local depolarization and repolarization phases during the tachycardia, discerning marked alterations in APD and take-off potentials of successive complexes. The first 2 to 5 tachycardia complexes show APD shortening, whereas the last tachycardia complex (# 9) is prolonged. Surprisingly, the APD of this last complex is even greater than during sinus rhythm although it is preceded by a much shorter diastolic interval.

Local Stimulus Response Latency During Premature Stimulation in the Human Atrium

Intra-atrial conduction time has been shown during programmed atrial stimulation to increase with premature stimulation.[11-13] An increased conduction time, however, can be caused either by a local atrial response delay to the pacing impulse at the stimulation site (local stimulus response latency) or by a slowing of the subsequent intra-atrial impulse propagation. With use of conventional clinical electrophysiologic pacing and recording techniques it is difficult to accurately differentiate between the local stimulus response latency and the propagation time of the atrial response. This results from two limitations in the design of conventional quadripolar catheters: 1) a relatively high pacing threshold, which causes large electrical stimulus artifacts with partial masking of the local response, and 2) a relatively large distance between the distal pacing electrode pair and the proximal recording electrode pair, making the distinction between local and distant electrical responses uncertain. As shown above, the MAP-pacing catheter produces a very small stimulus artifact with the upstroke of the elicited response following almost immediately. As will be shown, this allows one to identify local stimulus response latency during premature electrical stimulation and to distinguish local latency from intra-atrial propagation time.

In a study of 19 patients who underwent electrophysiologic testing for evaluation of documented or clinically suspected ventricular tachycardia,[14] two MAP-pacing combination catheters were positioned, one in the high right atrium and the other in the low right atrium. Stimulation in immediate vicinity to the MAP recording electrodes allowed us to differentiate the local stimulus response latency, and the propagation time of the atrial response to the remote recording site (Fig. 7). The interval between the local stimulus artifact and the sharpest deflection of the local MAP upstroke was defined as the local stimulus response latency. The interval between the sharpest deflection of the MAP at the stimulation site and that one at the distant recording site was defined as propagation time. Conduction time of the electrical impulse was the interval from the stimulus artifact to the sharpest deflection of the MAP at the distant recording site (ie, local stimulus response latency and propagation time). Proximity of extrastimulation was defined as the difference between the actual extrastimulus

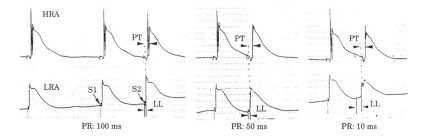

Figure 7. Simultaneous recordings of two MAP combination catheters from the high right atrium (HRA), and the low right atrium (LRA) during premature extrastimulation. Pacing is performed at the LRA; S1 denotes the stimulus artifact during basic cycle length of 600 milliseconds; S2 denotes the extrastimulus artifact. Proximity indicates the prematurity of the extrastimulus, which is referenced to the effective refractory period. At long coupling intervals (proximity 100 milliseconds), local stimulus response latency (LL) is small, but increases progressively with decreasing coupling intervals (proximity 50 milliseconds, and 10 milliseconds, respectively), while the propagation time (PT) of the evoked atrial response from the stimulation site (LRA) to the remote recording site (HRA) remains essentially unchanged. From Reference 14, with permission.

coupling interval and the ERP. The ERP was defined as the longest coupling interval between the upstroke of the MAP preceding the extrastimulus artifact and the extrastimulus artifact that failed to produce a ventricular response. The ERP was also referenced to the repolarization level of the preceding action potential.

Pacing was performed at twice diastolic threshold strength and at 2-millisecond pulse duration. The hearts were paced at a basic cycle length (S1-S1) of 600 milliseconds in a randomized fashion from the high right atrium and low right atrium, respectively. After every eighth stimulus at the basic cycle length, an extrastimulus was introduced. Extrastimulation was started with an S1-S2 coupling interval of 400 milliseconds and was shortened in 5-millisecond steps until the ERP was reached. The pause between the trains was 2 seconds.

Stimulation at the Basic Cycle Length

During regular pacing at a cycle length of 600 milliseconds, local latency was very small (3.8 ± 1.7 milliseconds). This was documented by the fact that the stimulus artifact either immediately preceded or was superimposed onto the upstroke phase of the MAP recording (Fig. 7). The propagation time of the electrical impulse from the stimulation site to the remote recording site at the basic cycle length of 600 milliseconds was on average 54.5 ± 14.3 milliseconds.

Effective Refractory Period

The ERP was determined with 5-millisecond precision in all 38 recordings and was 237.3 ± 25.4 milliseconds. The ERP occurred at a repolarization level of $74.4\pm12.2\%$ of the preceding action potential.

Effect of Premature Stimulation on Local Stimulus Response Latency and Propagation Time

During extrastimulation at wide coupling intervals (proximity ≥70 milliseconds), the local stimulus response latency remained essentially unchanged, with a maximal increase to 4.58 ± 0.22 milliseconds ($20.0\pm4.8\%$), compared to local stimulus response latency at the basic cycle length. With extrastimulation at tighter coupling intervals (proximity <70 milliseconds), local latency increased progressively. The most pronounced prolongation of local latency occurred with stimulation in close vicinity to the ERP, with local stimulus response latency increasing to 18.34 ± 1.44 milliseconds (an increase of $380\pm7.91\%$) at 10-millisecond proximity ($P<0.002$) and to

27.87±3.67 milliseconds (an increase of 630±13.18%) at 5-millisecond proximity, respectively ($P<0.0001$) (Fig. 8). Atrial propagation time remained essentially constant throughout the entire range of extrastimulus intervals. The maximal increase of the propagation time was 14.0±8.4%, which was not significant.

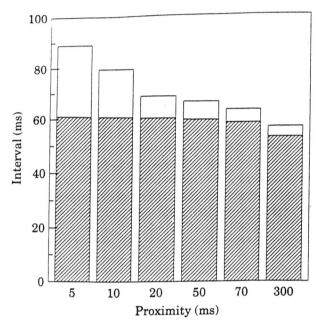

Figure 8. Local stimulus response latency (open bars) and propagation time (hatched bars) as a function of the extrastimulus proximity to the effective refractory period. Standard errors not shown for clarity. From Reference 14, with permission.

"Gap" Phenomenon Between Stimulus Intervals and Functional Atrial Response Intervals

The occurrence of local stimulus response latency with premature extrastimulation resulted in extrastimulus coupling intervals that were longer than the corresponding functional atrial response intervals. As local stimulus response latency increased progressively with premature extrastimulation, this "gap" phenomenon between the extrastimulus coupling intervals and the atrial coupling intervals became more pronounced. Therefore, the progressive shortening of the extrastimulus intervals was not paralleled by an equal shortening of the corresponding atrial response intervals (Fig. 9).

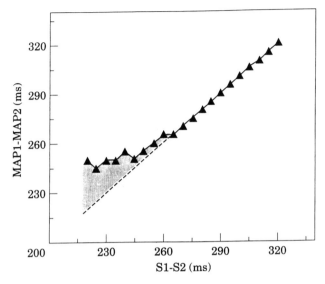

Figure 9. With progressively premature extrastimulation (S1-S2), local latency at the stimulation site increased. As a result, the shortening of the premature extrastimulus coupling interval (S1-S2) was no longer followed by a shortening of the corresponding atrial response interval (MAP1-MAP2) (shaded area). From Reference 14, with permission.

These data demonstrate that the local stimulus response latency may represent a substantial part of what is usually considered conduction time in the human atrium. They also show that local latency increases progressively with extrastimulation at successively decreasing coupling intervals while the propagation time between the elicited MAP and the remote MAP remains essentially unchanged during the entire range of premature stimulation.

Clinical Impact of Distinction Between Local Stimulus Response Latency and Propagation Time

The distinction between local stimulus response latency and propagation time in the human atrium showed that local latency increases progressively with premature extrastimulation whereas propagation time remains essentially unchanged. This has the following clinical implications: First, the increasing local latency during premature stimulation causes the atrial response coupling intervals to be longer than the corresponding extrastimulus intervals, ie, local latency curbs the targeted response interval. Second, local latency, and not an increase in propagation time, seems to be the main cause for differences between the functional refractory period and the ERP during programmed atrial stimulation. Finally, the contribution of local latency to conduction time should be considered in pace mapping for accurate comparison of the conduction time during pacing with that before pacing to avoid misinterpretations of conduction slowing as part of the reentry circuit (zone of slow conduction).

References

1. Franz MR, Chin MC, Sharkey HR, et al. A new single catheter technique for simultaneous measurement of action potential duration and refractory period in vivo. *J Am Coll Cardiol* 1990;16:878-886.
2. Franz MR, Bargheer K, Rafflenbeul W, et al. Monophasic action potential mapping in human subjects with normal electrocardiograms: Direct evidence for the genesis of the T wave. *Circulation* 1987;75:379-386.
3. Franz MR, Costard A. Frequency-dependent effects of quinidine on the relationship between action potential duration and refractoriness in the canine heart in situ. *Circulation* 1988;77:1177-1184.
4. Lee RJ, Liem LB, Cohen TJ, Franz MR. Relation between repolarization and refractoriness in the human ventricle: Cycle length dependence and effect of procainamide. *J Am Coll Cardiol* 1992;19:614-618.
5. Sager PT, Uppal P, Follmer C, et al. Frequency-dependent electrophysiologic effects of amiodarone in humans. *Circulation* 1993;88:1063-1071.
6. Costard-Jaeckle A, Liem LB, Franz MR. Frequency-dependent effect of quinidine, mexiletine, and their combination on postrepolarization refractoriness in vivo. *J Cardiovasc Pharmacol* 1989;14:810-817.
7. Costard-Jaeckle A, Franz MR. Frequency-dependent antiarrhythmic drug effects on postrepolarization refractoriness and ventricular conduction time in canine ventricular myocardium in vivo. *J Pharmacol Exp Ther* 1989;251:39-46.
8. Hondeghem LM. Antiarrhythmic agents: Modulated receptor applications. *Circulation* 1987;75:514-520.
9. Duff HJ, Gault NJ. Mexiletine and quinidine in combination in an ischemic model: Supra-additive antiarrhythmic and electrophysiologic actions. *J Cardiovasc Pharmacol* 1986;8:847-857.
10. Duff HJ, Mitchell LB, Manyari D, Wyse DG. Mexiletine-quinidine combination: Electrophysiologic correlates of a favorable antiarrhythmic interaction in humans. *J Am Coll Cardiol* 1987;10:1149-1156.
11. Buxton AE, Marchlinski FE, Miller JM, et al. The human atrial strength-interval relation. Influence of cycle length and procainamide. *Circulation* 1989;79:271-280.
12. Simpson R Jr, Amara I, Foster JR, et al. Thresholds, refractory periods, and conduction times of the normal and diseased human atrium. *Am Heart J* 1988;116:1080-1090.
13. Cosio FG, Palacios J, Vidal JM, et al. Electrophysiologic studies in atrial fibrillation. Slow conduction of premature impulses: A possible manifestation of the background for reentry. *Am J Cardiol* 1983;51:122-130.
14. Koller BS, Karasik PE, Solomon AJ, Franz MR. Prolongation of conduction time during premature stimulation in the human atrium is primarily caused by local stimulus response latency. *Eur Heart J* 1995;16:1920-1924.

6

The Monophasic Action Potential as a Guide and Clinical Teaching Tool During Routine Clinical Electrophysiology Studies

Pamela E. Karasik, MD, Mary E. Chavez, CVT, Ross D. Fletcher, MD and Michael R. Franz, MD, PhD

The contact electrode catheter that is capable of recording an intracardiac monophasic action potential (MAP) became available for widespread clinical use in the early 1990s.[1] Prior catheters were based on a suction electrode technique,[2] which was unwieldy and carried with it the risk of myocardial damage and air emboli. Although the MAP catheter was initially designed as a research tool, it has acquired a role in the clinical electrophysiology laboratory, and the indications for its use continue to expand.

Technical Aspects of Use

The catheter, as currently available (EP Technologies, San Jose, CA), is a 7F quadripolar combination pacing/recording catheter. The recording poles include a distal tip electrode coupled to a reference electrode recessed into the shaft, 5 mm proximal. The platinum pacing electrodes are oriented in an orthogonal fashion, 2.5 mm from the tip electrode. The

From Franz MR (ed): *Monophasic Action Potentials: Bridging Cell and Bedside.* ©Futura Publishing Company, Inc., Armonk, NY, 2000.

flexibility of the distal 7 cm of the catheter facilitates passage through the vascular tree and minimizes trauma to the endocardial surface. With this pacing electrode configuration, the capture threshold is low, on the order of 0.02 to 0.25 mA. This minimizes the stimulus artifact and its potential interference with the MAP recording.

Placement of the catheter in the heart is similar to placement of standard bipolar or quadripolar diagnostic catheters. The catheter is steerable within a 180° radius; this allows more control over the distal shaft and aids in crossing the tricuspid valve. To achieve stable MAP recordings, the tip of the catheter should be placed perpendicular to the endocardial surface, where it is held in place by the myocardial trabeculations. This may require placement of a "swan neck" in the distal 3 cm of the catheter (Fig. 1).

The recording poles of the catheter are identified as positive and negative. The distal pole is recorded as positive, and the proximal electrode is negative. The catheter can be connected through a standard intracardiac module or via a direct current (DC) input module, depending on the type of electrophysiology recorder in use. Recording via the DC module allows

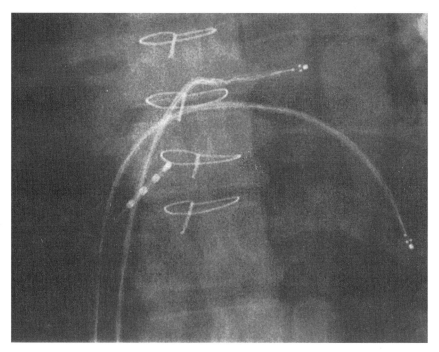

Figure 1. Radiograph in the PA projection demonstrating catheter placement for a diagnostic electrophysiology study. The narrow spaced quadripolar catheter is placed in the His bundle position. The upper MAP catheter is in the right ventricular outflow tract, and has a swan-neck curve to maintain perpendicular position in the myocardium. The lower MAP catheter is at the right ventricular apex.

for less electrical interference and provides clearer recordings during radio-frequency ablation or defibrillation. As the recording mode is different from that of standard quadripolar catheters (reversal of negative/positive), note that the correct lead configuration must be chosen on the electrophysiology recording system. The filter settings for the MAP catheter are open at 0 and 2500 Hz, while standard catheter settings are usually 30 Hz to 500 Hz. The gain is then adjusted so that the tracings are approximately the same size. The pacing poles are oriented opposite to one another and are connected to the intracardiac module in a standard fashion. If the MAP recording appears inverted, this may signal too much pressure on the endocardial surface, and the catheter should be pulled back until the tracing normalizes. Failure to do this may result in perforation. If the recording electrodes are not connected in the proper orientation, the signal will appear inverted as well. The catheter can be placed in both the atria and the ventricles. MAP recordings from the two chambers differ somewhat in their morphology. The atrial recording is more triangular in appearance, with a slower return to baseline. The ventricular recording has a more rounded, rapid descent to baseline (Fig. 2). Threshold measurements are obtained in a standard fashion. As previously mentioned, the threshold

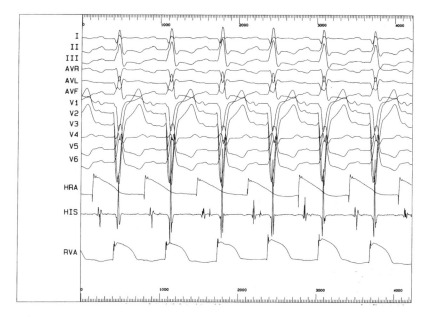

Figure 2. Tracing demonstrating the 12-surface electrocardiogram leads, the MAP recording from the high right atrium (HRA), the His bundle (HIS), and the right ventricular apex (RVA). Note the difference in the MAP recordings. The HRA is triangular in shape while the RVA has a more rounded plateau phase. The HIS is recorded on a standard quadripolar catheter.

current with the MAP catheter is on the order of 0.1 mA or less. If testing shows a high threshold, the catheter should be repositioned. Baseline perturbations can usually be attributed to catheter instability, and respond well to small advances in catheter position. On rare occasions the MAP recording can be contaminated by the electrocardiogram (ECG); this problem can usually be resolved by finding a new site.

During a diagnostic electrophysiology study in our laboratory, we routinely use two MAP catheters, and a narrow spaced (2-5-2 mm) quadripolar catheter. The first MAP catheter is placed in the high right atrium, the second in the right ventricular apex. The standard quadripolar catheter is placed across the tricuspid valve to record a His potential. After completion of the atrial and atrioventricular nodal parts of the study, the atrial catheter is placed in the right ventricular outflow tract (Fig. 3). The ventricular stimulation protocol is then performed in a standard fashion starting with programmed extrastimulation from the right ventricle. With proper placement, the catheters should maintain stable recordings for the duration of the electrophysiology study. Simultaneous recording from two sites in the ventricle provides additional information regarding local conduction velocity and latency. It also obviates the need to move the pacing catheter

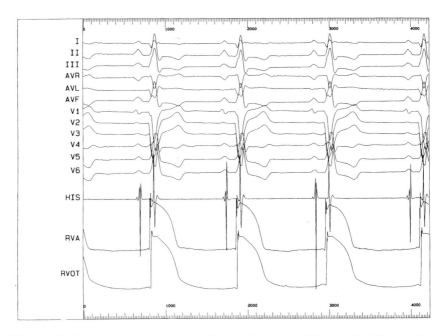

Figure 3. Twelve-surface electrocardiogram leads are followed by His bundle recording from a quadripolar catheter and the MAP recordings from the right ventricular apex (RVA) and right ventricular outflow tract (RVOT) after completion of the atrial study. Note the near simultaneous upstroke of the MAP recordings.

to a second site during the ventricular stimulation protocol. The close proximity of the pacing and recording electrodes minimizes conduction delay between the two sites (Fig. 4). Note that during pacing, the stimulus artifact coincides with the upstroke of the action potential.

As with any new technique, there is a learning curve to the use of the MAP catheter. Use of these catheters instead of standard quadripolar catheters may add 10 to 15 minutes to a diagnostic electrophysiology study.

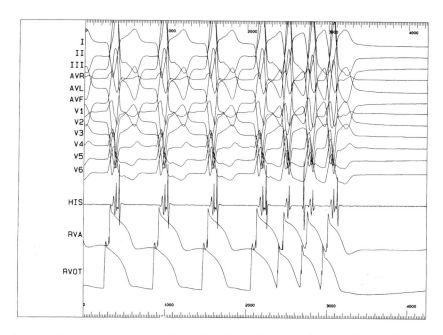

Figure 4. Tracing showing the 12-surface electrocardiogram leads, the His bundle (HIS) recording, and the MAP recordings from two sites in the right ventricle. The ventricle is paced from the right ventricular outflow tract (RVOT) catheter at a 600-millisecond drive, followed by 3 extrastimuli. Note the absence of a visible pacing spike, as well as the conduction time from one site to the other. Note also the shortening of the action potential duration with progressive extrastimuli.

Information Obtained from the MAP Catheter

Information regarding the effective refractory period (ERP) of the ventricle has been available since the beginning of clinical electrophysiology. The intracellular correlate of this, the action potential duration (APD), has been studied extensively in both the single-cell model and the animal model. The MAP catheter, with pacing and recording from nearly contiguous regions of the heart, allows one to measure both the APD and the ERP of a small group of myocytes in the living human heart. The ability to study changes in excitation, local repolarization, and conduction velocity may finally bridge the gap between cellular biology and human physiology. Although developed as a research tool, the MAP catheter can provide useful information to the clinician for the benefit of the patient.

Antiarrhythmic Drug Effect

One of the more obvious and clinically useful roles of the MAP catheter is its ability to asses the pharmacologic effect of antiarrhythmic agents. These drugs exert their effect by either extending refractoriness or pro-longing the action potential.[3] Traditionally, drug effect had been determined by the change in the ERP at a single site in the ventricle. Information regarding APD could only be inferred. The MAP catheter provides information regarding changes in repolarization and APD that are not available from a standard quadripolar catheter. When a patient is studied after 5 half-lives of a drug, the presumption is that they have reached a steady state. Use of MAP catheters will demonstrate very clearly if there has been the expected effect of lengthening of the APD and/or a change in postrepolariza-tion refractoriness. Studies have shown the effects of class I and class III agents on the duration of refractoriness. Lee et al[4] studied 32 patients receiv-ing sotalol and a class Ia antiarrhythmic. They found significant prolongation of the ERP and the APD, without changes in conduction velocity. In an earlier study, MAP recordings were taken in the right ventricle of 15 patients under-going routine diagnostic electrophysiologic testing.[5] The relationship be-tween cycle length and APD was clearly established. With increasing pacing rates, the action potential shortened as did the ERP. The patients then re-ceived procainamide intravenously, and a cycle length dependence in the ERP relative to the APD was demonstrated. Procainamide increased the ERP at each cycle length with greater effect seen at the shorter coupling intervals. This is consistent with known class I antiarrhythmic effects on sodium chan-nels, and provides an easy marker for pharmacologic effect. Confirming that there is a drug effect allows one to decide whether a clinical arrhythmia remains inducible because of inadequate dosing or because of true drug fail-ure. The ability to assess the drug effect on the electrical properties of the myocardium may allow more careful tailoring of a drug regimen for the indi-vidual patient.[6]

Ventricular Arrhythmias

The mechanism for the induction of ventricular tachycardia (VT) is not well understood, although clinical electrophysiology testing has been available for many years. The introduction of the MAP catheter may provide insight into the various mechanisms responsible for VT induction. While it is recognized that VT can be induced by introducing repetitive extrastimuli into the ventricle, and that the more premature the stimuli the more likely the induction, it is also well known that nonclinical arrhythmias can be induced with more premature stimulation.[7,8] There is a standard of practice that recommends keeping the coupling intervals to 200 milliseconds or greater to prevent induction of nonsignificant arrhythmias, although Josephson[9] suggests that the coupling interval during programmed electrical stimulation can be as low as 180 milliseconds. Koller et al[10] explored the relationship between APD and ERP, and how it changes with premature extrastimuli. They found that with each progressively closer extrastimulus, the ventricle could be captured at less complete levels of repolarization and, thus, the ERP was shortened. This was termed *encroachment* and was associated with a slowing of impulse propagation from the paced to the recording site. In the majority of instances, only when the ventricle was captured at less than 90% repolarization could VT be induced. Therefore, use of the MAP recording allows the investigator to assess APD and to more closely understand the tightness of coupling of extrastimuli. Some patients clearly have short APD and, at coupling intervals of 200 milliseconds, do not begin to show encroachment. These patients require more "aggressive" programmed stimulation protocols (Fig. 5). In our laboratory we do not set an arbitrary limit on coupling intervals of the premature stimuli. Rather, we guide our study by observing the amount of encroachment seen at progressively tighter intervals. We have not seen an increase in the number of "nonsignificant" arrhythmias, even when coupling intervals are as close as 170 milliseconds. Of note also is that when using the MAP catheter we frequently observe significant variability in APD at different sites in the ventricle. What may be considered a loose coupling interval at one site may cause significant encroachment at a second site. Often when we assess pharmacologic effects, we see significant APD prolongation at one site without apparent effect at a second site. In this situation the drug usually does not protect against VT induction (Fig. 6). Whether this represents underdosing of the drug or a true local difference in systemic effect is unknown.

Other mechanisms of tachycardia induction may be elucidated by use of the MAP catheter. Triggered arrhythmias due to early or late afterdepolarizations (EADs or DADs, respectively) can be a significant cause of clinical arrhythmias, but are usually only inferred. Use of the MAP recording catheter in the animal model has demonstrated these afterdepolar-

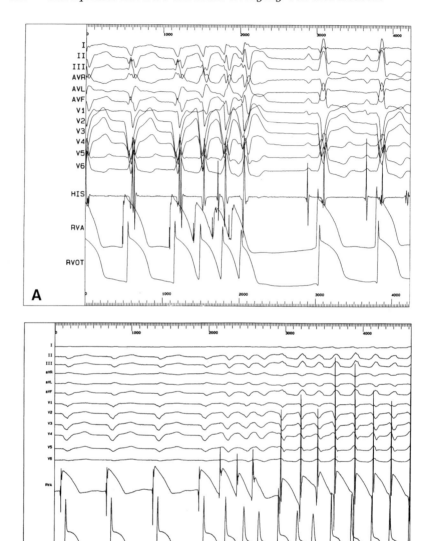

Figure 5. A. The ventricle is paced from the right ventricular apex (RVA) at 600 milliseconds, and 3 premature extrastimuli are delivered at 300, 240, and 205 milliseconds, respectively. Note the encroachment on phase 3 on the RVA MAP, as well as the local latency. There is also conduction delay between the two sites, such that there is no encroachment at the right ventricular outflow tract (RVOT) site. No ventricular tachycardia (VT) was induced with this drive train. **B**. In this patient, encroachment is seen at the second site but not at the pacing site. VT was induced.

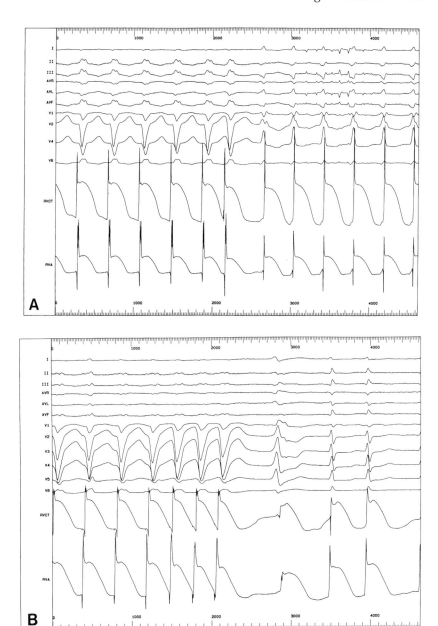

Figure 6. **A**. Ventricular tachycardia (VT) is induced at the baseline electrophysiologic study with a single premature ventricular contraction at a 400-millisecond drive, with 290-millisecond coupling interval. **B**. After treatment with procainamide, no sustained VT could be induced with up to 3 extrastimuli. Note the lengthening of the action potential duration as recorded by the MAP catheter.

izations.[11] Animals given ouabain and subject to pacing showed DADs and development of ectopic beats as well as VT. In patients with idiopathic VT, the MAP catheter may offer clues into the mechanism of the arrhythmia. In our laboratory a patient with a history of torsades de pointes and a single premature ventricular contraction focus was noted to have afterdepolarizations at the time of ablation (Fig. 7).

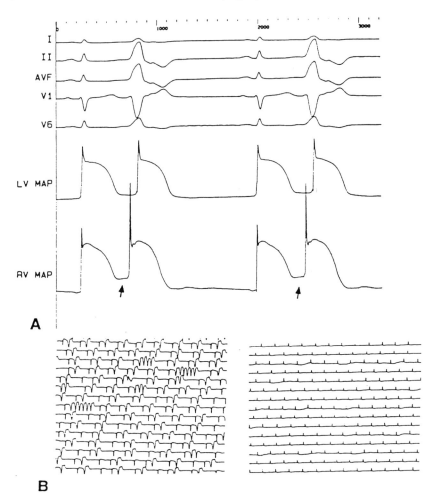

Figure 7. **A.** Surface electrocardiogram leads I, II, aVF, V_1, and V_6. The left ventricular (LV) catheter is positioned at the apex. The right ventricular (RV) catheter is positioned at the RV outflow tract (RVOT). The arrows indicate the beginning of afterdepolarizations originating at the RVOT at the site of ablation. **B.** This patient had multiple runs of nonsustained ventricular tachycardia and premature ventricular contraction (PVC)-induced torsades de pointes. After ablation, the PVCs were abolished.

Effect of Ischemia on Electrical Properties of Myocardium

Ischemia is well known to cause clinical arrhythmias, and use of the MAP catheter, in the cell, animal heart, and human, has offered new insights into the mechanisms of electrical instability.[12] At the cellular level, ischemia induces shortening of the APD, loss of amplitude, and a decrease in the upstroke velocity. Behrens et al[13] demonstrated in isolated rabbit hearts the effect of myocardial ischemia on APD. With ischemic times of up to 15 minutes, the action potential assumed a more triangular shape and there was shortening of the APD. These investigators also noticed an increase in dispersion of activation and repolarization, conditions thought to be associated with electrical instability.[14] These changes resolved with reperfusion. Similar findings were seen in the living human heart as described by John et al.[15] In 26 patients undergoing left heart angiography, they compared the changes in APD in zones of ischemic and normal myocardium. Ischemia was caused by rapid atrial pacing and confirmed by technetium-MIBI scanning. Significant APD shortening was seen in ischemic areas as compared to that seen in normally perfused areas. Taggart et al[16] extended these findings to the interventional laboratory. Twenty-one patients underwent percutaneous transluminal coronary angioplasty of either the left anterior descending artery or the right coronary artery. All patients received one or two MAP catheters in the right ventricle. Recordings were made during balloon inflation with atrial pacing at a fixed rate, to control for patient variability in heart rate. During balloon occlusion of the artery, there was shortening of the APD. What may be important clinically is a differential shortening between sites, as differential responses to ischemia have been seen when sites are compared between endocardium and epicardium.

Can the MAP Catheter Be Used to Asses Myocardial Viability in the Catheterization Laboratory?

The MAP catheter reflects ischemic changes in a small area of myocardium and therefore is a more sensitive tool than the surface ECG. The ability to demonstrate changes in APD during interventional procedures may aid the angiographer in choosing appropriate targets for intervention. With the addition of either incremental atrial pacing or dobutamine, it may be possible to demonstrate small areas of viability that would otherwise be inapparent.

Atrial Arrhythmias and the Use of the MAP Catheter

There have been a number of reports in the literature recently regarding the different intracardiac morphologies of atrial fibrillation and the possibility of pace-terminating the arrhythmia.[17] In the setting of type I atrial fibrillation, use of the MAP catheter can identify those patients with pace-terminable arrhythmia. These patients have discreet action potentials and regular isoelectric segments, which indicate the presence of an excitable gap. Normal sinus rhythm may often be restored in patients with atrial flutter, via burst pacing in the right atrium. A well known outcome of this procedure, however, is atrial fibrillation.[18] Use of the MAP catheter has been very helpful in determining the minimum cycle length that can safely be used when terminating atrial flutter. Moubarak et al,[19] in a series of 20 patients, showed that atrial fibrillation did not occur if the pacing rate was kept greater than 170 milliseconds.

In our laboratory we have found it helpful to use the MAP catheter during atrial pace-outs as well as during atrial flutter ablations. We have noted the occurrence of atrial flutter on the surface ECG while the local recordings demonstrate atrial fibrillation. As shown in panel A of Figure 8, the surface rhythm appears organized with a cycle length of 185 milliseconds. The recording from the high right atrium confirms this. Note, however the fragmented recording obtained from the low atrial catheter. This patient's arrhythmia could not be pace terminated. Another useful feature of the MAP recording is the rapidity with which atrial fibrillation can be detected during burst pacing. We have found that minimizing the delivery of pacing spikes once atrial fibrillation is induced increases the likelihood of conversion to sinus rhythm. This is shown in panel B of Figure 8.

In other instances we can use the information regarding atrial APD to avoid induction of arrhythmias. Koller et al[10] reported on the difference between stimulus response latency and delays in propagation of premature impulses. This information has proven useful in guiding appropriate management of the patient with atrial tachyarrhythmias.

Use of the MAP Catheter During Implantable Cardioverter Defibrillator Implants

In 1993, Swartz et al[20] were the first to show that there was often a discrepancy between the surface ECG and the intracardiac recordings during ventricular fibrillation (VF) in the human heart. They recorded MAPs from the right ventricle during nonthoracotomy implantable cardioverter

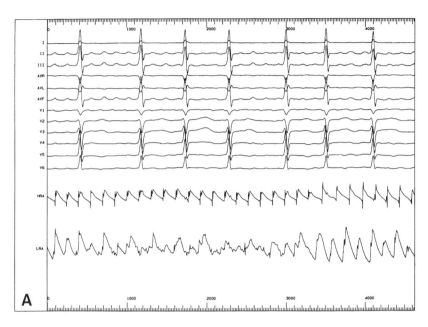

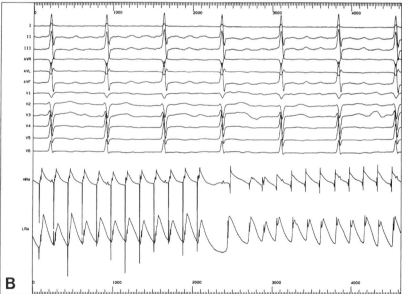

Figure 8. A. The 12-lead electrocardiogram is suggestive of atrial flutter with organized atrial activity. The top MAP recording is from the high right atrium (HRA) and also shows organized action potential durations. However, the lower tracing from the low right atrium (LRA) displays fragmented electrical activity most consistent with atrial fibrillation. **B**. Although atrial capture was possible in this patient, the arrhythmia was not pace-terminable.

defibrillator (ICD) implants in 22 patients. It was observed that most of the time VF was associated with nonfractionated MAP recordings. We have routinely used the MAP catheter in the right ventricle during ICD implants in our laboratory. With these catheters in place we are able to choose ideal coupling intervals for T wave shock induction of VF. Often the coupling interval measured via the surface ECG may not coincide with the optimal timing of the T wave shock. Observation of the timing of the defibrillation shock may also provide useful clinical information. We have noticed that there is frequently a discrepancy between the surface ECG and the intracardiac recordings. The surface may appear disorganized and fragmented, consistent with VF, but the MAP recording may show discrete action potentials suggestive of ventricular flutter (Fig. 9). This has significant ramifications for the determination of the accurate defibrillation threshold for the patient. We have encountered the unusual patient in whom VF is not easily induced but ventricular flutter is. When these patients subsequently have a true VF episode, the ICD may not defibrillate. The ability to confirm that the ICD has been shown to convert true VF is extremely important to the patient's clinical outcome.

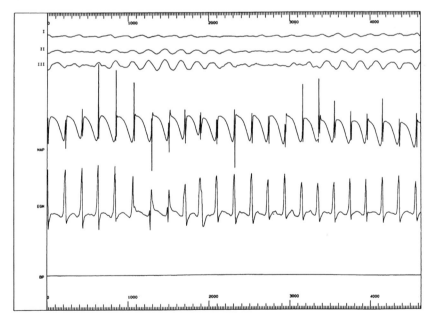

Figure 9. Three surface electrocardiogram leads are followed by a MAP recording in the right ventricular apex, an electrogram from a defibrillation lead (EGM), and the blood pressure (BP). Note the disorganization seen in the surface ECG consistent with ventricular fibrillation. The MAP recording, however, shows discrete organized action potentials with a cycle length of 200 milliseconds, more suggestive of ventricular tachycardia.

Conclusion

Use of the MAP catheter in the clinical electrophysiology laboratory has greatly expanded the amount of information available to the clinical electrophysiologist. With it, one can gather data regarding mechanisms of arrhythmia as well as pharmacologic effects of drug therapy. The ability to pace-terminate atrial flutter is enhanced, and appropriateness of ICD function can be confirmed. Routine use of the catheter in our laboratory has influenced patient care and continues to be the standard by which we treat the arrhythmia patient.

References

1. Franz MR, Chin MC, Sharkey HR, et al. A new single catheter technique for simultaneous measurement of action potential duration and refractory period in vivo. *J Am Coll Cardiol* 1990;16:878-886.
2. Olsson SB. Right ventricular monophasic action potentials during regular rhythm: A heart catheterization study in man. *Acta Med Scand* 1972;191:145-157.
3. Roden DM. Ionic mechanisms for prolongation of refractoriness and their proarrhythmic and antiarrhythmic correlates. *Am J Cardiol* 1996;78(suppl 4A):12-16.
4. Lee D, Newman D, Ham M, Dorian P. Electrophysiologic mechanisms of antiarrhythmic efficacy of a sotalol and class Ia drug combination: Elimination of reverse use dependence. *J Am Coll Cardiol* 1997;29:100-105.
5. Lee RJ, Liem LB, Cohen TJ, Franz MR. Relation between repolarization and refractoriness in the human ventricle: Cycle length dependence and effect of procainamide. *J Am Coll Cardiol* 1992;19:614-618.
6. O'Donoghue S, Platia EV. Monophasic action potential recordings: Evaluation of antiarrhythmic drugs. *Prog Cardiovasc Dis* 1991;34:1-14. Review.
7. Buxton AE, Waxman HL, Marchlinski RE, et al. Role of triple extrastimuli during electrophysiologic study of patients with documented sustained ventricular tachyarrhythmias. *Circulation* 1984;69:532-540.
8. Brugada P, Green M, Abdollah H, Wellens HJJ. Significance of ventricular arrhythmias initiated by programmed ventricular stimulation: The importance of the type of ventricular arrhythmia induced and the number of premature stimuli required. *Circulation* 1984;69:87-92.
9. Josephson ME. *Clinical Cardiac Electrophysiology: Techniques and Interpretations.* 2nd ed. Malvern, PA: Lea & Febiger; 1993:417-615.
10. Koller BS, Karasik PE, Solomon AJ, Franz MF. Relation between repolarization and refractoriness during programmed electrical stimulation in the human right ventricle. *Circulation* 1995;91:2378-2384.
11. de Groot SHM, Vos MA, Gorgels APM, et al. Combining monophasic action potential recordings with pacing to demonstrate delayed afterdepolarizations and triggered arrhythmias in the intact heart. *Circulation* 1995;92:2697-2704.
12. Mohabir R, Clusin WT, Lee H-C. Intracellular calcium alternans and the genesis of ischemic ventricular fibrillation. In Zipes D, Jalife J (eds): *Cardiac Electrophysiology: From Cell to Bedside.* Philadelphia: W. B. Saunders; 1990:448-456.
13. Behrens S, Li C, Franz M. Effects of myocardial ischemia on ventricular fibrillation inducibility and defibrillation efficacy. *J Am Coll Cardiol* 1997;29:817-824.

14. Watson RM, Schwartz JL, Maron BL, et al. Inducible polymorphic ventricular tachycardia and ventricular fibrillation in a subgroup of patients with hypertrophic cardiomyopathy at high risk for sudden death. *J Am Coll Cardiol* 1987;10:761-774.
15. John RM, Taggart PI, Sutton PM, et al. Endocardial monophasic acton potential recordings for the detection of myocardial ischemia in man: A study using atrial pacing stress and myocardial perfusion scintigraphy. *Am Heart J* 1991;122:1599-1609.
16. Taggart P, Sutton PMI, Boyett MR, et al. Human ventricular action potential duration during short and long cycles. *Circulation* 1996;94:2526-2534.
17. Pandozi C, Bianconi L, Villani M, et al. Local capture by atrial pacing in spontaneous chronic atrial fibrillation. *Circulation* 1997;95:2416-2422.
18. Waldo AL. Some observations regarding atrial flutter in man. *PACE* 1983; 6:1181-1189.
19. Moubarak J, Karasik P, Fletcher RD, Franz MR. Coversion of atrial flutter into fibrillation during overdrive pacing: Role of stimulus encroachment. *PACE* 1997;20:361.
20. Swartz JF, Jones JL, Fletcher RD. Characterization of ventricular fibrillation based on monophasic action potential morphology in the human heart. *Circulation* 1993;87:1907-1914.

7

How to Record High-Quality Monophasic Action Potential Tracings

Philip T. Sager, MD

Introduction

Monophasic action potential (MAP) recordings can provide pivotal data regarding in situ repolarization and the relationship between repolarization and refractoriness. These data are obtained by recording high-quality MAP tracings that faithfully reproduce repolarization and are without artifacts. Such high-fidelity recordings require a proper catheter, expertise in the proper positioning of the MAP catheter, appreciation of techniques for minimizing artifacts, and appropriate recording equipment.

Genesis of the MAP Recording

MAP tracings accurately reproduce the temporal sequence of myocyte repolarization, and the electrophysiologic explanation for the genesis of the MAPs[1,2] is discussed in detail in chapter 2. Briefly, the pressure contact of the MAP catheter locally depolarizes the cells at the catheter tip, and these cells form an electrical gradient with the adjacent, nondepolarized cells. Franz[2] has postulated that during diastole a sink current is formed

Supported, in part, from a Grant-in-Aid (G1117) from the Greater Los Angeles chapter of the American Heart Association.
From Franz MR (ed): *Monophasic Action Potentials: Bridging Cell and Bedside.*
©Futura Publishing Company, Inc., Armonk, NY, 2000.

from the adjacent normal cells to the depolarized cells at the MAP tip. This current reflects the relative changes in the potential of the normal cells during periodic cardiac depolarization and repolarization. Thus, the MAP tracing is highly dependent on the interface between the mechanically depolarized cells and the catheter tip, and it follows that the recording of high-quality tracings requires excellent stable catheter-tissue contact.

MAP Catheter Design

Early seminal recordings of MAPs were made by use of the suction electrode to create catheter contact with the myocardium.[3] Pioneering studies by Olsson et al[4-8] demonstrated alterations in human in situ repolarization during physiologic perturbations. However, due to concerns regarding suction-induced myocardial damage, the use of suction electrodes is not practical for recordings that last more than several minutes. In addition, the need for continuous suction has made the technique cumbersome and has raised concerns about the possibility of the development of an air embolus during left-sided recordings, should there be a malfunction in the equipment. Pivotal studies by Franz et al[9-15] propelled the field forward with the development of a contact electrode catheter that is safe, permits recordings of up to several hours, and results in high-fidelity stable MAP signals. Importantly, the MAP recordings of the time course of cardiac repolarization using this catheter have been validated against transmembrane action potential (TAP) recordings.[16]

The Franz electrode contact catheter[17] is a 6F catheter that permits recordings of MAP signals from the atria and ventricles. It has a hemispheric electrode at the catheter tip (1.5 mm in diameter) and a 1-mm reference (indifferent) electrode set back 5 mm from the distal tip of the catheter (Fig. 1). The proximal electrode is slightly recessed and is designed to come into contact only with blood, and not to have direct contact with the endocardium. The electrodes are formed from nonpolarizable silver/silver chloride powder placed within a polymeric compound, so that it is not possible for the silver ions to be denuded and deposited within the patient's endocardium or circulation.

It is essential that the catheter tip be maintained with constant contact against the endocardium throughout the cardiac cycle despite movement of the cardiac chambers during systole and diastole. Significant variations in tissue contact will result in changes in the MAP amplitude as well as the development of movement artifacts (see below). While earlier catheter designs dealt with this issue by using an internal stylet, more recently excellent tissue contact has been facilitated by the technical innovation of placing a metal spring intraluminal component in the distal aspect of the catheter. When the catheter is appropriately advanced against the

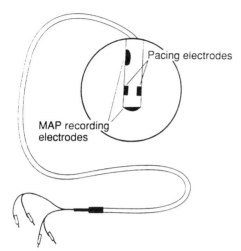

Figure 1. Schematic illustration of the pacing-MAP catheter, demonstrating the catheter's design. This catheter permits measurement of repolarization and refractoriness at the same ventricular site. Reprinted from Reference 15, with permission.

endocardium, the spring component maintains fairly constant pressure of the tip against the endocardium throughout the cardiac cycle. The distal tip of the catheter must oppose the endocardium with sufficient force so that contact is preserved but of an insufficient magnitude to cause catheter perforation or myocardial damage. More recently, two important technological advances, steerability and pacing capabilities, have significantly enhanced the catheter design.[15] Bidirectional steering permits easier catheter manipulation to the desired endocardial site and the addition of two pacing electrodes permits the ability to determine repolarization and refractoriness at the same myocardial site.[18-20] The latter modification includes the placement of two small platinum/iridium electrodes orthogonally 2 mm proximal from the tip electrode. The close spacing of these electrodes permits pacing to be performed at a very low pacing threshold (mean threshold = 0.09 mA).[15] The low pacing threshold reduces pacing artifacts seen in the MAP recordings to small or nondiscernible levels.

Catheter Placement

The catheter is advanced against the endocardial surface of the atria or the ventricle until tissue contact is optimized as evidenced by a change from an intracardiac electrogram signal or a local endocardial recording to a typical MAP signal. Once the catheter is firmly placed against the endocardial surface, a MAP is usually recorded after several beats (Fig. 2). The amount of tension on the catheter can then be increased or decreased in order to obtain a signal with an absolute minimum of artifact and with a flat diastolic baseline devoid of electrical activity. To a relative degree, the amplitude of the MAP recording is dependent on the degree of tissue contact and the best

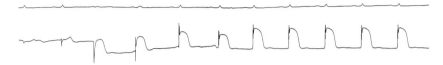

Figure 2. The left side of the figure shows the MAP catheter recording a local electrogram. Following advancement of the catheter, a partially formed MAP tracing is recorded which quickly matures into a high fidelity action potential recording.

recordings are those that have a constant degree of pressure throughout systole and diastole. As discussed below, varying tissue contact during the cardiac cycle can be a cause of movement artifacts. The most stable recordings are generally obtained when the distal end of the catheter opposes the endocardium in a perpendicular manner. While high-quality tracings can be obtained throughout the heart, we have found that the right ventricular midseptum or outflow tract is the easiest place at which to obtain high-quality right ventricular MAP recordings. The lateral right atrium is a particularly good site for atrial recordings. While a direct perpendicular catheter orientation is usually best, we have sometimes found that advancing the catheter against the myocardium with a curve on the distal end can result in stable recordings that are not possible with use of other techniques. Once a stable recording without artifacts is obtained, the recordings usually remain excellent for 1 to several hours. We usually use an introducer that can be locked down on the catheter once a stable position is obtained, and this helps maintain long-term recordings.

After a moderate amount of experience, the operator can expect to record high-quality MAP signals throughout the atria and the ventricles. In addition to placing the distal aspect of the catheter perpendicular to the endocardial surface, it is important that the distal 3 to 5 cm of the catheter be positioned so that it can flex freely as the atria or ventricles contract and relax, and that the catheter does not become entrapped or ensnared within the cardiac structure. This ability to flex and to maintain constant pressure throughout the cardiac cycle is an important feature of the catheter. The steerability feature of the MAP catheter permits careful positioning of the catheter tip into the desired position, allowing the more proximal aspect of the catheter shaft to remain free. It is important that the proximal electrode (the indifferent electrode) of the catheter not come into contact with myocardial tissue (which can cause major disruption of the MAP tracing), but rather that it records a reference voltage from the blood.

Criteria for Satisfactory Recordings

It is important that the operator pay close attention to the recording quality in order to make sure that meaningful signals are obtained that accurately reflect cardiac repolarization. With careful catheter positioning it is possible, with a minimum of time, to obtain high-quality, stable MAP recordings. Optimal recordings exhibit the following characteristics:

1. Recordings should be more than 10 mV when measured in the ventricle[2] and more than 3 mV when measured in the atrium.[8] The greater the MAP amplitude, the more minimized far-field electrical activity will be, resulting in a reduction in artifacts.
2. There should be a flat baseline both before and after the MAP recording without extra negative or positive deflections. If any extra signals are present during the diastolic interval, they should be less than 5% of the MAP amplitude.[2]
3. The action potential recordings should have the typical contour of an action potential, with a convex plateau, a smooth phase 3, and a rapid upstroke during phase 0. The upstroke during phase 0 will often overshoot the plateau, in contrast to TAP recordings, and this is intrinsic to the recording technique (the maximum amplitude of the MAP recording is thus measured from the plateau amplitude and not the maximum amplitude of phase 0). The upstroke phase of the MAP also contains a rapid biphasic deflection. This can appear as a notch or spike during phase 0, and represents the remnant of the intrinsic deflection.
4. In general, there will not be extra bumps or depolarizations during phase 3 or early following repolarization. If there are positive deflections during phase 3 or early during phase 4, the operator must be very diligent in making sure that these are part of repolarization and not artifacts before labeling them as afterdepolarizations. Changes in catheter contact during the cardiac cycle can result in deflections in the MAP recording secondary to movement artifacts. Specifically, relaxation can result in a reduction in tissue contact which can cause a positive deflection during phase 3 or during the early part of phase 4, that can be easily misinterpreted as an early afterdepolarization. Thus, it is essential to closely scrutinize the recordings and to ascertain whether afterdepolarizations disappear when the catheter is slightly advanced or slightly withdrawn.
5. The upstroke of the MAP should be clear and it should be rapid. Franz[2] has suggested that the upstroke should be completed within 5 milliseconds. There may be small negative or positive deflections just before the major upstroke, and these deflections most likely represent either remote electrical activity or the intracardiac QRS. These deflections, if small, should not interfere with accurate MAP measurements.
6. There should be no fluctuation in MAP amplitude, beat to beat. The presence of fluctuations suggests that there is a lack of stable catheter contact. The amplitude of the MAP signal is usually higher with greater tissue contact, and thus fluctuation in the amplitude

suggests that the contact is unstable. Similarly, the MAP signal should look basically identical beat to beat, and if there are changes in signal characteristics between beats this suggests that the tissue contact is not optimal.

7. When pacing from the MAP catheter at cycle lengths greater than 500 milliseconds, the MAP signal should appear identical beat to beat. During rapid pacing it is possible to have beat-to-beat alterations in the action potential duration at 90% repolarization (APD$_{90}$) that reflect true changes in cardiac electrophysiology.[21]

Filtering and Amplification

MAP recordings require amplification and high band filtering in order to reduce alternating current (AC) and high-frequency noise. The filter settings commonly used for standard electrophysiologic recordings (30 Hz/500 Hz) will result in electrogram recordings that are identical to those obtained with a bipolar catheter when the MAP catheter is used. In order to display a MAP signal, it is necessary to use a wider filtering bandwidth. For typical MAP recordings, filtering at 0.05 Hz to 1000 Hz allows satisfactory MAP recordings for most clinical purposes. Because the upstroke of the MAP is relatively slow compared to TAP recordings (mean of 7 V/s versus 200 to 300 V/s),[22] information can be lost and the upstroke signal can be artificially retarded at filter settings less than 2000 Hz.[2] Thus, for the highest fidelity recordings (commonly used primarily for research purposes), low-frequency filtering is not used, and the high-frequency filtering is performed at 5000 Hz.[2] Conventional electrophysiologic amplifiers use AC coupling and this can result in an upward drift of the MAP signal during diastole. Thus, the best recordings are obtained by using true direct current (DC) amplification. If a specific recording system does not have DC amplification, a specially designed, commercially available DC-coupled amplifier (EP Technologies Incorporated, San Jose, CA) can be used. This unit permits high-impedance filtering at 0 to 5000 Hz and also permits voltage calibration and automatic DC offset compensation. True DC coupling is necessary when one wants to record MAP signals during the application of internal or external electrical shocks, since the capacitive coupling in the standard AC-coupled recording system results in a large shock artifact, which is avoided when DC-coupled amplification is used (Fig. 3). When MAP signals are manually measured from recording paper, the paper speed should be a minimum of 100 mm/s, although rates in excess of 150 mm/s are optimal. MAP recordings can also be saved to tape or to optical disk for later processing.

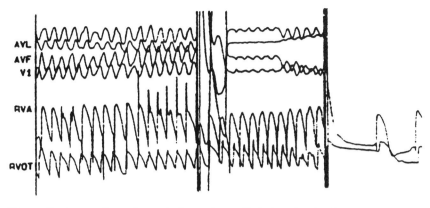

Figure 3. A recording of ventricular tachycardia being shocked by an implantable cardioverter defibrillator with resulting ventricular fibrillation that is then externally defibrillated. Because the MAP recording is DC-coupled, excellent MAP tracings are obtained immediately following the defibrillation shock, whereas the surface electrocardiographic signals are temporarily lost because they are AC-coupled.

MAP Measurements

MAP repolarization measurements made by use of the Franz catheter have been shown to follow a time course similar to that of TAP recordings.[16] The MAP duration is usually measured at 90% repolarization since the foot of the MAP makes clear differentiation of the end of repolarization very difficult or impossible (Fig. 4). The amplitude of the signal is determined from the diastolic baseline to the top of the phase 3 plateau. Importantly, the maximum deflection of phase 0 is not used, since this deflection includes the intrinsic deflection and often overshoots the plateau. The beginning of the MAP is defined as the moment of fastest rise of the upstroke during phase 0. Yuan et al[23] have suggested that a tangent line can be drawn during phase 3 and that the intersection of the baseline and the tangent line can be used to determine the end of repolarization; however most investigators have used the APD_{90}. While computer programs have been developed that permit automatic measurement of repolarization from MAP recordings,[24,25] it is essential that these be operator-reviewed to ascertain that there is accurate labeling of the beginning and end of MAP recordings.

As discussed above, maximum upstroke velocity is much slower on MAP recordings than on TAP recordings. The slower velocity of the MAP upstroke is the result of the fact that the MAP is a summation recording of a group of cells, and depolarization occurs sequentially over time in contrast to a TAP recording, in which it is measured from a single cell. Several studies have examined the *relative* changes in the upstroke veloc-

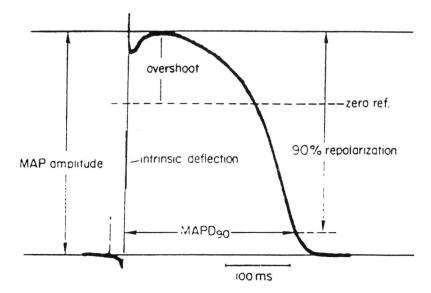

Figure 4. This figure demonstrates the method of MAP signal analysis. The amplitude of the MAP signal is measured as the distance from the diastolic baseline to the crest of the MAP plateau phase (not the peak of the upstroke). The duration of the MAP signal is measured as the interval along a line horizontal parallel to the diastolic baseline, from the fastest part of the MAP upstroke (or the intrinsic deflection, if visible) to the desired repolarization level. Example shows evaluation of the MAP duration at 90% repolarization. Reprinted from Reference 11, with permission.

ity, including the changes of this parameter during induction of ischemia[13] or administration of antiarrhythmic drugs.[26,27] Thus, while the absolute upstroke velocity is probably not very helpful, relative changes have been shown to correlate with physiologic perturbations in humans.

Since changes in tissue contact can result in significant changes in MAP amplitude, alterations in MAP amplitude in the beating heart is not a useful determinant of changes in local cardiac physiology.

Safety

In more than 500 recordings the author has observed 1 cardiac perforation and no other catheter-related sequela, demonstrating that careful catheter positioning and recording of MAP tracings can be performed with a high level of safety and an incidence of complications that is similar to those obtained with other electrophysiologic catheters.

Artifacts

Artifacts in the MAP recordings are the result of contamination of the recording with remote electrical activity or of variations in the contact pressure of the distal catheter against the endomyocardium. Small negative or positive deflections can occasionally be seen just prior to the MAP upstroke. While the exact mechanism of these deflections has not been conclusively determined, they are not present in TAP recordings and are most likely secondary to remote electrical activity. Such artifacts are often observed during sinus rhythm recordings (Fig. 5), but not when the patient is paced from the MAP-pacing catheter. This further suggests that these deflections are secondary to far-field signals and are not seen during ventricular pacing from the MAP catheter, since these distant signals would then be buried within the large MAP depolarizations. Some deflections may also arise from within the intracardiac QRS complex. Intracardiac QRS complex artifacts can be minimized by recording MAP tracings with relatively large amplitude (ie, more than 10 mV) in order to increase the ratio between the MAP signal and artifacts, as the intracardiac QRS potential is fixed.[2]

The upstroke of the MAP potential during phase 0 often has a biphasic notch, which represents the biphasic intrinsic deflection seen in the electrogram measured from the MAP catheter prior to applying further pressure, leading to development of MAP. This represents the local activation of the cells at the MAP catheter tip and is not an artifact but often results in an overshoot during phase 0. Examples of artifacts are demonstrated in Figures 5 through 9.

The MAP amplitude often increases during increased contact pressure of the distal tip against the endocardium. When pressure is not constant during systole and diastole, the changes in contact pressure can result in changes in MAP amplitude. Most typically, during diastole, relaxation of the ventricle can result in a decrease in contact pressure and this can result in a positive deflection, which can be misinterpreted as spontaneous diastolic depolarization (see Fig. 9). During systole the contact pressure may increase, occasionally causing a secondary increase in the MAP amplitude that results in positive deflections during phase 3 that could be misinterpreted as early afterdepolarizations. Thus, secondary oscillations in the MAP amplitude during phase 3 or early phase 4 must be carefully scrutinized before they are labeled as afterdepolarizations. Frequently, changing the amount of pressure exerted at the tip of the catheter by gently advancing (or sometimes withdrawing) the catheter can result in the disappearance of the "afterdepolarizations."

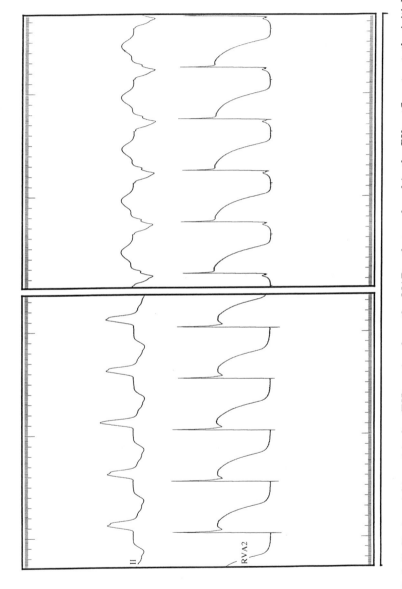

Figure 5. Left: During right ventricular (RV) pacing from the MAP catheter placed in the RV outflow tract, the initial upstroke of the MAP is rapid without artifact. Right: During RV pacing from a second catheter placed in the RV apex, the MAP has small deflections preceding phase 0, likely representing far-field electrical activity.

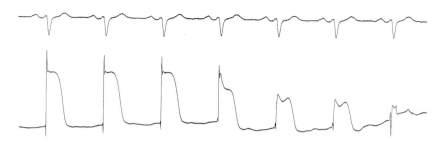

Figure 6. This figure shows deterioration of the MAP tracing secondary to loss of good MAP-endocardium tissue contact.

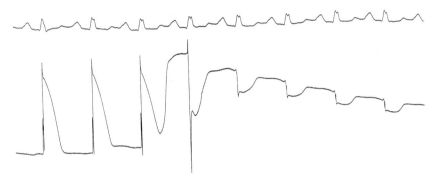

Figure 7. Inversion of the MAP tracing, which can occur secondary to buckling of the catheter with the proximal pole coming into contact with the endocardial surface, resulting in a reversal of the electrical potential and inversion of the recording. Another possibility for this artifact is that the catheter has perforated through the endocardial surface of the ventricle, causing a reversal in the electrical potential.

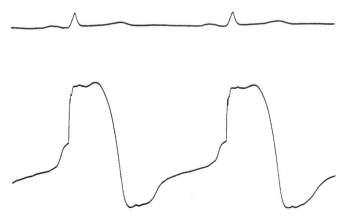

Figure 8. This is an example of poor tissue contact.

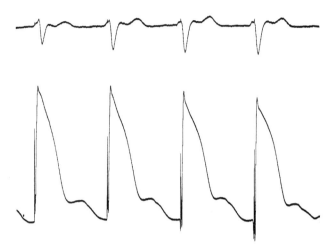

Figure 9. In this figure, varying tissue contact during systole and diastole causes positive deflections in the MAP tracing during phase 4 that could be erroneously ascribed to afterdepolarizations.

Conclusion

It is possible, with experience, to record high-quality MAP tracings from the atria and ventricles that faithfully follow the time course of cardiac repolarization and are virtually devoid of artifacts.

Acknowledgment The author greatly appreciates the excellent assistance of Ms. Elizabeth Corey in the preparation of this manuscript.

References

1. Franz MR, Bargheer K, Costard-Jäckle A, et al. Human ventricular repolarization and T wave genesis. *Prog Cardiovasc Dis* 1991;33:369-384.
2. Franz MR. Method and theory of monophasic action potential recording. *Prog Cardiovasc Dis* 1991;33:347-368.
3. Korsgren M, Leskinen E, Sjostrand U, et al. Intracardiac recording of monophasic action potentials in the human heart. *Scand J Clin Lab Invest* 1966;18:561-564.
4. Olsson SB, Varnauskas E, Korsgren M. Further improved method for measuring monophasic action potentials of the intact human heart. *J Electrocardiol* 1971;4:19-23.
5. Olsson SB. *Monophasic Action Potentials of Right Heart. Suction Electrode Method in Clinical Investigations* [PhD dissertation]. Göteborg: University of Göteborg, Elanders Boktryckeri AB; 1971.
6. Olsson SB, Varnauskas E. Right ventricular monophasic action potentials in man. Effect of abrupt changes of cycle length and of atrial fibrillation. *Acta Med Scand* 1972;191:159-166.

7. Olsson SB, Edvardsson N. Clinical electrophysiologic study of antiarrhythmic properties of flecainide: Acute intraventricular delayed conduction and prolonged repolarization in regular paced and premature beats using intracardiac monophasic action potentials with programmed stimulation. *Am Heart J* 1981;102:864-871.

8. Olsson SB, Brorson L, Edvardsson N, Varnauskas E. Estimation of ventricular repolarization in man by monophasic action potential recording technique. *Eur Heart J* 1985;6(suppl D):71-79.

9. Franz M, Schottler M, Schaefer J, Seed WA. Simultaneous recording of monophasic action potentials and contractile force from the human heart. *Klin Wochenschr* 1980;58:1357-1359.

10. Franz MR, Schaefer J, Schottler M, et al. Electrical and mechanical restitution of the human heart at different rates of stimulation. *Circ Res* 1983;53:815-822.

11. Franz MR. Long-term recording of monophasic action potentials from human endocardium. *Am J Cardiol* 1983;51:1629-1634.

12. Franz MR, Swerdlow CD, Liem LB, Schaefer J. Cycle length dependence of human action potential duration in vivo. Effects of single extrastimuli, sudden sustained rate acceleration and deceleration, and different steady-state frequencies. *J Clin Invest* 1988;82:972-979.

13. Franz MR, Flaherty JT, Platia EV, et al. Localization of regional myocardial ischemia by recording of monophasic action potentials. *Circulation* 1984;69:593-604.

14. Franz MR, Bargheer K, Rafflenbeul W, et al. Monophasic action potential mapping in human subjects with normal electrocardiograms: Direct evidence for the genesis of the T wave. *Circulation* 1987;75:379-386.

15. Franz MR, Chin MC, Sharkey HR, et al. A new single catheter technique for simultaneous measurement of action potential duration and refractory period in vivo. *J Am Coll Cardiol* 1990;16:878-886.

16. Franz MR, Burkhoff D, Spurgeon H, et al. In vitro validation of a new cardiac catheter technique for recording monophasic action potentials. *Eur Heart J* 1986;7:34-41.

17. Franz MR. Time for yet another QT correction algorithm? Bazett and beyond. *J Am Coll Cardiol* 1994;23:1554-1556. Editorial, comment.

18. Lee HC, Mohabir R, Smith N, et al. Effect of ischemia on calcium-dependent fluorescence transients in rabbit hearts containing indo 1. Correlation with monophasic action potentials and contraction. *Circulation* 1988;78:1047-1059.

19. Sager PT, Uppal P, Follmer C, et al. Frequency-dependent electrophysiologic effects of amiodarone in humans. *Circulation* 1993;88:1063-1071.

20. Franz MR, Costard-Jäckle A. Frequency-dependent effects of quinidine on the relationship between action potential duration and refractoriness in the canine heart in situ. *Circulation* 1988;77:1177-1184.

21. Sager PT, Eghbali H, Nguyen T, Follmer C. Kinetics of adaptation of the action potential duration during beta-adrenergic stimulation in humans. *PACE* 1994;17:829. Abstract.

22. Hoffman BF, Cranefield PF. *Electrophysiology of the Heart.* New York: Mc Graw Hill; 1960.

23. Yuan S, Blomstrom-Lundqvist C, Olsson SB. Monophasic action potentials: Concepts to practical applications. *J Cardiovasc Electrophysiol* 1994;5:287-308.

24. Franz MR, Kirchhof PF, Fabritz CL, Zabel M. Computer analysis of monophasic action potentials: Manual validation and clinically pertinent applications. *PACE* 1995;18:1666-1678.

25. Kanaan N, Jenkins J, Kadish A. An automatic microcomputer system for analysis of monophasic action potentials. *PACE* 1990;13:196-206.

26. Koller B, Franz MR. New classification of moricizine and propafenone based on electrophysiologic and electrocardiographic data from isolated rabbit heart. *J Cardiovasc Pharmacol* 1994;24:753-760.

27. Levine JH, Moore EN, Kadish AH, et al. The monophasic action potential upstroke: A means of characterizing local conduction. *Circulation* 1986;74:1147-1155.

8

Computer-Assisted Real-Time Monophasic Action Potential Analysis

Bjoern C. Knollman, MD

Monophasic action potentials (MAPs) are widely used in experimental and clinical settings to study the effects of electrophysiologic and pharmacologic interventions on the cardiac action potential. Unlike an electrocardiogram (ECG), the MAP provides a local measure of the voltage-time course of the underlying cellular action potential.[1] Therefore, the simultaneous recording of MAPs from several different sites can provide a spatial resolution of action potential changes induced by drug effects or ischemia.[2,3] However, precise manual analysis of hundreds of MAP recordings is cumbersome, and cannot be performed in real time. This limits the usefulness of spatial and temporal assessment of MAP recordings. Fortunately, the characteristics of the MAP signal (the sharp upstroke, the defined plateau phase, and the smooth monophasic repolarization phase) lend themselves to automated signal processing. Several computer algorithms designed to measure diverse parameters of the MAP signals have been developed and validated against manual MAP analysis.[4-9] This chapter illustrates the potential uses and the limitations of automated MAP analysis.

Quality Criteria for MAP Recordings

Since any analysis is only as good as the original data, automated MAP analysis should only be attempted from recordings that are consistent

From Franz MR (ed): *Monophasic Action Potentials: Bridging Cell and Bedside.* ©Futura Publishing Company, Inc., Armonk, NY, 2000.

and relatively noise free. MAP recordings are usually considered acceptable if the following criteria are fulfilled[10,11]: 1) Control MAP waveforms should show a uniform action potential contour with sharp upstroke, defined plateau, and smooth repolarization. 2) MAP amplitude and contour should be stable throughout the observation period. 3) The amplitude should exceed 15 mV under control conditions. 4) Phase 4 should be isoelectric. Criteria 1 and 2 are best evaluated by the observer, while criteria 3 and 4 can be incorporated in a computer algorithm. In addition, any computer program must account for several variations in the shape of the MAP waveform. Prepotentials or pacing spikes must be identified as such. If these requirements are met, automated MAP analysis can provide rapid and reliable information.

Development of a Computer Algorithm

One example of automated analysis of MAP signals is a computer algorithm developed in our laboratory and validated against manual measurement in a variety of experimental applications.[6] The algorithm is based on the manual MAP analysis developed by Franz[12] (Fig. 1, panel A) that had previously been validated by comparing MAP data with adjacently recorded transmembrane action potentials.[1] Our computer algorithm automatically determines the fastest point of the MAP upstroke phase (maximum dV/dt), finds the maximum amplitude of the MAP plateau, and measures the action potential duration (APD) at several user-selectable repolarization levels (eg, at 50% and 90% repolarization [APD_{50} and APD_{90}, respectively]). The program also returns the cycle length and the diastolic interval between APD_{90} and the next MAP upstroke. Up to 3 validation checks are performed at 5-millisecond intervals to reject prepotentials or pacing artifacts. The MAP plateau is determined as illustrated in panels B through D of Figure 1. Recordings with diastolic drifts that exceed 5% of the MAP amplitude are excluded from the analysis.

Particular emphasis was placed on obtaining accurate APD determinations under a variety of recording conditions or MAP waveforms. The two main causes for distortion of the MAP waveform are 1) superimposition of the intrinsic deflection that may mimic an overshoot ('spike') potential, and 2) "humps" and "wobbles" that may distort the diastolic baseline. The algorithm identified the total MAP amplitude as the distance between the diastolic baseline and the maximum *plateau* height of the MAP, regardless of variations in "spike-and-dome" appearance (Fig. 1). The diastolic baseline was the average potential between two consecutive MAP recordings, except for a 30-millisecond window before and after each MAP to minimize the influence of "prepotentials," local "QS complexes," or "afterdepolariza-

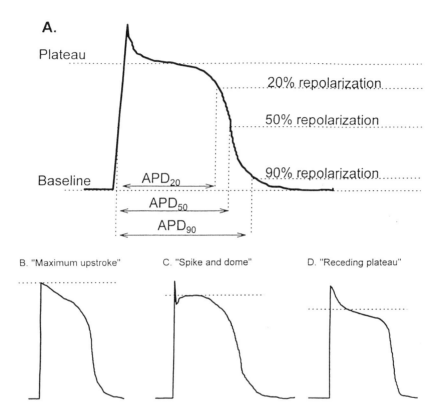

Figure 1. To analyze the MAP waveform, the computer algorithm automatically identifies the fastest point of the MAP upstroke phase. It then finds the interval between the fastest upstroke point and a user-selectable repolarization level to yield the action potential duration (APD) at their respective repolarization (eg, APD_{20}, APD_{50}, or APD_{90}) (**A**). The algorithm accounts for different shapes of the MAP, and automatically adjusts the MAP plateau height (**B** through **D**).

tions." Recordings with diastolic upslopes or downslopes exceeding 5% of the total MAP amplitude were excluded from analysis.

Technical Details

A convolution function was used to verify the fiduciary points of the MAP waveform without the need for user interaction. Up to 3 validation checks at 5-millisecond intervals were performed to eliminate prepotentials and to select the true rising edge and maximum amplitude of the MAP (Fig. 1, panel A). If an overshoot was present ('spike-and-dome" configuration, see Fig. 1, panel C), the overshoot amplitude was ignored and the crest of the plateau was assigned the value of the maximal MAP amplitude.

This was done because a spike on the MAP does not represent the true transmembrane overshoot potential but rather contamination from the local electrographic intrinsic deflection.[1] If no overshoot was present, no reassignment occurred. If the initial MAP downstroke (phase 2) converged gradually into the plateau phase (Fig. 1, panel B), the inflection point was used to set the value of the MAP plateau. The trailing edge of the MAP was defined by a return to less than 5% of the diastolic baseline potential. All data were accumulated into a value array from which the APD at the selected repolarization levels were calculated.

Manual Validation by Two Independent Observers

When the results of the computer algorithm were compared to the manual analysis by two blinded observers, the interobserver variability was consistently higher than the computer-observer variability. We found a greater than 97% agreement between the computer results and manual measurements of the cycle length or APD$_{90}$. Figure 2 compares manual and computer measurements of an electrical restitution curve. Note the smoother contour of the computerized measurement, which had a resolu-

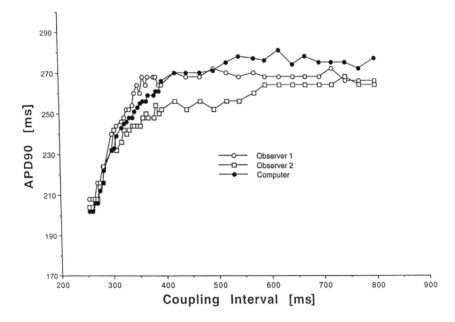

Figure 2. Electrical restitution curve (base drive cycle length 800 milliseconds) measured by two independent observers and the computer.

tion of 1 millisecond, compared to manual measurements obtained at a paper speed of 100 mm/s, with an associated measurement error of approximately 10 milliseconds. Faster paper speeds are difficult to obtain with use of standard chart recorders. Figure 3 shows other examples in which automated MAP analysis was validated against manual measurements: electrical APD alternans, an early marker of myocardial ischemia, occurred after introduction of global ischemia (panel A), and could be reliably detected. Adaptation curves after abrupt changes in paced cycle length are well tracked using the automated APD analysis, as shown in panel B of Figure 3.

Real-Time Analysis of MAP and Electrocardiographic Recordings

With the availability of faster microcomputers, the analysis of MAP signals can now be performed virtually at the same time that the recordings are being obtained. We recently reported a data acquisition system capable of recording up to 16 channels at 1 kHz and providing instantaneous measurements of cycle length, APD, and spatial dispersion.[8] Electrocardiographic data such as QT duration and dispersion could also be displayed together with the MAP recordings. However, the reliability of QT interval estimation by computer algorithms remains questionable,[13] and QT interval estimates are certainly more variable than APD measurements from MAP recordings. Figure 4 shows the front panel of the real-time analysis program. Ten MAP channels and 6 ECG channels were recorded simultaneously and the APD and QT duration analyzed. Shown are the events leading to the occurrence of torsades de pointes arrhythmia after infusion of d-sotalol in an isolated rabbit heart.[14] QT and APD were calculated for each beat in real time, and were plotted while the experiment was performed. An excessive action potential prolongation and increase in the dispersion of repolarization always preceded the onset of the tachyarrhythmias (Fig. 4, panel C). Note the marked APD alternans starting at beat number 75 in panel C, that occurred immediately prior to the onset of a polymorphic ventricular tachycardia with beat number 125 (original MAP/ECG tracings in panel A). Prominent early afterdepolarizations can be seen in several MAP tracings. This demonstrates how real-time MAP analysis could predict the occurrence of ventricular arrhythmias, at least in this experimental setting. More than generalized APD prolongation, the increased dispersion of ventricular repolarization is believed to play a role in genesis of ventricular arrhythmias.[15-17] The program therefore automatically calculates the dispersion of the APD_{90} and the QT interval. Figure 5 shows how an infusion of quinidine not only prolonged the APD_{90}, but dramatically increased the dispersion of repolarization in a Langendorff-perfused isolated rabbit heart.

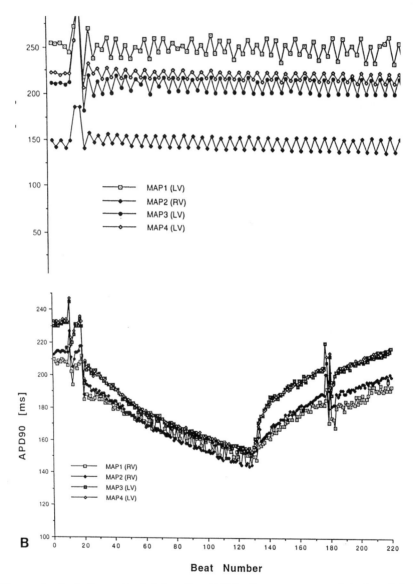

Figure 3. A. Action potential duration (APD) alternans occurred during global ischemia and pacing with a cycle length of 300 milliseconds. Significant alternans started after the introduction of an artificial pause. **B**. Automated analysis of APD$_{90}$ during a cycle length change from 800 to 300 milliseconds and back to 800 milliseconds. The spikes in the otherwise smooth curves represent spontaneous premature beats.

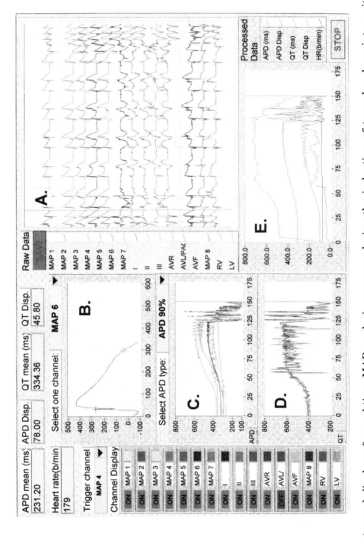

Figure 4. Front panel display of a real-time MAP analysis program during the induction of torsades de pointes with d-sotalol and low potassium. **A.** Original recordings from 10 MAP (top) and 6 electrocardiographic (ECG) leads. **B.** Enlarged MAP lead 6 with marks for the beginning and end of the action potential duration at 90% repolarization (APD₉₀) interval, measured for each beat. **C.** Beat-to-beat changes in APD₉₀ measurements from 10 MAP leads. Note the marked APD prolongation after approximately 25 beats and the progressively increasing APD alternans after 75 beats. **D.** QT measurements from 5 ECG leads (AVL display turned off). **E.** Display of mean APD₉₀, APD dispersion, mean QT duration, QT dispersion, and heart rate versus beat number. See color plate.

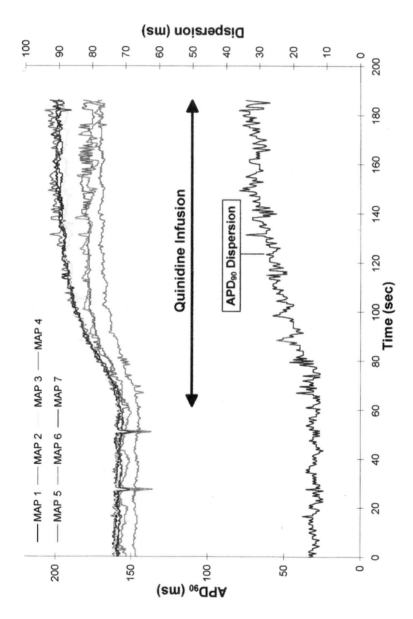

Figure 5. Real-time analysis of changes in APD$_{90}$ and dispersion of repolarization in response to perfusion with 20 µM quinidine in an isolated, perfused rabbit heart. See color plate.

Measuring the Repolarization Dispersion in the Voltage Domain

Dispersion of cardiac repolarization has been linked to ventricular arrhythmias both clinically and experimentally. Dispersion is usually determined from either ECG or MAP recordings.[2,17-19] Both approaches calculate spatial differences only from the *end* of repolarization. Such measurements provide information on dispersion only in one dimension—the time domain—and ignore spatial and temporal ventricular repolarization differences *during* the repolarization process itself. To address this question, we utilized the local nature of the MAP recording and calculated the voltage dispersion in repolarization from 10 simultaneously recorded epicardial and endocardial MAPs in an isolated, perfused rabbit heart.[20] Using modified MAP analysis software, all MAP waveforms were normalized to the individual MAP amplitude and then repolarization levels were calculated as shown in Figure 6. To test whether arrhythmia vulnerability for ventricular fibrillation is associated with dispersion in the voltage domain, we applied

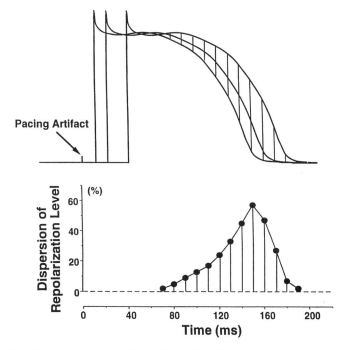

Figure 6. Schematic drawing of repolarization dispersion measurements in the voltage domain. Depicted are MAP waveforms recorded from 3 different epicardial sites. Vertical lines indicate the instantaneous voltage dispersion at various time points during repolarization. Lower image: the "dispersion curve" represents the voltage dispersion as a function of the repolarization time.

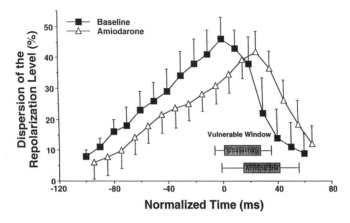

Figure 7. The peak of the voltage dispersion correlates with the vulnerable window for induction of ventricular fibrillation, both in normal and amiodarone-treated rabbits.

electrical field shocks to determine the vulnerable window for ventricular fibrillation inducibility, both in normal rabbits and in rabbits treated with amiodarone.[21] Figure 7 shows the relationship between voltage dispersion and susceptibility to ventricular fibrillation (= vulnerable window). The peak in voltage dispersion was closely correlated with the susceptibility to arrhythmia induction, in both the normal group and the amiodarone-treated group. The voltage dispersion was not significantly different in the amiodarone group; only the peak shifted toward longer action potentials, as expected from the QT prolongation. This shows that the peak of voltage dispersion is valuable for estimating the vulnerable window, at least in a rabbit model.

Future Directions

Automated analysis of MAP signals is feasible in real time, and allows rapid detection of changes in cardiac electrophysiology in response to pacing, field shock stimulation, drug interventions, or ischemia. What now is a useful tool for an investigator in a laboratory may someday become a routine procedure for the clinical electrophysiologist. The integration of MAP catheters and the appropriate MAP analysis algorithm in cardiac pacemakers or defibrillators can be envisioned. The ability to accurately measure cycle length and local APD would improve the detection and possibly the treatment of ventricular tachycardia or fibrillation. It may even become possible to treat atrial flutter or fibrillation with antitachycardia pacing or low-voltage defibrillation, before chronic electrical remodeling occurs.

References

1. Franz MR, Burkhoff D, Spurgeon H, et al. In vitro validation of a new cardiac catheter technique for recording monophasic action potentials. *Eur Heart J* 1986;7:34-41.

2. Zabel M, Portnoy S, Franz MR. Electrocardiographic indexes of dispersion of ventricular repolarization: An isolated heart validation study. *J Am Coll Cardiol* 1995;25:746-752.

3. Mohabir R, Franz MR, Clusin WT. In vivo electrophysiological detection of myocardial ischemia through monophasic action potential recording. *Prog Cardiovasc Dis* 1991;34:15-28.

4. Coulshed DS, Rudenski A, Cowan JC, et al. The use of a microcomputer to automate measurement of action potential duration for both transmembrane and monophasic action potentials. *Physiol Meas* 1993;14:347-358.

5. Dickenson DR, Davis DR, Beatch GN. Development and evaluation of a fully automated monophasic action potential analysis program. *Med Biol Eng Comput* 1997;35:653-660.

6. Franz MR, Kirchhof PF, Fabritz CL, Zabel M. Computer analysis of monophasic action potentials: Manual validation and clinically pertinent applications. *PACE* 1995;18:1666-1678.

7. Kanaan N, Jenkins J, Kadish A. An automatic microcomputer system for analysis of monophasic action potentials. *PACE* 1990;13:196-206.

8. Knollmann BC, Woosley RL, Franz MR. Real-time analysis of monophasic action potential and ECG recordings—a tool for monitoring acute drug effects on cardiac repolarization. *Clin Pharmacol Ther* 1996;59:164.

9. Cole PG, Dilly S, Lab M. A computerized method of cardiac action-potential duration analysis. *J Physiol* 1985;366:118P.

10. Xie JT, January CT. The monophasic action potential technique and its application in cardiac electropharmacology. *Methods Find Exp Clin Pharmacol* 1993;15:557-567.

11. Franz MR, Chin MC, Sharkey HR, et al. A new single catheter technique for simultaneous measurement of action potential duration and refractory period in vivo. *J Am Coll Cardiol* 1990;16:878-886.

12. Franz MR. Long-term recording of monophasic action potentials from human endocardium. *Am J Cardiol* 1983;51:1629-1634.

13. Woosley RL, Sale M. QT interval: A measure of drug action. *Am J Cardiol* 1993;72:36B-43B.

14. Zabel M, Hohnloser SH, Behrens S, Li YG, et al. Electrophysiologic features of torsades de pointes: Insights from a new isolated rabbit heart model [see comments]. *J Cardiovasc Electrophysiol* 1997;8:1148-1158.

15. Vassallo JA, Cassidy DM, Kindwall KE, et al. Nonuniform recovery of excitability in the left ventricle. *Circulation* 1988;78:1365-1372.

16. Kuo CS, Munakata K, Reddy CP, Surawicz B. Characteristics and possible mechanism of ventricular arrhythmia dependent on the dispersion of action potential durations. *Circulation* 1983;67:1356-1367.

17. Yuan S, Blomstrom-Lundqvist C, Pripp CM, et al. Signed value of monophasic action potential duration difference. A useful measure in evaluation of dispersion of repolarization in patients with ventricular arrhythmias [see comments]. *Eur Heart J* 1997;18:1329-1338.

18. Dinerman JL, Berger R, Haigney MC, et al. Dispersion of ventricular activation and refractoriness in patients with idiopathic dilated cardiomyopathy. *Am J Cardiol* 1997;79:970-974.
19. Behrens S, Li C, Fabritz CL, et al. Shock-induced dispersion of ventricular repolarization: Implications for the induction of ventricular fibrillation and the upper limit of vulnerability. *J Cardiovasc Electrophysiol* 1997;8:998-1008.
20. Behrens S, Li C, Knollmann BC, Franz MR. Dispersion of ventricular repolarization in the voltage domain. *PACE* 1998;21:100-107.
21. Behrens S, Li C, Franz MR. Effects of long-term amiodarone treatment on ventricular-fibrillation vulnerability and defibrillation efficacy in response to monophasic and biphasic shocks. *J Cardiovasc Pharmacol* 1997;30:412-418.

Section II

Rate-Dependent Modulation of Action Potential Duration in Normal and Ischemic Myocardium:
Introduction

It is well known that the duration of the cardiac action potential changes with the frequency from one beat to another, and with the prior heart beat history. Recently, new concepts emerged about how the cardiac action potential adapts to changes in heart rate, from short-term adaptation to long-term electrical remodeling following sustained tachycardia or bradycardia. These new data have given rise to new insights into the relationship between the heart's cycle length and its depolarization-repolarization intervals, while raising new questions. What are the processes that underlie short-term and long-term action potential duration changes? What shall we call rate adaptation, what cardiac memory, what electrical remodeling? What is the role of bradycardia in tachycardia-induced electrical remodeling?

Another action potential duration/heart rate aspect of currently renewed interest is the phenomenon of electrical alternans. Several chapters in this section present data on the mechanism of electrical alternans and its role in increasing dispersion of ventricular repolarization and initiating serious arrhythmias in the normal and ischemic heart. Monophasic action potential recordings undoubtedly have played a pivotal role in documenting these mechanisms including the role of electrical restitution in the intact heart in explaining electrical alternans and how it triggers ventricular fibrillation in the intact heart.

9

Activation-Repolarization Sequence Memory in the Isolated Rabbit Heart

Angelika Costard-Jaeckle, MD, Matthias Antz, MD and Michael R. Franz, MD, PhD

Thirty years ago, Chatterjee et al[1] showed that not only does pacing from an ectopic ventricular site produce electrocardiographic T wave changes during the time of pacing, but that T wave polarity changes persist long after pacing has been terminated. Such lasting modulation of T wave polarity by a change in the ventricular activation sequence challenges the traditional contention that myocardial repolarization follows a fixed pattern dictated by the action potential duration (APD) of individual cardiac cells. Studies of the human electrocardiogram by Rosenbaum et al[2] corroborated the original observation of Chatterjee et al, and further identified a very slow onset and offset of such pacing site-dependent modulation of myocardial repolarization. To explain these conspicuous findings, these authors suggested some form of cardiac "memory" by which myocardial cells "learn" to adjust to a new activation sequence, and by which they retain this new repolarization pattern long after normalization of ventricular activation. This cardiac memory hypothesis, however, has been strongly opposed, partly because of the novelty of such a concept for which no cellular electrophysiologic data have existed, and partly because similar T wave changes could result from extracardiac sources such as changes in autonomic innervation or regional myocardial injury.[3]

From Franz MR (ed): *Monophasic Action Potentials: Bridging Cell and Bedside.*
©Futura Publishing Company, Inc., Armonk, NY, 2000.

In 1989, we reported the first evidence that the heart's ability to adjust to a new activation sequence does in fact reside at the myocardial tissue level itself, and that no extracardiac factors are required to explain the phenomenon of cardiac memory[4]: in isolated Langendorff-perfused rabbit heart preparations, which lack neurohumoral control and were kept under stable metabolic conditions, we demonstrated that an alteration in the activation sequence of ventricular myocardium leads to a spatial reorientation of the APD, which can satisfactorily explain T wave changes in the concurrent body surface electrocardiogram.

A bipolar contact electrode[5] was used to map monophasic action potentials (MAPs) from 12 to 20 different right and left ventricular epicardial sites during pacing at a rate of 180 beats/min from 3 consecutive sites: during 45 minutes of right atrial pacing, during 120 minutes of right ventricular pacing, and again during 60 minutes of right atrial pacing. This bipolar contact electrode has been shown to reduce the activation time and the time course for repolarization of adjacent cells.[6] Recordings were made sequentially from each site with use of a detailed map of the epicardial surface to identify the locations from which each recording was made. Figure 1 shows a representative example of an epicardial map, in this case a left lateral view, with 7 original action potential recordings. When the

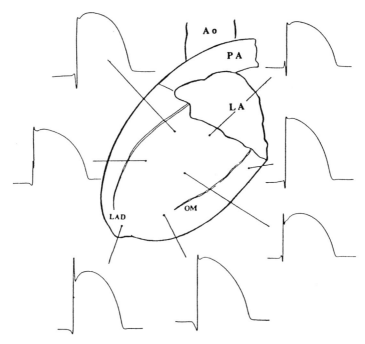

Figure 1. Map of epicardial surface with 7 original action potential recordings. See text for details.

center electrode was pressed slightly against the surface of the heart, MAPs developed and stabilized within 2 to 6 beats, allowing for the completion of action potential mapping at all recording sites within 5 minutes. When initial mapping studies after 45 minutes of atrial pacing were completed, pacing was switched to ventricular pacing and action potentials were recorded from the same epicardial sites as during atrial pacing at 5, 30, 60, 90, and 120 minutes after the onset of ventricular pacing. After 120 minutes of ventricular pacing, the stimulus output was switched back to the atrial pacing wires and action potential recordings were repeated 5, 30, and 60 minutes after resumption of atrial pacing. MAPs were analyzed for activation time (measured from the onset of the QRS complex in a continuously recorded electrocardiogram to the upstroke of the action potential), APD (measured from the intrinsic deflection of the upstroke to the level of 90% repolarization), and repolarization time (calculated as the sum of activation time and APD).

Figures 2 and 3 show representative data from one experiment.[4] If after 45 minutes of continuous atrial pacing, APD was plotted as a function of activation time, then a significant inverse correlation between activation time and APD was found, with sites activated earlier having longer APDs than sites activated later (Fig. 2, panel A). The slope (s) of the linear regression between activation time and APD, averaged for all experiments, was s=−1.63 (correlation coefficient: r=0.76), indicating that sites with

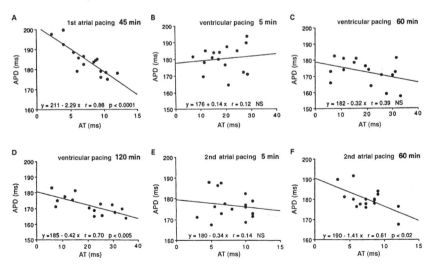

Figure 2. Linear regression analysis of the relationship between activation time (AT) and action potential duration (APD) at various times of the right atrial-right ventricular-right atrial pacing protocol in Langendorff-perfused rabbit hearts. Note loss of inverse correlation immediately after a change in pacing site and slow redevelopment of inverse correlation with continued pacing. See text for more details.

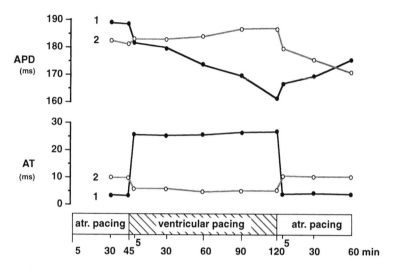

Figure 3. Time course of change in activation time (AT) and action potential duration (APD) at two different epicardial sites during a switch in pacing site from atrial to ventricular and vice versa.

later activation repolarized slightly before sites with earlier excitation (a slope of exactly 1 would indicate simultaneous repolarization). Five minutes after the switch to ventricular pacing, the inverse correlation between activation time and APD was lost (Fig. 2, panel B), indicating near random distribution of APD. Continued ventricular pacing, however, produced slow changes in APD which restored a significant linear and inverse relationship between activation time and APD (average of all experiments s=–0.71; r=0.68 at 120 minutes; *P*<0.0002 versus 5 minutes). Five minutes after resumption of atrial pacing, the previously obtained organization was lost again, but with continuing atrial pacing a significant inverse correlation was reestablished (s=–1.25; r=0.53; *P*<0.01 versus 5 minutes).

Switching the pacing site abruptly from an atrial site to a ventricular site causes an immediate change in ventricular excitation sequence, but, once changed, the activation sequence should remain stable. Accordingly, changes in the linear regressions during the period of pacing at a constant site should reflect changes in APD rather than changes in activation time. Figure 3 illustrates the time course of changes in activation time and APD during the atrial/ventricular/atrial pacing protocol for two different epicardial sites. These data confirm that switching the pacing site from atrial to ventricular, and vice versa, caused a sudden change in activation time, but, once changed, activation time remained constant for as long as the pacing site was kept constant. In contrast, during the period of continuous atrial or ventricular pacing, only APD changed. This occurred very slowly and in a direction opposite to the change in the corresponding activation time. After atrial pacing was resumed and activation times at both sites returned to their original values, APD again changed slowly, in a direction opposite to that before. Thus, the reestablished negative inverse correlation between activation time and APD during periods of pacing from the same site must be due to a slow adaptation of APD to the new excitation sequence.

An inverse correlation between activation time and APD should tend to make repolarization, the sum of both parameters, more uniform within the heart. Our experiments demonstrate that this is indeed the case. Figure 4 depicts the dispersion of repolarization throughout the pacing protocol expressed as the coefficient of variance of repolarization time between all recordings obtained in a given heart. Results averaged for all experiments demonstrate that immediately after the switch to ventricular pacing, the variability of repolarization time among the mapping sites increased markedly. Thus, the loss of the inverse correlation between activation time and APD leaves the repolarization sequence in a more dispersed state as compared to the original state. With continuous pacing from the ventricular site and resumption of the inverse relation between the activation time and the APD, variability of repolarization time decreased. With resumption

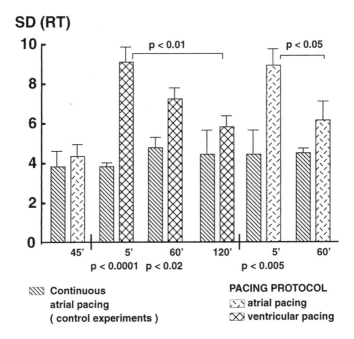

Figure 4. Bar graph of coefficient of variance of repolarization time at various times of the pacing protocol. Data represent mean from all experiments ($\pm$ standard deviation) and are compared with mean values from 5 control experiments of continuous atrial pacing.

of atrial pacing, dispersion of repolarization time again rose abruptly and, with continued right atrial pacing, again decreased. Both the increase in dispersion of repolarization with a sudden change in pacing site and the synchronization of repolarization during the periods of pacing from the same site were statistically significant.

These data support earlier findings that during normal ventricular excitation, APD is inversely correlated to activation time. The second intriguing finding is that the inverse relationship between activation time and APD is the result of a very slow mechanism that modulates ventricular repolarization according to the sequence of ventricular excitation. If ectopic ventricular pacing is sustained long enough, APD adjusts to the new excitation sequence and again correlates with activation time in an inverse fashion. We therefore conclude that the opposing direction of excitation and repolarization in the ventricle, which is the basis of the normal concordant T wave, is not an a priori relationship but is acquired by the heart over a period of constant excitation sequence.

How do myocardial cells "learn" to adjust their APD to a new excitation sequence? One possible mechanism is that artificial pacing affects autonomic innervation, which might in turn influence the time course of myocardial repolarization.[3] However, we demonstrated excitation-dependent modulation in an isolated heart preparation, which lacks neurohumoral control. This strongly suggests that the slow repolarization changes are intrinsic to the myocardial tissue. Another mechanism by which a change in ventricular excitation may modulate ventricular repolarization is electrotonic interaction.[3] Electrotonic current from cells activated later in the cardiac cycle may retard repolarization of cells activated earlier, and current from the first cells to repolarize may speed repolarization in cells not yet repolarized. Pure electrotonic interaction, however, should establish its effects instantaneously and not with a delay of hours. It is possible that a repeated current flow through low-resistance intercellular gap junctions modulates their resistance, thereby amplifying electrotonic effects. Further studies are needed to identify the exact cellular or molecular mechanism that underlies this conspicuous process of myocardial "learning" and "memory."

Clinical Implications of Electrotonic Modulation and Cardiac Memory

The observation that the APD depends on the sequence of activation, and that it requires time to establish such a close relationship, has several important implications. An inverse correlation between activation time and APD tends to compensate for the successive delay along the ventricular activation pathway and, consequently, tends to synchronize ventricular repolarization. Commensurate with this postulate, we found less dispersion of repolarization after prolonged pacing from the same site, when the inverse correlation between activation time and APD was highly significant, than shortly after a change in ventricular activation sequence, when the inverse correlation disappeared. Thus, a heart that is activated along the same activation pathway over a long time (as during sinus rhythm with activation of the ventricular myocardium via the His-Purkinje system) can be expected to have a well synchronized global ventricular repolarization. In contrast, ventricular extrasystoles or short runs of ventricular tachycardia would perturb the natural synchrony of ventricular repolarization. By the same rationale, short bursts of ventricular pacing, as commonly used during electrophysiologic testing, would result in an increase in dispersion of ventricular repolarization and thereby may add to the arrhythmia propensity of the ventricles.

Furthermore, electrocardiographic T wave abnormalities recorded after a period of aberrant conduction or ectopic activity may be explained by the modulation of ventricular repolarization induced by changes in the activation sequence. The prolonged T wave inversion upon resumption of normal excitation observed in patients with intermittent left bundle branch block may simply reflect adaptation of ventricular APD to the previous aberrant conduction pattern. Similarly, patients with intermittent ventricular pacemaker stimulation, ventricular tachycardia, repeated uniform extrasystoles, or ventricular preexcitation due to an accessory pathway, as in the Wolff-Parkinson-White syndrome, may demonstrate T wave changes long after spontaneous or ablative normalization of their ventricular activation sequence. Our data suggest that these persistent T wave changes do not necessarily imply pathophysiologic conditions such as automatic reflex alterations, ischemia, or pacing-induced myocardial injury, but could result exclusively from electrotonic modulation during the period of abnormal activation.

Finally, in concordance with the work of Rosenbaum and coworkers,[2] the activation time dependence of APD challenges the traditional categorization between primary and secondary T wave changes. *Primary* T wave changes have been defined as the result of uniform or nonuniform changes in APD occurring without changes in the sequence of activation. *Secondary* T wave changes are defined as those which reflect changes in the sequence of repolarization that results exclusively from changes in the sequence of activation, and are not associated with any changes in the duration and shape of action potentials. However, our data show that a change in activation sequence can produce changes in local APD over time in the absence of myocardial disease or change in innervation. Therefore, these T wave changes cannot be categorized as primary or secondary. Accordingly, a dogmatic categorization of T wave changes into "primary" and "secondary" can no longer be upheld.

References

1. Chatterjee K, Harris A, Davies G, et al. Electrocardiographic changes subsequent to artificial ventricular depolarization. *Br Heart J* 1969;341:770-779.
2. Rosenbaum MB, Blanco HH, Elizari MV, et al. Electrotonic modulation of the T wave and cardiac memory. *Am J Cardiol* 1982;50:213-222.
3. Hoffman BF. Electrotonic modulation of the T wave. *Am J Cardiol* 1982;50:361-362.
4. Costard-Jäckle A, Goetsch B, Antz M, Franz MR. Slow and long-lasting modulation of myocardial repolarization produced by ectopic activation in isolated rabbit hearts. *Circulation* 1989;80:1412-1420.
5. Franz MR. Long-term recording of monophasic action potentials from human endocardium. *Am J Cardiol* 1983;51:1629-1634.
6. Franz MR, Burkhoff D, Spurgeon H, et al. In vitro validation of a new cardiac catheter technique for recording monophasic action potentials. *Eur Heart J* 1984;7:34-41.

10

Tachycardia Superimposed on Bradycardia Prolongs Ventricular Refractoriness and Facilitates Arrhythmia Induction

Tadashi Satoh, MD and
Douglas P. Zipes, MD

Introduction

Bradycardia is a known cause of early afterdepolarization (EAD)[1-3] that may be the basis of torsades de pointes. For example, some patients with atrial fibrillation who are treated with quinidine develop torsades de pointes when they convert to sinus rhythm, and likely have a slower rate.[4] Also, torsades de pointes had been reported in patients who suddenly developed complete atrioventricular (AV) block after radiofrequency (RF) catheter ablation.[5] These clinical observations raise the question of whether the acute onset of bradycardia after a period of relative tachycardia facilitates the induction of ventricular tachyarrhythmias, including torsades de pointes. The purpose of the present study was to test, in animals, whether

This study was supported in part by the Herman C. Krannert Fund, Indianapolis; Grant HL-52323 from the National Heart, Lung, and Blood Institute, National Institutes of Health, Bethesda, MD.
From Franz MR (ed): *Monophasic Action Potentials: Bridging Cell and Bedside.* ©Futura Publishing Company, Inc., Armonk, NY, 2000.

the transient superimposition of a faster ventricular rate on a slower rate facilitated ventricular arrhythmia induction.

Experimental Method

Dogs weighing 20 to 30 kg were anesthetized and artificially ventilated. Catheters were placed in the left femoral artery and vein to monitor arterial blood pressure and to infuse drugs. A 6F electrode catheter was introduced into the AV junction via the right femoral vein and RF energy was delivered between the tip of the catheter and a backplate to produce complete AV block. Dogs were allowed to have a spontaneous ventricular escape rhythm and were studied 1 week later. At that time, monophasic action potentials (MAPs) were recorded via a 6F contact electrode catheter that was introduced into common carotid artery and positioned at the apical endocardium of the left ventricle (LV).[6] The signal was amplified and filtered at a frequency range of 0.04 to 500 Hz. MAPs were recorded simultaneously with surface electrocardiogram (ECG) leads I, II, and III.

Definition of EADs

EADs were defined as interruptions in the smooth contour during phase 3 repolarization of the MAPs. The magnitude of the EAD was calculated by a method that measured the area of the MAP and EAD. A line was drawn to extend the smooth sloping portion of phase 3 of the MAP to intersect a line drawn along the resting potential. The area enclosed by these two lines separated the EAD from the MAP. The area of the EAD was expressed as a percentage of the total MAP area. Previously, we[7,8] showed that this method correlated accurately with the amplitude of the EADs expressed as a percentage of the MAP amplitude. We also measured the QT interval from surface ECG lead II during constant LV pacing before and during cesium chloride (CsCl) injection.

Induction of Ventricular Arrhythmias

The purpose of this protocol was to examine whether a rapid ventricular rate superimposed on a bradycardia influenced the ability of CsCl, a potassium channel blocker, to induce ventricular tachyarrhythmias.[7-14] All dogs that had 1 week of complete AV block and established a ventricular escape rhythm of approximately 1200 milliseconds. During the study, the

LV was paced at a pacing cycle length of 1000 milliseconds except when rapid pacing was superimposed or spontaneous ventricular arrhythmias occurred. CsCl was injected intravenously at a incremental doses (0.25, 0.5, 0.625, 0.75, 1.0 mM/kg), spaced at 30-minute intervals, to determine the dose required to induce sustained ventricular tachycardia (VT). MAPs were recorded within 5 minutes of the completion of the CsCl injection when the maximal effect of the drug occurred. The area of MAPs and EADs was determined from the average of 3 consecutive ventricular complexes. The QT interval was measured from the same complexes from which the EAD values were obtained. To test the effects of bradycardia with and without superimposed tachycardia on VT induction by CsCl (Fig. 1, panel A), one group of 8 dogs did not undergo intervening rapid ventricular pacing before the injection of CsCl, while the second group of 7 dogs

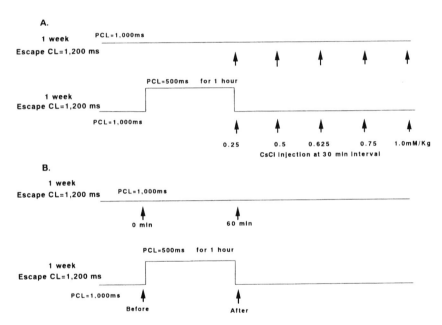

Figure 1. A. Protocol of induction of ventricular tachycardia. Arrows indicate injections of CsCl at 30-minute intervals in dogs with complete atrioventricular (AV) block for 1 week versus dogs that had complete AV block interrupted by 1 hour of rapid left ventricular (LV) pacing. Note that all measurements were made for both groups after return to a pacing cycle length of 100 milliseconds. **B**. Protocol of ventricular effective refractory period (VERP) measurements before and after rapid LV pacing. Arrows indicate when VERP was measured in dogs with complete AV block that underwent rapid LV pacing at a pacing cycle length of 500 milliseconds for 1 hour compared with dogs with complete AV block that were paced constantly at a pacing cycle length of 1000 milliseconds. VERP was measured at several basic cycle lengths (500, 700, 800, 1000 milliseconds). Escape CL indicates cycle length during the week of AV block before study.

underwent rapid LV pacing at a pacing cycle length of 500 milliseconds for 1 hour. The dose of CsCl that induced sustained VT was the endpoint of this experiment.

Response to CsCl of Dogs with and without Rapid Pacing

Early Afterdepolarizations

During 1 week of AV block before CsCl injection, the ventricular escape cycle lengths were similar for dogs that underwent rapid LV pacing (1209±111 milliseconds) and dogs that did not undergo rapid LV pacing (1216±116 milliseconds) (P=NS). However, the percent of developed EADs was greater in the dogs that underwent 1 hour of rapid LV pacing than in the dogs without rapid pacing at each dose of CsCl except 0.25 mM/kg (Table 1, Fig. 2). The dose-response curve of percentage of EAD to dose of CsCl for the dogs that did not receive rapid pacing was shifted downward and rightward compared with the dogs that did receive rapid pacing (Fig. 3).

QT Interval and MAP Duration

The QT interval and MAP duration at 90% repolarization were longer in controls and at each dose of CsCl except for 0.25 mM/kg in dogs that received 1 hour of rapid LV pacing compared with the dogs that did not receive rapid pacing (Fig. 4).

VT Prevalence

Ventricular bigeminy occurred at low doses of CsCl. As the dose of CsCl was increased, nonsustained VT or torsades de pointes was triggered by EADs that reached a sufficient magnitude (Fig. 5). Ventricular arrhythmias were more often induced at the same dose of CsCl in dogs that received rapid LV pacing than in dogs that did not receive rapid pacing. The prevalence of sustained VT at 0.75 mM/kg was greater in dogs that received rapid pacing than in the dogs that did not have rapid pacing (Fig. 6; P<0.05). Torsades de pointes was induced in 3 of 8 dogs that did not receive rapid pacing, and in 6 of 7 dogs that had rapid pacing (38% versus 86%; P=0.08).

Table 1
Effects of CsCl on EAD, QT, and MAPD$_{90}$ Repolarization

	0	0.25	CsCl dose 0.5	$mmol \cdot L^{-1} \cdot kg^{-1}$ 0.625	0.75	1
%EAD						
without 1 hour pacing (n×8)	0	7±2.5	11±3.5	18±4.9	29±4.8	37±5.0
with 1 hour pacing (n=7)	0	8±3.6	18±2.3	27±3.9	35±5.4	ND
P		ns	P<0.05	P<0.01	P<0.05	
QT interval						
without 1 hour pacing (n=8)	365±20.3	397±27.7	422±18.6	444±24.8	467±23.7	496±28.1
with 1 hour pacing (n=7)	383±8.9	413±9.0	439±9.4	471±17.5	490±13.1	ND
P	P<0.05	ns	P<0.05	P<0.05	P<0.05	
MAPD$_{90}$,ms						
without 1 hour pacing (n=8)	328±19.2	367±32.8	393±24.1	413±25.1	436±29.4	487±55.5
with 1 hour pacing (n=7)	345±6.7	390±18.2	415±11.6	441±20.1	466±18.3	ND
P	P<0.05	ns	P<0.05	P<0.05	P<0.05	

CsCl = cesium chloride; EAD = early afterdepolarization; MAPD$_{90}$ = monophasic action potential duration at 90% repolarization.

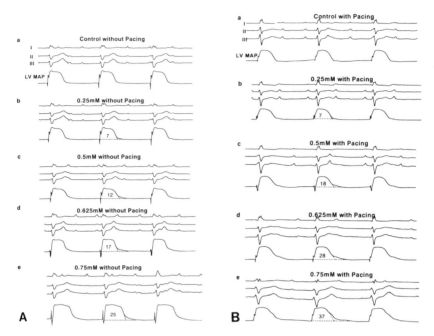

Figure 2. A. Examples of early afterdepolarization (EAD) induction with CsCl in a dog that did not receive rapid pacing. **B.** Example of EAD induction with cesium in a dog that received intervening rapid ventricular pacing for 1 hour. Numbers indicate % EAD.

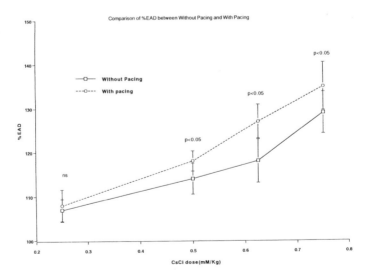

Figure 3. Dose-response curves of % early afterdepolarization (EAD) versus doses of CsCl. The curve in dogs without rapid pacing was shifted rightward and downward compared with that in dogs that underwent rapid left ventricular pacing.

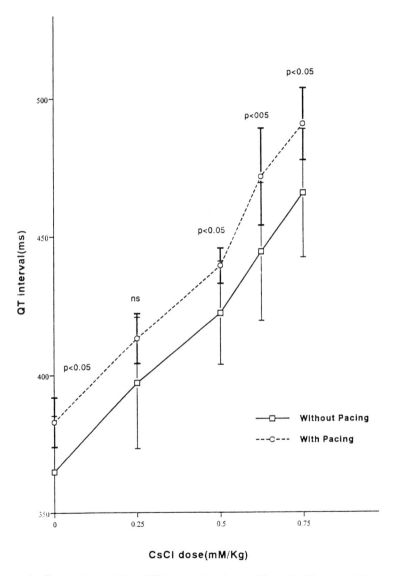

Figure 4. Comparison of the QT interval in dogs with and without rapid pacing for 1 hour before and after the administration of CsCl.

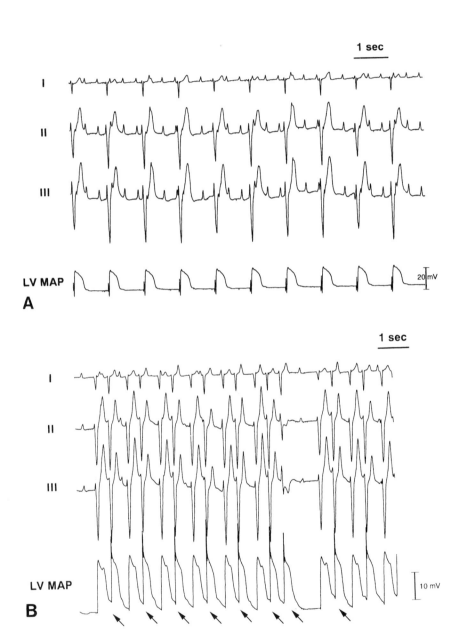

Figure 5. Recording of electrocardiogram and MAP before and during CsCl injection. **A**. Control MAP. **B**. Bigeminy that originated from early afterdepolarizations (EADs). *Continues.*

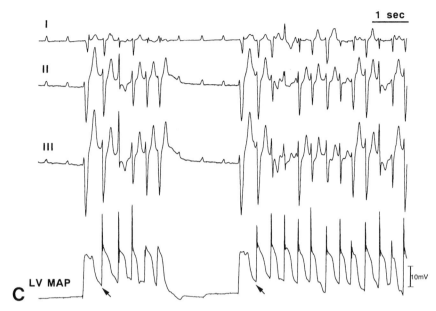

Figure 5 (*continued*). **C**. Example of polymorphic ventricular tachycardia, probably torsades de pointes, that originated from EADs. Arrows point to some EADs.

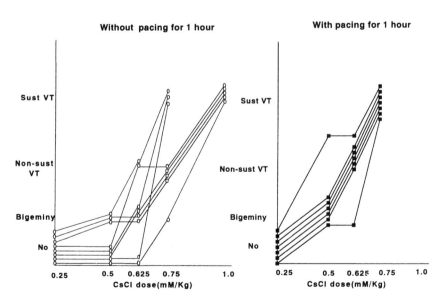

Figure 6. Prevalence of ventricular arrhythmias at various doses of CsCl in dogs with atrioventricular block that did not undergo (open circle) rapid pacing compared with those that underwent (filled square) rapid pacing. Sust VT = sustained ventricular tachycardia; Non-sust VT = nonsustained ventricular tachycardia; Bigeminy = ventricular bigeminy; No = no arrhythmia.

Ventricular Effective Refractory Periods

During this protocol we tested the effects on ventricular effective refractory period (VERP) of bradycardia alone and bradycardia with a superimposed rapid ventricular rate (Fig. 1, panel B). In dogs that had complete AV block for 1 week, VERP was measured at several pacing cycle lengths (500, 700, 800, 1000 milliseconds) before and immediately after 1 hour of rapid LV pacing at a pacing cycle length of 500 milliseconds. As a sham control, VERP was measured in 5 dogs that had complete AV block for 1 week and were paced as long as the above group but at a pacing cycle length of 1000 milliseconds throughout. VERP was also followed for 3 hours at 1-hour intervals in a group of 3 dogs that had complete AV block for 1 week and underwent rapid pacing for 1 hour. We also determined VERP in 3 dogs that had 1 week of complete AV block and received verapamil. In this group, after control VERP was measured, a loading dose of verapamil (0.015 mg/kg/min) was injected for 5 minutes, and a maintenance dose (0.003 mg/kg/min) was infused for 2 hours, beginning 60 minutes before and continuing during rapid ventricular pacing.

VERP values before and after 1 hour of rapid pacing at a pacing cycle length of 500 milliseconds are shown in Figure 7. VERPs were prolonged after rapid ventricular pacing compared with before pacing at each basic cycle length ($P<0.01$). The QT interval (basic cycle length = 1000 milliseconds) was 399 ± 26 milliseconds after and 380 ± 24 milliseconds before rapid pacing ($P<0.01$). In the sham group that did not undergo rapid pacing, VERP at the start of the hour was 249 ± 21 milliseconds, and it was 253 ± 24 milliseconds 60 minutes later ($P=NS$). The QT interval was 360 ± 9 milliseconds at the start of the hour and 361 ± 8 milliseconds at 60 minutes ($P=NS$). The difference in VERP at a basic cycle length of 1000 milliseconds after 1 hour in dogs that received rapid pacing (36 ± 9 milliseconds) compared with dogs that did not receive rapid pacing (4 ± 5 milliseconds) was significant ($P<0.01$). The duration of prolongation of VERP produced by 1 hour of rapid pacing continued for at least 3 hours. The VERP increase was 26 ± 6 milliseconds 1 hour after pacing, 29 ± 9 milliseconds at 2 hours, and 32 ± 6 milliseconds at 3 hours. These values were not statistically different from the value immediately after pacing (29 ± 2 milliseconds). The prolongation of VERP in dogs that had 1 week of AV block and received verapamil administration before and during rapid ventricular pacing was blunted but still prolonged ($P<0.01$) (Fig. 8).

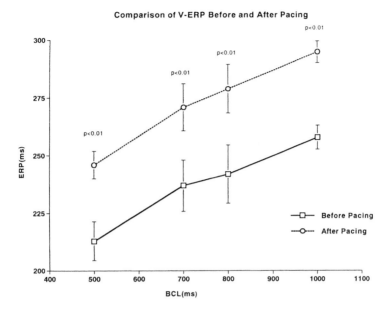

Figure 7. Comparison of ventricular effective refractory period (VERP) before and after rapid left ventricular (LV) pacing in dogs with atrioventricular block for 1 week. VERPs were prolonged after rapid LV pacing compared with before pacing at each pacing cycle length (P<0.01).

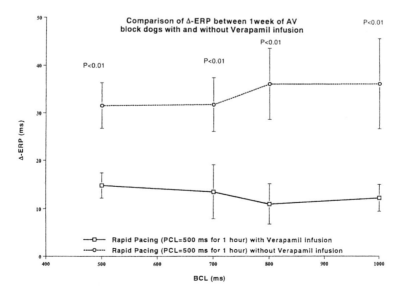

Figure 8. Effects of verapamil on Δ-VERP (change in ventricular effective refractory period) in dogs that underwent rapid ventricular pacing. Verapamil infusion significantly reduced the increase in the Δ-ERP produced by rapid pacing (P<0.01).

Mechanism

In this study we demonstrated that a rapid ventricular rate increase, even of short duration, can alter cardiac electrophysiologic properties, which in turn can influence the propensity for developing or sustaining ventricular arrhythmias in dogs. The transient superimposition of a fast ventricular rate on a slow rate was found to lengthen the QT interval and the duration of ventricular MAP and refractoriness, and to facilitate the induction of ventricular tachyarrhythmias, including torsades de pointes. Verapamil reduced, but did not entirely eliminate, the increase in refractoriness, and suggested that intracellular calcium overload mediated the changes, at least in part.

It is known that a gradual increase in stimulation of frequency causes an incremental increase in steady state muscle inotropy,[15] presumably as a result of voltage- and frequency-dependent potentiation of L-type calcium current,[16,17] which in turn augments calcium release from the sarcoplasmic reticulum stores during the action potential.[18] Elevated intracellular calcium concentration could also activate phospholipase C, which in turn could activate membrane-bound protein kinase C, ultimately leading to phosphorylation of ion channel/ion pumps,[19,20] which could also mediate changes in refractoriness. Because the refractory period changes lasted so long, alterations in the proteins that regulate the potassium and other channels appeared to be the most likely explanation.

References

1. Roden DM, Hoffmann BF. Action potential prolongation and induction of abnormal automaticity by low dose quinidine concentration in canine Purkinje fibers: Relations to potassium and cycle length. *Circ Res* 1985;56:857-867.
2. El-Sherif N, Zeiler RH, Craelius W, et al. QTU prolongation and polymorphic ventricular tachyarrhythmias due to bradycardia-dependent early afterdepolarizations: Afterdepolarizations and ventricular arrhythmias. *Circ Res* 1988;63:286-305.
3. January CT, Shorofsky S. Early afterdepolarizations: Newer insights into cellular mechanisms. *J Cardiovasc Electrophysiol* 1990;1:161-169.
4. Roden DM, Woosley RL, Primm PK. Incidence and clinical features of the quinidine-associated long QT syndrome: Implications for patient care. *Am Heart J* 1986;111:1088-1093.
5. Brandt RR, Shen W-K. Bradycardia-induced polymorphic ventricular tachycardia after atrioventricular junction ablation for sinus tachycardia-induced cardiomyopathy. *J Cardiovasc Electrophysiol* 1995;6:630-633.
6. Franz MR. Bridging the gap between basic and clinical electrophysiology: What can be learned from monophasic action potential recordings? *J Cardiovasc Electrophysiol* 1994;5:669-710.
7. Ben-David J, Zipes DP. Differential response to right and left ansae subclaviae stimulation of early afterdepolarizations and ventricular tachycardia induced by cesium in dogs. *Circulation* 1988;78:1241-1250.

8. Ben-David J, Zipes DP. α-Adrenoceptor stimulation and blockade modulates cesium-induced early afterdepolarizations and ventricular tachycardias in dogs. *Circulation* 1990;82:225-233.

9. Isenberg G. Cardiac Purkinje fibers: Cesium as a tool to block inward rectifying potassium current. *Pflügers Arch* 1975;365:98-106.

10. Brachmann J, Scherlag B, Rosenshtraukh LV, Lazarra R. Bradycardia-dependent triggered activity: Relevance to drug-induced multiform ventricular tachycardia. *Circulation* 1983;68:846-856.

11. Damiano BP, Rosen MR. Effects of pacing on triggered activity induced by early afterdepolarizations. *Circulation* 1984;69:1013-1025.

12. Levine JH, Guarnieri T, Weisfeldt ML, et al. Cesium chloride-induced long QT syndrome: Demonstration of afterdepolarizations and triggered activity in vivo. *Circulation* 1985;77:1149-1161.

13. Satoh T, Hirao K, Hiejima K. The relationship between early afterdepolarization and the occurrence of torsades de pointes: An in vivo canine model study. *Jpn Circ J* 1993;57:543-552.

14. Satoh T, Zipes DP. Rapid rates during bradycardia prolong ventricular refractoriness and facilitates ventricular tachycardia induction with cesium in dogs. *Circulation* 1996;94:217-227.

15. Bouchard RA, Bose D. Analysis of the interval-force relationship in rat and canine ventricular myocardium. *Am J Physiol* 1989;257:H2036-H2047.

16. Sculptoreanu A, Rotman E, Takahashi M, et al. Voltage-dependent potentiation of the activity of cardiac L-type calcium channel α1 subunits due to phosphorylation by cAMP-dependent protein kinase. *Proc Natl Acad Sci U S A* 1993;90:10135-10139.

17. Cannell MB, Cheng H, Lederer WJ. Spatial non-uniformities in $[Ca^{2+}]_i$ during excitation-contraction coupling in cardiac myocytes. *Biophys J* 1994; 67:1942-1956.

18. Lopez-Lopez JR, Shacklock PS, Bake CW, Wier WG. Local calcium transients triggered by single L-type calcium channel currents in cardiac cells. *Science* 1995;268:1042-1045.

19. Harding DP, Virschenlohr HL, Metcalf JE, et al. The effect of stimulation frequency on end-diastolic $[Ca^{2+}]_i$ in isolated ferret heart. *J Physiol (Lond)* 1989;417:519. Abstract.

20. Szabo B, Sweiden R, Rajagopalan CV, Lazzara R. Role of $Na^+:Ca^{2+}$ exchange current in Cs^+-induced early afterdepolarization in Purkinje fibers. *J Cardiovasc Electrophysiol* 1994;5:933-944.

11

Cardiac Memory in the Atria

Mark A. Wood, MD

The phenomenon of cardiac repolarization memory in ventricular tissue has been well described in preceding chapters. Despite the relevance of repolarization memory to ventricular arrhythmias, very few studies have explored repolarization memory in atrial tissue.[1,2] In fact, even the most fundamental question—does atrial repolarization memory exist?—has not been fully answered. A host of related questions awaits the clear documentation of the presence or absence of atrial repolarization memory. If atrial memory exists, what are the mechanisms? If atrial memory is absent, why does it not exist? What is the role of atrial memory (existent or nonexistent) in atrial arrhythmogenesis? Finally, questions can be raised concerning the relationship between atrial electrical remodeling that follows atrial tachyarrhythmias and atrial repolarization memory. Is remodeling a form of "memory"? Are these distinct entities or manifestations of the same physiologic process?

These fundamental questions assume increasing importance during a period of growing interest in nonpharmacologic therapies for the management of atrial arrhythmias. For example, permanent multisite atrial pacing may prevent recurrent atrial fibrillation by modifying atrial electrical activation and repolarization.[3] Exploration of the memory phenomenon on the atrial level may lead to insights into atrial electrophysiology and may provide a better understanding of evolving antiarrhythmia therapies. This chapter reviews the current data on atrial repolarization memory and addresses these basic questions on atrial memory. Special emphasis is given to the use of monophasic action potential (MAP) recordings in this research.

From Franz MR (ed): *Monophasic Action Potentials: Bridging Cell and Bedside.* ©Futura Publishing Company, Inc., Armonk, NY, 2000.

Does Atrial Memory Exist?

Given the paucity of data on atrial memory, this question cannot be definitively answered at this time. However, insights are available from basic animal studies.[1,2] To this author's knowledge, only one study has specifically sought to demonstrate if atrial repolarization memory exists. In this study Wood et al[1] used the isolated Langendorff rabbit heart model to map left and right atrial activation times (ATs) and corresponding local action potential durations (APDs). This model replicated that used by Costard-Jäckle et al[4] to demonstrate ventricular repolarization memory in the isolated rabbit heart. For the study of atrial memory, each of 39 rabbit hearts underwent epicardial mapping of 3 right atrial and 3 left atrial sites (Fig. 1) at baseline (time 0) and then following 45, 90, 135, and 180 minutes of either right (n=13), left (n=13), or biatrial (n=13) pacing. All MAP recordings were made during pacing at 250-millisecond cycle lengths, with use of custom made suction MAP probes. The recording sites were chosen to sample the widest range of ATs during atrial pacing. Twenty-five MAP tracings were recorded from each site at each time (sampling rate 4000 Hz) with use of custom software for personal computer. For each site, the 25 MAP tracings were computer averaged to generate a single composite MAP tracing for analysis of AT (interval from stimulus artifact to MAP upstroke) and APD (time from MAP upstroke to 90% repolarization) (Fig. 2). The statistical analysis compared the relationship between values of AT and APD at each sampling time. Right atrial appendage pacing was used to simulate the normal atrial activation sequence in one group of

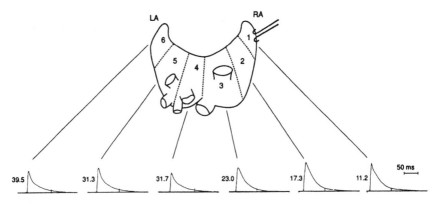

Figure 1. Diagram showing the location of the 6 recording sites from each rabbit heart. RA = right atrium; LA = left atrium. The figures at the bottom show MAP recordings from each site after 180 minutes of continuous right atrial pacing (location of pacing wires shown). The numbers to the left of the MAP tracings denote activation time to each site. Note the prolongation of activation time from site 1 to site 6. Reproduced from Reference 1, with permission of the American Heart Association.

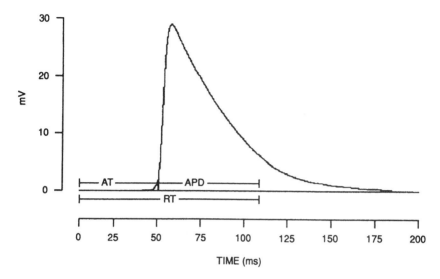

Figure 2. MAP recordings from a single epicardial atrial site after 180 minutes of continuous atrial pacing. The intervals measured to determine activation time (AT) and action potential duration to 90% repolarization (APD) are shown. The pacing stimulus occurs at time 0. Repolarization time (RT) is sum of AT and APD. Reproduced from Reference 1, with permission of the American Heart Association.

hearts. Left atrial appendage pacing and biatrial pacing were used to produce an ectopic atrial activation sequence in the remaining 2 groups.

If atrial repolarization memory exists and is analogous to ventricular memory, then an inverse relationship between AT and APD would be expected at baseline and during continuous right atrial pacing. This inverse relationship would not be expected initially with left atrial pacing but should develop during continuous left atrial or biatrial pacing to conform to the new activation sequences. Three statistical approaches were used to analyze the data for the relationships between AT and APD at each site. First, separate regression analyses were performed for each of the 39 hearts at each of the 5 sampling times. At no time for any of the 3 pacing groups was a statistically significant relationship between AT and APD demonstrated. This finding is in direct contrast to the demonstration of ventricular memory in the same model in which an inverse AT-APD relationship was noted as baseline, was lost within 5 minutes of ventricular pacing, and was reestablished for the new activation sequence after 1 hour of continuous ventricular pacing.[4] Such a relationship was not seen in atrial tissue despite 3 hours of continuous pacing. Second, regression analysis was performed after all data points from each heart were pooled at each time to evaluate the relations between AT and APD. Even when comparing absolute values of AT and APD, as well as normalized values for each heart (to minimize between subject variations), no significant relationships could be identified at any of the 5 sampling times. This pooled analysis also failed to demonstrate significant relationships between AT and APD when analysis of right and left atrial data were performed separately. Third, the relationship between APD and activation sequence was analyzed by analysis of variance using anatomic distance from the pacing site as an index of activation sequence. Again, no relationship between activation sequence and APD could be demonstrated at any time. To ensure that undersampling of data points did not mask a relationship between AT and APD, 6 additional hearts underwent sampling of 20 atrial sites at time 0 and after 3 hours of right (n=3) or left (n=3) atrial pacing. Again, no statistically significant relationships between AT and APD were found for this group. These data are interpreted to demonstrate the absence of atrial memory in the isolated rabbit heart model. This finding occurred despite a high statistical power of 0.95 to detect its presence and despite the ability to demonstrate ventricular memory in a similar preparation.[4]

Other findings from this study included the demonstration of a longer average left atrial APD than right atrial APD and a shorter dispersion of atrial repolarization times during left atrial pacing compared to right atrial pacing at each of the 5 sampling times. (Figs. 3 and 4). The reduced dispersion of atrial repolarization with left atrial pacing was believed to result from early activation of left atrial sites with the longest APDs coupled with later activation of the right atrium with shorter APDs.

The lack of influence of changes in activation sequence on local atrial APD has also been demonstrated by Spach et al[2] with use of an isolated dog right atrial preparation. In this study, with use of microelectrode MAP recordings, local APDs were unchanged by separation of adjacent muscle bundles from the recording site or by alteration in activation sequence by changes in the atrial pacing sites. These findings suggest the absence of rapidly acting electrotonic influences on atrial APD and possibly the absence of atrial memory, although the duration of ectopic pacing was not reported. Throughout these perturbations the relative relationships of APDs between adjacent atrial sites remained fairly constant, ie, sites with APDs that were longer than those of adjacent sites maintained longer APDs relative to adjacent sites despite global changes in APD.

To this author's knowledge, detailed information about the relationship between AT and APD in humans has not been described. Early efforts to provide such information are under way in this author's laboratory. In patients with normal hearts who are undergoing clinically indicated electrophysiologic studies, the right atrium is mapped with a steerable Ag-AgCl electrode MAP catheter. The local APD at each site is compared to the local AT during sinus rhythm and before any atrial pacing or arrhythmia induction. In a limited number of patients, no relationship between AT and APD has been demonstrated (M.A. Wood, unpublished observations, October 1997) (Fig. 5).

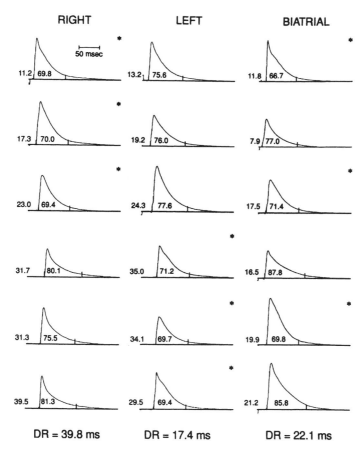

Figure 3. Vertical columns of tracings showing MAP recordings from 6 recording sites after 180 minutes of pacing from 3 different rabbit hearts. Right: heart undergoing right atrial pacing; Left: heart undergoing left atrial pacing; Biatrial: heart undergoing simultaneous right and left atrial pacing. For columns "Right" and "Left," the recording sites are arranged vertically from the site closest to the pacing stimulus (top) to that furthest away (bottom). For the "Biatrial" pacing heart the paired right and left atrial sites are arranged vertically from closest pacing site (top) to farthest away (bottom). The asterisks denote the right atrial recordings for each heart. DR = dispersion of repolarization (longest repolarization time minus shortest repolarization time). Note the longer left atrial APD compared to right atrial APD regardless of site of pacing. The DR is shortest during left atrial pacing. Reproduced from Reference 1, with permission of the American Heart Association.

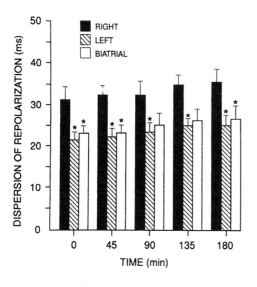

Figure 4. Average dispersion of repolarization at each of the 5 recording times from hearts undergoing right, left, and biatrial pacing. The asterisks denote $P<0.05$ compared to the right atrial pacing group at each time. Reproduced from Reference 1, with permission of the American Heart Association.

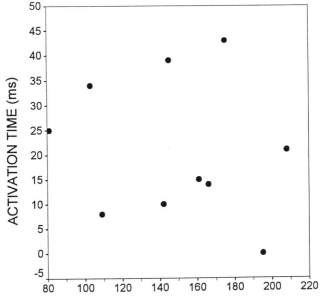

Figure 5. Graph of action potential duration (APD) versus activation time (AT) during sinus rhythm from 10 right atrial sites in a patient with no heart disease. AT was determined from the start of the surface electrocardiographic P wave to the upstroke of the MAP tracing made with a steerable Ag-AgCl tipped catheter. Recording sites included the atrial appendage, crista terminals, lateral free wall, and septum. No relationship exists between AT and APD in this data set by linear regression analysis (R=0.18; $P=0.62$).

Why Not Atrial Memory?

An absence of atrial memory should in no way be confused with a lack of spatial organization or complexity of atrial repolarization. The absence of memory suggests only that this organization may not be adaptable to new sequences of activation or that memory is not present on a global atrial scale. Spach et al[2] demonstrated an inverse relationship between atrial APD and anatomic distance from the sinus node in isolated sections of dog right atrium, a relationship analogous to the inverse relations of AT and APD maintained by ventricular memory. As noted, however, this relation was not influenced by electrotonic modulation or by changes in activation sequence. Instead, the relative APDs between adjacent atrial sites remained fairly constant, suggesting a relatively "fixed" organization of atrial repolarization at this anatomic level. Histologically, the site of longest APDs also had the greatest intercellular spaces, but no association between APD and myocyte structure could be detected. Also in this study, regional differences in APD were associated with variations in troponin T isoforms. These findings suggest that regional atrial repolarization patterns may be relatively fixed in relation to adjacent atrial regions. This could result from a dependence of atrial repolarization on spatially heterogenous intrinsic myocyte electrical properties, regional intercellular architecture, heterogeneous protein expression, regional wall tension, or influences of regional contractile properties.[5,6] These influences may be incompatible with the expression of repolarization memory.

The absence of atrial memory in these studies may result from a variety of factors. Given the extreme complexity of the atrial geometry, prevention of reentry at the regional level rather than the global level may be of paramount importance. As noted by Spach et al[7] in the isolated atrial model, local reentry is "amazingly complex," with different mechanisms of reentry occurring over different anatomic scales of size and in relation to local anatomy. The relativity constant patterns of repolarization between adjacent atrial structures may prevent local reentry at some increased risk of global atrial reentry.[2,7] The seemingly unadaptable patterns of atrial repolarization may also reflect the demands of coordinating atrial contraction and mechanical function throughout a very complex anatomic structure.

While the mechanism of ventricular repolarization memory is not known, theories include the effects of electrotonic forces and transmural current gradients, both of which may be sufficiently lacking in atrial tissue to allow for memory.[8-10] The effects of electrotonic currents may be highly dependent on type and quantity of membrane currents, tissue mass, tissue geometry, fiber orientation, and intercellular connections, all of which differ markedly from ventricular tissue. In canine ventricular tissue the I_{to}

blocker 4-aminopyridine prevents the memory phenomenon, possibly by abolishing the transmural gradient in the magnitude of this current.[10] While I_{to} is also important to atrial repolarization and demonstrates regional heterogeneity in rabbit atria, the reduced mass and wall thickness of the atria may preclude memory.[11] To summarize, the geometry, architecture, membrane currents, and cellular organization of the atria are all markedly different from those of the ventricles. Given their dissimilarities it should not be surprising that the memory phenomenon may be expressed differently or not at all in atrial tissue.

Atrial Memory and Arrhythmogenesis

The potential role of the memory phenomenon in atrial arrhythmogenesis is purely speculative. Numerous studies have correlated an increased dispersion of atrial refractoriness with an enhanced vulnerability to atrial arrhythmias, in both humans and animal models.[12-14] Given this vulnerability, mechanisms to maintain atrial repolarization synchrony would seem desirable. Conceivably, the absence of a protective memory phenomenon may contribute to the great prevalence of atrial fibrillation in clinical practice. While the true consequences of the absence of atrial memory are not known, the importance of minimizing the dispersion of atrial activation and repolarization is assumed in new therapies for atrial fibrillation, such as multisite atrial pacing.[3] The apparent success of such therapy may be due in part to a better global synchronization of atrial repolarization during multisite atrial pacing for atrial fibrillation than can be achieved by the diseased atria during sinus rhythm.

If atrial repolarization memory is critical to suppression of atrial arrhythmias, one may ask why this protective mechanism did not evolve for the atria as it has for ventricular tissue. As discussed, this phenomenon may not be possible given the mass, architecture, and electrophysiology of atrial tissue. The demonstrated patterns of atrial repolarization may be the best 'compromise" between prevention of local reentry and global reentry. Finally, the evolutionary drive for prevention of atrial arrhythmias may be less than that for the prevention of lethal ventricular arrhythmias.

Limitations

The cited studies all have limitations. These studies derive from isolated animal heart models, and marked interspecies differences are known to exist. No thorough study of atrial repolarization memory in humans is available. It is possible that the atrial memory process is slow to develop and is missed by these studies. The possibility of local repolarization memory in the atria cannot be excluded.

Is Atrial Remodeling Atrial Memory?

Finally, consideration should be given to the relationship between atrial repolarization memory and atrial electrical remodeling, because both phenomena involve the continued expression of specific repolarization patterns after the inciting stimulus is removed. Atrial electrical remodeling is described in detail elsewhere in this text but refers to a shortening of atrial refractoriness and APD following the termination of atrial fibrillation or flutter.[15-17] Clear definitions of memory and remodeling have not been established, but in current usage, repolarization memory implies a protective physiologic adaption and remodeling implies a detrimental pathologic process.[9,18] Whether either process is truly adaptive or detrimental is unknown. The question can reasonably be raised whether remodeling represents a maladaptive expression of atrial memory. In ventricular tissue the expression of repolarization memory is both rate- and duration-dependent.[19] Conceivably, the rapid rates of atrial fibrillation combined with the altered activation sequence could accelerate a slowly developing atrial memory. This could result in the shortening of atrial repolarization that persists after the restoration of normal atrial rates. In these studies it is not possible to separate the potential influence of rapid rates and abnormal sequence of activation in this process.

The true differences between atrial remodeling and atrial memory have not been well explored. However, insights into the distinct nature of the processes are again provided by the use of MAP recordings in the isolated heart model. Despite the absence of atrial memory in response to abnormal sequences of atrial activation at a physiologic heart rate in the isolated rabbit heart, Wood et al[20] have demonstrated the presence of atrial remodeling after rapid atrial pacing in this same model. In this study, atrial APDs measured with suction MAP probes were significantly shortened after completing 90 minutes of biatrial pacing at 80-millisecond cycle lengths compared to control hearts undergoing biatrial pacing at 250-millisecond cycle lengths (n=10 each group) (Fig. 6). Of note, this remodeling was prevented by the presence of 0.1 mM verapamil or by 1 mM 4-aminopyridine during the rapid pacing. It is of interest that 4-aminopyridine also abolishes the memory phenomenon in ventricular tissue. While not conclusive, this set of experiments demonstrates the capability of the rabbit atria to undergo electrical remodeling despite the absence of atrial memory in the rabbit heart preparation. While these findings

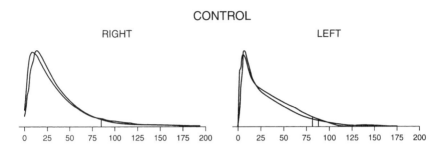

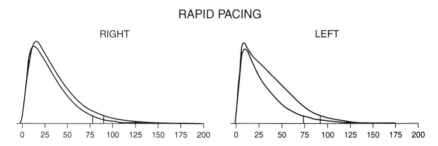

Figure 6. Changes in atrial MAP in response to 90 minutes of atrial pacing at physiologic heart rates (250 milliseconds, CONTROL) or rapid rates (80 milliseconds, RAPID PACING) in 2 isolated rabbit heart preparations. Each of the 4 panels shows superimposed MAP tracings from before and after the pacing period. All recordings were made at 250-millisecond paced cycle lengths. RIGHT = right atrial recordings; LEFT = left atrial recordings. The vertical markers indicated action potential duration (APD) at 90% repolarization in each tracing. For the control heart, left atrial APD decreased by 4 milliseconds and right atrial APD did not change. For the rapid atrial pacing heart, the APDs decreased by 12 milliseconds and 19 milliseconds for the right and left atria, respectively. Reproduced from Reference 20, with permission.

suggest distinct processes, additional research is needed to clarify the relationship of these entities in humans.

Conclusions

Global atrial repolarization memory is not demonstrable in the isolated rabbit heart model. In canine studies, local atrial APD does not appear to be altered by electrotonic modulation or by the sequence of atrial activation. The patterns of atrial repolarization are complex but appear to have spatial organization without the ability to modify these patterns in response to short-term changes in activation sequence. These spatial patterns of repolarization may be important for the prevention of local reentry, while the prevention of global reentry is of secondary importance. The absence of atrial memory may result from many factors including atrial mass and wall thickness, atrial geometry, fiber organization, and membrane currents, all of which differ markedly from ventricular tissue. The relationship between atrial memory and atrial electrical remodeling is not clear. The demonstration of electrical remodeling, but not atrial memory in the same rabbit heart model, suggests distinct processes.

References

1. Wood MA, Mangano RA, Scheiken RM, et al. Modulation of atrial repolarization by site of pacing in the isolated rabbit heart. *Circulation* 1996;94:1465-1470.
2. Spach MS, Dolber PC, Anderson PAW. Multiple regional differences in cellular properties that regulate repolarization and contraction in the right atrium of adult and newborn dogs. *Circ Res* 1989;65:1594-1611.
3. Prakash A, Saksena S, Hill M, et al. Prevention of recurrent atrial fibrillation with chronic dual-site atrial pacing. *J Am Coll Cardiol* 1996;28:687-694.
4. Costard-Jäckle A, Goetsch B, Antz M, et al. Slow and long-lasting modulation of myocardial repolarization produced by ectopic activation in isolated rabbit hearts. *Circulation* 1989;80:1412-1420.
5. Satoh T, Zipes DP. Unequal atrial stretch in dogs increases dispersion of refractoriness conducive to developing atrial fibrillation. *J Cardiovasc Electrophysiol* 1996;7:833-842.
6. Saffitz JE, Davis LM, Darrow BJ, et al. The molecular basis of anisotropy: Role of gap junctions. *J Cardiovasc Electrophysiol* 1995;6:498-510.
7. Spach MS, Dolber PC, Heigdloge JF. Interaction of inhomogeneities of repolarization with anisotropic propagation in dog atria. A mechanism for both preventing and initiating reentry. *Circ Res* 1989;65:1612-1631.
8. Malik M, Camm AJ. Effects of myocardial electrotonic interaction on the sequence of excitation and repolarization and on T wave polarity. Computer modeling experiments. *Clin Phys Physiol Meas* 1992;13:365-387.
9. Geller JC, Rosen MR. Persistent T-wave changes after alteration of the ventricular activation sequence. New insights into cellular mechanisms of "cardiac memory.' *Circulation* 1993;88:1811-1819.
10. del Balzo V, Rosen MR. T wave changes persisting after ventricular pacing in canine heart are altered by 4-aminopyridine but not by lidocaine. Implications with respect to phenomenon of cardiac "memory." *Circulation* 1992;85:1464-1472.
11. Yamashita T, Nakajima T, Hazama H, et al. Regional differences in transient outward current density and inhomogeneities of repolarization in rabbit right atrium. *Circulation* 1995;92:3061-3069.
12. Leitch JW, Basta M, Fletcher PJ. Effect of phenylephrine infusion on atrial electrophysiologic properties. *Heart* 1997;78:166-170.
13. Liu L, Nattel S. Differing sympathetic and vagal effects on atrial fibrillation in dogs: Role of refractoriness heterogeneity. *Am J Physiol* 1997;273:H805-H816.
14. Tsuji H, Fujiki A, Tani M, et al. Quantitative relationship between atrial refractoriness and the dispersion of refractoriness in atrial vulnerability. *PACE* 1992;15:403-410.
15. Goette A, Honeycutt C, Langberg JJ. Electrical remodeling in atrial fibrillation. *Circulation* 1996;64:2968-2974.

16. Daoud EG, Bogun F, Goyal R, et al. Effect of atrial fibrillation on atrial refractoriness in humans. *Circulation* 1996;94:1600-1606.

17. Wijffels MCEF, Kirckhof CJHJ, Dorland R, et al. Atrial fibrillation begets atrial fibrillation. A study in awake chronically instrumented goats. *Circulation* 1995;92:1954-1968.

18. Zipes DP. Electrophysiological remodeling of the heart owing to rate. *Circulation* 1997;95:1745-1748.

19. Rosenbaum MB, Blanco HH, Elizari MV, et al. Electrotonic modulation of the T wave and cardiac memory. *Am J Cardiol* 1982;50:213-222.

20. Wood MA, Caponi D, Sykes AM, et al. Atrial electrical remodeling by rapid pacing in the isolated rabbit heart: Effects of Ca^{++} and K^+ channel blockade. *J Interv Card Electrophysiol* 1998;2:15-23.

12

Use of Cardiac Action Potentials to Investigate Cardiac Memory:

From Bedside to Computer Model

Rajiva Goyal, MD, FACC and
Fred Morady, MD

Introduction

The term *cardiac memory* has been used to describe primary T wave changes following minutes to several hours of right ventricular (RV) pacing.[1] The term has also been used to describe different types of T wave changes, including those following intermittent left bundle branch block, ventricular tachycardia, and ventricular preexcitation.[2-4] For this temporal change in repolarization to be present, two components are necessary, namely memory and accumulation.[1,5-7] A true memory component is present when repeated episodes of an altered activation sequence exert a cumulative effect on repolarization during normal activation. Accumulation is the occurrence of progressively greater repolarization change during normal activation following progressively longer durations of an altered activation sequence. The time required for the primary repolarization changes to develop is dependent on the duration of the altered activation sequence.

Previous work has suggested that at least 15 minutes of an altered activation is necessary for primary ventricular repolarization abnormality

From Franz MR (ed): *Monophasic Action Potentials: Bridging Cell and Bedside.*
©Futura Publishing Company, Inc., Armonk, NY, 2000.

to become manifest.[1] The resolution of this primary change can take place from hours to several days following the altered activation sequence and is also dependent on the duration of the altered activation sequence.[1,6,7] It has been suggested that changes that take hours to days to become manifest and to resolve are probably mediated through changes in gene expression and protein synthesis.[8] However, primary T wave changes that develop and resolve over minutes rather than hours are probably not mediated through these mechanisms and are the focus of our research.

Ventricular Memory: Effect of Short Periods of an Altered Activation Sequence

Traditionally, the memory phenomenon has been evaluated by the analysis of visually apparent T wave changes on the surface electrocardiogram.[1] Other studies have evaluated the phenomenon using either transmembrane action potential recordings or monophasic action potential (MAP) recordings in tissue or animal preparations.[6,7,9]

In the present study, MAP recordings were used to evaluate changes in primary ventricular repolarization, cardiac memory.[10-16] The MAP recordings for each patient at baseline were used as the patient-specific template for the subsequent comparisons.[16] A MAP catheter (model 1675P, EP Technologies, San Jose, CA) was positioned at the RV septum in 13 patients. High right atrial (RA) pacing was performed to simulate the normal activation pattern, and a catheter, positioned in the RV apex, was used for ventricular pacing, to simulate an altered sequence of activation. The cardiac action potential is affected by changes in rate and by changes in autonomic tone; these factors were held constant.[17,18] All pacing was performed at an uninterrupted cycle length of 500 milliseconds and during pharmacologic autonomic blockade.[19]

Root Mean Square Analysis of MAP Recordings

APD_{90}, defined as the time interval from the rapid upstroke (phase 0) to the time for the action potential amplitude to decrease to 10% of the peak plateau amplitude, has been used to quantify MAP recordings.[10,11,13] A different percentage change in the peak plateau amplitude could have been used for the analysis. Therefore, to incorporate all of the different percentage changes and, in essence, to get a quantitative analysis of the MAP morphology, the MAP recordings were analyzed by use of a root mean square (RMS) of the difference between two recordings.

Previous work has suggested that the initial deflection of the MAP recordings is subject to variability.[13,14] Therefore, in the morphology comparison, the first 15 milliseconds of the MAP recordings were not included in the RMS of the difference analysis. The subsequent 230 milliseconds of digitized data were analyzed. Signal averaging was also used to increase the signal-to-noise ratio. It is known that the amplitude of MAP recordings decreases over time; however, this has little impact on the APD_{90} values.[12,15] The morphology comparison using RMS of the difference, however, is affected by changes in amplitude. Therefore, the amplitudes of the signal-averaged MAP recordings were normalized prior to RMS evaluation. An RMS of the difference value greater than 4 mV is indicative of visually apparent changes in MAP morphology. The RMS of the difference analysis comparing baseline MAP recordings with recordings taken at 1, 5, 10, and 15 minutes during atrial pacing demonstrated no significant temporal change in morphology (3.5 ± 0.9, 3.3 ± 0.1, 3.6 ± 0.1, and 3.4 ± 0.1 mV, respectively; $P=0.4$).

Demonstration of Ventricular Memory

To evaluate the memory phenomenon, baseline MAPs were recorded for 1 minute during RA pacing. RV pacing was then performed for 1 minute followed by RA pacing for 2 minutes. This pacing sequence was repeated for a total of 4 RV pacing sequences. Compared to baseline, after each minute of RV pacing there was a progressive shortening in APD_{90} (226 ± 5 versus 223 ± 4, 216 ± 6, 211 ± 4, and 207 ± 5 milliseconds, respectively; $P<0.05$). The RMS of the difference between the baseline MAP recordings and the signal average of the first 50 beats following each RV pacing train demonstrated a difference in morphology (6.3 ± 0.3, 7.7 ± 0.3, 9.0 ± 0.5, and 9.4 ± 0.6 mV, respectively). Regression analysis demonstrated a progressively greater change in RMS of the difference after each of the 4 RV pacing trains ($r=0.96$, $P=0.02$). Also important to note was the fact that there was no difference in the APD_{90} or the RMS of the difference between baseline and MAP recordings just prior to the second, third, and fourth period of RV pacing. This indicated that the repolarization changes had reverted back to normal during the 2 minutes of RA pacing.

Demonstration of Accumulation

After acquisition of baseline MAP recordings for 1 minute during RA pacing, different durations of RV pacing were performed prior to returning to RA pacing, during which data acquisition and comparisons were performed. Compared to baseline, progressively greater durations of RV pacing (1, 5, 10, and 15 minutes) resulted in greater maximum APD_{90} shortening (225 ± 5 versus 222 ± 4, 220 ± 7, 215 ± 8, and 213 ± 7, respectively; $P<0.02$). The change in repolarization did not return to baseline during the 6 minutes of RA pacing. Regression analysis demonstrated a progressively greater change in the RMS of the difference after progressively longer durations of RV pacing ($r=0.97$, $P<0.01$).

Summary

This study demonstrated that 1 minute of an altered activation sequence is sufficient to create a transient change in ventricular repolarization after resumption of a normal activation sequence. The RMS of the difference analysis is more sensitive and specific in quantifying changes in MAP recordings. Moreover, both criteria for cardiac memory are demonstrated by using comparisons of endocardial recordings before and after ventricular pacing.[16]

Atrial Memory?

The term *cardiac memory* has been applied to ventricular repolarization; however, similar phenomena may be present in atrial tissue. Wood et al,[20] in a Langendorff rabbit heart preparation, evaluated the effect of RA, left atrial, and biatrial pacing on APD_{90}. Cardiac memory, defined as the inverse relationship between the activation time of the MAP recording and APD_{90}, was not demonstrated in this study. Possible reasons for this negative result may be that altered activation of the atrium was not achieved, or that the rabbit atrium does not demonstrate this phenomenon.

To investigate this further, we evaluated the effect of short episodes of coronary sinus pacing on the atrial repolarization using MAP recordings.[21] Coronary sinus pacing was used to simulate an altered activation sequence. In 20 patients, a quadripolar catheter was positioned at the high RA and in the coronary sinus, and a MAP catheter (model 1675P, EP Technologies) at the interatrial septum. All pacing was performed at 500 milliseconds and during autonomic blockade, similar to the protocol outlined above.

Accumulation Phenomenon in the Atrium

The temporal stability of atrial MAP recordings during RA pacing was evaluated in a group of 5 control subjects. When comparing the first minute to that after 20 minutes of RA pacing, no difference in the APD_{90} was noted (269 ± 24 versus 268 ± 19, respectively; $P=0.3$). The 15 study subjects underwent one of two pacing protocols which involved 5 minutes of RA pacing (baseline), followed by either 5 or 15 minutes of coronary sinus pacing, followed by 10 minutes of RA pacing. MAP recordings were compared only during RA pacing before and after coronary sinus pacing.

There was no significant change in the APD_{90} when comparing values before to those after 5 minutes of coronary sinus pacing (248 ± 12 versus 247 ± 13, respectively; $P=0.4$). However, in comparison to baseline, there was a significant decrease in APD_{90} after 15 minutes of coronary sinus pacing (228 ± 3 versus 202 ± 4 milliseconds; $P<0.05$). This change persisted during the 10 minutes of RA pacing. In summary, a change in the site of atrial pacing that results in altered atrial activation can result in a change in repolarization despite a stable pacing cycle length and constant autonomic tone. This change appears to be proportional to the duration of the altered activation sequence and therefore demonstrates properties of accumulation. However, further work is needed to document the second component of the memory phenomenon.

Simulation of Cardiac Memory in a Computer Model

As demonstrated above, repolarization changes that are compatible with cardiac memory can be reproduced in a matter of a few minutes. A change in cellular coupling kinetics might explain the rapid onset and offset of the memory phenomenon. However, it is not possible to study cellular coupling changes in more than two cells at a time in either an in vivo or an in vitro preparation. Therefore, a mathematical approach was used to study the role of cellular kinetics on the phenomenon of cardiac memory. The Drouhard-Roberge modifications of the Hodgkin-Huxley equations were used to represent ionic currents in the individual cells.[22]

Description of the Model

A 2-dimensional propagation model similar to that used by other investigators was implemented on Hewlett Packard (Palo Alto, CA) work station (HP-735).[22-26] However, unlike previously described models, in this model the coupling between cells was expressed by a resistor in parallel with a capacitor. In essence, each cell was coupled to 4 neighboring cells by a resistor and a capacitor in parallel (Fig. 1). Anisotropic conduction was maintained in this mathematical matrix by having the resistance greater in the direction perpendicular to the fiber

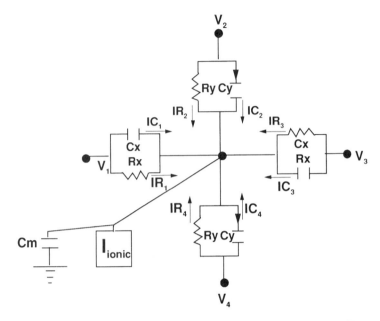

Figure 1. Diagrammatic representation of 5 cells from the model. Four cells (surrounding black circles) surround one cell (central black circle). I_{ionic} = the current generated by the modified Beeler-Reuter equations for each cell. The center cell is connected to 4 surrounding cells with a resistor and capacitor in parallel. Cx and Cy = capacitors in parallel and perpendicular to the fiber axis, respectively; Rx and Ry = resistors in parallel and perpendicular to the fiber axis, respectively; IR_n and IC_n = current flow through the resistor and capacitor; V_n = voltage of the surrounding cells; Cm = membrane capacitance.

axis compared to the direction parallel to this axis. Both the capacitive and resistive components of the coupling could be varied independently for the different simulations.

Protocol

To simulate normal activation, pacing was performed in a direction parallel to the fiber axis and pacing perpendicular to this axis simulated altered activation. Geller and Rosen[6] used a similar definition in their in vitro study. Pacing was performed for 3 beats in a direction parallel to the fiber axis, followed by pacing perpendicular to this axis for either 25 or 50 beats, followed by pacing parallel to the fiber axis for 5 beats. Action potential durations were compared during pacing parallel to the fiber axis before and after pacing perpendicular to this axis. A simulated electrocardiogram, produced by comparing the derived action potential with a template,[27] was used to display the quantitative change in action potential morphology (ie, the T wave).

Cellular Coupling Kinetics and Cardiac Memory

In the model with solely resistive coupling between cells, repolarization changes compatible with the memory phenomenon could not be reproduced. In a second set of simulations the coupling kinetics between cells were dependent on both a capacitor and resistor in parallel. To maintain anisotropic conduction, the values of the resistors in parallel to the fiber axis were set to 5000 Ω.cm and those perpendicular to this axis were 10,000 Ω.cm. The values of the capacitive coupling in the directions perpendicular to and parallel to the fiber axis were varied for different simulations. There was a significant increase in the mean APD_{90} when comparing baseline action potentials to those following pacing for 25 beats perpendicular to the fiber axis (439 ± 34 versus 453 ± 30; $P<0.001$). When there was no directional difference in capacitance in relation to the fiber axis, the primary repolarization change could not be demonstrated (438 ± 10 versus 439 ± 9 milliseconds). Therefore, capacitive anisotropy was essential in this mathematical model to reproduce the memory phenomenon.

Pacing perpendicular to the fiber axis modified the morphology of the action potential. An upright T wave was present during pacing parallel to the fiber axis prior to pacing perpendicular to this axis (Fig. 2). Of note

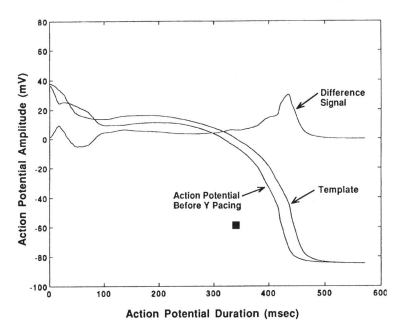

Figure 2. Action potential during pacing parallel to the fiber axis before pacing perpendicular to this axis, template, and the difference signal. An upright T wave is present in the difference signal.

is that after pacing perpendicular to the fiber axis for 25 beats, the T wave was inverted during pacing parallel to this axis (Fig. 3). The model demonstrated the phenomenon of accumulation, such that 50 beats of pacing perpendicular to the fiber axis resulted in a greater change in APD_{90} compared to pacing for 25 beats (Fig. 4).

Summary

This study demonstrated that the phenomenon of cardiac memory can be simulated in a mathematical model of cells coupled by a resistor in parallel with a capacitor, but not when coupling is only resistor-based. The memory phenomenon reproduced in the mathematical model demonstrates properties of accumulation, such that a longer duration of an altered activation results in greater repolarization changes during normal activation.

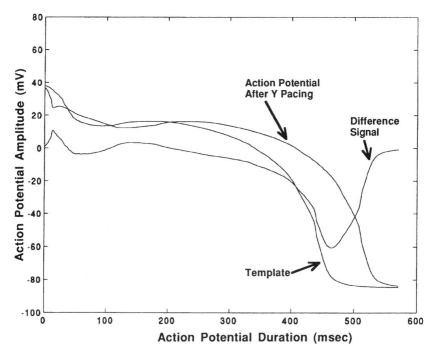

Figure 3. Action potential of the first beat during pacing parallel to the fiber axis after pacing perpendicular to this axis, template, and the difference signal. Note that an inverted T wave is present in the difference signal.

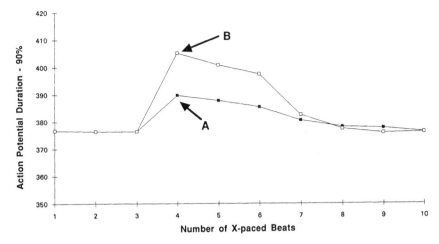

Figure 4. Plot of action potential duration at 90% repolarization (APD_{90}), in milliseconds, versus the number or beats paced in the direction parallel to the fiber axis (x-paced beats). Beat 3 is before pacing and beat 4 is after pacing perpendicular to the fiber axis. The duration of pacing perpendicular to the fiber axis was 25 beats for experiment A and 50 beats for experiment B. Note that the increase in APD_{90} is greater during experiment B compared to experiment A.

Implications

In conclusion, the results of these studies demonstrate that very short periods of an altered activation sequence may exert lingering effects on the repolarization process once normal activation resumes, both in the ventricle and the atrium. Previous studies have suggested that atrial fibrillation produces electrophysiologic changes in the atrium that predispose to recurrent atrial fibrillation.[28,29] It is known that the longer the duration of atrial fibrillation, the greater the shortening in atrial refractory period (electrical remodeling).[29,30] A number of possible mechanisms have been evoked to explain this electrical remodeling, including a change in autonomic tone, mechanoelectrical feedback, rate-dependent changes, ischemia, and cytosolic calcium overload.[29,31-33] The phenomenon of cardiac memory might offer an additional explanation for the electrical remodeling noted after episodes of atrial fibrillation, in which multiple wavelets activate the atria in different directions (altered activation). This altered activation may result in shortening of atrial repolarization once sinus rhythm has been restored, and hence predispose the atrium to further episodes of fibrillation. Similarly the cardiac memory phenomenon might result in changes in ventricular repolarization, whereby an episode of ventricular tachycardia may predispose to early recurrences of the arrhythmia.

References

1. Rosenbaum MB, Blanco HH, Elizari MV, et al. Electrotonic modulation of the T wave and cardiac memory. *Am J Cardiol* 1982;50:213-222.
2. Luy G, Bahl OP, Massie E. Intermittent left bundle branch block: A study of the effects of left bundle branch block on ECG patterns of MI and ischemia. *Am Heart J* 1944;28:332-347.
3. Engel JR, Shah R, DePodesta LA, et al. T wave abnormalities of intermittent left bundle branch block. *Ann Intern Med* 1978;89:204-206.
4. Kalbfleisch SJ, Sousa J, El-Atassi R, et al. Repolarization abnormalities after ablation of accessory atrioventricular connections with radiofrequency current. *J Am Coll Cardiol* 1991;18(7):1761-1766.
5. Autenrieth G, Surawicz B, Kuo CS, et al. Primary T wave abnormalities caused by uniform and regional shortening of ventricular monophasic action potential in dog. *Circulation* 1975;51:688-676.
6. Geller JC, Rosen MR. Persistent T wave changes after alteration of ventricular activation sequence: New insights into cellular mechanisms of "cardiac memory." *Circulation* 1993;88(I):1811-1819.
7. del Balzo U, Rosen MR. T wave changes persisting after ventricular pacing in canine hearts are altered by 4-aminopyridine but not by lidocaine: Implications with respect to phenomenon of cardiac "memory." *Circulation* 1992; 85:1464-1472.
8. Katz MK. T wave "memory": Possible causal relationship to stress-induced changes in cardiac ion channel? *J Cardiovasc Electrophysiol* 1992;3:150-158.
9. Costard-Jaeckle A, Goetsch B, Antz M, et al. Slow and long-lasting modulation of myocardial repolarization produced by ectopic activation in isolated rabbit hearts: Evidence for cardiac 'memory." *Circulation* 1989;80:1412-1420.
10. Franz MR, Bargheer K, Rafflenbeul W, et al. Monophasic action potential mapping in human subjects with normal electrocardiograms: Direct evidence for the genesis of the T wave. *Circulation* 1987;75:379-386.
11. Hoffman BF, Cranefield PF, Lepeschkin E. Comparison of cardiac monophasic action potentials recorded by intracellular and suction electrodes. *Am J Physiol* 1959;196:1297-1299.
12. Franz MR, Burkhoff D, Spurgeon H, et al. In vitro validation of a new cardiac catheter technique for recording monophasic action potentials. *Eur Heart J* 1986;7:34-41.
13. Ino T, Karagueuzian HS, Hong K, et al. Relation of monophasic action potential recorded with contact electrode in underlying transmembrane action potential properties in isolated cardiac tissues: A systematic microelectrode validation study. *Cardiovas Res* 1988;22:255-264.
14. Franz MR. Method and theory of monophasic action potential recording. *Prog Cardiovasc Dis* 1991;33:347-368.
15. Franz MR. Long term recording of monophasic action potentials from human endocardium. *Am J Cardiol* 1983;51:1629-1634.
16. Goyal R, Syed ZA, Mukhopadhyay PS, et al. Changes in cardiac repolarization following short periods of ventricular pacing. *J Cardiovasc Electrophysiol* 1998;9:269-280.
17. Denes P, Wu D, Dhingra R, et al. The effects of cycle length on cardiac refractory periods in man. *Circulation* 1974;49:32-41.
18. Morady F, Kadish AH, Toivonen LK, et al. The maximum effect of an increase in rate on human ventricular refractoriness. *PACE* 1988;11:2223-2234.

19. Jose AD, Taylor RR. Autonomic blockade by propranolol and atropine to study intrinsic myocardial function in man. *J Clin Invest* 1969;48:2019-2031.
20. Wood MA, Mangano RA, Schieken RM, et al. Modulation of atrial repolarization by site of pacing in the isolated rabbit heart. *Circulation* 1996;94:1465-1471.
21. Goyal R, Morady F. Atrial cardiac memory: Fact or fiction? *J Electrocardiol* 1997,30:S11.
22. Drouhard JP, Roberge FA. Revised formulation of the Hodgkin-Huxley representation of the sodium current in cardiac cells. *Comp Biomed Res* 1987;20:333-350.
23. Roberge FA, Vinet A, Victorri B. Reconstruction of propagated electrical activity with a two dimensional model of anisotropic heart muscle. *Circ Res* 1986; 58:461-475.
24. Lesh MD, Pring M, Spear JF. Cellular uncoupling can unmask dispersion of action potential duration in ventricular myocardium: A computer modeling study. *Circ Res* 1989;65:1426-1440.
25. Barr RC, Plonsey R. Propagation of excitation in idealized anisotropic two-dimensional tissue. *Biophys J* 1984;45:1191-1202.
26. Spach MS, Heidlage JF. A multidimensional model of cellular effects on the spread of electronic currents and on propagating action potentials. *Crit Rev Biomed Eng* 1992;20:141-169.
27. Wohlfart B. Simulation of ECG from two pairs of action potentials. *Clin Physiol* 1993;13:453-467.
28. Kopecky SL, Gersh BJ, McGoon MD, et al. The natural history of lone atrial fibrillation: A population based study over three decades. *N Engl J Med* 1987;317:669-674.
29. Wijffels MCEF, Kirchhof CJHJ, Dorland R, et al. Atrial fibrillation begets atrial fibrillation: A study in awake chronically instrumented goats. *Circulation* 1995;92:1954-1968.
30. Daoud EG, Bogun F, Goyal R, et al. Effect of atrial fibrillation on atrial refractoriness in humans. *Circulation* 1996;94:1600-1606.
31. Calkins H, El-Atassi R, Kalbfleisch S, et al. Effect of an acute increase in atrial pressure on atrial refractoriness in humans. *PACE* 1992;15:1674-1680.
32. Akay M, Craelius W. Mechanoelectrical feedback in cardiac myocytes from stretch-activated ion channels. *IEEE Trans Biomed Eng* 1993;40:811-816.
33. Goette A, Honeycutt C, Langberg JJ. Electrical remodeling in atrial fibrillation: Time course and mechanisms. *Circulation* 1996;94:2968-2974.

13

Action Potential Alternans, Electrical Restitution, Repolarization Dispersion, and Arrhythmia Vulnerability in the Isolated Ischemic Rabbit Heart

Robert W. Kurz, MD and
Michael R. Franz, MD, PhD

One of the earliest electrophysiologic signs of myocardial ischemia is alternation of the T wave in duration and magnitude from beat to beat. Although ischemia-induced T wave alternans (TWAs) has been reported previously in clinical[1] and experimental settings,[2] this phenomenon has recently achieved particular significance through the demonstration that the TWA is a powerful predictor of ventricular fibrillation.[3,4] Because the electrocardiographic T wave is the body surface reflection of spatial and temporal differences in ventricular repolarization, a meaningful pathophysiologic approach to TWAs must address the electrophysiologic mechanisms at the myocardial tissue level, specifically abnormalities of the action potential duration (APD) response. This approach will also help to understand why ischemic TWAs increase dispersion of repolarization and facilitate ventricular tachyarrhythmias (VTAs). The concept that APD alternans

From Franz MR (ed): *Monophasic Action Potentials: Bridging Cell and Bedside.*
©Futura Publishing Company, Inc., Armonk, NY, 2000.

set up the conditions for VTA is based on the assumption of different APDs in adjacent myocardial regions that result in substantial inhomogeneities of cellular repolarization. Such differences in APD can induce regional conduction block due to regionally disparate refractoriness or can result in flow of injury current, both of which may facilitate VTA.[5,6]

These authors studied, in intact Langendorff-perfused rabbit hearts, the relationship between APD alternans and different degrees of global ischemia. Simultaneous recordings of monophasic action potentials (MAPs) at various distinct locations of the intact heart allowed us to detect heterogeneity of the electrophysiologic parameters during global ischemia. The methods used in these studies and the obtained data have been previously described in detail.[7-9] In brief, Langendorff-perfused rabbit hearts were submitted to global ischemia by lowering of the perfusion by 60% to 100%. The left ventricle (LV) was loaded with a fluid-filled balloon adjusted to 5 mm Hg end-diastolic pressure, while the right ventricle (RV) was left unloaded. With use of Franz Ag-AgCl contact electrodes,[10] MAPs were recorded simultaneously from 3 distinct epicardial sites: the anterior portion of the RV and the lateral and anterior surface of the LV. The APD was determined as the interval from the steepest upstroke of the MAP to its 70% repolarization level, with the distance from the MAP plateau to its diastolic baseline taken as the total amplitude. The onset, magnitude, and pattern of APD alternans were evaluated by measurements of beat-to-beat differences in APD.[8]

APD Alternans During Ischemia: Interdependence of Flow, Preload, and Cycle Length

Dependence of APD Alternans on the Duration of Ischemia

There was an initial transient *increase* in APD before APD *shortened* below baseline values. This transient APD increase was best seen in the RV recording where, presumably, the development of ischemia progressed with a slower time course (see below). With ongoing ischemia and during the shortening phase of APD, MAP recordings began to alternate in duration and amplitude from one beat to another. APD alternans appeared either "in phase" or "out of phase" (*discordant* versus *concordant* alternans) between different recording sites. With perfusion kept constant at a low level, APD alternans progressed, and the difference in APD and the degree of alternans between the 3 recording sites became more pronounced (Fig. 1). Thus, both *temporal* APD dispersion (beat-to-beat alternans) and *spa-*

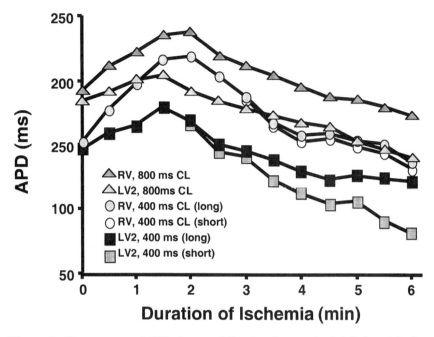

Figure 1. Time course of APD changes following the onset of global ventricular flow reduction. The graph displays APD changes in 3 different pacing rates. There was an initial prolongation of ADP that was most obvious in RV recordings, followed by progressive APD shortening. At a later time, APD curves split into one of longer and one of shorter values. This split indicates APD alternans by absolute APD values on a beat-to-beat basis. APD = action potential duration; CL = cycle length; RV = right ventricle; LV1 = left lateral ventricle; LV2 = left anterior ventricle. Reproduced from Reference 8, with permission.

tial dispersion (site-to-site differences in APD) occurred and progressed with ongoing time of reduced flow.

Dependence of APD Alternans on the Recording Site

The onset and time course of MAP changes recorded after myocardial flow reduction differed markedly between the 3 recording sites. APD shortening and alternans always occurred first at the LV recording sites (anterior LV wall before lateral LV wall) and only later and to a lesser degree at the RV recording site (Figs. 1 and 2). This may be explained by the fact that only the LV was hemodynamically loaded by an intracavitary fluid-filled balloon, while the RV was unloaded. This suggests that, under ischemic conditions, ventricular loading makes an essential contribution to the development of APD alternans.

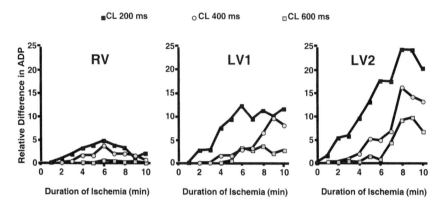

Figure 2. Development of ischemic APD alternans during 6 minutes of total ischemia at 3 different recording sites at a constant CL of 400 m. The values represent the relative differences in APD between two consecutive, alternating MAPs, expressed as percentage of the longer one. At the 3 recording sites, EA commenced at different time points, continously increased thereafter, and reached different maxima after 6 minutes of total ischemia (values are means; SEM<4% are not shown for clarity of the illustration; n=8) EA = electrical alternans; APD = action potential duration; MAP = monophasic action potential; CL = cycle length; RV = right ventricle; LV1 = left lateral ventricle; LV2 = left anterior ventricle. Reproduced from Reference 8, with permission.

Dependence of APD Alternans on the Pacing Rate

APD alternans was highly sensitive to heart rate. At any of the 3 recording sites, while of different magnitudes between these sites, alternans developed earlier and were much more pronounced at shorter cycle lengths than at longer ones (Fig. 2). A higher heart rate may increase the metabolic demand of the myocardium, thereby aggravating existing ischemia. The following data, however, suggest that cycle length may in itself be a determinant of alternans, without being secondary to rate-induced increase of the ischemic burden. At long cycle lengths (600 milliseconds), APD alternans could not be detected within 6 minutes of complete ischemia (100% flow reduction). When the paced cycle length was shortened abruptly (eg, to 200 milliseconds), APD alternans developed within the first 2 beats following the rate increase. Conversely, when, during persistent ischemia, the cycle length was lengthened again, APD alternans was immediately abolished (Fig. 3). This immediate onset and offset of APD alternans could be consistently reproduced. Thus, a longer cycle length (ie, 600 milliseconds) not only prevented spontaneous APD alternans but also abolished APD alternans induced by a shorter cycle length (ie, 200 or 400 milliseconds).[8] It is highly unlikely that the metabolic situation deteriorates significantly within a single beat after the rate increase and recovers equally fast after the rate decrease. Instead, these

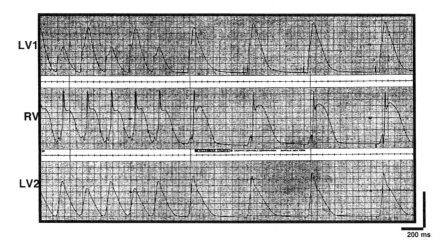

200 ms

Figure 3. Original tracings of 3 MAPs recorded from different epicardial sites during global ischemia. The severe out-of-phase EA at 200m CL pacing where longer and shorter APDs coincide at the different recording sites is completely dampened after the rate switch to 600-ms CL. Abbreviations are same as in Figure 1. Reproduced from Reference 8, with permission.

observations underscore the importance of a shorter cycle length for APD alternans development, and suggest that cycle length itself is a contributor to ischemic alternans independent of the degree of ischemia.

Dependence of APD Shortening and Alternans on the Degree of Flow Reduction

Figures 1 and 2 depict the development of MAP changes not only as a function of recording site, paced cycle length, and duration of ischemia, but also by degree of flow reduction (ranging from 80% to 100%). The more severe the myocardial flow reduction was, the earlier the above-described MAP changes (and their temporal and spatial dispersion) occurred and the more rapidly they progressed.

Time Course and Spatial (In)Congruence of Electrical Restitution Curves Before and During Ischemia

To further elucidate the role of cycle length in ischemic APD alternans development, we determined the normal and ischemic interbeat dependence of APD by determining the electrical restitution curve (ERC). The ERC describes the APD dependence over a range of single cycle length changes, from the most premature beat to the one following a long pause.[11] The ERC therefore is a useful means to describe the immediate effects of cycle length changes on the subsequent APD. As shown previously,[12] the ERC relates not only to changes in cycle length but more specifically to changes in the electrical diastolic interval, which is important to consider for understanding the beat-to-beat changes in APD during electrical alternans.

Normal ERCs showed a steep initial recovery phase which turned into a plateau at premature cycle lengths of approximately 300 milliseconds and thereafter remained fairly constant. During normal perfusion, ERCs at the 3 different recording sites were nearly superimposable (Fig. 4). Global ischemia induced significant changes in ERCs. Ischemia produced a flattening of the initial ERC slope and this flattening progressed with continuing ischemia (Fig. 5). Furthermore, with progressing ischemia, ERCs were shifted rightward (toward longer cycle lengths) and downward (toward shorter APDs). Thus, the shortening response of APD to ischemia

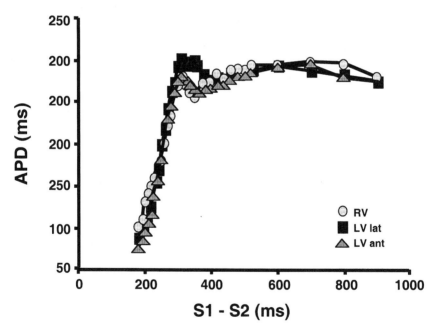

Figure 4. Example of ERCs recorded simultaneously at 3 different epicardial sites during normal perfusion at a basic CL of 500 m. The ERCs exhibit a steep initial recovery phase with complete APD recovery at an S1-S2 interval of approximately 300 m. APD remained stable for the entire range of S1-S2 intervals up to 900 m. APD = action potential duration; ERC = electrical restitution curve; BCL = basic cycle length; RV = right ventricle; LV lat = left lateral ventricle; LV ant = left anterior ventricle; S1-S2 = test cycle length. Reproduced from Reference 9, with permission.

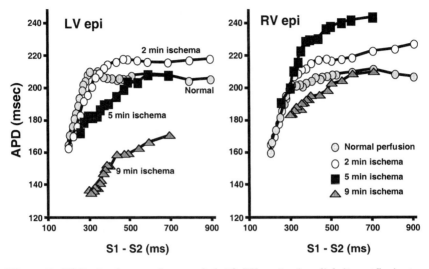

Figure 5. ERCs simultaneously recorded at 3 different epicardial sites at 5 minutes of ischemia. The time coiurses of the ERCs diferend significantly from each other. The disparity between of the ischemic ERCs increased tooward shorter S1-S2 intervals and ws most pronounced between the RV and either LV recording sites. APD = action potential duration; ERC = electrical restitution curve; S1-S2 = test cycle length; RV = right ventricle; LV ;lat = left lateral ventricle; LV ant = left anterior ventricle. Reproduced from Reference 9, with permision.

increased and also began at longer cycle lengths. Importantly, during ischemia, the time courses of the ERCs at the 3 recording sites differed significantly from each other, providing grounds for the increased spatial dispersion seen in APD and alternans during regular pacing.[9]

Link Between Impaired Electrical Restitution and APD Alternans

The occurrence of APD alternans during myocardial ischemia coincided with a flattening of the time course of the ERC.[9] The decreased slope of the initial phase of the ERC indicates incomplete recovery of APD, which fell short significantly of the APD reached at the same cycle length under nonischemic conditions. Thus, more time is needed for APD to reach its steady state value and, therefore, APD recovery becomes more dependent on the duration of the preceding diastolic interval. Since the ERC is a function of the electrical diastolic interval,[12] the ischemia-induced delay in electrical restitution can explain the development of persistent APD alternans (Fig. 6). While the rapid time course of the normal ERC ensures complete APD recovery from one beat to the next, even at fast heart rates, incomplete recovery of APD during ischemia sets the stage

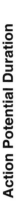

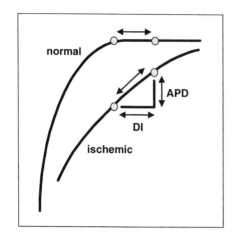

Action Potential Duration

Diastolic Interval

Figure 6. Suggested mechanism of electrical alternans based on the flattening of the ERC. The rapid time course of the normal ERC ensures complete APD recovery from one beat to the next. Incomplete recovery of APD during ischemia sets the stage for alternating longer and shorter action potentials. Because electrical restitituon is a function of the preceding diastolic interval, shortening of APD at a given CL entails reciprocal lengthening of the subsequent diastolic interval, which in turn legthens the subsequent APD and shortens the following diastolic interval. The slow recovery time course during ischemia perpetuates the alternans of APD and diastolic interval as the APD moves up and down the slope of ERC without ever reaching full recovery. ERC = electrical restitution curve; APD = action potential duration; CL = cycle length. Reproduced from Reference 9, with permission.

for alternating longer and shorter action potentials. Shortening of APD at a given cycle length entails reciprocal lengthening of the subsequent diastolic interval which, in turn, lengthens the subsequent APD and shortens the following diastolic interval. The slow recovery time course during ischemia, with an ERC slope of near unity, perpetuates the alternans of APD and diastolic interval as the APD moves up and down the slope of the ERC without ever reaching full recovery (Fig. 6).

Possible Ionic Mechanisms

Ischemia produced flattening of the slope of the ERC, indicating a slowed recovery of membrane gating variables from previous excitation and inactivation. In addition, ischemia caused a downward shift of the ERC. The downward shift could be due to extracellular potassium ion accumulation, which is increased during ischemia,[13] as APD bears an inverse relationship to the extracellular potassium ion concentration. Ischemia also causes an increase in the intracellular calcium ion concentration that may shorten the APD by activation of the potassium outward current or by an electrogenic Na^+-Ca^{++} exchange.[14] The downward shift of the ERC during ischemia likewise may reflect increases in intracellularly stored calcium ions. Other means of increasing intracellular activator calcium, such as increasing the extracellular calcium ion concentration or rapid pacing, also shift the ERC downward and flatten its time course.[15]

Clinical Importance of APD Alternans During Ischemia

Electrical alternans in the setting of ischemia was first demonstrated by Hellerstein and Liebow[16] and confirmed by others.[17] These authors documented a high incidence of ST segment and TWAs of the electrocardiogram occurring early upon coronary occlusion. Investigations of the intracellular electrical activity have demonstrated alternans of both duration and amplitude of ischemic action potentials that accompany ST segment and TWAs.[18-20] The clinical and electrophysiologic significance of APD alternans lies in its close relationship to ischemia-induced arrhythmias. Several groups have shown that VTA during acute myocardial ischemia is preceded immediately by a period of APD alternans, suggesting a causal relationship between the two.[1,18-20] Abe and coworkers[1] were able to show in canine hearts that the occurrence of arrhythmias during single coronary occlusion was much more common when there was a greater magnitude of alternans and regional dispersion of repolarization.

Ischemia-Induced Dispersion of Repolarization and its Relation to the Inducibility of Ventricular Tachyarrhythmias

To gain further insight into the relationship between ischemia-induced APD alternans and the overall effect on dispersion of ventricular repolarization, hearts were paced continuously with regular stimuli at a cycle length of 500 milliseconds. During normal perfusion and ischemia, conduction time and APD were measured sequentially and the developing disparities were calculated as the differences between simultaneous recordings. The sum of conduction time and APD was defined as the total repolarization time (TRT). Dispersion of conduction time, APD, and TRT was defined as the greatest difference between the respective parameter, and was calculated by subtracting the smallest value from the greatest value of 3 simultaneous recordings. In addition, the effect of programmed extrastimulation on the generation of VTA, defined as an episode of 3 or more successive ventricular depolarizations, was studied.

Effect of Global Ischemia on Dispersion of Conduction Time, APD, and TRT

Under normal perfusion, the dispersion for the measured parameters conduction time, APD, and TRT, was negligible. During ischemia, however, the dispersion of conduction time and APD increased markedly (Fig. 7). The contributions of conduction time and APD to dispersion of TRT were variable, depending on their different time courses. The dispersion of conduction time and APD could either partially compensate or further augment the dispersion of the other single parameter. Overall, the dispersion of TRT increased in a nearly linear fashion during a 10-minute period of complete ischemia (Fig. 7).[7]

Inducibility of Ventricular Tachyarrhythmias

Spontaneous VTA did not occur during normal conditions or during global ischemia in any preparation and could not be induced by extrastimulation during normal perfusion. Under ischemic conditions, however, VTA

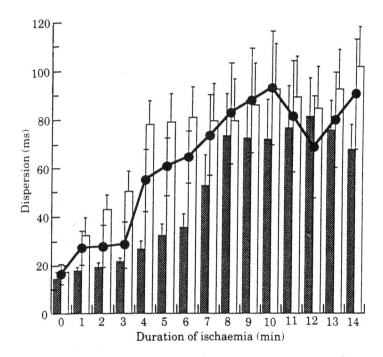

Figure 7. Development of dispersion of CT, APD, and TRT between the 3 recording sites during 14 minutes of global ischemia. Dispersion was calculated as the maximum difference of the respective parameter between two recording sites. Dispersion of TRT remained within the range of the dispersion of the single parameters CT and APD, indicating that dispersion of CT and APD are not adding up but rather partially compensating for each other, depending on their different time course during ischemia. CT = conduction time (filled bars); APD = action potential duration at 70% of repolarization (open bars); TRT = total repolarization time (filled circles with lines). Reproduced from Reference 7, with permission.

could be induced by extrastimulation. The dispersion in TRT of the last regular beat preceding VTA was significantly greater compared to normal conditions. A highly significant correlation was found between the inducibility of arrhythmias and the effects of extrastimulation on the dispersion of conduction time. Extrastimulation that failed to induce VTA resulted in a small increase in dispersion of conduction time compared to the preceding steady state beat. However, extrastimulation that triggered VTA showed a more than 2-fold increase of dispersion of conduction time compared to the last steady-state beat, indicating marked slowing of conduction at 1 of the 3 recording sites.[7]

An increased dispersion in repolarization within ischemic myocardium was suggested as early as 1958 and has been proposed to be causally related to VTA.[21] Marked dispersion of the refractory periods has been observed in adjacent regions during the early phase of ischemia.[22] The vulnerability of ventricular myocardium to arrhythmias increases with the rise in temporal and spatial dispersion of refractoriness.[23] In our experiments of global ischemia, dispersion of TRT increased in a relatively linear fashion after perfusion stop. Extrastimulation could induce VTA only during ischemia, when preparations were characterized by a significantly increased dispersion of TRT.[7] Comparable data were provided by Kuo and coworkers[24] who have used regional cooling to produce dispersion of repolarization. These authors also showed that VTA could be induced by extrastimulation, in the settings of increased heterogeneity of repolarization.[7,24]

Conclusions and Clinical Implications

While global ischemia as in these experiments is not a common manifestation of coronary artery disease, our results may be relevant to clinical conditions such as low-output heart failure, dilative cardiomyopathy, or diffuse coronary artery disease. As in our experimental model, in these clinical conditions of global reduction in coronary perfusion, inhomogeneous myocardial ischemia may result from differences in ventricular wall thickness, transmural perfusion pressure, ventricular strain, and ventricular geometry.

We found APD alternans to be a sensitive parameter for ischemia, depending on both duration and severity of underperfusion and preload. The effect of cycle length on APD alternans seems to be functionally separate from the effect of cycle length on the ischemic burden. A considerable delay in electrical restitution has been found during ischemia and may constitute a pivotal factor for a disturbed relationship between APD and cycle length and for the generation of ischemic APD alternans. The arrhythmogenic potential of the temporal and spatial heterogeneity of electrophysiologic properties of the ischemic heart was further corroborated in our experiments by the demonstration that VTA induction by extrastimulation was greatly facilitated by the ischemia-induced dispersion of repolarization and conduction.

Acknowledgments The author is indebted to his mentors, in particular KH Tragl.

References

1. Abe S, Nagamoto Y, Fukuchi Y, et al. Relationship of alternans of monophasic action potential and conduction delay inside the ischemic border zone to serious ventricular arrhythmia during acute myocardial ischemia in dogs. *Am Heart J* 1989;117:1223-1233.
2. Dilly SG, Lab MJ. Electrophysiological alternans and restitution during acute regional ischaemia in myocardium of anaesthetized pig. *J Physiol (Lond)* 1988;402:315-333.
3. Nearing BD, Huang AH, Verrier RL. Dynamic tracking of cardiac vulnerability by complex demodulation of the T wave. *Science* 1991;252:437-440.
4. Verrier RL, Nearing BD. Electrophysiologic basis for T wave alternans as an index of vulnerability to ventricular fibrillation. *J Cardiovasc Electrophysiol* 1994;5:445-461.
5. Janse MJ, van Capelle FJL, Morsink H, et al. Flow of "injury" current and patterns of excitation during early ventricular arrhythmias in acute regional myocardial ischemia in isolated porcine and canine hearts. Evidence for 2 different arrhythmogenic mechanisms. *Circ Res* 1980;47:151-165.
6. Janse MJ, Wit AL. Electrophysiological mechanisms of ventricular arrhythmias resulting from myocardial ischemia and infarction. *Physiol Rev* 1989; 69:1049-1069.
7. Kurz RW, Xiao-Lin R, Franz MR. Increased dispersion of ventricular repolarization and ventricular tachyarrhythmias in the globally ischaemic rabbit heart. *Eur Heart J* 1993;14:1561-1571.
8. Kurz RW, Mohabir R, Ren XL, Franz MR. Ischaemia induced alternans of action potential duration in the intact heart: Dependence on coronary flow, preload and cycle length [see comments]. *Eur Heart J* 1993;14:1410-1420.
9. Kurz RW, Ren XL, Franz MR. Dispersion and delay of electrical restitution in the globally ischaemic heart. *Eur Heart J* 1994;15:547-554.
10. Franz MR. Long-term recording of monophasic action potentials from human endocardium. *Am J Cardiol* 1983;51:1629-1634.
11. Bass BG. Restitution of the action potential in cat papillary muscle. *Am J Physiol* 1975;228:1717-1724.
12. Franz MR, Schaefer J, Schottler M, et al. Electrical and mechanical restitution of the human heart at different rates of stimulation. *Circ Res* 1983;53:815-822.
13. Weiss J, Shine KI. Efects of heart rate on extracellular [K+] accumulation during myocardial ischemia. *Am J Physiol* 1986;250:H982-H991.
14. Lee HC, Mohabir R, Smith N, et al. Effect of ischemia on calcium-dependent fluorescence transients in rabbit hearts containing ino 1. Correlation with monophasic action potentials and ontraction. *Circulation.* 1988;78:1047-1059.
15. Boyett MR, Jewell BR. A study of the factors responsible for rate-dependent shortening of the action potential in mammalian ventricular muscle. *J Physiol* 1978;285:359-380.

16. Hellerstein HK, Liebow IM. Electrical alternation in experimental coronary artery occlusion. *Am J Physiol* 1950;160:366-374.
17. Hoffman BF, Suckling EE. Effect of heart rate on cardiac membrane potentials and the unipolar electrogram. *Am J Physiol* 1954;179:123-130.
18. Downar E, Janse MJ, Durrer D. The effect of acute coronary artery occlusion on subepicardial transmembrane potentials in the intact porcine heart. *Circulation* 1977;56:217-224.
19. Lab MJ, Woollard KV. Monophasic action potentials, electrocardiograms and mechanical performance in normal and ischaemic epicardial segments of the pig ventricle in situ. *Cardiovasc Res* 1978;12:555-565.
20. Hashimoto H, Nakashima M. Effects of calcium antagonists on the alternation of the ST-T complex and associated conduction abnormalities during coronary occlusion in dogs. *Br J Pharmacol* 1981;74:373-380.
21. Cranefield PF, Hoffman BF. Propagated repolarization in heart muscle. *J Gen Physiol* 1958;41:633-649.
22. Kimura S, Bassett AL, Kohya T, et al. Simultaneous recrding of action potentials from endocardium during ischemia in the isolated cat ventricle: Relation of temporal electrophysiologic heterogeneities to arrhythmias. *Circulation* 1986;74:401-409.
23. Kuo CS, reddy CP. Manukata K, Surawicz B. Mechanism of ventricular arrhythmias caused by increased dispersion of repolarization. *Eur Heart J* 1985;6(Suppl D):63-70.
24. Kuo CS, Munakata K, Reddy CP, Surawicz B. Characteristics and possible mechanisms of ventricular arrhythmia dependent on the dispersion of action potential durations *Circulation* 1983;67:1356-1367.

14

The Role of Cytosolic Calcium in Electrical and Mechanical Alternans During Ischemia

William T. Clusin, MD, PhD

APD Alternans During Ischemia

A major factor leading to the genesis of ventricular fibrillation (VF) during ischemia is spatial and temporal nonuniformity of the ventricular action potential from beat to beat. Action potential duration (APD) alternans during experimental coronary artery occlusion was first observed in 1977, in floating microelectrode recordings from in situ hearts.[1-5] All of these studies reported alternans in the duration and/or amplitude of action potentials during ischemia.

Action potential alternans is correlated with and is an important cause of T wave alternans on the surface electrogram (the other cause is 2:1 conduction block). T wave alternans directly precedes the onset of VF during experimental ischemia. T wave alternans is known to occur in the region of myocardium where blood flow is compromised, and can be confined to small regions within the ischemic zone.[6] Whenever T wave alternans occurs, there is dispersion of refractoriness that is believed to be an important precondition for development of VF.

Figure 1 shows simultaneous recordings of the epicardial electrogram and transmembrane potential obtained with a floating microelectrode in an ischemic pig heart. At 3.5 minutes of ischemia there is marked beat-to-beat alternation in APD, without any change in action potential upstroke

From Franz MR (ed): *Monophasic Action Potentials: Bridging Cell and Bedside.* ©Futura Publishing Company, Inc., Armonk, NY, 2000.

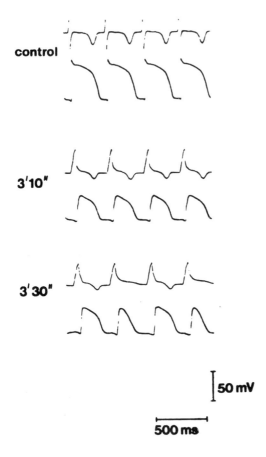

Figure 1. Representation of T wave alternans and action potential duration (APD) alternans recorded with a floating microelectrode in a porcine heart during coronary artery occlusion. Transmembrane potentials are shown in the lower trace, and local extracellular electrograms in the upper trace. Marked T wave alternans and APD alternans are evident at 3 minutes and 30 seconds of ischemia. From Reference 1.

control

3'10"

3'30"

50 mV

500 ms

or amplitude. This is associated with T wave alternans on the surface electrogram. The type of result shown in Figure 1 suggests that ischemia has altered the transmembrane currents that control repolarization in individual myocardial cells. This type of result would not be indicative of conduction block.

Recent research on the genesis of VF has suggested an additional mechanism by which the result shown in Figure 1 could lead to VF. It is known that onset of VF is caused by the development of rotors, which break up at the periphery due to 2:1 conduction block. Creation of multiple subsidiary rotors (daughter rotors) leads to chaos on the electrocardiogram. Conduction block in a reentry circuit is often preceded by period alternans, which is a manifestation of APD alternans. APD alternans can also lead to R wave alternans, which reflects variations in conduction velocity due to variation in sodium channel availability. Both of these phenomena have been described in an experimental model of ischemic VF.[7]

Measurement of $[Ca^{++}]_i$ During Experimental Ischemia

In the mid 1970s it was discovered that ionic currents in excitable cells can be controlled (ie, gated) by free calcium acting at the inner surface of the cell membrane.[8] This observation led to the hypothesis that effects of ischemia on the action potential could be mediated by abnormalities of cytosolic calcium ($[Ca^{++}]_i$). Measurement of $[Ca^{++}]_i$ in myocardial cells first became practical around 1980, when it became possible to inject aequorin into the cytoplasm of cardiac myocytes. Measurement of $[Ca^{++}]_i$ in cardiac cells became much easier with the development of tetracarboxylate calcium indicators that can be loaded into cells as cell-permeant acetoxymethyl esters. The first recordings of $[Ca^{++}]_i$ transients from intact, arterially perfused hearts were obtained using indo-1 AM and reported in 1987.[9] Nine laboratories have now used this technique and more than 25 papers on the subject have been published.

Effects of stop-flow ischemia on the $[Ca^{++}]_i$ transient in a saline-perfused rabbit heart loaded with indo-1 are shown in Figure 2. The top trace is the monophasic action potential (MAP) recorded with the Franz MAP electrode, and the lower trace is the ratio of fluorescence emissions at 400 and 550 nm (F_{400} and F_{550}, respectively). An increase in $[Ca^{++}]_i$ increases fluorescence at 400 nm and decreases fluorescence at 550 nm. The F_{400} to F_{550} ratio is therefore especially sensitive to $[Ca^{++}]_i$. The normal $[Ca^{++}]_i$ transient has a brisk upstroke, and decays throughout the interval between beats. After 90 seconds of ischemia (right panel) there is a reduction in resting membrane potential, shown by the MAP recording, and an upward shift in the systolic and diastolic level of the $[Ca^{++}]_i$ transient. Broadening of the $[Ca^{++}]_i$ transient is also observed. An increase in the systolic and diastolic level of $[Ca^{++}]_i$, together with broadening of the $[Ca^{++}]_i$ transient have been observed during comparable periods of low-flow ischemia in rat hearts loaded with indo-1.[10,11]

The effects of longer periods of ischemia on $[Ca^{++}]_i$ are shown in Figure 3, which shows averaged data from 5 hearts, all paced at 150 to 180 beats/min. Values shown represent peak systolic $[Ca^{++}]_i$. There is an initial increase in $[Ca^{++}]_i$, which reaches a peak at 90 seconds. Between 2 and 5 minutes of ischemia, there is a fall in systolic $[Ca^{++}]_i$, which is probably due to conduction block, and a resultant fall in action potential frequency. Between 5 and 10 minutes of ischemia, there is a secondary increase in $[Ca^{++}]_i$. An increase in $[Ca^{++}]_i$ by 10 minutes of ischemia has been reported in all studies that used a $[Ca^{++}]_i$ indicator.

A major drawback of the indo-1 technique is that it cannot be used in the presence of blood, due to absorption of the ultraviolet illumination and blue-green emission light by hemoglobin. This problem has recently

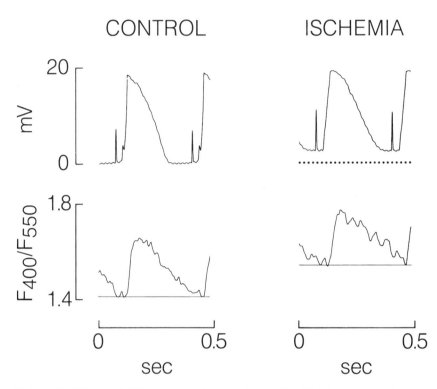

Figure 2. Effects of 90 seconds of ischemia on the $[Ca^{++}]_i$ transient (bottom trace) and MAP (top trace). Ischemia caused reduction of the resting potential and broadening of the action potential. Ischemia also increased both the peak systolic and end-diastolic level of the $[Ca^{++}]_i$ transient and caused broadening of the peak. From Reference 29.

been solved by the development of long wavelength fluorescent $[Ca^{++}]_i$ indicators that can also be loaded into cardiac cells as cell-permeant acetoxymethyl esters. Recordings of high-quality $[Ca^{++}]_i$ transients during baseline and ischemic conditions were recently obtained in blood-perfused rabbit hearts, with use of the long wavelength $[Ca^{++}]_i$ indicator Fura Red (Molecular Probes, Eugene, OR).[12] In contrast to indo-1, Fura Red fluorescence is measured at a single emission peak (>645 nm), and decreases as a result of an increase in $[Ca^{++}]_i$ (Fig. 4, middle trace). The bottom trace in Figure 4 shows reflected excitation light (F_{546}). The degree of motion artifact is small, and can be corrected by electronic computation of the $F_{>645}/F_{546}$ ratio (top trace). The value of this ratio (and hence $[Ca^{++}]_i$) does not change when the perfusate is switched from blood to saline and back.

The methodology for recording $[Ca^{++}]_i$ transients with Fura Red has recently been adapted to the open chest in vivo porcine heart through the invention of special apparatus for limiting motion of the probe with respect

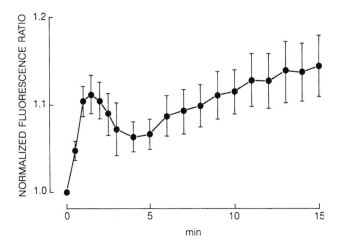

Figure 3. Effect of ischemia on peak systolic $[Ca^{++}]_i$ in 5 hearts loaded with indo-1. Data points show the peak systolic value of the $[Ca^{++}]_i$-dependent fluorescence emission ratio (F_{400}/F_{550}). The ratio value from each heart is normalized to the corresponding ratio at the onset of ischemia. Ischemia produces a prompt increase in peak systolic $[Ca^{++}]_i$ by about 2 minutes of ischemia. This is followed by a gradual decline in $[Ca^{++}]_i$ between 2 and 5 minutes, and then a progressive secondary rise between 5 and 15 minutes. From Reference 30.

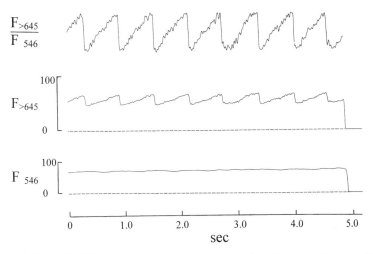

Figure 4. Fura Red fluorescence transients from a blood perfused heart. Blood is oxygenated and diluted 30%. Heart is illuminated at 546 nm. Middle trace shows fluorescence at greater than 645 nm ($F_{>645}$). Fluorescence levels are reduced from preblood values by absorbance of excitation light (preblood end-diastolic value = 100%). Bottom trace shows reflected excitation light F_{546}. Motion artifact is seen to be very small. Top trace shows the $F_{>645}/F_{546}$ ratio. Ratio is unchanged on switching from saline to blood. This indicates that there is no associated change in $[Ca^{++}]_i$. From Reference 12.

to the heart surface.[13] Recordings obtained from the in vivo heart were not qualitatively different from those in Langendorff-perfused rabbit hearts. This technology should permit measurement of $[Ca^{++}]_i$ during regional ischemia produced by coronary artery occlusion.

$[Ca^{++}]_i$ Transient Alternans During Ischemia

Beat-to-beat $[Ca^{++}]_i$ transients remain uniform throughout the first minute of ischemia. However, during the second or third minute of ischemia, a characteristic pattern of alternans develops, in which the amplitude of every other transient is diminished, and arises from a higher end-diastolic level. The smaller transients are therefore followed by a more complete decay. Panel A of Figure 5 shows the pattern of alternans recorded from the epicardial surface of a saline-perfused rabbit heart loaded with indo-1. The duration of ischemia is 3 minutes A similar recording, obtained in a blood-perfused heart with Fura Red, is shown in panel B. This result is qualitatively very similar, except that a rise in $[Ca^{++}]_i$ produces a decrease in the fluorescence ratio.

The pattern of alternans is stable at any given site on the ventricular epicardial surface. However, if the fiber optic probe is moved rapidly to a different site during a continuous recording, the pattern may reverse, so that if odd-numbered transients were larger at the first site, they are smaller at the second site. This observation indicates that the alternans behavior of the Ca transients in a particular region is independent of the behavior in other regions, which results in spatial heterogeneity of the $[Ca^{++}]_i$ transient during ischemia.

Effect of Blood Perfusion on $[Ca^{++}]_i$ Transient Alternans

With use of Fura Red, Wu and Clusin[12] recently compared the effects of ischemia in saline-perfused versus blood-perfused rabbit hearts. Effects of ischemia in blood-perfused hearts were similar to those in saline-perfused hearts. However, the incidence and magnitude of $[Ca^{++}]_i$ transient alternans was much greater in the blood-perfused hearts. To quantify the magnitude of $[Ca^{++}]_i$ transient alternans in saline-perfused versus blood-perfused hearts, an alternans ratio was defined as $1 - B/A$, where A is the net amplitude (end-diastolic value to peak systolic value) of the taller transient, and B is the net amplitude of the smaller transient. To determine the alternans ratio, the 8 consecutive beats with the largest degree of alternans (ie, 4 consecutive pairs of beats) were identified, and the resulting

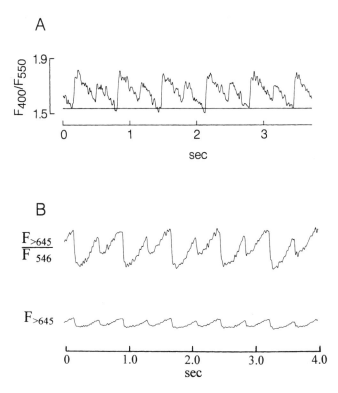

Figure 5. **A**. Alternans of $[Ca^{++}]_i$ transients after 3 minutes of ischemia. Recording is from a saline-perfused rabbit heart loaded with indo-1. Even-numbered beats had smaller $[Ca^{++}]_i$ transients that arose from a higher end-diastolic level and were followed by a more complete decay. From Reference 29. **B**. Similar recording obtained from a blood-perfused heart loaded with Fura Red. Transients are downgoing because a $[Ca^{++}]_i$ increase causes a decrease in Fura Red fluorescence.

alternans ratios were averaged. Alternans occurred in 9 of 11 blood-perfused ischemic hearts (82%) and in 6 of 14 saline-perfused hearts (43%). The mean alternans ratio was 22.8±4.5% in the blood-perfused hearts versus 7.3±2.6% in the saline-perfused hearts ($P<0.005$). These results indicate that occurrence of alternans is greatly potentiated by the presence of blood. This result highlights the importance of studying ischemia-induced VF in a blood-perfused heart.

The fact that blood perfusion greatly increases the incidence and magnitude of $[Ca^{++}]_i$ transient alternans during ischemia suggests that some substance released from blood cells might mediate the development of alternans. Several substances present in blood that are capable of increasing $[Ca^{++}]_i$ in cardiac myocytes have been identified. These include thrombin,[14] endothelin,[15] and platelet-release products.[16] Of these substances, platelet-release products may produce $[Ca^{++}]_i$ transient alternans when applied to spontaneously beating embryonic myocardial cells.

Figure 6 shows an experiment in which a spontaneously beating chick embryonic myocardial cell aggregate has been exposed to a filtrate of platelet-release products produced by activation of the platelets with thrombin. The thrombin inhibitor PPACK was added to prevent direct action of thrombin on the myocardial cells. The platelet filtrate caused an increase in both the systolic and end-diastolic levels of the transients, along with spontaneous $[Ca^{++}]_i$ transient alternans.

The specific platelet release product responsible for the effects on $[Ca^{++}]_i$ was partly characterized by Chien et al.[16] The effects on $[Ca^{++}]_i$ were not mimicked by a thromboxane analog, or by several substances known to be released from platelets, including ADP, serotonin, or platelet-activating factor. The responsible product was heat-sensitive, trypsin-sensitive, and partitioned into the aqueous phase of a chloroform suspension. Its molecular weight was less than 3 kD. Protease inhibitor appeared to prolong its activity. These results suggest that trypsin-sensitive peptide(s) released from platelets can cause $[Ca^{++}]_i$ transient alternans in cardiac myocytes.

In general, the phenomenon of alternans is very prominently described in studies involving blood-perfused or in vivo hearts, especially during ischemia. While APD alternans can be observed in saline-perfused hearts, superfused papillary muscles, or dissociated cardiac cells, the phenomenon is much less readily observed in such settings. These observations underscore the limitations of various ex vivo models of cardiac ischemia, and the possible role of blood elements in the pathogenesis of VF.

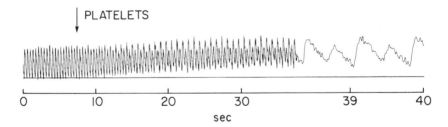

Figure 6. Effect of platelet filtrate on calcium transients in a spontaneously beating chick heart cell aggregate loaded with indo-1. Cell free platelet release products were obtained from rabbit platelets activated with thrombin. A thrombin inhibitor (PPACK) was then added to block direct effects of thrombin on the platelets. The platelet filtrate caused an increase in both systolic and end-diastolic levels of the transients. In addition, there was development of spontaneous $[Ca^{++}]_i$ transient alternans, resembling what occurs in the indo-1 or Fura Red-loaded rabbit heart during stop-flow ischemia. Chien et al, unpublished observations. Methods described in Reference 17.

Mechanical Alternans During Ischemia

[Ca^{++}]$_i$ transient alternans during ischemia is manifested physiologically as *both* APD alternans and contraction alternans. Contraction alternans can be recorded using an intracavitary balloon in the left ventricle, or using an epicardial strain gauge transducer. Examples of both types of recordings, obtained simultaneously, are shown in Figure 7.

Ischemia produces a rapid reduction in contraction strength that begins within seconds of cessation of perfusion. Developed pressure falls to half of the normal amount in approximately 20 seconds. This reduction in contraction strength must be due to reduced sensitivity of the myofilaments to calcium, because there is no associated diminution of the [Ca^{++}]$_i$ transient.

Very weak contractions (10% to 15% of normal) typically persist for several minutes and usually exhibit alternans. As seen in Figure 7, this

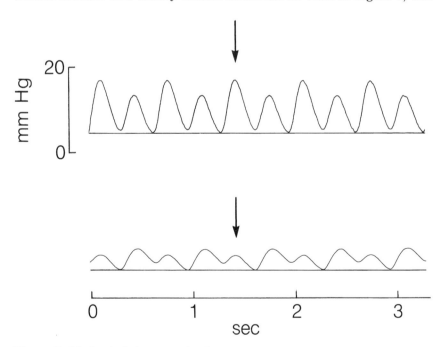

Figure 7. Mechanical alternans after 3 minutes of ischemia. Contractions recorded by an intracavitary balloon (top trace) have been displayed on the same time scale as local contractions recorded by an epicardial strain gauge transducer (bottom trace). The alternans pattern was similar in the two recordings, but was out of phase, so that strong contractions recorded by the balloon (top arrow) coincided with weak contractions recorded by the strain gauge (bottom arrow). From Reference 29.

alternans involves both the peak systolic and end-diastolic levels of force. Alternans of diastolic force is much more prominent in the epicardial recording obtained with the strain gauge. These alternations in diastolic force are almost certainly reflective of the alternations in end-diastolic $[Ca^{++}]_i$ that have been discovered through the use of fluorescent $[Ca^{++}]_i$ indicators.

As noted above, alternans of $[Ca^{++}]_i$ transients can exhibit spatial nonuniformity. The nonuniformity of the $[Ca^{++}]_i$ transients is associated with similar variations in contraction strength. In Figure 7, alternans is observed in both the left ventricular pressure recording (top trace) and in contractions recorded by the epicardial strain gauge transducer (bottom trace), which has an interpin distance of 4 mm. However, as indicated by the arrows, the pattern of alternans is out of phase in the two recordings so that the weak contractions recorded by the strain gauge correspond to strong contractions recorded from the entire ventricle. This result indicates that fluctuations in contraction strength during alternans occur independently in localized regions of the heart so that the pattern recorded by the intracavitary balloon represents a net imbalance in the summated activity of different regions. This interpretation has been confirmed by simultaneous recordings with two strain gauge transducers.

Ionic Basis of APD Alternans

The presumptive connection between $[Ca^{++}]_i$ transient alternans, action potential alternans, and VF is that $[Ca^{++}]_i$ regulates membrane currents that control APD. As discussed below, two types of calcium-activated currents have been described in the heart: calcium-activated inward currents, which would tend to lengthen the action potential, and calcium-activated outward currents, which would tend to abbreviate the action potential. The first step in determining which type of currents are involved is to establish, in the same population of cells, whether the alternans is concordant or discordant. Concordant alternans, in which the longer action potentials coincide with the larger calcium transients, implies that fluctuations in $[Ca^{++}]_i$-activated inward current are predominantly involved. Discordant alternans, in which the briefer action potentials coincide with the smaller calcium transients, implies that fluctuations in $[Ca^{++}]_i$-activated outward current are involved.

The relationship between calcium transient and action potential alternans can be studied by combined use of fluorescent calcium indicators and the MAP technique. Figure 8 shows MAPs recorded from a rabbit heart after 2 minutes of ischemia. MAPs alternate between long duration and brief duration, with no change in amplitude or upstroke. As in Figure 1,

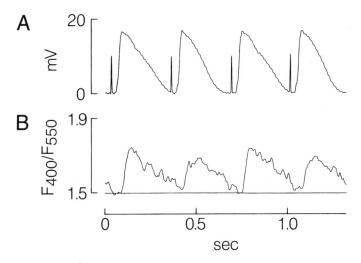

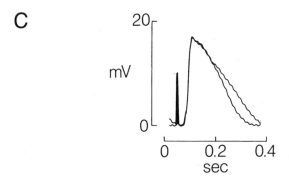

Figure 8. A. Simultaneous [Ca^{++}]$_i$ transients and MAPs after 2 minutes of ischemia. MAP duration and the amplitude of the [Ca^{++}]$_i$ transient both alternate from beat to beat. **C.** Photographic superimposition of long and short action potentials from A. Action potentials were nearly identical during the first 80 milliseconds and did not diverge until after the [Ca^{++}]$_i$ transient had reached its peak. **B.** [Ca^{++}]$_i$ transients from the same experiment as A. Transients are simultaneous with the MAPs in A, but the MAPs are obtained from a small region of myocardium centered 3 mm outside the illuminated region. Action potential duration and [Ca^{++}]$_i$ transient alternans are concordant, but this has not been established at the cellular level. From Reference 29.

this result indicates that there is no conduction block at this stage of ischemia.

Panel B of Figure 8 shows $[Ca^{++}]_i$ transients recorded from the same ischemic heart as in panels A and C. Recordings were obtained at the same time as those in panel A, except that the MAP catheter was 3 mm from the edge of the illuminated region from which the transients were obtained. As a result, the two recordings are not from the same population of cells. Alternans in Figure 8 is concordant: the more prolonged action potentials accompany the larger $[Ca^{++}]_i$ transients. However, to be certain that this relationship holds at the cellular level, the apparatus must be modified so that both signals can be recorded from the same population of cells. An apparatus with this capability is currently being developed.[17]

At least 3 types of calcium-activated ion currents are known to exist in cardiac cells and have been studied extensively at the cellular level. These are as follows: 1) An outward calcium-activated chloride current definitely contributes to early (phase 1) repolarization.[18,19] 2) An electrogenic sodium/calcium exchange causes inward current in cells at diastolic membrane potentials. 3) Nonselective calcium-activated cation channels have been described that are equally permeant to sodium and potassium.[20,21] Activation of these channels would depolarize resting cells and would produce action potential prolongation.

Which of the above currents has the predominant action depends on experimental conditions. Calcium-activated inward currents are best demonstrated when the membrane potential is close to the resting potential. The best examples of such currents are the transient inward currents induced by caffeine[22] or digitalis toxicity.[23] In these situations, there is abnormal release of calcium from the sarcoplasmic reticulum when the membrane potential is close to the resting level. This results in a phasic inward current carried by either nonselective cation channels or electrogenic sodium calcium exchange. In contrast, calcium-activated outward currents have the greatest influence when the membrane is in the plateau range. Activation of such a current will produce marked shortening of the action potential plateau.

An experiment in which a calcium-activated outward current is elicited in a rabbit ventricular cell is depicted in Figure 9. For this experiment, dissociated rabbit ventricular myocytes were loaded with the photo-sensitive calcium chelator Nitr-5. Flash-induced photolysis of Nitr-5 leads to an increase in $[Ca^{++}]_i$, which also augments the stores of calcium that are released from the sarcoplasmic reticulum with each beat. In Figure 9, the calcium released by flash photolysis of Nitr-5 is monitored with the fluorescent $[Ca^{++}]_i$ indicator, fluo-3 (lower trace). As shown in the upper trace, flash photolysis of Nitr-5 produces immediate abbreviation of APD, with subsequent relengthening as $[Ca^{++}]_i$ declines. This abbreviation of the action potential is very likely due to opening of calcium-activated chloride

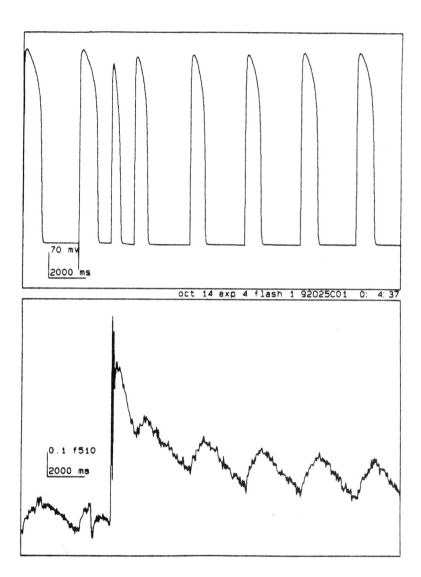

Figure 9. Effects of flash photolysis of Nitr-5 on the action potential and calcium transient as recorded with fluo-3 in an isolated rabbit ventricular myocyte. The action potential, recorded by a whole cell patch pipette, is shown in the upper trace, and the $[Ca^{++}]_i$ transient, recorded by fluo-3, is shown in the lower trace. The abbreviation of the action potential that occurs with photolysis of Nitr-5 may reflect the operation of calcium-activated chloride channels. Courtesy of Mark Anderson. Methods described in Reference 31.

channels, which carry outward current during the action potential plateau, and would accelerate repolarization.[18,19] This hypothesis can be tested in the future by using various anions that are known to block calcium-activated chloride channels. Such experiments could reveal whether phasic activation of specific calcium activated currents is responsible for APD alternans during ischemia.

Clinical Implications

The most important clinical implication of this work is that therapeutic strategies that ameliorate myocardial ischemia, or calcium overload during ischemia, should reduce the incidence of death from VF and produce a corresponding reduction in *overall mortality*. That this can occur in specific groups of patients is well established for coronary bypass surgery, cholesterol biosynthesis inhibitors, and β-adrenergic blockers. Proving such effects with calcium channel blockers has been more difficult because, by unknown mechanisms, these drugs can increase mortality in patients who have poor ventricular function. Giving verapamil or diltiazem to patients who have good ventricular function does not increase overall mortality, and may prevent some episodes of VF, as is known to occur in animals. Whether β-blockers are superior in this group of patients has not been established.

It is important to distinguish between patients who die of VF due to acute ischemia and those who have chronic ventricular arrhythmias due to healed myocardial infarction. The latter arrhythmias are due to slowed conduction at the boundary of the healed infarct, which leads to reentry. Such patients have inducible arrhythmias during programmed stimulation, and slow potentials on signal-averaged electrocardiograms. It was recently shown that such patients have microvolt level T wave alternans that is detectable by spectral analysis of computerized electrocardiograms.[24] This T wave alternans is not due to acute ischemia and probably results from 2:1 conduction block in specific regions of myocardium that are involved by scar. A 2:1 conduction block would lead to absence of calcium transients during blocked beats, but calcium transients during *conducted* beats should remain uniform. Alternation of APD in specific myocardial cells (Fig. 1) is probably not involved.

Patients with recurrent ventricular tachycardia are normally treated with implantable defibrillators, which produce a dramatic reduction in mortality. These patients are different from the much larger group of patients in whom coronary thrombosis and primary VF are the mode of arrhythmic death, to which they are immediately susceptible.

Conclusion

The hypothesis that $[Ca^{++}]_i$ plays a role in the genesis of ischemic VF was originally based on pharmacologic evidence. Pretreatment of animals with either β-adrenergic blockers[25] or calcium channel blockers[26,27] can prevent VF during experimental coronary artery occlusion. These drugs are known to, or can be presumed to, diminish the effects of ischemia on $[Ca^{++}]_i$. In the case of verapamil, suppression of $[Ca^{++}]_i$ transient alternans and its physiologic manifestations has been specifically demonstrated. Conversely, prevention of ischemic VF by diltiazem has been shown not to result from reduction in cardiac work or changes in collateral coronary blood flow.[28]

The above observations suggest that effects of ischemia on calcium-activated membrane current are a direct and perhaps obligatory cause of VF during the acute phase of coronary artery occlusion. Experiments to show which specific ion currents are responsible for APD alternans and to delineate the molecular events that lead to $[Ca^{++}]_i$ transient alternans during ischemia are now more feasible than ever.

References

1. Downar E, Janse MJ, Durrer D. The effects of acute coronary artery occlusion on subepicardial transmembrane potentials in the intact porcine heart. *Circulation* 1977;56:217-224.
2. Kleber AG, Janse MJ, van Capelle FJL, et al. Mechanism and time course of S-T and T-Q segment changes during acute regional myocardial ischemia in pig heart determined by extracellular and intracellular recordings. *Circ Res* 1978;42:603-613.
3. Russell DC, Smith HJ, Oliver MF. Transmembrane potential changes and ventricular fibrillation during repetitive myocardial ischemia in the dog. *Br Heart J* 1979;42:88-96.
4. Cinca J, Janse MJ, Morena H, et al. Mechanism and time course of the early electrical changes during acute coronary occlusion. An attempt to correlate the early ECG changes in man to the cellular electrophysiology in the pig. *Chest* 1980;77:499-505.
5. Penny WJ, Sheridan D. Arrhythmias and cellular electrophysiological changes during myocardial "ischemia" and reperfusion. *Cardiovasc Res* 1983;17:363-372.
6. Carson DL, Cardinal R, Savard P, et al. Characterization of unipolar waveform alternation in acutely ischaemic porcine myocardium. *Cardiovasc Res* 1986;20:521-527.
7. Garfinkle A, Chen P-S, Walker DO, et al. Quasiperiodicity and chaos in cardiac fibrillation. *J Clin Invest* 1997;99:305-314.
8. Clusin W, Spray DC, Bennett MVL. Activation of a voltage insensitive conductance by inward calcium current. *Nature* 1975;256:425-427.
9. Lee H-C, Clusin WT. Cytosolic calcium transients from the beating mammalian heart. *Proc Natl Acad Sci U S A* 1987;84:7793-7797.

10. Figueredo VM, Brandes R, Weiner MW, et al. Endocardial versus epicardial differences of intracellular free calcium under normal and ischemic conditions. *Circ Res* 1993;72:1082-1090.

11. Camacho SA, Figueredo VM, Brandes R, Weiner MW. Ca^{++}-dependent fluorescence transients and phosphate metabolism during low-flow ischemia in rat hearts. *Am J Physiol* 1993;265:H114-H122.

12. Wu Y, Clusin WT. Calcium transient alternans in blood-perfused ischemic hearts: Observations with fluorescent indicator Fura Red. *Am J Physiol* 1997;273:H2161-H2169.

13. Clusin WT, Vriens P, Qian Y-W. Cytosolic calcium transients from in vivo porcine hearts. *J Investig Med* 1998;46:193A.

14. Chien WW, Mohabir R, Clusin WT. Effect of thrombin on calcium homeostasis in chick embryonic heart cells. *J Clin Invest* 1990;85:1436-1443.

15. Lauer MR, Gunn MD, Clusin WT. Endothelin activates voltage-dependent Ca^{2+} current by a G protein-dependent mechanism in rabbit cardiac myocytes. *J Physiol* 1992;448:729-747.

16. Chien WW, Mohabir R, Newman D, et al. Effects of platelet release products on cytosolic calcium in cardiac myocytes. *Biochem Biophys Res Commun* 1990;170:1121-1127.

17. Clusin WT, Han J, Qian YW. Simultaneous recordings of calcium transients and action potentials from small regions of the perfused rabbit heart. *PACE* 1999;22:834. Abstract.

18. Zygmunt AC, Gibbons WR. Calcium-activated chloride current in rabbit ventricular myocytes. *Circ Res* 1991;68:424-437.

19. Zygmunt AC. Intracellular calcium activates a chloride current in canine ventricular myocytes. *Am J Physiol* 1994;267:H1984-H1995.

20. Colquhoun D, Neher E, Reuter H, et al. Inward current channels activated by intracellular Ca^{++} in cultured cardiac cells. *Nature* 1981;294:752-754.

21. Ehara T, Noma A, Ono K. Calcium-activated non-selective cation channels in ventricular cells isolated from adult guinea-pig hearts. *J Physiol* 1988;403:117-133.

22. Clusin WT. Caffeine induces a transient inward current in cultured cardiac cells. *Nature* 1983;301:248-250.

23. Lederer WJ, Tsien RW. Transient inward current underlying arrhythmogenic effects of cardiotonic steroids in Purkinje fibers. *J Physiol* 1976;263:73-100.

24. Estes MA, Michaud G, Zipes DP, et al. Electrical alternans during rest and exercise as predictors of vulnerability to ventricular arrhythmias. *Am J Cardiol* 1997;80:1314-1318.

25. Fearon RE. Propranolol in the prevention of ventricular fibrillation due to experimental coronary artery occlusion. Observations on the mode of action. *Am J Cardiol* 1967;20:222-228.

26. Kaumann AJ, Aramendia P. Prevention of ventricular fibrillation induced by coronary ligation. *J Pharmacol Exp Ther* 1968;164:326-332.

27. Clusin WT, Bristow MR, Baim DS, et al. The effects of diltiazem and reduced serum ionized calcium on ischemic ventricular fibrillation in the dog. *Circ Res* 1982;50:518-526.

28. Clusin WT, Buchbinder M, Ellis AK, et al. Reduction of ischemic depolarization by the calcium channel blocker diltiazem: Correlation with improvement of ventricular conduction and early arrhythmias in the dog. *Circ Res* 1984;54:10-20.

29. Lee H-C, Mohabir R, Smith N, et al. Effect of ischemia on calcium-dependent fluorescence transients in rabbit hearts containing indo-1. *Circulation* 1988;78:1047-1059.
30. Mohabir R, Lee H, Clusin WT. Effects of ischemia and hypercarbic acidosis on calcium transients, contraction and pH_i in perfused rabbit hearts containing indo-1 and BCECF. *Circ Res* 1991;69:1525-1537.
31. Anderson ME, Braun AP, Schulman H, Premack BA. Multifunctional Ca^{++}/calmodulin-dependent protein kinase mediates Ca^{++} induced enhancement of L-type Ca^{++} current in rabbit ventricular myocytes. *Circ Res* 1994;75:854-861.

15

Action Potential Duration Restitution and Graded Response Mechanisms of Ventricular Vulnerability to Reentry and Fibrillation:

Role of Monophasic Action Potential Recordings

Hrayr S. Karagueuzian, PhD,
Young-Hoon Kim, MD, Masaaki Yashima, MD,
Tsu-Juey Wu, MD and Peng-Sheng Chen, MD

Introduction

It is known that ventricular vulnerability to fibrillation is increased during *repetitive* extrastimulation, ie, application of two consecutive premature stimuli (S2-S3). Similarly, vulnerability is also increased when a

This study was supported in part by an NIH Specialized Center of Research (SCOR) Grant for Sudden Death (HL52319), and a FIRST Award (HL50259), from the National Institutes of Health, UC Tobacco Related Disease Research Program (6RT-0020) (H.S.K.) the Electrocardiographic Heartbeat Organization (H.S.K.), an AHA National Center Grant-in-Aid (9750623N) (H.S.K.) the Ralph M. Parsons Foundation, Los Angeles CA, and an AHA Wyeth-Ayerst Established Investigatorship Award (P.-S. C.).

From Franz MR (ed): *Monophasic Action Potentials: Bridging Cell and Bedside.* ©Futura Publishing Company, Inc., Armonk, NY, 2000.

single *strong* premature stimulus (S2) is applied at a critical coupling interval. The onset of fibrillation under these two conditions is triggered by the initiation of reentry. While the cellular mechanism by which a strong S2 initiates a functional reentry in the ventricle, leading to ventricular fibrillation (VF), has been described by us,[1] much work remains to be done in order to elucidate the cellular basis of reentry formation during repetitive extrastimulation by two consecutive S2-S3 stimuli. Using monophasic action potential (MAP) recordings, we provide a tentative mechanism of vulnerability to reentry based on the dynamics of uniform dispersion of repolarization using MAP duration (MAPD) restitution curve kinetics[2,3] and computer simulation of excitable media.[4-6] The steeper the slope of the MAPD restitution curve, the greater the beat-to-beat (dynamic) changes in the repolarization.[7] A short-term increase in the dispersion increases vulnerability to reentry and VF in the normal ventricle without the need for a fixed, preexisting functional, and/or anatomic dispersion or inhomogeneity.[1,4-6,8,9]

"Vulnerability," in the setting of isolated tissue studies, is defined as the ability of the stimulus to initiate reentry. In the in situ heart, vulnerability is defined as the ability of the same stimulus to induce reentry leading to VF.

Methods and Materials

Studies for the testing of the two proposed mechanisms of ventricular vulnerability to reentry (dispersion of repolarization and graded response) were tested in the intact in situ ventricles of open-chest anesthetized dogs and in isolated, superfused canine ventricular tissues. In addition, a computer simulation study on the effects of increased dispersion (gradient) of repolarization on the dynamics of induced reentrant wave fronts (spiral waves) was evaluated based on the Fitz-Hugh Nagumo model of excitation by using the massively parallel connection machine.[4,6]

Dispersion and Vulnerability

Figure 1 shows simultaneous MAP recordings in a representative dog from the right ventricle (RV) and the left ventricle (LV) during S2 (panel A) and S3 (panel B) stimulation, with the S2 fixed 50 milliseconds outside the refractory period of the S1. In both cases, premature stimulation is applied at progressively longer diastolic intervals starting just outside the refractory period. From these recordings we construct MAPD restitution curves of S2 and S3 and compute the temporal and spatial dispersion of MAPD.[2,3]

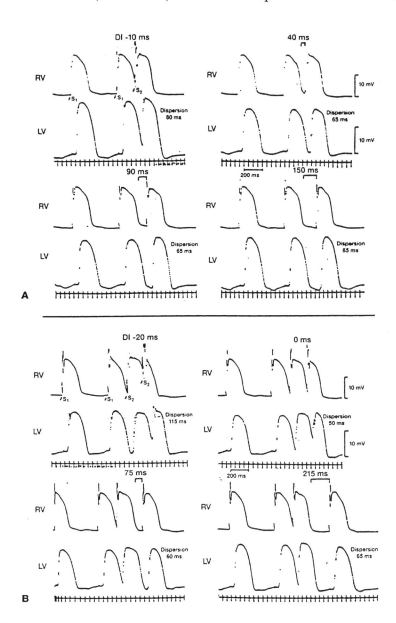

Figure 1. Simultaneous MAP recordings from the endocardium of the right ventricle near the outflow tract (RV) and from the left ventricular apex (LV). **A.** Effects of S2 at progressively longer coupling intervals starting at −10-millisecond diastolic interval (DI) up to 150 milliseconds. **B.** Effects of premature stimulation with an S3 while the S1-S2 coupling interval is fixed. See text for details. From Reference 2, with permission.

Temporal Dispersion of MAPD

At a given site, variations of the MAPD during a given change in the diastolic interval reflect the temporal dispersion at that site in response to a change in activation time (ie, diastolic interval). Figure 2 illustrates MAPD restitution of S2 and S3 at both the RV site (panel A) and the LV site (panel B). As can be seen during the restitution of S3, the range of

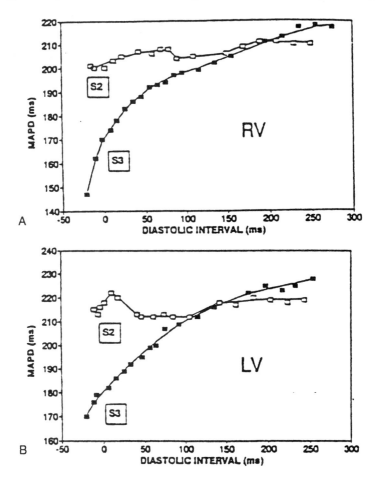

Figure 2. Comparison of monophasic action potential duration (MAPD) restitution curves in the right ventricular endocardium (RV) and the left ventricular apex (LV) in a representative dog. **A.** Restitution of S2 and S3 in the RV. **B.** Restitution of S2 and S3 in the LV. These plots are obtained from recordings such as shown in Figure 5. Note that the steeper slope of the restitution curve during S3 in both the RV and the LV causes a large difference in the MAPD (temporal) with each slight increase in the diastolic interval. For mean quantitative values see Table 1. From Reference 2, with permission.

MAPD changes, at both RV and LV sites, was significantly larger than during S2. The variations of the MAPD were most apparent during the early part of the restitution. For example, during the initial increment of 100 milliseconds of the diastolic intervals, the MAPD lengthened by a mean of 47 milliseconds, while during the restitution of S2 it lengthened only by 16 milliseconds ($P<0.001$) (Table 1).[2,3]

Spatial Dispersion of MAPD

At a given coupling premature stimulus interval, the difference in the MAPD between the RV and the LV is taken as a measure of spatial dispersion of MAPD. The recordings shown in Figure 1 and the graphic plot shown in Figure 3 illustrate the spatial variations of repolarization between the RV and the LV sites. The dispersion between these two sites is caused by the combined differences in activation times between the RV (pacing site) and the LV, and by the intrinsic MAPD restitution kinetics at the two sites. This combined effect, labeled as *Dispersion (total)*, along with the dispersion caused solely by differences in activation time, are shown in Figure 3. In contrast, however, during the restitution of S3 the total dispersion of the MAPD between the RV and the LV sites is not caused only by the differences in the activation time but also by the steeper slope of the MAPD restitution during S3. In the example of Figure 3, at a coupling interval of 165 milliseconds, the MAPD difference between the RV and the LV was higher than the differences caused by differential activation time. [2,3]

In Vitro Isolated Tissue Studies

The ability of our contact electrode catheter to truly reflect the underlying cellular repolarization kinetics was confirmed by using the combined

Table 1
Comparison of MAPD Restituion Parameters
of S2 and S3 in Closed-Chest Dog

Parameters	S2	S3
MAPD restitution (N = 10)		
APD minimum	189±16	144±18*
maximum	213±15	216±15
Total APD change	24±12	72±18*
Dispersion (100 ms)	16±5	47±13*
Amplitude	0.11±0.06	0.33±0.08*

Dispersion (100 ms) = dispersion of repolarization during initial 100 ms of diastolic interval; MAPD = monophasic action potential duration.
*$P<0.001$; basic cycle length = 500 ms. N = number of dogs.

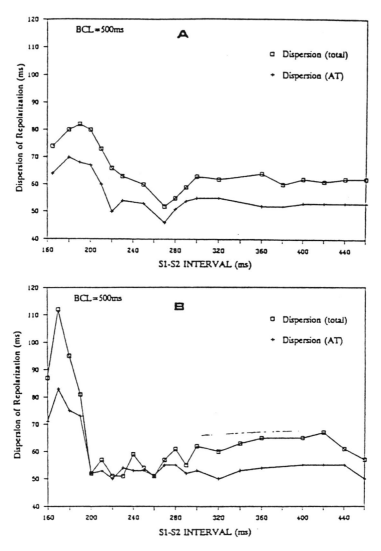

Figure 3. Difference (dispersion) of monophasic action potential duration (MAPD) between the right ventricular endocardium (RV) and the left ventricular apex (LV). **A.** Dispersion caused by the difference in activation time (AT) and total dispersion caused by activation difference and by the intrinsic restitution properties. During the restitution of S2, the difference in MAPD is 10 to 15 milliseconds, caused mainly by difference in the activation time at the two sites. **B.** Difference in MAPD during the restitution of S3. Note that the total peak dispersion of 115 milliseconds difference in the MAPD between the RV and the LV is caused by the sum of differences in activation time (85 milliseconds) and by the intrinsic restitution kinetics (30 milliseconds). Total dispersion (difference) is 115 milliseconds. BCL = basic cycle length. From Reference 1, with permission.

single microelectrode and MAPD recording approach. Figure 4 illustrates 5 cell layers of epicardial transmembrane action potential recordings (panel A) followed by contact MAP recordings from the same site (panel B) during regular pacing at 800-millisecond cycle length. It is apparent that all 5 cell layers had uniform action potential duration (APD) and that the MAPD fairly accurately reflected the underlying transmembrane APD. Similar concordance in APD was observed in the free-running Purkinje fiber bundle (Fig. 5, panel C). However, at endocardial sites, MAP was longer than the underlying muscle cell APD but shorter than the most superficial endocardial Purkinje fiber APD (Fig. 5, panels A and B). It is apparent in cases of mixed cell population that the MAPD reflects the average duration of the underlying cell population. Figure 6 is a comparative graphic plot of APD during premature stimulation (upper panels) obtained with simultaneous microelectrode and contact MAP electrode catheter recordings (lower panels) during premature stimulation, in isolated canine endocardial, epicardial, and Purkinje fiber bundle.

Simulation Studies

The importance of the steepness of the slope of the APD restitution curve in ease of reentry induction and instability of the induced reentrant wave front was investigated in a 125 by 125 interconnected cell model of

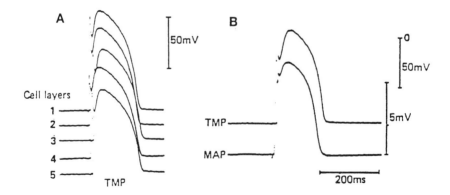

Figure 4. Comparison of epicardial transmembrane action potential (TMP) and monophasic action potential (MAP) in a representative canine thin epicardial slice during regular pacing at 800-millisecond cycle length. **A**. TMP recordings from 5 consecutive cell layers as the microelectrode was progressively advanced downward. Similar mapping of superficial cell layers within 1 cm^2 also yielded uniform TMP morphology (not shown). **B**. Simultaneous epicardial TMP and MAP recordings within 5 mm of each other. Reproduced from Reference 20, with permission.

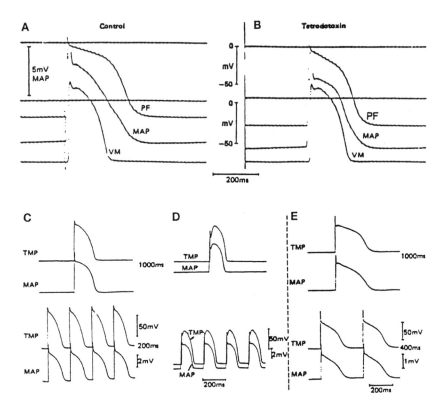

Figure 5. Comparative simultaneous monophasic action potential (MAP) and transmembrane action potential (TMP) recordings from isolated canine subendo-cardial Purkinje fiber (PF) and subendocardial ventricular muscle cell (VM) (**A**, **B**). The 3 recordings are made within 5 mm of each other during regular drive at 800-millisecond cycle length in a representative isolated canine right ventricular endocardial tissue. During control, the MAPD is shorter than the duration of PF but longer than the underlying TMP duration of the VM. With 5 μM of tetrodotoxin, a substantial shortening of the of the PF APD occurs while the APD of the VM slightly lengthens. The duration of the MAP still remains intermediate between the durations of the both fiber types. (See text for more discussion). Panels **C** through **E** show simultaneous TMP and MAP recordings of isolated canine endocardial (A), epicardial (B), and free-running Purkinje (C) fibers within 5 mm of each other. In all panels, the last of 8 regularly driven beats at 800-millisecond cycle length (S1) and a premature stimulus (S2) are shown. Note the similarities of the APD in the epicardial and free-running Purkinje preparation and a the longer MAPD than the TMP duration in the endocardium as in A and B. Recordings such as these were used to plot Figure 10. Reproduced from Reference 20, with permission.

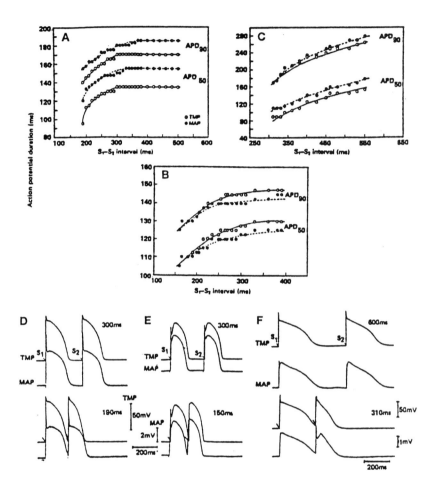

Figure 6. Effects of premature stimulation on isolated canine endocardial (**A**) epicardial (**B**) and free-running Purkinje (**C**) fibers. The duration of the 90% (APD90) and 50% (APD50) repolarization are shown for both transmembrane action potential (TMP) and monophasic action potential (MAP) recordings. Panels A through C show actual simultaneous TMP and MAP recordings during the last regularly driven S1 and a premature stimulus S2. Note the relative similarities of both types of recordings except at the endocardium, where MAPD is much larger than the duration of TMP of the underlying ventricular muscle cell. This larger difference is due to the longer APD of the most superficial subendocardial Purkinje fibers that are in contact with the endocardial MAP electrode. Reproduced from Reference 20, with permission.

the Fitz-Hugh Nagumo equations uses the massively parallel connection machine.[4,6] Nonstationary spiral waves can more easily be induced in a matrix with steeper kinetics of APD restitution kinetics. In addition, larger gradients in excitability, a characteristic manifestation of a steeper slope of APD restitution curve, promotes meandering of wave fronts (nonstationarity). Such meandering results in a complex distribution of excitability (ie, nonuniform recovery of excitability), a phenomenon known to promote wavebreaks and fibrillationlike (ie, polymorphic) activity in ventricular tissue[8,10] and in simulation studies.[8,11]

The Graded Responses and Vulnerability to Reentry

The Relationship Between the S2 and the Graded Responses

The properties of the graded responses, defined as depolarizing responses that are evoked during phase 3 repolarization (incomplete recovery) and that manifest continuously variable configuration as a function of the S2 stimulating current, were evaluated near the cathodal and the anodal sides of the S2 stimulus.[1]

Effects of the Current Strength

An increase in the strength of the S2 current from 5 to 100 mA, at a fixed interval (effective refractory period [ERP] 20 milliseconds), caused a progressive increase in the amplitude (2 ± 0.8 mV to 63 ± 13 mV) and duration (5 ± 2 milliseconds to 87 ± 23 milliseconds) of the induced graded responses (n=6).[1] Figure 7, panel A illustrates an example of increased amplitude and duration of the graded response by increasing the S2 current strength. No graded responses could be induced during the entire phase 2 (plateau) of the action potential no matter how strong the S2 was (see below). These findings are compatible with those of Kao and Hoffman,[12] seen on subendocardial fibers.

Effects of the Coupling Interval

Similarly, an increase in the coupling interval of the S2, at a fixed current strength, caused a progressive increase in the amplitude and the duration of the graded responses (Fig. 7, panel B). The mean shortest and longest coupling intervals during which graded responses could be induced

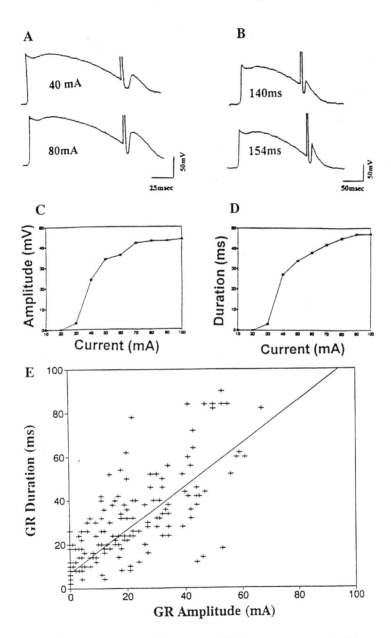

Figure 7. Relation of the graded response (GR) properties to the S2 stimulus characteristics. **A.** Effects of increasing the S2 current strength from 40 mA to 80 mA. **B.** Effects of S2 increasing the coupling intervals from 140 milliseconds to 154 milliseconds in a different tissue. An increase in the amplitude and the duration of the graded response occurs in both cases. **E.** Correlation between the graded response amplitude and its duration (see text for details).

at pacing cycle length of 600 milliseconds were 115±8 milliseconds and 170±12 milliseconds, respectively (n=12).[1]

Graded Response Amplitude-Duration Relationship

A regression analysis of 187 induced graded responses (Fig. 7, panel E) in 8 tissue samples showed a significant ($P<0.01$, r=0.79) positive linear correlation between the graded response amplitude and the graded response duration.

$$\text{Duration (milliseconds)} = 0.98 \text{ ms/mV} \qquad (1)$$
$$\times \text{amplitude (mV)} + 8.41 \text{ ms.}^{1}$$

Graded Response and ERP Prolongation

Figure 8 shows the relationship between the total APD and the ERP. In 6 tissue samples, a regression analysis of 78 different measurements showed a significant positive correlation ($P<0.01$, r=0.96) between the ERP and the total APD over 100 milliseconds of APD prolongation.[1]

$$\text{ERP (ms)} = 1.067 \times \text{APD (ms)} - 24.51 \text{ ms} \qquad (2)$$

Voltage Dependency of the Graded Responses

The graded response amplitude was voltage dependent. As the take-off potential became more negative (ie, −15 mV to −65 mV), the amplitude of the graded response induced by a given S2 current strength grew progressively.[1] Similarly, for a given take-off potential, the amplitude of the graded responses increased with increasing S2 current strength, consistent with the results of Knisley et al.[13]

Graded Responses Near the Anodal Pole

Graded responses were also observed near the anodal pole of the S2 stimulus, with characteristics that depended on the S2 stimulus parameters. No graded responses could be induced at distances greater than 3 mm for the anode or during the entire plateau range of the action potential for current strengths up to 100 mA. S2 applied at a slightly later part of the plateau induced small amplitude (2 to 4 mV) graded responses with a net shortening of the total APD. However, with relatively late-coupled S2 stimuli (ie, >110 milliseconds), a graded response with a net prolongation of the total APD occurs, consistent with previous studies on Purkinje fibers[14]

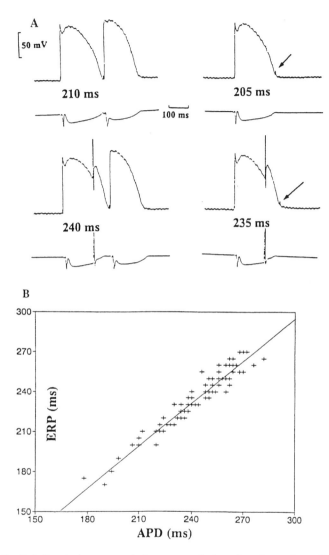

Figure 8. Relation between graded response-induced prolongation of the action potential duration (APD) and the effective refractory period (ERP). **A.** Top recordings show induction of the earliest premature stimulus with an S1-S2 coupling interval of 210 milliseconds and a block with an S1-S2 of 205 milliseconds. After the induction of a graded response (lower left recording) the earliest premature response is now initiated at an S1-S2 coupling interval of 240 milliseconds with block occurring at an S1-S2 interval of 235 milliseconds, reflecting a 30-millisecond increase in the ERP. Action potentials are recorded along the fiber 1 mm away from the cathode pole of the S2. The lower recording is a bipolar electrogram. **B.** Relation between the graded response-induced prolongation of the total APD (abscissa) and the resultant increase in the ERP (ordinate). Used with permission from the American Heart Association: *Circulation*, Reference 1.

and on endocardial ventricular muscle cells.[15] At equal distances from the two poles of the S2 along the fiber (analysis done 2 mm away from each pole and with an S2 of 80 mA), the amplitude and the duration of the graded responses were significantly lower ($P<0.01$) in the cells at the anodal side than in the cells at the cathodal side (6 ± 2 mV versus 28 ± 9 mV and 16 ± 4 milliseconds versus 36 ± 10 milliseconds, respectively).[1]

The Extent and Velocity of Graded Response Propagation

The induced graded responses propagated in a decremental and anisotropic fashion from near the S2 stimulus site to more distant sites. In order to determine the distance over which the graded responses can propagate before dying out, we sequentially recorded action potentials at increasing distances from S2 toward the S1 stimulus site. The S2 strength (50 mA) and coupling interval (180 milliseconds) were fixed, a timing that coincided to ERP 15 milliseconds. Transmembrane recordings were then made along and across the long axis of the fiber orientation at increasing distances (steps of 0.5 mm) from the S2 stimulus site. The propagation of the graded responses was anisotropic; they propagated for longer distances along the fiber than across it. The longitudinal extent of propagation, however, was higher (up to 5 mm) than in the transverse direction (up to 3 mm).[1]

Comparative Conduction Velocities of the Graded and the Regenerative Responses

The graded responses propagate in both longitudinal and transverse directions. The longitudinal velocity of the spread, estimated as the time interval between the peaks of two graded responses recorded over a known distance, was 5 to 6 times slower than the velocity of propagation of regular impulses. The mean conduction velocity of the graded responses was significantly slower ($P<0.001$) than the velocity of the regenerative responses (18.2 ± 3.8 cm/s versus 60 ± 10.9 cm/s, respectively, n=6)[1] (Fig. 9).

Propagation of the Graded Responses and Initiation of Action Potentials

When the amplitude of the propagated graded responses in the recovering cells toward the S1 site reached threshold, an action potential was initiated (Fig. 9). Threshold potential could be reached by the propagated graded responses either by increasing the coupling intervals of the S1-S2 or by increasing the S2 current strength.[1]

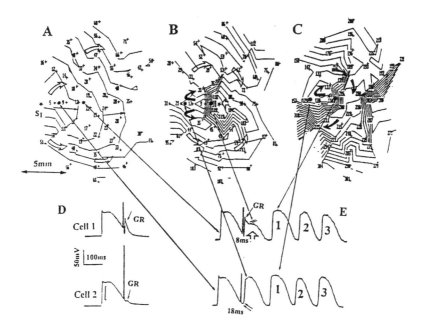

Figure 9. Sequential activation map and two simultaneous action potential recordings. A 56-channel bipolar electrode array was used in this study. **A**. Isochronal activation map (10-millisecond isochrone interval) during regular S1-S1 pacing at 600-millisecond cycle length (*). The crosses (+) represent electrode locations and the numbers give the time of activation, with the onset of S1 as time zero. The two dots represent the two sites from which subsequent simultaneous action potentials are recorded. The arrows in panels A through C point to the direction of wave front propagation. The horizontal double-headed arrow indicates the fiber orientation and also serves as length scale. **B**. Isochronal activation map of an S2 stimulus (40 mA at 136-millisecond interval) applied in the center of the tissue (asterisk pointed to by an open arrow). The site of earliest activation is located 3 mm away from the S2 toward the S1 site (isochrone encircling 9-millisecond site). The S2-initiated wave front propagates first toward the S1 site then rotates (double curved arrows) around the site of block and reaches proximal to the site of block in 104 milliseconds, forming a figure-eight. Panel **C** shows that activation continues through the initial site of block as in Figure 2. **D**. Two simultaneous action potential recordings from sites indicated in A. An S2 stimulus (40 mA, 122-millisecond interval) induces a graded response in Cell 1 (arrow) that propagates to Cell 2 with decrement in amplitude (35 mV to 5 mV) (single arrows). Panel **E** shows that an S2 (40 mA, 136-millisecond interval) initiates a graded response in Cell 1 with an 8-millisecond delay, and an action potential in Cell 2 with an 18-millisecond delay that arises from the graded response (double arrows). The action potential initiated in Cell 2 blocks at the site of Cell 1 (large open arrow with double horizontal lines in Cell 1) with an electrotonic depolarization as in Figures 8, 9, and 10. The reentrant wave front in C excites Cell 1 then Cell 2 as shown in E with action potential number 1. Two subsequent reentrant action potentials are also shown (2 and 3). Used with permission from the American Heart Association: *Circulation*, Reference 1.

Graded Responses and Initiation of Reentry

In 5 tissues, after an initial activation map was constructed, we recorded with one microelectrode from the area of the earliest activity and with a second from the area of local conduction block. Figure 9 shows one such example. Figure 9, panel A shows activation during regular pacing. Panel B shows that an S2 of 35-mA strength applied with a coupling interval of 150 milliseconds caused a local block and distal early activation (two curved arrows) leading to the first reentrant wave front (Panel C) as in Figure 2. Subsequent simultaneous recordings of two transmembrane potentials (TMPs; site of block and site of earliest activation, 2 dots in panels A through C) are shown in Figure 9, panels D and E. The distally originated front (panel B) rotates around the site of block then reenters (panel C), initiating the first action potential (#1 in panel E).[1]

Activation Pattern After a Super-Strong S2 Stimulus That Does Not Induce Reentry

Activation map with 480 electrodes showed that currents above the upper limit of vulnerability (ULV) induce bidirectional conduction block near the S2 site that prevents reentry. Figure 10 describes the scenario

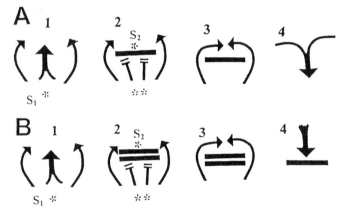

Figure 10. Diagrammatic illustration of the propagated graded response hypothesis of vulnerability. **A.** Initiation of figure-eight reentry according to the graded response hypothesis. Fiber orientation is north-south. Numbers 1 in both rows show wave front propagation during regular S1 pacing (*). Number 2 in **A** shows response after an S2 stimulus (*) with the earliest site of activity arising between the S1 and S2 (**). The front then blocks at the S2 site (A2, horizontal line), rotates around the area of block (A3) then reenters (A4) when this area recovers its excitability as the first figure-eight reentry cycle. **B.** Same scenario but with an S2 strength that is above the upper limit of vulnerability. In this case excess prolongation of the refractory period (double horizontal lines in B2 and B3) prevents reentry (B4).

leading to the formation of functional reentry by critical S2 stimulus. An increase in the strength of the S2 converts the local unidirectional block to bidirectional block that prevents the formation of reentry. This represents the well known phenomenon of the ULV.[16]

The Role of MAP Recordings During VF

While MAP recordings provide valuable information on the repolarization kinetics during regular pacing at relatively fast rates of stimulation (Figs. 5 and 6), the value of MAP recordings becomes progressively lost as the rate further accelerates and during VF. The disorganized and chaotic[17] nature of activation wave front dynamics during VF seem to prevent extraction of reliable information on the kinetics of local myocardial repolarization. Furthermore, MAP recordings cannot detect the slowly rising low-amplitude graded responses despite the fact that these graded responses play an important role in the initiation of reentry.[1] These two important limitations are made clear during simultaneous MAP and cellular TMP recordings with a glass microelectrode in the isolated, perfused swine RVs. MAP recordings during ventricular tachycardia-flutter caused by a single stationary reentrant wave front can provide useful information; however, MAP recordings during flutter or VF caused by multiple reentrant and nonreentrant wave fronts become distorted and difficult to interpret.

Figure 11 shows simultaneous recordings of TMP and MAP during an accelerating ventricular flutter caused by a single reentrant wave front in an isolated swine RV model.[18] During a relatively slower rate (initial 11 beats), both types of recordings show regular beat-to-beat repolarization. However, when the rate accelerates (subsequent 14 beats), only the TMP recordings show distinct beat-to-beat repolarization that can be measured, while the MAP recording becomes distorted. In addition to distorting the repolarization, the contact MAP electrode cannot record graded responses. Figure 12 shows simultaneous TMP and MAP recordings during VF sustained by multiple reentrant and nonreentrant wave fronts.[17,18] While TMP recordings clearly show the presence of graded responses during VF, no such information can be obtained from the MAP recordings. In addition, with TMP recordings it is easier to identify and detect the presence of an excitable gap (Fig. 12) that is difficult to show on the MAP recordings. Figure 13 shows that during VF, MAP can, at certain times, show intermittent regular and irregular activity during accelerated ventricular rhythms (ventricular flutter and VF) without detection of graded responses or an excitable gap. These observations indicate that distinct beat-to-beat activation and repolarization during rate acceleration and changes in activation

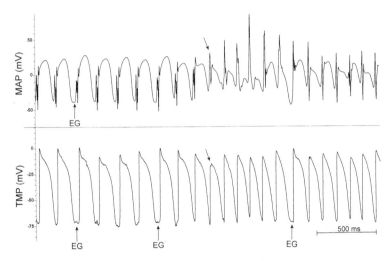

Figure 11. Simultaneous recordings of monophasic action potential (MAP) and cellular transmembrane potential (TMP) in an isolated, perfused swine right ventricle. Transition from ventricular tachycardia to ventricular fibrillation (downward pointing arrows) is shown. Note that during fibrillation multiple wave fronts are present (not shown) and the activation sequence becomes erratic. EG = excitable gap. The distance between the MAP and TMP recordings are about 1 cm (previously unpublished).

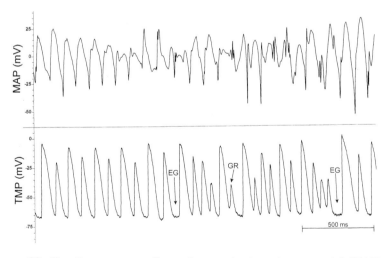

Figure 12. Simultaneous recordings of monophasic action potential (MAP) and cellular transmembane potential (TMP) in an isolated, perfused swine right ventricle. Recordings are made during ventricular fibrillation. While excitable gap (EG) and graded responses (GR) could be detected on the cellular TMP recordings, no such feature could be detected on the MAP recordings. The distance between the MAP and TMP recordings is about 1 cm (previously unpublished).

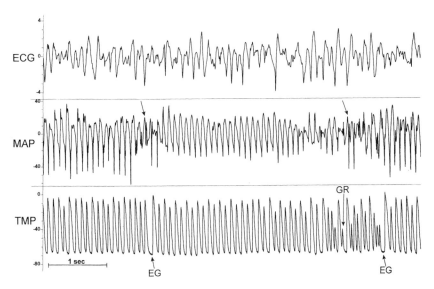

Figure 13. Simultaneous recordings of pseudoelectrocardiogram (ECG), monophasic action potential (MAP), and cellular transmembane potential (TMP) in an isolated, perfused swine right ventricle during ventricular fibrillation. While the TMP consistently shows distinct repolarization, the presence of excitable gap (EG) and graded responses (GR) can only be seen on the TMP recordings. The distance between the MAP and TMP recordings is about 1 cm (previously unpublished).

sequence, excitable gap, and graded responses can only be detected using single-cell microelectrode recordings.

Discussion

The Slope of the APD Restitution Curve as an Index of Ventricular Vulnerability to Reentry

The in situ and in vitro studies show that double premature stimulation increases in the slope of the APD restitution curve. Such an effect is known in simulation studies to ease induction of nonstationary reentrant wave fronts in the form of figure-eight.[4,6,7] It is important to note that increases in slope promote larger gradients in excitability, a phenomenon known to enhance meandering,[4,6,8] which amplifies the nonuniformity of the tissue, leading to wavebreaks. It is still unclear how a uniform dispersion of APD can lead to the formation of the first reentrant wave front. It is possible that in regions of the myocardium where a steep gradient in excitability is present, wavebreak (conduction block) may occur, in turn leading to spiral wave formation.[8] Furthermore, once a reentrant wave front is induced, the presence of a steep excitability gradient, which occurs in cases with steeper slopes of APD restitution curves, facilitates drift or meandering of the reentrant wave front,[8] a phenomenon that further increases tissue nonuniform recovery of excitability (nonuniform dispersion of APD), leading to wavebreak and polymorphic activity.[8,11] Increased slope of APD restitution curves may also induce sudden directional difference in the repolarization gradient.[19] Directional difference in the sequence of repolarization may alter the activation sequence leading to wavebreak and reentry. Directional difference in the APD (repolarization) gradient might result from differences of the APD restitution curves in different cell types,[20] or might result from regional differences at different ventricular myocardial sites.[19] During early premature stimulation, if a region shows a slight delay in the activation time, the APD of this same area will be significantly longer than that in areas showing earlier activation times.[19] This reversal of APD distribution occurs because sites with steep slopes of APD restitution will manifest a large increase in their APDs when a slight increase in their diastolic interval occurs, relative to sites that are activated at a shorter diastolic interval.[19] An alternative mechanism for the induction of reentry caused by increased slope of the APD restitution curve is the induction of APD oscillations in the form of alternans or chaotic APD dynamics.[7] These oscillatory behaviors cause temporal and spatial heterogeneities in excitability.[7] It has been shown that when the slope of the APD restitution curve becomes greater than 1, the APD starts to oscillate on a beat-to-beat basis.[7,21-25] Initially, the oscillation is in the form of alternans (period 2), then as the drive rate increases, more irregular TMP dynamics (chaos) arise.[21] The APD oscillations need not be in phase with each other at different myocardial sites[7] and, thus, by virtue of the out-of-phase oscillation, increased nonhomogeneity in excitability may develop that greatly facilitates the induction of wavebreaks (conduction block) and reentry. Clearly, more work is needed to elucidate the role of uniform and nonuniform dispersion of APD in the induction of the first functional reentrant wave front in the ventricle.

Propagated Graded Responses and Ventricular Vulnerability to Reentry

The need for a critical current strength—one that is neither too high nor too low—to induce VF was recognized by Battelli before the turn of the century.[26] Since then, it has been shown that the critical stimulus must be applied during a finite period of the cardiac cycle, the vulnerable period.[27-31] The lower and the upper levels of current strengths needed for VF induction, recently reconfirmed to be present in humans,[32] were termed the *lower limit of vulnerability* (or VF threshold) and the *ULV*, respectively.[16] Now, still, no quantitative cellular descriptors of excitability and precise patterns of transmembrane voltage distribution have been provided to explain the chain of cellular events that lead to functional reentry formation in the normal ventricle after a strong S2 stimulus. Although theory has predicted and proposed the existence of critical-stimulus point (singularity) hypothesis of vulnerability, no clear cellular descriptors of the critical point hypothesis have ever been offered.[33] The chain of trans-membrane cellular events in the critical point hypothesis of vulnerability to reentry remains unknown.[33] Is the critical point the site at which block occurs, as proposed by Winfree,[33] or it is the site of the earliest activation? According to the graded response hypothesis, the intersection of the propagated graded responses (stimulus-related parameter) with the recovering cells toward the S1 stimulus (recovery-related parameter) corresponds to the site of earliest activation and *not* to the site of conduction block. This intersection site therefore cannot be the site of the critical point or phase singularity as proposed by Winfree.[33] It is, however, clear that in the critical point hypothesis proposed by Frazier et al,[34] the propagating graded responses play no role in the induction of reentry. In this way our proposed graded response hypothesis of reentry formation differs in a major way from the critical point hypothesis proposed by Frazier et al.[34] Furthermore, the propagated graded response phenomenon, in addition to its vulnerability hypothesis, can also provide a reasonable cellular mechanistic explanation for the phenomenon of the ULV and the protective effect of a second stimulus S3. With critical timings of the S3, graded responses can be induced at the site of the S3 that causes increased prolongation of the ERP that leads to conduction block, thus preventing the formation of reentry or promoting its termination, depending on the timing of the S3.

The findings of the present studies provide for the first time, 4 quantitative cellular electrophysiologic descriptors that explain the mechanism of ventricular vulnerability to functional reentry and the ULV, in normal ventricular myocardium with uniform anisotropy and initial uniformity in repolarization[1,35]:

1. origination of action potentials at a site distal to the S2 stimulus site;
2. local unidirectional conduction block near the S2 site;
3. slow retrograde conduction from the site of earliest activation toward the initial site of conduction block, allowing recovery of excitability and the opportunity for reentry (the timely juxtaposition of an early site of activation to a region or prolonged refractoriness causes a wavebreak that may lead to reentry);
4. higher S2 current strengths further prolong the duration of the ERP at the S2 site and convert unidirectional conduction block to bidirectional conduction block preventing reentry.

The conversion of unidirectional conduction block to bidirectional block explains the phenomenon of the ULV that occurs with strong S2 stimuli.

What Does a Critical Premature Stimulus (S2) Do at the Macroscopic Scale Size?

Using computerized mapping in the in situ ventricles, we have shown[36,37] that VF induced by a critical point S2 stimulus is initiated by a figure-eight reentry around the S2 site that acts as the site of the unidirectional conduction block. With extracellular recordings, we speculated[37] that the mechanism of the S2-induced reentry at the onset of VF in the intact in situ hearts was caused by the ability of S2-induced graded responses to first prolong refractoriness near the S2 site and second, propagate away from the S2 site and initiate activation at a site distant from the S2 site.[38,39] According to this hypothesis, the propagated graded response hypothesis, or the graded response hypothesis,[37] the distally initiated wave front propagates around both sides of the functional conduction block and reenters through the site of the initial block when it recovers its excitability, completing the first figure-eight reentry cycle (Figs. 9 and 10). However, this early version of the graded response hypothesis suggested the presence of an area of direct excitation near the strong S2 stimulus electrode. Because extracellular recordings were used in these studies, it was impossible to differentiate the active regenerative responses (direct excitation) from high-amplitude passive graded responses. Therefore, in these early studies, the mechanism of block near the S2 site could not be ascertained. Specifically, it was not known how block (refractoriness) was developed near the S2 site: was it caused by the graded responses or by the refractoriness left behind by the premature direct excitation? Furthermore, it was also not known how distal activation away from the S2 site first originated. The demonstration of the lack of virtual electrode effect (rise time in the distal cell graded response *significantly lags behind* the rise time of the proximal cell graded response) provided strong argument for the existence of a propagation rather than direct S2 electrode stimulus effect (virtual electrode effect).

What Does a Critical Premature Stimulus (S2) Do at the Microscopic (Cellular) Scale Size?

According to the graded response hypothesis, an S2-induced reentry should arise from the interaction of the propagated graded responses with the recovered cells distant from the S2 site. If the S2 strength is too low, the depolarizing graded response it induces may be too small to propagate toward recovering cells and/or too weak (subthreshold) to evoke a regenerative response at a distal site.[1] Alternatively, with low currents the prolongation of the refractory period near the S2 site may not be sufficient to result in unidirectional conduction block. Either mechanism may prevent reentry.

On the other hand, if the S2 strength is too high, bidirectional conduction block may occur due to increased prolongation of the refractoriness by the graded responses near the S2. In this case reentry is also prevented. The results presented in this chapter provide cellular evidence, using microelectrode recordings, that the graded response hypothesis of vulnerability is indeed operative.

Conclusions

The graded response hypothesis offers an adequate quantitative cellular description to explain the vulnerability hypothesis (ie, the mechanism of the formation of the first functional reentrant wave front). This same hypothesis can further explain the cellular basis of the ULV. The presence of a ULV for reentry in our in vitro model mimics the presence of a ULV in in situ canine hearts[16,31] and in humans.[32] Because the values of the ULV and the defibrillation energy requirements are closely related,[32] the graded response mechanism of ventricular vulnerability to reentry may also have relevance to the mechanism of ventricular defibrillation. In addition, much strong suggestive evidence supports the notion of increased ventricular vulnerability to reentry by increased dispersion (uniform and nonuniform) of excitability. At present, however, there is a need to develop a hypothesis to unequivocally explain in a quantitative manner (ie, at the cellular level) how a dispersion leads to the formation of the first reentrant wave front. It is suggested that the slope of the APD restitution curve may be used as a marker for cardiac dispersion and may therefore measure cardiac vulnerability to reentry and fibrillation. MAP recordings can provide useful information for determining the slope of the APD restitution curve and local repolarization kinetics during relatively slow rates. However, MAP recordings cannot detect graded responses, and they become distorted during faster rates of activation (flutter and fibrillation) that are maintained by multiple reentrant and nonreentrant wave fronts. Finally, MAP recordings often fail to detect the presence of an excitable gap, which is clearly identified during TMP recordings.

References

1. Gotoh M, Uchida T, Mandel WJ, et al. Cellular graded responses and ventricular vulnerability to reentry by a premature stimulus in isolated canine ventricle. *Circulation* 1997;95(8):2141-2154.
2. Kobayashi Y, Gotoh M, Mandel WJ, Karagueuzian HS. Increased temporo-spatial dispersion of repolarization during double premature stimulation in the intact ventricle. *PACE* 1992;15:2194-2199.
3. Kobayashi Y, Peters W, Khan SS, et al. Cellular mechanisms of differential action potential duration restitution in canine ventricular muscle cells during single versus double premature stimuli. *Circulation* 1992;86:955-967.

4. Karagueuzian HS, Kogan BY. Action potential duration restitution dynamics and its relation to spiral wave formation: An experimental and computer simulation study. In Shenasa M, Borggrefe M, Breithardt G (eds): *Cardiac Mapping*. Mount Kisco, New York: Futura Publishing Co., Inc.; 1993:627-645.

5. Kogan BY, Karplus WJ, Billett BS, et al. The role of diastolic outward current deactivation kinetics on the induction of spiral waves. *PACE* 1991;14:1688-1693.

6. Kogan BY, Karplus WJ, Billett BS, et al. The simplified FitzHugh-Nagumo model with action potential duration restitution: Effects on 2-D wave propagation. *Physica D* 1991;50:327-340.

7. Karagueuzian HS, Khan SS, Hong K, et al. Action potential alternans and irregular dynamics in quinidine-intoxicated ventricular muscle cells. Implications for ventricular proarrhythmia. *Circulation* 1993;87:1661-1672.

8. Pertsov AM, Davidenko JM, Salomonsz R, et al. Spiral waves of excitation underlie reentrant activity in isolated cardiac muscle. *Circ Res* 1993;72:631-650.

9. Davidenko JM, Salomonsz R, Pertsov AM, et al. Effects of pacing on stationary reentrant activity. Theoretical and experimental study. *Circ Res* 1995; 77:1166-1179.

10. Davidenko JM, Pertsov AM, Salomonsz R, et al. Stationary and drifting spiral waves of excitation in isolated cardiac tissue. *Nature* 1991;355:349-351.

11. Starmer CF, Romashko DN, Reddy RS, et al. Proarrhythmic response to potassium channel blockade. Numerical studies of polymorphic tachyarrhythmias. *Circulation* 1995;92:595-605.

12. Kao CY, Hoffman BF. Graded and decremental response in heart muscle fibers. *Am J Physiol* 1958;194:187-196.

13. Knisley SB, Smith WM, Ideker RE. Effect of field stimulation on cellular repolarization in rabbit myocardium. Implication for reentry induction. *Circ Res* 1992;70:707-715.

14. Weidmann S. Effects of current flow on the membrane potential of cardiac muscle. *J Physiol* 1951;115:227-236.

15. Cranefield PF, Hoffman BF. Propagated repolarization in heart muscle. *J Gen Physiol* 1958;41:633-649.

16. Chen P-S, Shibata N, Dixon EG, et al. Comparison of the defibrillation threshold and the upper limit of ventricular vulnerability. *Circulation* 1986;73:1022-1028.

17. Garfinkel A, Chen P-S, Walter DO, et al. Quasiperiodicity and chaos in cardiac fibrillation. *J Clin Invest* 1997;99:305-314.

18. Kim YH, Garfinkel A, Ikeda T, et al. Spatiotemporal complexity of ventricular fibrillation revealed by tissue mass reduction in isolated swine right ventricle. Further evidence for the quasiperiodic route to chaos hypothesis. *J Clin Invest* 1997;100:2486-2500.

19. Laurita KR, Girouard SD, Rosenbaum DS. Modulation of ventricular repolarization by a premature stimulus: Role of epicardial dispersion of repolarization kinetics demonstrated by optical mapping of the intact guinea pig heart. *Circ Res* 1996;79:493-503.

20. Ino T, Karagueuzian HS, Hong K, et al. Relation of monophasic action potential recorded with contact electrode to underlying transmembrane action potential properties in isolated cardiac tissues: A systematic microelectrode validation study. *Cardiovasc Res* 1988;22:255-264.

21. Chialvo DR, Jalife J. Non-linear dynamics of cardiac excitation and impulse propagation. *Nature* 1987;330:749-752.

22. Chialvo DR, Michaels DC, Jalife J. Supernormal excitability as a mechanism of chaotic dynamics of activation in cardiac Purkinje fibers. *Circ Res* 1990;66:525-545.

23. Vinet A, Chialvo DR, Michaels DC, Jalife J. Nonlinear dynamics of rate-dependent activation in models of single cardiac cells. *Circ Res* 1990;67:1510-1524.

24. Lewis TJ, Guevara MR. Chaotic dynamics in an ionic model of the propagated cardiac action potential. *J Theor Biol* 1990;146:407-432.

25. Kaplan DT, Cohen RJ. Is fibrillation chaos? *Circ Res* 1990;67:886-892.

26. Battelli F. Le mécanisme de la mort par les courants électriques chez l'homme. *Revue Médicale de la Suisse Romande* 1899;10:605-618.

27. King BG. *The Effect of Electric Shock on Heart Action with Special Reference to Varying Susceptibility in Different Parts of the Cardiac Cycle* [PhD thesis]. New York: Aberdeen Press; Columbia University; 1934.

28. Ferris LP, King BG, Spence PW, Williams HB. Effect of electric shock on the heart. *Electrical Engineering* 1936;55:498-515.

29. Wiggers CJ, Wegria R. Ventricular fibrillation due to single, localized induction and condenser shocks applied during the vulnerable phase of ventricular systole. *Am J Physiol* 1940;128:500-505.

30. Moe GK, Harris S, Wiggers CJ. Analysis of the initiation of fibrillation by electrographic studies. *Am J Physiol* 1941;134:473-492.

31. Shibata N, Chen P-S, Dixon EG, et al. Influence of epicardial shock strength and timing on the induction of ventricular arrhythmias in dogs. *Am J Physiol* 1988;255:H891-H901.

32. Hwang C, Swerdlow CD, Kass RM, et al. Upper limit of vulnerability reliably predicts the defibrillation threshold in humans. *Circulation* 1994;90:2308-2314.

33. Winfree AT. Electrical instability in cardiac muscle: Phase singularities and rotors. *J Theor Biol* 1989;138:353-405.

34. Frazier DW, Wolf PD, Wharton JM, et al. Stimulus-induced critical point: Mechanism for electrical initiation of reentry in normal canine myocardium. *J Clin Invest* 1989;83:1039-1052.

35. Gotoh M, Karagueuzian HS, Chen PS. Anisotropic repolarization in ventricular tissue. *J Am Coll Cardiol* 1995;170A. Abstract.

36. Chen P-S, Wolf P, Dixon EG, et al. Mechanism of ventricular vulnerability to single premature stimuli in open chest dogs. *Circ Res* 1988;62:1191-1209.

37. Chen P-S, Cha Y-M, Peters BB, Chen LS. Effects of myocardial fiber orientation on the electrical induction of ventricular fibrillation. *Am J Physiol* 1993;264:H1760-H1773.

38. Van Dam RT, Moore NE, Hoffman BF. Initiation and conduction of impulses in partially depolarized cardiac fibers. *Am J Physiol* 1963;204:1133-1144.

39. Ino T, Fishbein MC, Mandel WJ, et al. Cellular mechanisms of ventricular bipolar electrograms showing double and fractionated potentials. *J Am Coll Cardiol* 1995;4:1080-1089.

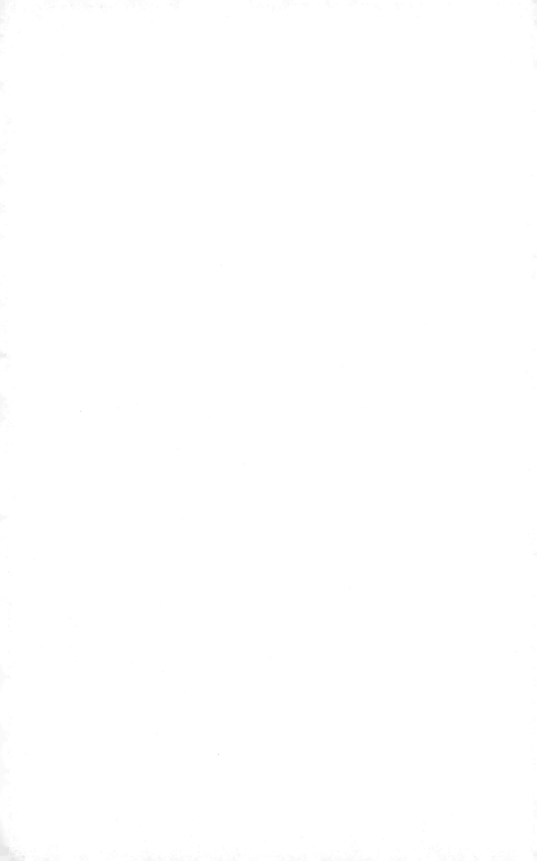

16

Physiologic Mechanisms Underlying the Link Between T Wave Alternans and Vulnerability to Ventricular Fibrillation

Richard L. Verrier, PhD, FACC and
Bruce D. Nearing, PhD

Introduction

The physiologic processes that have an impact on repolarization are manifold and highly interactive. For example, during exercise there are numerous independent and countervailing influences which summate to inscribe the morphology of action potential repolarization and the T wave. Among the most significant are heart rate, autonomic changes, myocardial temperature, and blood constituents. These distinct influences are discussed in this chapter, first independently and then in the context of typical daily activities, including exercise, emotional responses, hyperventilation, orthostasis, and eating.

Particular emphasis is placed on the phenomenon of T wave alternans, a beat-to-beat fluctuation in the amplitude and morphology of the T wave,

Supported by grant HL50078 from the National Heart, Lung, and Blood Institute and ES 08129 from National Institute of Environmental Health, National Institutes of Health, Bethesda, MD.

for several reasons. First, this phenomenon may be far more prevalent than has been previously appreciated. This is probably due to the fact that detection has relied on a qualitative approach and only the more macroscopic manifestations of alternans have been described in the limited context of exercise stress testing,[1-3] severe classic and Prinzmetal's angina,[4,5] and the long QT syndrome.[6-9] Recently, however, more subtle forms of the phenomenon that are detectable by signal processing techniques have been reported under diverse physiologic and pathophysiologic conditions, including sympathetic nervous system stimulation and behavioral stress in the normal heart,[6,10] and during exercise in patients with myocardial ischemia and infarction, cardiomyopathy, and heart failure.[11-15]

Importantly, there is growing experimental and clinical evidence that T wave alternans may be a useful predictor of risk for life-threatening arrhythmias.[16,17] Finally, alternation in repolarization dynamics, the ST segment, and T wave duration can have a significant impact on the measurement of QT and T. In fact, investigators have commented that T wave alternation can corrupt the measurement of ST segment level.[18] The case is made in this chapter that alternating behavior of repolarization may be more signal than noise, and that the phenomenon is relatively ubiquitous and is manifold in its expression depending on the underlying physiologic basis (Figs. 1 through 4). The putative electrophysiologic mechanisms are discussed.

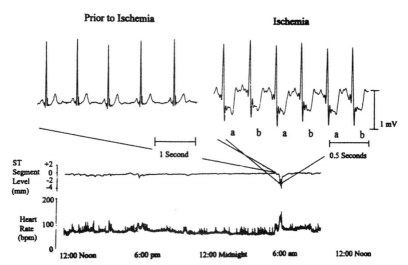

Figure 1. Representative ambulatory ECG recordings of ST segment level, heart rate, and electrocardiogram in a patient from the Angina and Silent Ischemia Study (ASIS), recorded with use of an ACS ambulatory recorder. In the absence of significant ST segment depression, there is no visible T wave alternans. During a bout of ischemia, as indicated by a drop in ST segment level, there is marked T wave alternans in the absence of R wave alternans or other notable changes in the activation waveform. From Reference 55, with permission.

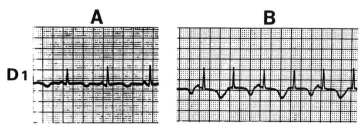

Figure 2. Electrocardiogram of 9-year-old patient affected by long QT syndrome.
A. At rest. **B**. Alternation of T wave appeared during unintentionally induced
fear. Reprinted from Reference 33, with permission from the American Heart
Association.

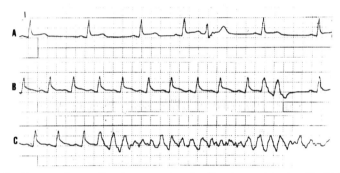

Figure 3. Sinus tachycardia after atropine, leading to ventricular fibrillation. Patient with anterior infarction, lead I. **A**. Sinus bradycardia (rate 55 beats/min) with
ventricular ectopics. **B**. Recording 2 minutes after atropine, 0.6 mg, i.v. Sinus
tachycardia (rate 110/min) with consecutive ventricular ectopics. **C**. Recording 3
minutes after atropine, showing development of ventricular fibrillation. Reprinted
from Reference 56, with permission from Raven Press.

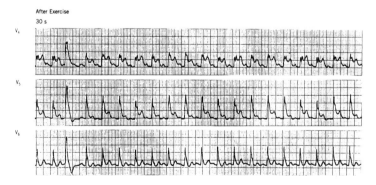

Figure 4. Immediate postexercise tracing, leads V_4 through V_6. ST segment elevation and ST-T alternans, best seen in lead V_5, became most prominent at 30 seconds
after exercise, and isolated ventricular premature beats appeared (third complex
from left). Reproduced from Reference 1, with permission from the American
Medical Association.

Basic Influences on the T Wave

Heart Rate

In the normal heart, accelerations in sinus rate shorten repolarization and the QT interval.[19,20] Except for extremely rapid rates, when the T wave flattens, its morphology and amplitude are relatively unaffected. However, under pathophysiologic conditions, most notably myocardial ischemia, elevations in heart rate can lead to drastic changes in ST segment and T wave morphology. Depending on whether the ischemia is subepicardial or subendocardial, elevated heart rate can enhance the magnitude of ST elevation or depression, respectively.[21] Elevated heart rates can predispose to increased heterogeneity of repolarization and exacerbation of myocardial ischemia. Sinus tachycardia can also induce T wave alternans during acute myocardial ischemia, a response which is thought to be due, in large part, to disruption of intracellular cycling of calcium.[22-27]

In terms of measurement, it has been argued that heart rate confounds the quantification of T wave alternans. In fact, the increase in T wave alternans magnitude associated with increased heart rate,[13,28,29] especially during myocardial ischemia, reflects an increase in cardiac vulnerability. Thus, the variations in the T wave are a measure of the true physiologic change, and should not be interpreted as an error in measurement.

Sympathetic Stimulation

Stimulation of the stellate ganglia markedly hastens repolarization and shortens the QT interval.[21,30] The direct effect of catecholamines on the myocardium, as evidenced by intracoronary infusion of epinephrine or norepinephrine, is a marked increase in the amplitude of the T wave.[31] These effects of adrenergic activation are independent of changes in heart rate, as they are not replicated by comparable accelerations in rate by atrial pacing or by administration of atropine. Intense sympathetic stimulation, even in the normal heart, can lead to quantifiable levels of T wave alternans.[6,10] Sympathetic stimulation superimposed on myocardial ischemia greatly enhances the magnitude of T wave alternans.[10,29,32] This effect is thought to result largely from disruption of intracellular cycling of calcium, as it is abolished by calcium channel blockade.[22-27] In the long QT syndrome, adrenergic stimulation prolongs the QT interval due to genetically based derangements in ion channel function.[33] Furthermore, marked alternation of the T wave has been observed in long QT patients, who are susceptible to recurrent episodes of syncope and torsades de pointes.[6-9] A cellular basis in action potential morphology and duration has been established.[34-38] Rosenbaum and Acunzo[35] have proposed that the rate dependency of T wave alternans in patients with the long QT syndrome is due to disparities in action potential duration in response to rate of stimulation and in electrical restitution characteristics in subendocardial versus subepicardial fibers.

Parasympathetic Stimulation

Stimulation of the parasympathetic nerves generally exerts an effect on repolarization and T wave morphology that is opposite to that of sympathetic stimulation.[39] Vagal action antagonizes the effects of sympathetic activity according to two mechanisms. First, vagally released acetylcholine inhibits norepinephrine release presynaptically. Second, acetylcholine stimulates the muscarinic receptors to inhibit adrenergically mediated formation of second messenger.[40] Acetylcholine also affects excitable properties by altering the acetylcholine-sensitive potassium channel.[41] In experimental animals, vagal stimulation has been shown to be capable of suppressing ischemia-induced T wave alternans independent of a rate change.[16] In a patient with recurring ventricular fibrillation, Navarro-Lopez and coworkers[42] showed that activation of the vagus nerve by carotid sinus massage could suppress recurring T wave alternans. The effect could also have been due in part to baroreceptor-mediated withdrawal of sympathetic tone.

Temperature

Temperature exerts a significant influence on electrophysiologic properties of the heart, because of the impact on ion fluxes and various metabolic processes.[20] Increase in heart temperature generally results in accelerated repolarization and shortening of the QT interval. Decrease in temperature exerts essentially an opposite effect. Hypothermia is frequently associated with the appearance of a J wave, also referred to as an Osborne wave, which is a slow, upright deflection between the end of the QRS complex and the early portion of the ST segment. Severe hypothermia results in drastic changes in repolarization and frank T wave alternans is observed, correlating with a reduction in ventricular fibrillation threshold and increased propensity for ventricular fibrillation.[28]

In humans, the response to hyperthermia is complex, as it is often associated with physical, behavioral, and autonomic changes. Taggart and coworkers[43] documented pronounced ST and T wave changes in humans in a sauna. It is unknown whether the hyperthermic effects of fever produce any specific influence on repolarization independent of the accompanying tachycardia.

Electrolytes

Disturbances in electrolyte balance exert profound changes in repolarization, QT interval, and T wave morphology.[20] The most significant are those associated with disruption in plasma potassium and calcium. The electrocardiographic changes are complex and are strongly related to the magnitude of the electrolyte imbalance. Elevated extracellular potassium abbreviates the duration of the action potential, increases the velocity of phase 3, and decreases the resting membrane potential. The first two effects, which have been attributed to an enhanced membrane permeability to potassium, are probably responsible for the reduction in the QT interval and the narrow, peaked T wave. Peaking occurs when the plasma K concentration exceeds 5.5 mEq/L. Only extremely high or low calcium concentrations produce electrophysiologic abnormalities that are of clinical significance. Hypokalemia results in generally reciprocal changes. Hypocalcemia substantially prolongs the action potential plateau and increases the QT interval. It has also been shown to induce T wave alternans. The role of pH has been difficult to elucidate because acidosis and alkalosis are usually associated with abnormal concentrations of potassium and ionized calcium.

Integrated Responses

Exercise and Recovery

Even in normal subjects, vigorous exercise can lead to striking changes in ST segment and T wave, which can be readily misinterpreted as pathologic. These changes, including alterations in ST segment slope, shortening of the QT interval, and flattening of the T wave, are due to the complex nature of the physiologic responses to exercise, which include heart rate elevation, sympathetic nervous system activation, increases in body temperature, and alterations in blood composition including osmolality, potassium, and pH, as well as alterations in chest impedance and cardiac dynamics.[44,45] In a classic study of 40 low-risk normal male subjects, Froelicher and colleagues[45] characterized the repolarization changes associated with treadmill exercise. During exercise, they observed depression of the J junction and tall, peaked T waves at maximal exercise and at 1 minute of recovery. They commented that the changes were similar to early signs of ischemia, although the subjects were normal. Together with J junction depression, rapid ST segment upsloping was observed. T wave alternans has not been reported in normal subjects during exercise. However, there have been several reports of exercise-induced, sizeable T wave alternans in patients with severe coronary artery disease.[2,3] The phenomenon has also been reported in the postexercise recovery phase in these patients (Fig. 4).[1] More recently, the application of signal processing techniques has revealed that the phenomenon, in its more subtle but prognostically significant forms, is more prevalent during exercise than has been anticipated. Low-level T wave alternans during moderate exercise has also been reported in patients with cardiomyopathy[14] and heart failure.[15] Perhaps the most dramatic form of exercise-induced T wave alternans has been observed over many years in patients with the long QT syndrome.[6,7] Provocation of T wave alternans by exercise has been suggested as a suitable means to disclose latent propensity to lethal arrhythmias.[13-15,46]

Emotions

Intense emotion can produce significant T wave abnormalities in individuals without heart disease.[47] The behavioral states of fear, especially fear of operation, anxiety, worry, or longing, under hypnotic suggestion, result in repolarization changes consistent with enhanced sympathetic activation, tachycardia, and altered respiration. In a classic series of studies, Taggart and coworkers[48,49] demonstrated that the tension and stress associated with automobile driving in congested traffic can lead to flattening or inversion of the T wave. They commented that although the abnormalities occurred during tachycardia, they were probably not due to tachycardia per se, because elevation to comparable heart rates by atropine administration did not replicate the changes associated with stress.

It has long been known in patients with long QT syndrome that intense emotions can elicit alternating behavior of the T wave which may progress to torsades de pointes (Fig. 2). Recently, we demonstrated that induction of an anger-like state in canines during a confrontation paradigm produced marked shortening of QT interval, peaking of T waves, and T wave alternans even in the normal heart.[16] When anger was induced during coronary artery occlusion, there was an apparent synergistic effect in which alternans was more marked than the sum of the independent effects of anger and ischemia.

Hyperventilation

Excessive respiratory activity may produce abnormally low or inverted T waves in healthy individuals. Biberman and coworkers[50] have shown that these changes are probably not due to the previously invoked mechanisms of alkalosis, to alterations in plasma electrolytes, or to changes in the position of the heart in the chest. They demonstrated that the T wave abnormalities induced by hyperventilation, although consistently accompanied by tachycardia, could not be solely attributed to a critical increase in heart rate. This inference is consistent with the demonstration that the T wave becomes inverted after hyperventilation but remains upright when tachycardia is provoked by exercise.

The transient T wave inversion associated with hyperventilation is comparable to that observed during infusion of isoproterenol.[50] This observation suggests that the effect of hyperventilation may be due to asynchronous shortening of ventricular repolarization during the early phase of sympathetic activation. Furthermore, the T wave changes associated with hyperventilation can be prevented by propranolol administration.

Orthostasis

The transient orthostatic alterations in T wave morphology have also been attributed largely to increased sympathetic nerve activity. It has been shown that adrenergic blockade increases the ventricular gradient and decreases the QRS/T angle in the upright position; this is the purported basis for orthostatically induced electrocardiographic abnormalities.[51] There is evidence to suggest that rate change alone is not sufficient to account for orthostatically induced T wave changes. Again, the primary determinant appears to be direct adrenergic influences on cardiac repolarization properties.

Postprandial Changes

A diminution in the amplitude of the T wave, or inversion in leads I, II, and V_2 through V_4, commonly occurs within 30 minutes of the consumption of approximately 1200 calories.[52] Sears and Manning[53] reported that postprandial T wave changes occurred in 3.9% of 2000 young, healthy airmen. The putative mechanisms included lowering of plasma potassium concentration, sinus tachycardia, and possibly sympathetic nerve activation. Conversely, it has been demonstrated that a variety of nonspecific T wave abnormalities frequently vanish with short-term fasting.[54]

Electrophysiologic Mechanisms Underlying T Wave Alternans as an Index of Vulnerability to Fibrillation During Myocardial Ischemia

Although T wave alternans is a distinct phenomenon, the particular pattern of oscillation varies considerably as a function of the underlying pathophysiologic state.[8,16,17] For example, in the long QT syndrome, the T wave frequently alternates above and below the isoelectric line without concomitant ST segment change.[7,9] In ambulatory patients with stable coronary disease, in whom ischemia is usually subendocardial, there is ST segment depression with discrete T wave alternation primarily in the first half of the T wave, without evident R wave changes (Fig. 1).[55] In the setting of Prinzmetal's angina[4,5] or acute myocardial infarction,[17,56] both of which are characterized by transmural ischemia, the entire ST-T segment is elevated and alternates (Fig. 3). In the general electrophysiologic patient population, including those with chronic coronary disease, dilated coronary myopathy, and heart failure, there may be subtle, nonvisible alternation in the T wave that is detectable by spectral analytical techniques and has predictive value in terms of arrhythmia-free survival.[11,12,16,17] Collectively, these observations indicate that the physiologic basis for alternans differs considerably as a function of the pathophysiologic state, and this is a paramount consideration in the evaluation of the electrophysiologic mechanism, as has been discussed in a number of recent reviews.[8,16,17]

Dispersion of Repolarization

The weight of evidence indicates that regional disturbances in repolarization rather than in activation sequence form the basis for the linkage between ischemia-induced T wave alternans and susceptibility to cardiac arrhythmias.[57,58] This conclusion is drawn from diverse studies employing a wide variety of methodologic approaches ranging from intracellular recordings in isolated ischemic tissue to intracellular and extracellular recordings in intact preparations both with and without isopotential maps. Kurz and colleagues demonstrated that both the amplitude and the duration of action potentials alternate within the region of ischemia and exhibit regional heterogeneity.[59] Using finite element analysis, Smith and Cohen[60] demonstrated that dispersed subpopulations of cells could give rise to macroscopic electrical alternans by creating transitory barriers to conduction that lead to wave front fractionation and reentry.

Konta and associates[57] investigated the pattern of regional ST segment alternans during left anterior descending coronary artery occlusion in dogs. They employed epicardial mapping of electrograms and found that the amplitude of ST segment alternans, determined as the difference in ST segment elevation in two consecutive electrograms, was significantly larger in animals that fibrillated as compared to those that did not. Alternans was localized within the ischemic and border zones and was not evident in normal tissue. The area and magnitude of ST segment elevation did not correlate with the occurrence of ventricular fibrillation. Based on these observations, the investigators concluded that increased magnitude of ST segment alternans during acute ischemia constitutes a measure of risk for ventricular fibrillation because alternans is a reflection of temporal and spatial unevenness of ventricular repolarization, properties which are integrally linked to ventricular vulnerability.

Disturbances in recovery of excitability have also been implicated as a potential basis for the connection between T wave alternans and vulnerability to ventricular fibrillation. The underlying mechanisms appear to be postrepolarization refractoriness resulting in unidirectional block and reentry and the precipitation of ventricular tachycardia. Other investigators have proposed that triggered activity due to early afterdepolarizations is a basis for T wave alternans.[8]

MAP Recordings During Ischemia-Induced T Wave Alternans

Sutton and coworkers[61] recorded monophasic action potentials from the left ventricular epicardium in 36 patients undergoing cardiopulmonary bypass surgery. They observed that electrical alternans of action potential configuration and duration during coronary occlusion was a frequent event, being present in 14 (39%) of patients even with short duration occlusions lasting approximately 90 seconds. The phenomenon could be elicited by slight increases in heart rate in the absence of occlusion, and was enhanced further during occlusion and release of the graft (Fig. 5). The investigators commented on the regional nature of action potential alternans, as it was not detectable when the exploring electrode was positioned in an adjacent site approximately 1 cm away. None of the patients exhibited alternans

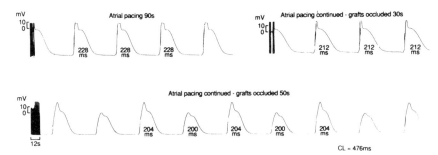

Figure 5. Monophasic action potentials during atrial pacing. Top left: immediately before graft occlusion after 90-second pacing. Top right: grafts occluded for 30 seconds. The lower trace shows alternans after 50-second graft occlusion, and the progressive development is shown in the slow playout at the beginning of the strip. Interbeat duration shows only a small variation while amplitude changes are striking. Zero mV calibration of the MAP signal is shown in the slow playout in both upper traces. Reprinted from Reference 61, with permission from the European Society of Cardiology.

in the surface electrocardiogram, but since they were studied during open chest bypass surgery, standard precordial electrocardiograms were not obtained. Moreover, the occlusions were of less than 1 minute duration, whereas in experimental models, nearly 2 minutes of occlusion are typically required to elicit visible alternans in surface leads. The authors concluded that *"the clinical electrocardiogram may be silent to this potentially prearrhythmic situation in many cases."*

Ionic Basis for Ischemia-Induced T Wave Alternans

Alterations in transmembrane or intracellular calcium movement appear to play a major but nonexclusive role in the initiation of T wave alternans during acute myocardial ischemia. This is based on investigations involving calcium channel blockers, including verapamil, diltiazem, and nexopamil, that suppress T wave alternans and prevent ventricular tachyarrhythmias during myocardial ischemia and reperfusion.[22-27] The role of calcium in T wave alternans is discussed in detail by Dr. Clusin in chapter 14 of this volume. Salerno and colleagues[4] reported that, in patients with Prinzmetal's variant angina, pretreatment with diltiazem abolished both ischemia-induced T wave alternans and ventricular arrhythmias. Whereas these agents affect myocardial perfusion as well as cardiac excitable properties, TQ-segment data suggest that their capability to suppress T wave alternans is independent of the influence of the drug on the extent of the ischemic insult. With use of the fluorescent calcium indicator Indo 1, Lee and colleagues[24] demonstrated that alternans in the ischemic area is associated with spatial heterogeneity of calcium transients (Fig. 6).[24] In addition, ryanodine, a drug that blocks calcium release from the sarcoplasmic reticulum, has been shown to suppress ischemia-induced alternans and the accompanying transients in calcium ion flux. The precise mechanisms whereby ionized calcium induces alternans, the specific intracellular compartments involved, and the role of sodium-calcium exchange require further exploration.

Potassium may also play an important role in ischemia-induced T wave alternans. This assertion is based on the fact that extracellular accumulation of this ion is thought to be responsible for postrepolarization refractoriness and is likely to contribute to the well established depression of electrical restitution of action potential duration. Lukas and Antzelevitch[62] demonstrated that the transient outward current is prominent mainly in epicardial and not endocardial tissue, and suggested that this divergence may contribute to differences in action potential morphology. Electrical alternans of epicardial action potential with a 2:1 or 3:1 pattern was evident during ischemia. This observation further emphasizes that the observed pattern of T wave alternans may result from changes in ion

A

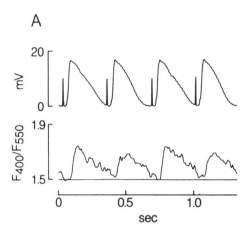

B

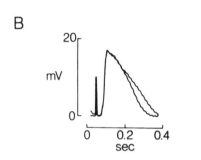

Figure 6. A. Recordings of simultaneous calcium transients and action potentials after 2 minutes of ischemia. Duration of the action potential alternates from beat to beat, as does the peak amplitude of the calcium transient. End-diastolic level of the calcium transient also exhibits fluctuations so that the lower amplitude transients (2nd and 4th) arise from a higher starting point. **B**. Photographic superimposition of long- and short-duration action potentials from A. Action potentials are nearly identical during the first 80 milliseconds, and do not diverge until after the calcium transient has reached its peak. This observation indicates that variations in the amplitude of the calcium transient are not a direct consequence of variations in membrane potential. Fluctuations of the calcium transient in A are not an artifact of motion, as can be shown by comparison of the F_{400}/F_{550} ratio with recordings at single wavelengths. Calcium transients in A all reach a peak systolic value that exceeds the preischemic value of 1.6. Reprinted from Reference 23, with permission of the American Heart Association.

channel kinetics, which are determined by density or number of channels and by the time needed for channel opening. In a pilot study, it was shown that blockade of the ATP-sensitive potassium channel by glibenclamide prevents reperfusion- as well as ischemia-induced shortening of action potential and reentrant arrhythmias.

Microvolt versus Millivolt Alternans: Are They Different Entities?

There has been considerable confusion concerning the difference between microvolt alternans and millivolt alternans. On first principles, there is no rationale for inferring mechanisms based on the magnitude of alternans. As discussed above, in most cases alternans is a continuum, and the greater the magnitude of alternans, the higher the likelihood of impending ventricular tachycardia and fibrillation. This is particularly evident in acute myocardial ischemia, when large amplitude alternans culminates in ventricular tachycardia/ventricular fibrillation. Thus, the terms "covert," 'nonvisible," and "microvolt" alternans are unfortunate, as they convey an erroneous impression of a phenomenon discrete from larger, visible, or millivolt alternans. The essential issue is whether the continuous function, alternans, has prognostic significance during the nonacute phase of disease, when its magnitude is less than when the condition worsens and leads to more sizeable alternans, a greater level of instability, and a higher likelihood of crossing the threshold for an arrhythmia.

The physiologic factors and proposed electrophysiologic bases for T wave alternans as an index of vulnerability to ventricular fibrillation are summarized in Table 1.

Table 1
Electrophysiologic Basis for T Wave
Alternans as a Function of Disease State

Disease or Condition	Putative Mechanism
Acute ischemia 1A phase: 2–10 min. of ischemia	Reentrant mechanisms: • alternation in action potential morphology • postrepolarization refractoriness • dispersion of repolarization in subpopulations of cells
1B phase: 10–30 min of ischemia	Nonreentrant mechanisms: • 2:1 activation block • derangements in impulse formation (frequently triggered by abrupt changes in cycle length)
Acute myocardial infarction	combination of reentrant and nonreentrant mechanisms: • action potential morphology alternation • conduction abnormalities
EP patient population Stable, nonischemic, but damaged cardiac substrate due to chronic coronary disease, cardiomyopathy, heart failure	• Reentry around nonviable tissue • Dispersion of repolarization in subpopulations of cells
Long QT syndrome	• Disparity in action potential duration in response to rate of stimulation and electrical restitution in subendocardial versus subepicardial fibers

Adapted from Verrier in Oto 1996 with permission from Kluwer Academic Press.

Conclusions

The repolarization phase of the electrocardiogram is extremely labile and highly responsive to diverse physiologic influences. In many cases, the normal response to intense physical or emotional stress is difficult to separate from pathophysiology on the basis of the ECG alone. Thus, an in-depth appreciation of normal physiology is essential for accurate measurement and interpretation of the QT interval and T wave characteristics. T wave alternation appears to be a more prevalent phenomenon than has been heretofore appreciated, and can have an impact on measurement of repolarization indexes, particularly as the QT interval duration and ST segment level are fluctuating on a beat-to-beat basis during T wave alternans. In fact, repolarization alternans should be perceived as more signal than noise, and appears to have significant promise as a predictor of vulnerability to life-threatening arrhythmia.

References

1. Belic N, Gardin JM. ECG manifestations of myocardial ischemia. *Arch Intern Med* 1980;140:1162-1165.
2. Wayne VS, Bishop RL, Spodick DH. Exercise-induced ST segment alternans. *Chest* 1983;83:824-825.
3. Ring ME, Fenster PE. Exercise-induced ST segment alternans. *Am Heart J* 1986;111:1009-1011.
4. Salerno JA, Previtali M, Panciroli C, et al. Ventricular arrhythmias during acute myocardial ischaemia in man. The role and significance of R-ST-T alternans and the prevention of ischaemic sudden death by medical treatment. *Eur Heart J* 1986;7:63-75.
5. Turitto G, El-Sherif N. Alternans of the ST segment in variant angina. Incidence, time course and relation to ventricular arrhythmias during ambulatory electrocardiographic recording. *Chest* 1988;93:587-591.
6. Schwartz PJ, Malliani A. Electrical alternation of the T-wave: Clinical and experimental evidence of its relationship with the sympathetic nervous system and with the long Q-T syndrome. *Am Heart J* 1975;89:45-50.
7. Schwartz PJ, Zaza A, Locati E, et al. Stress and sudden death. The case of the long QT syndrome. *Circulation* 1991;83(suppl 4):II71-II90.
8. Surawicz B, Fisch C. Cardiac alternans: Diverse mechanisms and clinical manifestations. *J Am Coll Cardiol* 1992;20:483-499.
9. Zareba W, Moss AJ, le Cessie S, et al. T wave alternans in idiopathic long QT syndrome. *J Am Coll Cardiol* 1994;23:1541-1546.
10. Nearing BD, Huang AH, Verrier RL. Dynamic tracking of cardiac vulnerability by complex demodulation of the T wave. *Science* 1991;252:437-440.
11. Rosenbaum DS, Jackson LE, Smith JM, et al. Electrical alternans and vulnerability to ventricular arrhythmia. *N Engl J Med* 1994;330:235-241.
12. Rosenbaum DS, Albrecht P, Cohen RJ. Predicting sudden cardiac death from T wave alternans of the surface electrocardiogram: Promise and pitfalls. *J Cardiovasc Electrophysiol* 1996;7:1095-1111.

13. Hohnloser SH, Klingenheben T, Zabel M, et al. T wave alternans during exercise and atrial pacing in humans. *J Cardiovasc Electrophysiol* 1997;8:987-993.

14. Murda'h MA, Nagayoshi H, Albrecht P, et al. T-wave alternans as a predictor of sudden death in hypertrophic cardiomyopathy. *Circulation* 1996;94:II669. Abstract.

15. Zabel M, Siedow A, Klingenheben T, et al. Noninvasive risk stratification in patients with congestive heart failure: Comparison of traditional risk markers and T-wave alternans. *J Am Coll Cardiol* 1997;29:515A. Abstract.

16. Verrier RL, Nearing BD. Electrophysiologic basis for T-wave alternans as an index of vulnerability to ventricular fibrillation. *J Cardiovasc Electrophysiol* 1994;5:445-461.

17. Verrier RL, Nearing BD. T-wave alternans as a harbinger of ischemia-induced sudden cardiac death. In Zipes DP, Jalife J (eds): *Cardiac Electrophysiology: From Cell to Bedside*. Philadelphia: W. B. Saunders; 1995:467-477.

18. Williams RR, Wagner GS, Peter RH. ST-segment alternans in Prinzmetal's angina. A report of two cases. *Ann Intern Med* 1974;81:51-54.

19. Surawicz B. The pathogenesis and clinical significance of primary T wave abnormalities. In Schlant RC, Hurst JW (eds): *Advances in Electrocardiography*. New York: Grune & Stratton, Inc.; 1972:377-421.

20. Surawicz B. *Electrophysiologic Basis of ECG and Cardiac Arrhythmias*. Baltimore: Williams & Wilkins; 1995.

21. Surawicz B, Saito S. Exercise testing for detection of myocardial ischemia in patients with abnormal electrocardiograms at rest. *Am J Cardiol* 1978;41:943.

22. Clusin WT, Bristow MR, Baim DS, et al. The effects of diltiazem and reduced serum ionized calcium on ischemic ventricular fibrillation in the dog. *Circ Res* 1982;50:518-526.

23. Hashimoto H, Suzuki K, Miyake S, et al. Effects of calcium antagonists on the electrical alternans of the ST segment and on associated mechanical alternans during acute coronary occlusion in dogs. *Circulation* 1983;68:667-672.

24. Lee H-C, Mohabir R, Smith N, et al. Effect of ischemia on calcium-dependent fluorescence transients in rabbit hearts containing indo 1. Correlation with monophasic action potentials and contraction. *Circulation* 1988;78:1047-1059.

25. Mohabir R, Clusin WT, Lee H-C. Intracellular calcium alternans and the genesis of ischemic ventricular fibrillation. In Zipes DP, Jalife J (eds): *Cardiac Electrophysiology: From Cell to Bedside*. Philadelphia: W. B. Saunders; 1990:448-456.

26. Nearing BD, Hutter JJ, Verrier RL. Potent antifibrillatory effect of combined blockade of calcium channels and 5-HT$_2$ receptors with nexopamil during myocardial ischemia and reperfusion in canines: Comparison to diltiazem. *J Cardiovasc Pharmacol* 1996;27:777-787.

27. Wu Y, Clusin WT. Calcium transient alternans in blood-perfused ischemic hearts: Observations with fluorescent indicator fura red. *Am J Physiol* 1997;273:H2161-H2169.

28. Adam DR, Smith JM, Akselrod S, et al. Fluctuations in T-wave morphology and susceptibility to ventricular fibrillation. *J Electrocardiol* 1984;17:209-218.

29. Euler DE, Guo H, Olshansky B. Sympathetic influences on electrical and mechanical alternans in the canine heart. *Cardiovasc Res* 1996;32:854-860.

30. Schwartz PJ, La Rovere MT, Vanoli E. Autonomic nervous system and sudden cardiac death: Experimental basis and clinical observations for post-myocardial infarction risk stratification. *Circulation* 1992;85(suppl I):I77-I91.

31. Sparks HV, Hollenberg M, Carriere S, et al. Sympathomimetic drugs and repolarization of ventricular myocardium of the dog. *Cardiovasc Res* 1970;4:363-370.

32. Nearing BD, Oesterle SN, Verrier RL. Quantification of ischaemia-induced vulnerability by precordial T-wave alternans analysis in dog and human. *Cardiovasc Res* 1994;28:1440-1449.

33. Schwartz PJ, Priori SG, Locati EH, et al. Long QT syndrome patients with mutations of the SCN5A and HERG genes have differential responses to Na^+ channel blockade and to increases in heart rate. Implications for gene-specific therapy. *Circulation* 1995;92:3381-3386.

34. Sakurada H, Tejima T, Hiyoshi Y, et al. Association of humps on monophasic action potentials and ST-T alternans in a patient with Romano-Ward syndrome. *PACE* 1991;14:1485-1491.

35. Rosenbaum MB, Acunzo RS. Pseudo 2:1 atrioventricular block and T wave alternans in the long QT syndromes. *J Am Coll Cardiol* 1991;18:1363-1366.

36. Shimizu W, Yamada K, Arakaki Y, et al. Monophasic action potential recordings during T-wave alternans in congenital long QT syndrome. *Am Heart J* 1996;132:699-701.

37. El-Sherif N, Caref EB, Yin H, et al. The electrophysiological mechanism of ventricular arrhythmias in the long QT syndrome. Tri-dimensional mapping of activation and recovery patterns. *Circ Res* 1996;79:474-492.

38. Shimizu W, Antzelevitch C. Cellular and ionic basis for T wave alternans under long QT conditions. *Circulation* 1999;99:1499-1507.

39. Levy MN, Schwartz PJ (eds): *Vagal Control of the Heart*. Mt. Kisco, NY: Futura Publishing Company, Inc.; 1994.

40. Levy MN, Warner MR. Autonomic interactions in cardiac control: Role of neuropeptides. In Zipes DP, Jalife J (eds): *Cardiac Electrophysiology and Arrhythmias*. Philadelphia: W. B. Saunders; 1990:305-311.

41. Sicilian Gambit. Task Force of the Working Group on Arrhythmias of the European Society of Cardiology. A new approach to the classification of antiarrhythmic drugs based on their actions on arrhythmogenic mechanisms. *Circulation* 1991;84:1831-1851.

42. Navarro-Lopez F, Cinca J, Sanz G, et al. Isolated T wave alternans. *Am Heart J* 1978;95:369-374.

43. Taggart P, Parkinson P, Carruthers M. Cardiac responses to thermal, physical, and emotional stress. *Br Med J* 1972;3:71-76.

44. Wolthuis RA, Froelicher VF, Hopkirk A, et al. Normal electrocardiographic waveform characteristics during treadmill exercise testing. *Circulation* 1979;60:1028-1035.

45. Froelicher VF, Wolthuis R, Fisher J, et al. Variations in normal electrocardiographic response to treadmill testing. *Am J Cardiol* 1981;47:1161-1187.

46. Verrier RL, Stone PJ. Exercise stress testing for T wave alternans to expose latent electrical instability. *J Cardiovasc Electrophysiol* 1997;8:994-997.

47. Surawicz B. ST-T abnormalities. In MacFarlane PW, Lawrie TD (eds): *Comprehensive Electrocardiology*. New York: Pergamon Press; 1989.

48. Taggart P, Gibbons D, Somerville W. Some effects of motor-car driving on the normal and abnormal heart. *Br Med J* 1969;4:130-134.

49. Taggart P, Carruthers M, Joseph S, et al. Electrocardiographic changes resembling myocardial ischaemia in asymptomatic men with normal coronary arteriograms. *Br Heart J* 1979;41:214-225.

50. Biberman L, Sarma RN, Surawicz B. T wave abnormalities during hyperventilation and isoproterenol infusion. *Am Heart J* 1971;81:166.

51. Schweitzer P, et al. Der Einfluss der adrenergen Blockade auf die orthostatischen Veraenderungen der Integralvektoren von QRS. *Z Kreislaufforsh* 1967;56:316.

52. Simonson E, McKinlay CA. The meal test in clinical electrocardiography. *Circulation* 1950;1:1006.

53. Sears GA, Manning GW. Routine electrocardiography. Postprandial T wave changes. *Am Heart J* 1958;56:591.

54. Sleeper JC, Orgain ES. Differentiation of benign from pathologic T waves in the electrocardiogram. *Am J Cardiol* 1963;11:338.

55. Verrier RL, Nearing BD, MacCallum G, et al. T-wave alternans during ambulatory ischemia in patients with stable coronary disease. *Ann Noninvasive Electrocardiol* 1996;1:113-120.

56. Pantridge JF. Autonomic disturbance at the onset of acute myocardial infarction. In Schwartz PJ, Brown AM, Malliani A, Zanchetti A (eds): *Neural Mechanisms in Cardiac Arrhythmias*. New York: Raven Press; 1978:7-17.

57. Konta T, Ikeda K, Yamaki M, et al. Significance of discordant ST alternans in ventricular fibrillation. *Circulation* 1990;82:2185-2189.

58. Green LS, Fuller MP, Lux RL. Three-dimensional distribution of ST-T wave alternans during acute ischemia. *J Cardiovasc Electrophysiol* 1997;8:1413-1419.

59. Kurz RW, Mohabir R, Ren X-L, et al. Ischaemia induced alternans of action potential duration in the intact heart: Dependence on coronary flow, preload, and cycle length. *Eur Heart J* 1993;14:1410-1420.

60. Smith JM, Cohen RJ. Simple finite-element model accounts for wide range of ventricular dysrhythmias. *Proc Natl Acad Sci U S A* 1994;81:233-237.

61. Sutton PMI, Taggart P, Lab M, et al. Alternans of epicardial repolarization as a localized phenomenon in man. *Eur Heart J* 1991;12:70-78.

62. Lukas A, Antzelevitch C. Differences in the electrophysiologic response of canine ventricular epicardium and endocardium to ischemia: Role of the transient outward current. *Circulation* 1993;88:2903-2915.

17

Changes in Monophasic Action Potential Configuration and Prevalence of Ventricular Fibrillation During Regional Ischemia and Reperfusion in the Intact Canine Heart:

Effects of Preconditioning Ischemia and Potassium Channel Modulators

Toshihisa Miyazaki, MD, Satoshi Ogawa, MD and Douglas P. Zipes, MD

Introduction

Ventricular arrhythmias occur frequently after acute occlusion of a coronary artery, and often degenerate into ventricular fibrillation (VF). VF can also be easily induced by rapid reflow of an occluded artery. Such ischemic and reperfusion VF are believed to be major causes of sudden cardiac death in humans.[1,2] The electrophysiologic mechanisms of ischemia and reperfusion-induced arrhythmias have been studied in animal models mainly by mapping of the activation sequence of depolarization. According to these studies, most of ischemic ventricular arrhythmias occur due to

From Franz MR (ed): *Monophasic Action Potentials: Bridging Cell and Bedside.*
©Futura Publishing Company, Inc., Armonk, NY, 2000.

reentry in the ischemic myocardium,[3-5] while a focal mechanism, perhaps precipitated by injury current that flows from ischemic to boundary zone, is also involved in some of the ischemic arrhythmias.[4] In contrast to acute ischemia, more than half of the reperfusion arrhythmias are initiated by nonreentrant mechanisms.[6]

Only a few studies[7] have been done to determine the changes in the local repolarization process induced by regional ischemia and reperfusion and their relation to arrhythmogenesis in the intact hearts; this is probably because it is difficult to record transmembrane action potentials. It is easier, however, to record monophasic action potentials (MAPs) from the beating heart and to characterize the repolarization process of the regionally ischemic myocardium.[8]

This chapter presents our data showing correlation between temporal MAP changes and arrhythmogenesis during regional ischemia and reperfusion in the intact canine hearts and the electrophysiologic basis of antiarrhythmic action of preconditioning ischemia, and offers plausible ion channels responsible for regional ischemia-induced MAP shortening.

Experimental Model and MAP Recording

In pentobarbital-anesthetized, open-chest dogs, the left anterior descending coronary artery (LAD) was dissected free at a site distal to the first or second diagonal branch. A silk suture was positioned around the LAD, passed through a plastic tube, and used as a noose to obtain complete occlusion and reperfusion of the LAD by tightening and releasing the suture. Five-minute occlusion of the LAD was repeated up to 4 times, separated by 30-minute intervals of reperfusion. Heart rate was maintained constant by atrial pacing at a cycle length slightly shorter than the individual sinus cycle length (300 to 400 milliseconds). If VF occurred during LAD occlusion, the occlusion was discontinued and the heart was defibrillated with a direct-current shock of 5 to 20 J applied with paddles to the ventricles. If VF occurred upon reperfusion, direct-current shock was applied immediately.

Because 5-minute coronary occlusion causes reversible electrophysiologic changes, and repeated occlusions do not affect collateral blood flow to the ischemic myocardium, this model has an advantage in terms of assessing the effects of an intervention on the electrophysiologic changes and arrhythmogenesis within the same animal with a constant area at risk and a comparable degree of ischemia.[9]

The MAP was recorded from the epicardium by use of a hand-held pressure contact electrode probe (model 200, EP Technologies, San Jose, CA). In some experiments, endocardial MAP was also recorded simultaneously by use of a catheter with silver-silver chloride electrode (EP Technologies model 1675), which was introduced via the left carotid artery. These MAP recording probes were positioned at the anticipated center of the ischemic zone of the left ventricle, and signals were amplified with direct current coupled differential amplifiers at a frequency range of 0.04 to 500 Hz. MAPs were accepted if they fulfilled the following criteria: 1) constant configuration and stable resting membrane potential, and 2) stable amplitude of phase 2 greater than 10 mV during the baseline recording. The MAP amplitude was measured as the potential difference between phase 2 and the maximal diastolic potential during phase 4; then the MAP duration at 90% repolarization (APD_{90}) was measured.

Relation of Temporal MAP Changes to VF and the Effects of Preconditioning Ischemia

Suppression of ischemia- and reperfusion-induced arrhythmias by preconditioning ischemia has been reported in animals[10-12] and humans.[13] We[14] have suggested that suppression of heterogeneous development of autonomic denervation may account at least in part for its antiarrhythmic action. However, the electrophysiologic basis of preconditioning effects is not fully understood, especially with respect to the effects on repolarization process.

Therefore, in the first protocol we studied the temporal relationship between the changes in epicardial MAP configuration and the occurrence of VF during the first coronary occlusion-reperfusion sequence, and we examined the effects of preconditioning ischemia on MAP changes and arrhythmias during the following ischemia and reperfusion episodes by comparing the second sequence data with the first sequence data in 32 animals.[15]

The prominent changes in configuration of the epicardial MAP observed during the first coronary occlusion-reperfusion sequence were as follows: 1) progressive shortening of MAP duration after coronary occlusion, and quick recovery of the MAP duration immediately after reperfusion, with some overshoot lengthening as compared to the baseline duration before occlusion (Fig. 1); 2) alternans of MAP duration (Fig. 2); and 3) transient appearance of humps that resembled early afterdepolarizations (EADs) or delayed afterdepolarizations (DADs) during coronary occlusion (Fig. 3) as well as after reperfusion. Among these changes, a marked alternans of the MAP duration was the best predictor of the following development of VF (ie, the prevalence of VF was significantly higher in animals with the maximal difference in APD_{90} between the two consecutive beats ≥20 milliseconds than in animals with less than 20 milliseconds [46% versus 11%; $P<0.05$]) (Figs. 2 and 4). Such alternans of MAP duration increased as a function of time after

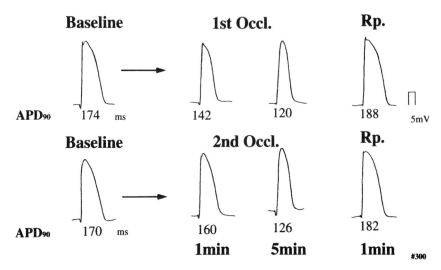

Figure 1. Progressive shortening of epicardial MAP duration after left anterior descending coronary artery occlusion and quick recovery after reperfusion with some overshoot lengthening. Note that the extent of shortening is reduced during the second occlusion as compared to the first. Measured duration at 90% repolarization (APD_{90}) is indicated at the bottom of each MAP.

acute coronary occlusion (Fig. 5). The prevalence of VF also tended to be higher in animals with a greater shortening rate of APD_{90}, and with appearance of EAD- or DAD-like humps (Fig. 4).

Interestingly, each of these MAP changes observed during the first coronary occlusion-reperfusion sequence was suppressed markedly during the second sequence (Figs. 1 through 3 and Fig. 5). Mean shortening rate of APD_{90} during coronary occlusion was reduced ($22\pm2\%$ versus $18\pm2\%$; n=31; $P<0.01$). The increase in alternans was eliminated almost completely (Figs. 2 and 5). The incidence of EAD- or DAD-like humps was reduced (14/31 versus 3/31; $P<0.05$). Consistent with these changes, the incidence of VF during the second occlusion-reperfusion sequence was significantly reduced as compared with the first sequence (9/32 versus 3/32; $P<0.05$). This temporal correlation suggests that suppression of MAP shortening, alternans, and the afterdepolarizations by preconditioning ischemia may contribute to its antifibrillatory action during subsequent ischemia and reperfusion. We speculate further that improvement of intracellular Ca^{++} handling may be involved in the electrophysiologic and antiarrhythmic effects of preconditioning ischemia.

Appearance of EAD-like hump was common during the first sequence, although triggering of arrhythmias from the hump could not be demonstrated. Of note, the EAD-like hump was recorded commonly during the first coronary occlusion (8/31 dogs; 26%) (Fig. 3), as well as during reperfu-

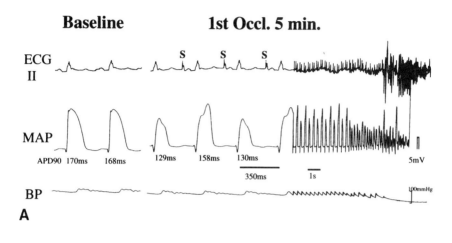

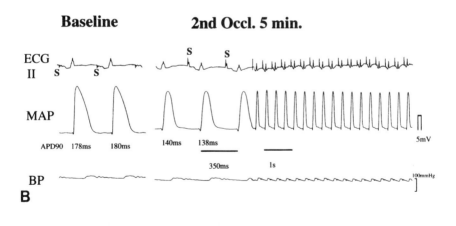

Figure 2. Appearance of a marked alternans of epicardial MAP duration that preceded ventricular fibrillation (VF) at 5 minutes after the first left anterior descending coronary artery occlusion (**A**), and suppression of the alternans and VF during the second occlusion (**B**). S denotes the stimuli from atrial pacing.

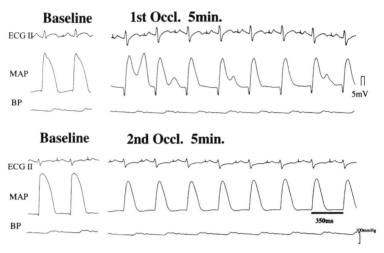

Figure 3. Appearance of early-afterdepolarization-like humps at 5 minutes after the first left anterior descending coronary artery occlusion, and elimination of the humps during the second occlusion.

Prevalence of VF

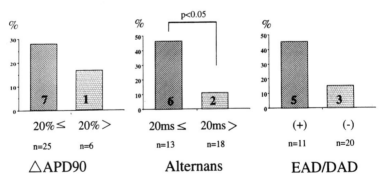

Figure 4. Correlation between temporal MAP changes and the prevalence of ventricular fibrillation (VF) during the first left anterior descending coronary artery (LAD) occlusion and reperfusion. Relation of the mean shortening rate of action potential duration at 90% repolarization during 5-minute coronary occlusion (ΔAPD90), alternans of epicardial MAP duration (ie, the maximal difference in APD_{90} between the two consecutive beats [Alternans]), and the presence of EAD-/DAD-like humps to the prevalence of VF during the first LAD occlusion and reperfusion is shown. The actual number of dogs that developed VF is indicated in each bar graph. The prevalence of VF was higher in dogs with ΔAPD90 $\geq$20%, alternans $\geq$20 milliseconds, or the presence of EAD-/DAD-like humps than in dogs without each change. VF occurred in 5 of 8 dogs (63%) with all of these changes. Among these changes, alternans $\geq$20 milliseconds was the best predictor of the development of VF.

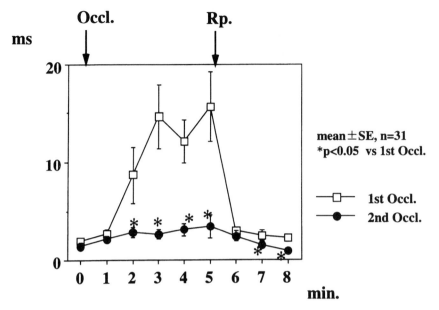

Figure 5. Increase of alternans of epicardial MAP duration after the first left anterior descending coronary artery occlusion, and suppression of the alternans during the second occlusion.

sion (6/24; 25%). It is known that EADs are induced by reperfusion of the ischemic myocardium[16] or on recovering from ischemia-like conditions.[17] Our findings suggest that EADs also develop during early ischemia. Extracellular accumulation of potassium during acute ischemia may inhibit the development of EADs; however catecholamines increased in the ischemic myocardium,[18] and abnormal handling of intracellular Ca^{++} may facilitate EADs. The results of this study are consistent with an earlier one in which we recorded apparent EADs during acute coronary occlusion in dogs.[19]

Effects of Drugs on Regional Ischemia-Induced MAP Shortening

The most consistent change observed in the epicardial MAP during regional ischemia was shortening of its duration (Fig. 1). To determine the plausible ion channels that were causing this change, we examined the effects of various potassium channel modulators.[20-23] In this protocol, we used the data obtained during the second occlusion-reperfusion sequence as control, and the drugs were administered before the third or fourth occlusion. This is based on the findings that the first occlusion causes a greater shortening of the epicardial MAP duration than does the second occlusion as described above, whereas the occlusions that follow cause similar MAP shortening in control group animals.[20]

Different MAP Changes in the Epicardium and Endocardium

By the simultaneous recording of epicardial and endocardial MAPs during the control occlusion, we found that the extent of MAP shortening was greater at the epicardium than at the endocardium.[22] This finding is consistent with previous studies in isolated ventricular tissue,[24] in isolated cat ventricle,[25] and in the intact canine hearts.[26] Figure 6 shows an example of simultaneous MAP recordings. The epicardial MAP was shortened, whereas endocardial MAP was rather lengthened after LAD occlusion, which increased the time lag of repolarization between the two layers. Consistent with these changes, the unipolar electrogram recorded from epicardium of the ischemic zone exhibited ST segment elevation and increase in T wave amplitude. Because endocardial and epicardial potential difference contributes to electrocardiographic ST-T waves,[27] it is likely that such differential change in epicardial and endocardial action potential configurations can be one of the causes of electrocardiographic ST-T changes immediately after acute coronary occlusion.

Effects of K$_{ATP}$ Channel Modulators

We have suggested that activation of epicardially dominant ATP-sensitive potassium (K$_{ATP}$) channels plays a major role in such differential

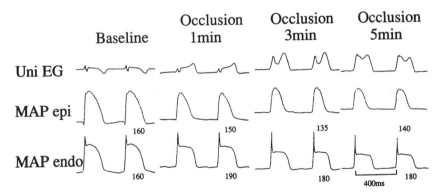

Figure 6. Simultaneous recordings of epicardial (epi) and endocardial (endo) MAPs, and unipolar electrogram (Uni EG) from epicardium of the ischemic zone. See text for details.

change in epicardial and endocardial action potential configurations.[22] 5-Hydroxydecanoate (5-HD), a blocker of K$_{ATP}$ channels, suppressed the shortening of epicardial MAP preferentially[20,22] (Fig. 7, panel A), (as did glibenclamide[20]), and reduced the difference of MAP duration between the two layers.[22] In contrast, nicorandil, an opener, augmented the shortening preferentially at the epicardial layer and increased the difference[22] (Fig. 7, panel B). Glibenclamide has also been shown to enhance, and pinacidil to reduce, attenuation in sympathetic responsiveness after acute coronary occlusion.[28]

Furukawa and colleagues[29] have demonstrated that epicardial myocytes have a lower threshold of K$_{ATP}$ channel activation than endocardial myocytes, ie, K$_{ATP}$ channels of the epicardial myocytes are activated with less reduction of intracellular ATP concentration. The epicardially dominant activation of K$_{ATP}$ channels during regional ischemia as suggested by the present data may be attributed to such lower activation threshold and/or a denser distribution at the epicardial layer, although the latter possibility remains to be proved.

The finding that action potential change during ischemia is greater at the epicardial layer than at the endocardial layer[22,24-26] appears contradictory in light of the findings that the endocardial layer is subjected to a greater reduction of myocardial blood flow[9,14,30] and to earlier development of myocardial necrosis[31,32] than the epicardial layer during regional ischemia. However, epicardially dominant activation of K$_{ATP}$ channels may explain, at least in part, a greater action potential change and preferential survival of the epicardial myocardium. It is possible that activation of K$_{ATP}$ channels protects the myocardium against ischemia/reperfusion damage and helps it survive during prolonged ischemia.[33,34]

In addition, activation of epicardially dominant K$_{ATP}$ channels and a resultant difference of action potential configurations can be a cause of electrocardiographic ST-T changes observed immediately after acute coronary occlusion. Kubota et al[35] have reported that ST segment elevation during acute coronary occlusion is suppressed by the pretreatment with glibenclamide. Also, we have found that ST segment elevation and increase in T wave amplitude of the epicardial unipolar electrograms are suppressed by the pretreatment with glibenclamide but are augmented by nicorandil.[36]

K$_{ATP}$ Channel Dilemma: Is it Clinically Important?

Spatially different activation of cardiac K$_{ATP}$ channels leads to concerns about its proarrhythmic action during the early phase of regional ischemia, because action potentials would be shortened heterogeneously and spatial dispersion of repolarization time would be increased, which may facilitate reentrant arrhythmias. In fact, profibrillatory action of K$_{ATP}$

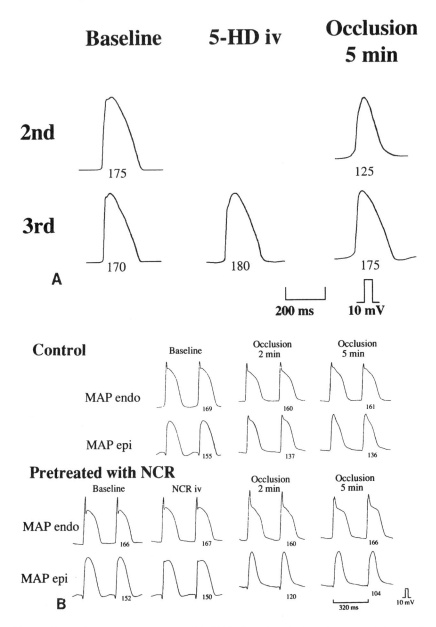

Figure 7. A. Shortening of epicardial MAP duration during the second (control) left anterior descending coronary artery (LAD) occlusion and suppression of the shortening during the third occlusion by pretreatment with 5-hydroxydecanoate (5-HD), a blocker of KATP channels. **B.** Simultaneous recordings of endocardial and epicardial MAPs during the second LAD occlusion (Control) and preferential augmentation of epicardial MAP shortening during the following occlusion by pretreatment with KATP channel opener nicorandil (NCR).

channel openers has been reported in a variety of experimental models (ie, in isolated myocardial tissue,[37] in isolated hearts,[38] and in a conscious canine model of sudden death.[39] On the other hand, antifibrillatory action of glibenclamide was reported in isolated rat hearts.[40]

In the intact canine model of regional ischemia, however, the incidence of VF during coronary occlusion and reperfusion was reduced by the pretreatment with K_{ATP} channel openers nicorandil (0.2 to 0.5 mg/kg, i.v.)[21] and lemakalim (3 to 15 µg/kg, i.v.),[41] but was increased by K_{ATP} channel blockers 5-HD (30 mg/kg, i.v.)[42] and glibenclamide (0.15 to 0.3 mg/kg, i.v. [S. Ito, T. Miyazaki, unpublished data, October 1997]). There are several possible explanations for these somewhat unexpected results. First, although they augmented MAP shortening, K_{ATP} channel openers nicorandil and lemakalim, at clinical doses, do not have an influence on the effective refractory periods of the ischemic myocardium.[41] Second, augmentation of ischemia-induced MAP shortening by K_{ATP} channel openers would reduce voltage-dependent inward Ca^{++} current and Ca^{++} entry via Na^+-Ca^{++} exchange mechanism (shortened action potential plateau limits Ca^{++} entry via the exchange mechanism), thereby inhibiting intracellular Ca^{++} overloading during ischemia and reperfusion. This might suppress a variety of arrhythmogenic mechanisms including triggered activity, enhanced automaticity, and even reentry related to the conduction disturbances. K_{ATP} channel blockers may exhibit an opposite action. Finally, K_{ATP} channel openers improve ischemia per se, whereas blockers worsen the degree of ischemia because they suppress hypoxic vasodilation of coronary arterioles[43] and inhibit the autoregulation mechanism in coronary circulation.[44] Finally, reduction in regional sympathetic dysfunction may be antiarrhythmic.[28]

The data suggest that activation of K_{ATP} channels and the effects of K_{ATP} channel openers are clinically important in terms of cardioprotection against ischemia/reperfusion damage.[21,33,34,45,46] On the other hand, antidiabetic sulfonylureas may worsen cardiac function by abolishing the protection afforded by K_{ATP} channels in patients with coronary artery disease who are subjected to ischemia. In fact, increased mortality rate due to cardiovascular causes has been reported in diabetic patients who received tolbutamide.[47]

Effect of a Class III Antiarrhythmic Drug

Activation of K_{ATP} channels plays an important role in action potential shortening and potassium efflux during metabolic inhibition or hypoxia in vitro,[33,45,48,49] global ischemia,[50] and regional ischemia.[20-22,51] However, little is known about the involvement of delayed rectifier potassium currents (I_K), which are physiologically important repolarization currents, in action potential shortening during ischemia, although their involvement appears likely because catecholamines are increased in the ischemic myocardium,[18] which may facilitate a slow component of I_K.[52,53] Also, the mode of action of class III antiarrhythmic drugs during regional ischemia is not fully understood.

We[23] therefore examined the effect of MS-551, a new class III antiarrhythmic drug that inhibits I_K at a clinical concentration.[54] In the absence of myocardial ischemia, MS-551 (0.3 mg/kg i.v. followed by 0.05 mg/kg/min d.i.v.) prolonged MAP duration significantly in a reverse use-dependent manner; however this effect was eliminated completely by 5-minute coronary occlusion, ie, MAP duration was shortened to the same level observed during control occlusion, and the difference between preocclusion and postocclusion MAP durations was increased as compared to the control occlusion. Figure 8 shows such an example. After the pretreatment with intravenous propranolol, MS-551 had no effect on occlusion-induced MAP shortening, but increased the difference between preocclusion and postocclusion MAP durations.

These results suggest that I_K does not play an important role in regional ischemia-induced MAP shortening. Also, this finding appears important in terms of a possible increase by a class III drug in spatial dispersion of

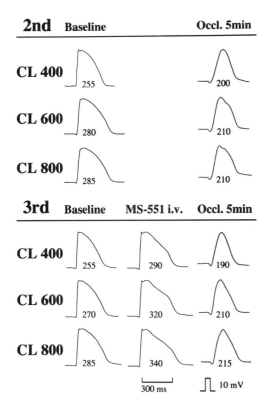

Figure 8. Disappearance of the class III effect of MS-551 on epicardial MAP duration during 5-minute left anterior descending coronary artery occlusion. See text for details.

repolarization between normal and ischemic myocardium, which may not be prevented by combined administration of a β-adrenoceptor—blocking agent.[23] Our results are concordant with previous studies[55,56] showing that the class III action of d,l-sotalol, a class III antiarrhythmic drug with β-blocking property on repolarization, was eliminated by 20 to 30 minutes of ischemia.

Effect of Gadolinium, a Blocker of Stretch-Activated Channels

The mechanoelectrical feedback phenomenon is the concept that myocardial stretch modulates electrophysiologic properties, ie, shortens ventricular action potential duration[57] and reduces action potential amplitude[58] and resting membrane potential.[59] Acute stretch has been shown to lengthen atrial refractoriness.[60,61] The ion channels that mediate these changes remain to be clarified, however, stretch-activated channels (SACs) are speculated.[62] Activation of SACs generates cationic currents including sodium, potassium, and calcium currents. At more negative potentials than the reversal potentials (−40 to 0 mV), SACs generate net inward cationic currents and thereby depolarize the resting membrane potential, whereas SACs shorten action potential duration by generating net outward cationic currents at more positive potential, ie, at plateau phase. Because action potential shortening and depolarization of the resting membrane potential are the same changes as those seen in the mechanoelectrical feedback phenomenon, involvement of SACs in this phenomenon is strongly suspected. In fact, we have found that gadolinium, a blocker of SACs,[63] suppresses mechanoelectrical feedback and arrhythmias induced by transient cross-clamping of the ascending aorta in the intact dogs.[64]

Also, it is likely that SAC-mediated mechanoelectrical feedback occurs during regional ischemia, because the ischemic myocardium is stretched by passive bulging motion. To address this hypothesis, we examined the effect of gadolinium on repolarization time of the ischemic myocardium (S. Takagi, T. Miyazaki, unpublished data, March 1997). Unipolar and bipolar electrograms were recorded from 47 epicardial sites of the anticipated ischemic zone. QT interval and activation time were measured on unipolar and bipolar electrograms, respectively. The QT index, a QT minus activation time interval, was used as a measure of local repolarization time.

During control occlusion, QT index was shortened and ST segment of the unipolar electrogram was elevated significantly. Gadolinium (500 μmol, 2500 μmol) injected into the left atrium before the ensuing coronary occlusions suppressed QT index shortening, ST segment elevation, and premature ventricular complexes in a dose-related manner. In a separate group, gadolinium also suppressed these changes in the presence of glibenclamide. Plasma level of gadolinium after the 2500-μmol injection ranged from 1 to 4 μM, which is known to inhibit SACs selectively.[65]

These data suggest that SACs are involved in the shortening of repolarization, in ST segment elevation, and in some arrhythmias during early phase of acute coronary occlusion, independent of K_{ATP} channels.

Summary

In order to characterize the changes in repolarization process of the regionally ischemic myocardium, we recorded MAPs in the intact canine hearts. Epicardial MAP recording during 5-minute LAD occlusion and reperfusion demonstrated reversible shortening and alternans of MAP duration, and transient appearance of EAD- or DAD-like humps during ischemia as well as upon reperfusion. Among these changes, a marked alternans of the MAP duration was the best predictor of the development of VF that followed. Preconditioning ischemia suppressed all these changes as well as the occurrence of VF, suggesting that improvement of repolarization abnormalities may be related to its antifibrillatory action.

Simultaneous recording of epicardial and endocardial MAPs showed that the extent of regional ischemia-induced MAP shortening was greater at the epicardium than at the endocardium. We have suggested that epicardially dominant activation of K_{ATP} channels plays a major role in creating such a difference and causing the electrocardiographic ST-T changes, because K_{ATP} channel blockers suppressed the preferential epicardial MAP shortening, reduced the MAP difference between the two layers, and suppressed the ST-T changes whereas K_{ATP} channel opener nicorandil had opposite effects. Gadolinium also suppressed the shortening of repolarization and ST segment elevation, even in the presence of glibenclamide, suggesting that SACs are involved, independent of K_{ATP} channels, in repolarization and electrocardiographic ST-T changes observed immediately after acute coronary occlusion. In contrast, MS-551, a new class III antiarrhythmic drug that inhibits I_K, had no effect on epicardial MAP shortening, suggesting that I_K does not play an important role in regional ischemia-induced repolarization change.

References

1. Kuller LH. Sudden death—definition and epidemiologic considerations. *Prog Cardiovasc Dis* 1980;23:1-12.
2. Goldstein S. The necessity of a uniform definition of sudden coronary death: Witnessed death within 1 hour after the onset of acute symptoms. *Am Heart J* 1982;103:156-159.
3. Kaplinsky E, Ogawa S, Balke W, Dreifus L. Two periods of early ventricular arrhythmia in canine acute myocardial infarction model. *Circulation* 1979;60:397-403.

4. Janse MJ, van Capelle FLJ, Morsink H, et al. Flow of injury current and patterns of excitation during early ventricular arrhythmias in acute regional myocardial ischemia in isolated porcine and canine hearts. Evidence for two different arrhythmogenic mechanisms. *Circ Res* 1980;47:151-165.

5. Pogwizd SM, Corr RB. Reentrant and nonreentrant mechanisms contribute to arrhythmogenesis during early myocardial ischemia: Results using three dimensional mapping. *Circ Res* 1987;61:352-371.

6. Pogwizd SM, Corr RB. Electrophysiologic mechanisms underlying arrhythmias due to reperfusion of ischemic myocardium. *Circulation* 1987;76:404-426.

7. Downar E, Janse MJ, Durrer D. The effect of acute coronary occlusion on subepicardial transmembrane potentials in the intact porcine heart. *Circulation* 1977;56:217-224.

8. Franz MR, Flaherty JT, Platia EV, et al. Localization of regional myocardial ischemia by recording of monophasic action potentials. *Circulation* 1984;69:593-604.

9. Miyazaki T, Zipes DP. Pericardial prostaglandin biosynthesis prevents the increased incidence of reperfusion-induced ventricular fibrillation produced by efferent sympathetic stimulation in dogs. *Circulation* 1990;82:1008-1019.

10. Vegh A, Komoro S, Szekeres L, et al. Antiarrhythmic effects of preconditioning in anesthetized dogs and rats. *Cardiovasc Res* 1992;26:487-495.

11. Shiki K, Hearse GJ. Preconditioning of ischemic myocardium: Reperfusion-arrhythmias. *Am J Physiol* 1987;253:H1470-H1476.

12. Hager JM, Hale SL, Kloner RA. Effects of preconditioning ischemia on reperfusion arrhythmias after coronary artery occlusion and reperfusion in the rat. *Circ Res* 1991;68:61-68.

13. Anzai T, Yoshikawa T, Asakura Y, et al. Effect on short-term prognosis and left ventricular function of angina pectoris prior to first Q-wave anterior wall acute myocardial infarction. *Am J Cardiol* 1994;74:755-759.

14. Miyazaki T, Zipes DP. Protection against autonomic denervation following acute myocardial infarction by preconditioning ischemia. *Circ Res* 1989;64:437-448.

15. Ito S, Miyazaki T, Miyoshi S, et al. Ventricular fibrillation and shortening, alternans, and afterdepolarizations of epicardial monophasic action potentials during coronary occlusion and reperfusion: Effect of repetition of ischemia. *Jpn Circ J* 1999;63:201-208.

16. Priori S, Mantica M, Napolitano C, Schwartz PJ. Early afterdepolarizations induced in vivo by reperfusion of ischemic myocardium. A possible mechanism for reperfusion arrhythmias. *Circulation* 1990;81:1911-1920.

17. Rozanski GJ, Witt RC. Early afterdepolarizations and triggered activity in rabbit cardiac Purkinje fibers recovering from ischemia-like conditions. Role of acidosis. *Circulation* 1991;83:1352-1360.

18. Hirsche HJ, Franz CHR, Bos L, et al. Myocardial extracellular K^+ and H^+ increase and noradrenalin release as possible cause of early arrhythmias following acute coronary artery occlusion in pigs. *J Mol Cell Cardiol* 1980;12:579-593.

19. Vera Z, Pride HP, Zipes DP. Reperfusion arrhythmias: Role of early afterdepolarizations studied by monophasic action potential recordings in the intact canine heart during autonomically denervated and stimulated states. *J Cardiovasc Electrophysiol* 1995;6:532-543.

20. Moritani K, Miyazaki T, Miyoshi S, et al. Blockade of ATP-sensitive potassium channels by 5-hydroxydecanoate suppresses monophasic action potential

286 • *Monophasic Action Potentials: Bridging Cell and Bedside*

shortening during regional myocardial ischemia. *Cardiovasc Drugs Ther* 1994;8:749-756.

21. Miyazaki T, Moritani K, Miyoshi S, et al. Nicorandil augments regional ischemia-induced monophasic action potential shortening and potassium accumulation without serious proarrhythmia. *J Cardiovasc Pharmacol* 1995;26:949-956.

22. Miyoshi S, Miyazaki T, Moritani K, Ogawa S. Different responses of epicardium and endocardium to KATP channel modulators during regional ischemia. *Am J Physiol* 1996;271:H140-H147.

23. Moritani K, Miyazaki T, Miyoshi S, et al. Acute myocardial ischemia interferes with class III action of MS-551. *Jpn J Electrocardiol* 1997;17:55-61.

24. Gilmour RF Jr, Zipes DP. Different electrophysiological responses of canine endocardium and epicardium to combined hyperkalemia, hypoxia, and acidosis. *Circ Res* 1980;46:814-825.

25. Kimura S, Bassett AL, Kohya T, et al. Simultaneous recording of action potentials from endocardium and epicardium during ischemia in isolated cat ventricle: Relation of temporal electrophysiologic heterogeneities to arrhythmias. *Circulation* 1986;86:401-409.

26. Taggart P, Sutton PMI, Spear DW, et al. Simultaneous endocardial and epicardial monophasic action potential recordings during brief periods of coronary artery ligation in dog: Influence of adrenalin, beta blockade and alpha blockade. *Cardiovasc Res* 1988;22:900-909.

27. Spach MS, Barr RC. Origin of epicardial ST-T wave potentials in the intact dog. *Circ Res* 1976;39:475-487.

28. Ito M, Pride HP, Zipes DP. Glibenclamide enhances but pinacidil reduces attenuation in sympathetic responsiveness after acute coronary artery occlusion. *Circ Res* 1994;75:379-392.

29. Furukawa T, Kimura S, Furukawa N, et al. Role of cardiac ATP-regulated potassium channels in differential responses of endocardial and epicardial cells to ischemia. *Circ Res* 1991;68:1693-1702.

30. Griggs DJ, Nakamura Y. Effects of coronary constriction on myocardial distribution of iodoantipyrine-[131]. *Am J Physiol* 1968;215:H1082-H1086.

31. Fujiwara H, Ashraf M, Sato S, Millard RW. Transmural cellular damage and blood flow distribution in early ischemia in pig hearts. *Circ Res* 1982;51:683-693.

32. Lowe JE, Cummings RG, Adams DH, Hull RE. Evidence that ischemic cell death begins in the subendocardium independent of variations in collateral flow or wall tension. *Circulation* 1983;68:190-202.

33. Cole WC, McPherson CD, Sontag D. ATP-regulated K⁺ channels protect the myocardium against ischemia/reperfusion damage. *Circ Res* 1991;69:571-581.

34. Grover GJ, Dzwonczyk S, Parham CS, et al. The protective effects of cromakalim and pinacidil on reperfusion function and infarct size in isolated rat hearts and anesthetized dogs. *Cardiovasc Drugs Ther* 1990;4:465-474.

35. Kubota I, Yamaki M, Shibata T, et al. Role of ATP-sensitive K⁺ channels on ECG ST segment elevation during a bout of myocardial ischemia: A study on epicardial mapping in dogs. *Circulation* 1993;88:1845-1851.

36. Miyoshi S, Miyazaki T, Ito S, et al. Different epicardial and endocardial activation of KATP channels might cause peaked T-waves during acute coronary occlusion. *Eur Heart J* 1996;20(suppl):3093.

37. Di Diego JM, Antzelevitch C. Pinacidil-induced electrical heterogeneity and extrasystolic activity in canine ventricular tissues. Does activation of ATP-regulated potassium current promote phase 2 reentry? *Circulation* 1993;88:1177-1189.

38. Wolleben CD, Sanguinetti MC, Siegel PKS. Influence of ATP-sensitive potassium channel modulators on ischemia-induced fibrillation in isolated rat hearts. *J Mol Cell Cardiol* 1989;21:783-788.

39. Chi L, Uprichard ACG, Lucchesi BR. Profibrillatory action of pinacidil in a conscious canine model of sudden coronary death. *J Cardiovasc Pharmacol* 1990;15:452-464.

40. Kantor PF, Coetzee WA, Carmeliet EE, et al. Reduction of ischemic K⁺ loss and arrhythmias in rat hearts. Effect of glibenclamide, a sulfonylurea. *Circ Res* 1990;66:478-485.

41. Asanagi M, Miyazaki T, Moritani K, et al. Effects of lemakalim, an ATP-sensitive potassium channel opener on monophasic action potential duration and refractoriness of the ischaemic myocardium. A comparative study with nicorandil. *Eur Heart J* 1995;16(suppl):367.

42. Miyazaki T, Asanagi M, Moritani K, et al. Comparative effects of ATP-sensitive potassium channel opener and blocker on ischaemia-induced action potential shortening, conduction delay, and ventricular fibrillation in dogs. *Eur Heart J* 1994;15(suppl):136.

43. Von Beckerath N, Cyrys S, Dischner A, Daut J. Hypoxic vasodilatation in isolated, perfused guinea-pig heart: An analysis of the underlying mechanisms. *J Physiol* 1991;442:297-319.

44. Narishige T, Egashira K, Akatsuka Y, et al. Glibenclamide, a putative ATP-sensitive K⁺ channel blocker, inhibits coronary autoregulation in anesthetized dogs. *Circ Res* 1993;73:771-776.

45. Noma A. ATP-regulated K⁺ channels in cardiac muscle. *Nature* 1983;305:147-148.

46. Yao Z, Cavero I, Gross GJ. Activation of cardiac K_ATP channels: An endogenous protective mechanism during repetitive ischemia. *Am J Physiol* 1993; 264:H495-H504.

47. Meinert CL, Knatterud GL, Prout TE, et al. A study of the effects of hypoglycemic agents on vascular complications in patients with adult-onset diabetes: II. Mortality results. *Diabetes* 1970;19:789-830.

48. Fosset M, De Weille Jr, Green RD, et al. Antidiabetic sulfonylureas control action potential properties in heart cells via high affinity receptors that are linked to ATP-dependent K⁺ channels. *J Biol Chem* 1988;263:7933-7936.

49. Nakaya H, Takeda Y, Tohse N, Kanno M. Effects of ATP-sensitive K⁺ channel blockers on the action potential shortening in hypoxic and ischaemic myocardium. *Br J Pharmacol* 1991;103:1019-1026.

50. Wilde AAM, Escande D, Schumacher CA, et al. Potassium accumulation in globally ischemic mammalian heart. A role for the ATP-sensitive potassium channel. *Circ Res* 1990;67:835-843.

51. Bekheit S, Restivo M, Boutjdir M, et al. Effects of glyburide on ischemia-induced changes in extracellular potassium and local myocardial activation: A potential new approach to the management of ischemia-induced malignant ventricular arrhythmias. *Am Heart J* 1990;119:1025-1033.

52. Sanguinetti MC, Jurkiewicz NK. Two components of cardiac delayed rectifier K⁺ currents. Differential sensitivity to block of class III antiarrhythmic agents. *J Gen Physiol* 1990;96:195-215.

53. Yazawa K, Kameyama M. Mechanism of receptor-mediated modulation of the delayed outward potassium current in guinea-pig ventricular myocytes. *J Physiol (Lond)* 1990;421:135-150.

54. Nakaya H, Takeda Y, Tohse N, Kanno M. Effects of MS-551, a new class III antiarrhythmic drug, on action potential and membrane currents in rabbit ventricular myocytes. *Br J Pharmacol* 1993;109:157-163.

55. Culling W, Penny WJ, Sheridan DJ. Effects of sotalol on arrhythmias and electrophysiology during myocardial ischaemia and reperfusion. *Cardiovasc Res* 1984;18:397-404.

56. Cobbe SM, Manley BS, Alexopoulos D. The influence of acute myocardial ischaemia on the class III antiarrhythmic action of sotalol. *Cardiovasc Res* 1985;19:661-667.

57. Lab MJ. Contraction-excitation feedback in myocardium. Physiological basis and clinical relevance. *Circ Res* 1982;50:757-766.

58. Franz MR, Burkoff D, Yue DT, Sagawa K. Mechanically induced action potential changes and arrhythmia in isolated and in situ canine hearts. *Cardiovasc Res* 1989;23:213-223.

59. Stacy GP, Jobe RL, Taylor LK, Hansen DE. Stretch-induced depolarizations as a trigger of arrhythmias in isolated canine left ventricles. *Am J Physiol* 1992;263:H613-H621.

60. Kaseda S, Zipes DP. Contraction-excitation feedback in the atria: A cause of changes in refractoriness. *J Am Coll Cardiol* 1988;11:1327-1336.

61. Klein LS, Miles WM, Zipes DP. Effect of atrioventricular interval during pacing or reciprocating tachycardia on atrial size, pressure, and refractory period. Contraction-excitation feedback in human atrium. *Circulation* 1990;82:60-68.

62. Lab MJ. Mechanoelectric feedback (transduction) in heart: Concepts and implications. *Cardiovasc Res* 1996;32:3-14.

63. Yang X-C, Sachs F. Block of stretch-activated ion channels in Xenopus oocytes by gadolinium and calcium ions. *Science* 1989;243:1068-1071.

64. Takagai S, Miyazaki T, Furukawa Y, et al. Involvement of stretch-activated cation channels in spatial difference of ventricular monophasic action potential duration and arrhythmias during acute pressure overload. *Circulation* 1996;94(suppl I):I-528.

65. Hansen DE, Borganelli M, Stacy GP, Taylor LK. Dose-dependent inhibition of stretch-induced arrhythmias by gadolinium in isolated canine ventricles. Evidence for a unique mode of antiarrhythmic action. *Circ Res* 1991;69:820-831.

Section III

Dispersion of Repolarization and Refractoriness:
Introduction

Dispersion of ventricular repolarization and, consequently, of refractoriness has become known as a harbinger of serious arrhythmias and sudden cardiac death. The body surface electrocardiogram (ECG) has been proposed as a tool to assess dispersion of ventricular repolarization noninvasively, by calculating the difference between the shortest and longest QT interval in the 12-lead ECG (known as QT dispersion). This approach is limited because the ECG is probably not capable of discerning the actual dispersion of myocardial repolarization. Nonetheless, correlations between the ECG and direct measurements of ventricular repolarization dispersion by MAP recordings exist, and are explored in this section. The reports in this section range from basic studies of repolarization dispersion in an isolated heart preparation to those obtained in the human heart, including the role of left ventricular hypertrophy as an important substrate for increased dispersion and possibly arrhythmogenesis. Specific insight into dispersion of repolarization is given by experts using classic microelectrode or novel optical mapping techniques, providing the basic foundation of the dispersion of repolarization during regular and premature heart beats.

Cardiac disease, most notably myocardial ischemia, may adversely affect dispersion of ventricular repolarization. This is especially true for the dependence of repolarization dispersion on heart rate and antiarrhythmic drugs. Thus, this section also reviews timely information on whether heart rate and drugs attenuate or enhance dispersion of ventricular repolarization.

18

High-Resolution Measurement of Ventricular Repolarization Using Voltage-Sensitive Dyes

Imad Libbus, MS, Kenneth R. Laurita, PhD and David S. Rosenbaum, MD

Introduction

Sudden cardiac death due to reentrant ventricular arrhythmias is among the most devastating manifestations of heart disease in adults. The structural and electrophysiologic changes that predispose chronically diseased hearts to ventricular arrhythmias have been studied extensively, yet relatively little is known of the complex sequence of events that incite malignant arrhythmias in some patients but not in others. Consequently, sudden cardiac death remains a major unresolved public health problem. In recent years, there has been increased interest in the possible role of cardiac repolarization in the mechanisms of reentrant arrhythmias. This interest was undoubtedly fueled by greater awareness of the molecular and ionic determinants of abnormal repolarization in human diseases such as the long QT syndrome.[1,2]

Inhomogeneity in refractoriness and action potential duration (APD) has been widely recognized as an important factor underlying the initiation of ventricular fibrillation.[3] It is thought that nonuniform recovery favors the fractionation of impulses arising during the relative refractory period, and gives rise to reentrant arrhythmias. Presumably, any increase in disper-

From Franz MR (ed): *Monophasic Action Potentials: Bridging Cell and Bedside.* ©Futura Publishing Company, Inc., Armonk, NY, 2000.

sion would increase the likelihood of reentry. An early premature stimulus applied at a site with shortened APD gives rise to block and reentry, while a stimulus at a site with long APD does not induce an arrhythmia.[4] Because there are important heterogeneities in functional expression and distribution of ionic currents between cells spanning the transmural[5] and epicardial[6] surfaces of the ventricle, the mechanisms and factors responsible for generating and maintaining spatial dispersion of repolarization are complex and poorly understood. In this chapter we review techniques used to measure dispersion of repolarization in the heart, and focus on new approaches for assessing dispersion using optical mapping with voltage-sensitive dyes.

Conventional Techniques for Measuring Dispersion of Repolarization

Glass microelectrode recordings have been used extensively to record the cardiac action potential in single cells. Allessie[7] recorded action potentials from up to 10 simultaneous atrial sites with microelectrode techniques. Using a concentrically and radially adjustable holder for 10 microelectrodes, maps of activation and recovery were obtained in rabbit atria during periods of sustained tachycardia. Successive recordings were made and time-aligned to yield an effective map from 94 sites. This innovative approach was used to develop the "leading circle" concept of reentry.[7] However, this experiment also highlights the limitation of microelectrode mapping. It is difficult to maintain stable impalements from multiple sites simultaneously, making it difficult to use microelectrode techniques to map regional inhomogeneities of repolarization, particularly as they change rapidly during perturbations of heart rate at the onset of tachycardia. It is particularly difficult to obtain multisite action potential recordings from the intact heart using glass microelectrodes, although floating microelectrodes have been successfully employed in intact heart preparations to measure action potentials from a single recording site.[8]

Measurement of effective refractory period (ERP) with extracellular electrodes is another method that has been used extensively to assess recovery of excitability in the heart. The ERP is measured by stimulating the preparation at a baseline cycle length (S1) and introducing a premature extrastimulus (S2) at progressively shorter S1-S2 intervals until the premature stimulus fails to capture the tissue. The ERP is defined as the longest S1-S2 interval that fails to induce a propagated response, and has been widely used to measure dispersion of ventricular[3,9,10] and atrial[11,12] recovery in vivo by sequentially repeating the measurement from multiple sites. As early as 1964, Han and Moe[3] used an array of 12 unipolar electrodes to measure dispersion of refractoriness in the dog. There are several important limitations to ERP mapping. First, the ERP provides no direct information about the time course of the transmembrane potential. Furthermore, because ERP measurements are made sequentially and not simultaneously, the measurement of dispersion of repolarization assumes that the electrophysiologic conditions remain stable and unaffected by the procedure over long time periods.[13] Finally, there is an inherent limitation of the spatial resolution with which dispersion of repolarization can be measured with electrode techniques. It is difficult, if not impossible, to use electrode techniques to assess electrical heterogeneities on a size scale that approaches the cardiac myocyte.

Recently, investigators have attempted to estimate spatial dispersion of repolarization from unipolar electrograms recorded from multiple simultaneous extracellular electrodes using high-speed computers and multiplexing technology.[14,15] Because extracellular electrograms do not measure transmembrane potential, the activation and recovery of the cardiac tissue can only be estimated indirectly by this technique.[16] The activation-recovery interval (ARI) has been proposed as a measure of the duration of local repolarization.[16-18] It is commonly defined as the time between the most rapid decrease in voltage of the QRS and the maximum rate of voltage increase in the T wave, and has been correlated with APD and ERP to within 6 milliseconds during steady state pacing conditions.[17,18] During graded ischemia, variability of ARI increases further due to the rapidly changing electrophysiologic state.[17] The strength of ARI mapping lies in the simultaneous nature of the recordings, permitting beat-by-beat measurement of dispersion of repolarization. However, Haws and Lux[17] warned that the ARI may not accurately measure recovery time in the presence of nonuniform membrane properties. Furthermore, it is not clear that ARI mapping can be applied to transient electrophysiologic conditions, such as during a premature stimulus or the initiation of tachycardia.

An extracellular electrode applied to the myocardium with suction or firm contact can record a monophasic action potential (MAP), which reproduces the time course of cellular repolarization and depolarization with considerable accuracy.[19] MAP duration correlates with ERP when both are measured simultaneously at multiple sites in the human ventricle.[20] Therefore, the MAP is presently the most reliable method for measuring dispersion of repolarization in humans.[21-25] The MAP has also been applied to numerous investigations of dispersion of repolarization in animal models.[21,23-25] Like microelectrodes, it is difficult to obtain multiple simultaneously stable recordings,[13] which limits the spatial resolution that can be achieved with contact electrodes. Spatial resolution is further limited because the MAP is derived from a region of myocardium of approximately 5 mm in diameter, which also implies that the MAP is derived from an aggregate of cells and is not identical to a single-cell action potential recording. Furthermore, motion artifacts due to contraction of the heart can make it difficult to identify and interpret small deflections (ie, early afterdepolarizations) during the repolarization phase of the MAP.[19]

Optical Action Potential Mapping

Voltage-sensitive dyes have been used for several decades to measure transmembrane potential in excitable cells. These dyes bind the cell membrane with high affinity, exhibit changes in fluorescence that vary linearly with transmembrane potential, and closely reproduce the time course of the cardiac action potential.[26-28] When the dye is excited at a specific wavelength, it emits light at a longer wavelength,[29] which allows fluoresced light to be distinguished from reflected light using appropriately selected optical filters and a photodetector.

Voltage-sensitive dyes can be divided into two classes, distributive dyes and electrochromic dyes, according to their response to membrane potential.[29] Electrochromic dyes have a response time on the nanosecond time scale, respond directly to the membrane's electrical field, and are therefore suitable for recording the action potential. One of the most widely used electrochromic dyes is di-4-ANEPPS, a styryl dye whose fluorescence response varies linearly with membrane potential.[30] Although the change in fluorescence is fairly small (8% to 10% per 100 mV), it is almost instantaneous, making it ideal for detecting the rapid changes within the action potential. As with most styryl dyes, di-4-ANEPPS exhibits good photostability and no apparent toxicity in intact heart preparations.[29] With use of a video camera or an array of photodetectors, it is possible to record action potentials from hundreds to thousands of cardiac sites simultaneously.[31-35] Therefore, in many respects, optical mapping combines the advantages of microelectrode recording techniques and multisite simultaneous extracellular mapping.

We have developed an optical system to map cardiac action potentials with high resolution from the intact beating heart (Fig. 1).[36,37] After staining with the voltage-sensitive dye, the preparation is illuminated with a 250-W tungsten-halogen lamp at the excitation wavelength (540±5 nm). Fluoresced light from the preparation is focused onto a 16×16 element photodetector array using a high numerical aperture Nikon camera lens, which can be moved along an optical rail to provide a wide range of magnifications. Each of the 256 photodetector elements is a silicon photodiode, which features a fast response time and high sensitivity in the visible to near-infrared range. The output of the photodiode is coupled to several amplifier stages, which are used to amplify and filter the optical action potential. A computer algorithm developed by Rosenbaum et al[33] is used

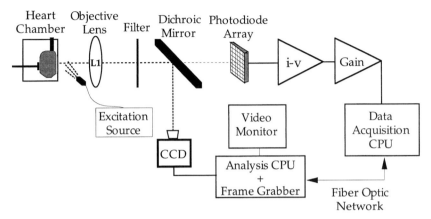

Figure 1. Schematic diagram of the optical mapping system. The preparation is illuminated with a tungsten-halogen lamp at a wavelength of 540±5 nm. Magnification is adjusted by moving the objective lens along an optical rail. The fluoresced light is filtered to remove reflected light, and projected onto the photodiode array. The signals from the photodiode array are amplified with variable gain (1× to 1000×) and filtered with variable high-pass (0 to 0.56 Hz) and low-pass (500 to 1000) cutoff frequencies. Optical action potentials are then multiplexed, sampled at up to 3500 Hz per channel, and stored on a data acquisition computer. To record the position of the optical action potentials on the heart, a snapshot of the preparation is taken with a CCD camera. Reproduced from Reference 38, with permission.

to assign activation and recovery times to each action potential. Depolarization is defined as the time of maximum first derivative of the action potential, and repolarization is defined as the time of maximum second derivative during the downstroke of the action potential. APD is the difference between the time of cellular depolarization and repolarization.

A fundamental difference between microelectrode and optical action potential recordings relates to the source of the signal. The microelectrode records an action potential from a single cell while an optical signal is derived from a small aggregate of cells, whose size and number are dependent on optical magnification, detector size, and the light transmission properties of cardiac tissue. As magnification increases, spatial resolution increases and fewer cells contribute to the optical signal.[38] To determine how closely the optical action potential approximates the transmembrane action potential, optical and microelectrode action potential recordings were compared in an intact beating heart. The rise time of optical action potentials was measured as a function of magnification (Fig. 2). As expected, the optical action potential upstroke approximates the single cell at high magnifications. At low magnifications, more cells contributed to the optical action potentials, and the rise time was slightly prolonged due to a spatial averaging effect.[38] With increased magnification, fewer cells contribute to the optical action potential, and signal quality decreases.

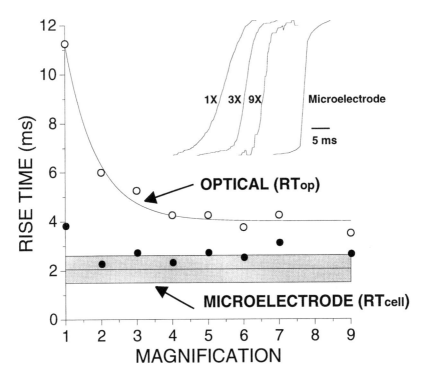

Figure 2. Rise time of optical action potentials as a function of magnification (open circles). The mean ($\pm$ SD) rise time measured with glass microelectrodes is shown by the shaded bar. At low magnifications, the rise time of the optical action potential is prolonged due to spatial averaging. At high magnifications, the rise time of the optical action potential approaches the rise time measured with glass microelectrodes. At all magnifications, single-cell rise times estimated from the optical action potentials (filled circles) closely approximate the rise times measured with microelectrodes.[38] As magnification increases, signal quality decreases (see inset). Reproduced from Reference 38, with permission.

The resolution required to measure optical action potentials is, in part, dictated by the experimental question being addressed. However, it is clear that optical mapping techniques can be used effectively to measure dispersions of repolarization on a microscopic size scale.[37] If the experiment requires mapping from a larger area, then spatial resolution must be sacrificed. However, each optical recording pixel should correspond to an area on the heart that is no larger than the electrical space constant of cardiac muscle (1×1 mm). Otherwise it is theoretically possible that one optical recording site might contain various cell types with heterogeneous action potential characteristics, making it difficult to interpret the optically recorded action potential.

In addition to mapping area, it is important to consider the contribution of deeper cell layers to the optical action potential. We characterized the light transmission properties of guinea pig ventricle using a spectrophotometer and found that myocardial tissue preferentially absorbs wavelengths below 600 nm.[38] Ninety-five percent of the optical signal originates from a depth of less than 500 μm, and the greatest contribution comes from within 100 μm of the epicardial surface. For magnifications ranging from 1× to 4×, action potentials are measured from spots of 950 to 240 μm, corresponding to sample volumes of 0.090 to 0.0056 mm^3. Again, it is important to assure that the population of cells that contribute to the optical action potential is homogenous with regard to their function and structure. Because fiber orientation changes between myocardial layers, the depth of the optical recording should be minimized so that the optical map is not confounded by the rotational anisotropy of the layers. In most cases this is not a problem, because the optical recording essentially arises from cells within 200 μm of the epicardial surface whereas the orientation of fibers begins to change significantly at depths exceeding 1000 μm.

As is the case with MAP recordings, the optical action potential is vulnerable to motion artifacts associated with cardiac contraction. Cardiac motion can distort the optical action potential and obscure the time course of membrane repolarization.[38] Motion can be reduced significantly by reducing calcium concentration or by inhibiting contraction with use of drugs that inhibit excitation-contraction coupling. Unfortunately, these interventions can significantly alter the electrophysiologic properties of cardiac cells and influence the measurement of repolarization.[38] There are alternatives, such as mechanical stabilization of contraction, that have been successful in eliminating apparent motion artifacts without altering the electrophysiologic properties of the heart.[38,39]

Optical Mapping of Repolarization Heterogeneities in the Heart

Optical mapping with voltage-sensitive dyes is uniquely suited for measuring dispersion of repolarization, especially when repolarization gradients change dynamically from beat to beat. Previously, we used a multisite optical mapping system to determine the effect of cycle length shortening on dispersion of repolarization in Langendorff-perfused guinea pig hearts.[33] This paradigm was selected because it simulates the paroxysmal onset of reentrant tachycardia. The heart was stimulated at a cycle length of 500 milliseconds for 5 minutes before the cycle length was abruptly shortened and maintained at 300 milliseconds. APD was calculated for each of 128 mapping sites spanning the epicardial surface of the heart, and plotted as a function of the site's distance from the apex (Fig. 3). Note

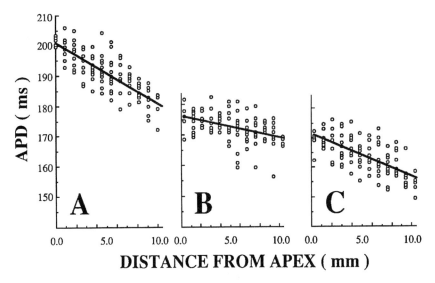

DISTANCE FROM APEX (mm)

Figure 3. Action potential duration (APD) at each ventricular site, plotted as a function of distance from apex. Optical action potentials were recorded simultaneously from multiple sites on the epicardial surface of an intact guinea pig heart. Maps were recorded from a 1×1 cm area encompassing the anterior left ventricular surface. APD gradients, indicated by the slope of the regression line, are shown during baseline pacing at a cycle length (CL) of 500 milliseconds (**A**), after an abrupt CL shortening to 300 milliseconds (**B**), and as dispersion recovers to baseline (**C**). At baseline pacing, a steep apex-to-base APD gradient is evident (**A**). After abrupt CL shortening, the APD gradient diminishes (**B**). By the 24th cardiac cycle, the APD gradient is restored to baseline levels, although absolute APDs have shortened substantially from their baseline levels (**C**). Reproduced from Reference 33, with permission.

first that during baseline steady state stimulation (Fig. 3, panel A) multisite simultaneous optical action potential recordings revealed a uniform apex-to-base gradient in APD. Therefore, it is possible to not only detect dispersions of repolarization, but to also derive detailed information on the nature, characteristics, and stability of such dispersion. For example, after stimulus cycle length was abruptly shortened the dispersion gradient was dynamically attenuated as evidenced by flattening in the slope of the regression line (Fig. 3, panel B). By the 24th cardiac cycle, the APD gradient is restored near baseline, even though APDs at each site shorten substantially from their baseline values.[33]

Dispersion index, defined as the variance of APDs recorded simultaneously across the mapping field, was used as a beat-to-beat index of repolarization inhomogeneity (Fig. 4). During baseline pacing, the dispersion of repolarization was largely due to an APD gradient caused by progressive lengthening of the APD from apex to base. Under control conditions, a reduction in cycle length was accompanied by a characteristic decrease

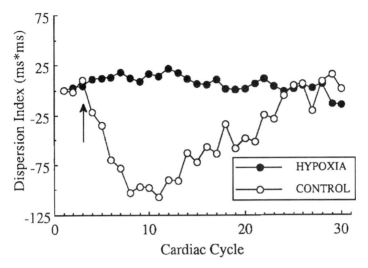

Figure 4. Plots of repolarization dispersion index (DI) as a function of cardiac cycle. DI is defined as the action potential duration variance across the entire array, and is shown as the stimulation cycle length (CL) is shortened from 500 to 300 milliseconds (vertical arrow). DI decreases rapidly in oxygenated myocardium (control) as a transient response to CL shortening and returns to baseline. DI fails to decrease in hypoxic ventricle. Reproduced from Reference 33, with permission.

in dispersion index. This response was transient, and dispersion returned to its baseline value after approximately 25 beats at the faster cycle length. The transient reduction of the apex-to-base APD gradient can be attributed to a rapid lowering of APD in the apex relative to the base. Under hypoxic conditions, a change in cycle length did not result in a decreased dispersion.

These findings suggest that dispersion of repolarization is not a static property of myocardial tissue but rather it changes dynamically with changes in heart rate. A transient reduction in dispersion appears to be a physiologic response of the normal heart to cycle length shortening. A change in cycle length attenuates the normally occurring apex-to-base APD gradient. Such a change in the spatial heterogeneity of APD in response to abrupt cycle length changes may alter electrophysiologic vulnerability to reentrant arrhythmias. Under control conditions, dispersion is actively modulated in a manner that is expected to decrease vulnerability to reentry. Under hypoxic conditions, the protective response is absent.

It is clear that voltage-sensitive dye techniques are useful for tracking dynamic beat-to-beat changes in spatial dispersion of repolarization. However, it is also possible to investigate cellular mechanisms that underlie the spread of repolarization of the heart using optical action potential mapping. Using an array of photodiode detectors, it is possible to record the details of membrane potential change from multiple simultaneous sites with high spatial, voltage, and temporal resolutions. Such studies are particularly useful when the kinetics of membrane repolarization processes vary significantly between cells across a region of interest. Laurita et al[6] used optical mapping techniques to measure the kinetics of APD restitution between cells across the epicardial surface of guinea pig heart, to determine if heterogeneities of cellular repolarization could explain the complex patterns of global ventricular repolarization observed during perturbations in heart rate. APD restitution was measured simultaneously from 128 epicardial sites by introducing a premature stimulus after a basic drive train, and measuring the relationship between APD of the premature beat and the diastolic interval that preceded it.

We hypothesized that changes in the pattern and distribution of repolarization at the level of the whole heart could be explained by spatial heterogeneity of repolarization properties between cells. Contour maps of depolarization and APD were analyzed for a broad range of premature S1-S2 coupling intervals (Fig. 5). During baseline steady state stimulation, the impulse propagated uniformly from the site of pacing, and a significant gradient of APD was evident. When the S1-S2 interval was shortened over a broad range of intermediate values (205 milliseconds in Fig. 5), there was no significant change in the activation pattern. However, the APD gradient vanished as APD became much more homogeneous across the mapping field. When the S1-S2 interval was further shortened approaching the ventricular refractory period (175 milliseconds in Fig. 5), the activation pattern remained essentially unchanged, but APD dispersion changed significantly. The APD gradient reappeared, but the orientation of the gradient was inverted compared to baseline. Therefore, APD dispersion exhibited a biphasic dependence on coupling interval, decreasing to a minimum at intermediate coupling intervals, and increasing at short coupling intervals.[6]

Unlike repolarization, the pattern of depolarization is not significantly affected by the premature stimulus, indicating that the changes in the gradient of repolarization are not due to conduction slowing. There are substantial gradients of cellular repolarization in guinea pig epicardium, and the magnitude and orientation of these gradients are highly sensitive to the timing of a premature stimulus. Therefore, dispersion of repolarization is modulated in a predictable coupling-interval–dependent manner. In the absence of a premature stimulus, the magnitude and orientation of APD gradients remained constant over a wide range of steady-state cycle lengths. Therefore, rapid pacing alone is not responsible for the modulation of repolarization gradients.

To test the hypothesis that heterogeneity of restitution kinetics can explain modulated dispersion of repolarization, an empirical restitution rate constant (R_K), defined as the maximum change in APD over a given change in diastolic interval, was used to characterize the time course of restitution at each mapping site.[6] From Figure 6, it is evident that restitution

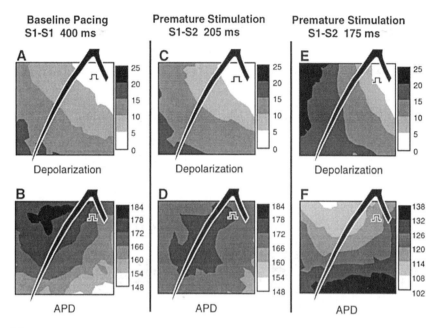

Figure 5. Depolarization and action potential duration (APD) contour maps during baseline pacing (**A, B**), a premature beat at an intermediate coupling interval (**C, D**), and a premature beat at a coupling interval near the refractory period (**E, F**). A gray scale is shown to the right of each contour map, and indicates time in milliseconds. Action potentials were recorded from a 1×1 cm area on the epicardial surface of an intact guinea pig heart, and a representation of the left anterior descending coronary artery is superimposed for visual reference. Depolarization is not significantly affected by S1-S2 coupling interval (**A, C, E**), but APD dispersion is highly sensitive (**B, D, F**). APD dispersion decreases from baseline (400 milliseconds; **A**) to a minimum at an intermediate coupling interval (205 milliseconds; **D**) and increases at a short coupling interval (175 milliseconds; **F**). The APD gradient at a short coupling interval is inverted compared to baseline. Reproduced from Reference 6, with permission.

properties are indeed heterogeneously distributed between cells across the epicardial surface of the heart. Moreover, regional heterogeneities in the restitution rate constant are not random, but vary systematically across the epicardial surface. Cells in proximity to the base of the ventricle exhibited relatively fast restitution, while cells near the apex of the ventricle exhibited relatively slow restitution (Fig. 6). This pattern closely mirrors the distribution of APD observed between cells during baseline steady-state conditions (APD$_b$ in Fig. 6).

It is important to note that the close correlation between R_K and APD$_b$ can completely explain modulation of dispersion in response to a premature stimulus. In response to a premature stimulus delivered at an intermediate coupling interval, cells near the base having the longest APD$_b$

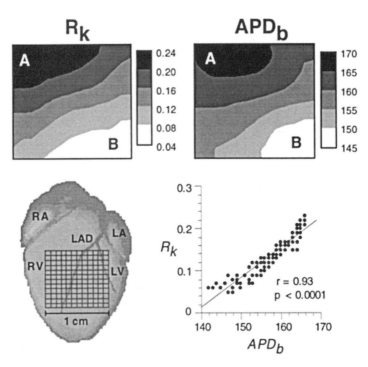

Figure 6. Spatial dispersion of restitution rate constant (R_K) and action potential duration (APD) during baseline pacing (APD$_b$). A gray scale is shown to the right of each contour map, and indicates normalized units (R_K) or milliseconds (APD$_b$). Pacing was performed from the upper left corner (site A) of the mapping field for all measurements. Diagram shows the mapping field and its position relative to the intact heart preparation (lower, left). RA = right atrium; LA = left atrium; RV = right ventricle; LV = left ventricle; LAD = left anterior descending coronary artery. R_K is heterogeneously distributed between cells across the epicardial surface of the heart (upper, left). R_K is plotted as a function of APD$_b$ for each mapping site (lower, right), demonstrating their linear relationship. Reproduced from Reference 6, with permission.

underwent the greatest degree of APD shortening because they possessed the fastest R_K. Therefore, a premature stimulus in this range effectively synchronizes repolarization across the heart. When the premature coupling interval was further shortened, APD of the cells that previously had the longest APD$_b$ (near the base of the heart) now had the shortest APD, whereas cells near the apex of the heart had relatively long APDs after the premature coupling interval, since they possessed the slowest R_K. Spatial heterogeneity of R_K, and the relationship between R_K and APD$_b$, fully explain both phases of the modulated dispersion response. First, marked reduction of dispersion over a broad range of intermediate premature coupling intervals, and second, restoration of repolarization gradients of equal magnitude but opposite orientation after very short premature coupling intervals.

Coupling-interval–dependent modulation of dispersion gradients is expected to significantly influence the state of electrical vulnerability in the heart. For example, it is well recognized that the conditions for reentry are not necessarily present at baseline but form dynamically in response to a provocative stimulus. Modulated dispersion gradients may provide a mechanism by which a reentrant substrate forms, disappears, or reforms after a change in cycle length. These findings may have important implications for our understanding of the factors that determine why sustained versus nonsustained ventricular tachycardia develops under apparently similar conditions in the same patient.

Summary

A variety of mapping techniques have been used to measure dispersion of repolarization in the heart. Glass microelectrodes accurately measure transmembrane potential in the single cell, but it is difficult to maintain multiple stable impalements. ERP mapping can accurately assess recovery of excitability in the heart, but because ERP recordings are obtained sequentially, they are not suitable for electrophysiologically unstable preparations. MAP mapping is most suitable for measuring dispersion of repolarization in humans, but spatial resolution is limited by the size of the electrode and by the sequential nature of the recordings.

Optical mapping with voltage-sensitive dyes offers unique advantages for mapping repolarization. It conveys direct information on the time course of membrane potential. In addition, cellular repolarization can be mapped from multiple simultaneous sites with spatial resolution approaching the size scale of the cardiac myocyte.[37] No other technique currently offers these advantages. In this regard, optical mapping provides an important tool for integrating our understanding of the molecular and biophysical basis for the cardiac action potential with a comprehensive knowledge of arrhythmia mechanisms at the level of the whole heart. Further work is required to overcome several important limitations of optical mapping. For example, motion artifacts and the absence of information regarding absolute transmembrane potential remain problematic in some experimental situations. In addition, it is difficult to record optical maps from tissue layers that lie beneath the surface of the heart. It is essential to overcome this problem in order to elucidate the role of transmural electrical heterogeneities in the mechanism of arrhythmias.[5] Preliminary work from our laboratory indicates that in the near future it will be possible to assess transmural heterogeneities using optical mapping techniques.[40]

References

1. Curran ME, Splawski I, Timothy KW, et al. A molecular basis for cardiac arrhythmia: *HERG* mutations cause long QT syndrome. *Cell* 1995;80:795-803.

2. Wang Q, Shen J, Splawski I, et al. *SCN5A* mutations associated with an inherited cardiac arrhythmia, long QT syndrome. *Cell* 1995;80:805-811.

3. Han J, Moe G. Nonuniform recovery of excitability in ventricular muscle. *Circ Res* 1964;14:44-60.

4. Allessie MA, Bonke FI, Schopman FJG. Circus movement in rabbit atrial muscle as a mechanism of tachycardia: The role of nonuniform recovery of excitability in the occurrence of unidirectional block as studied with multiple microelectrodes. *Circ Res* 1976;39:169-177.

5. Antzelevitch C, Sicouri S, Litovsky SH, et al. Heterogeneity within the ventricular wall: Electrophysiology and pharmacology of epicardial, endocardial and M cells. *Circ Res* 1991;69:1427-1449.

6. Laurita KR, Girouard SD, Rosenbaum DS. Modulation of ventricular repolarization by a premature stimulus: Role of epicardial dispersion of repolarization kinetics demonstrated by optical mapping of the intact guinea pig heart. *Circ Res* 1996;79:493-503.

7. Allessie MA. Circus movement in rabbit atrial muscle as a mechanism of tachycardia. III. The "leading circle" concept: A new model of circus movement in cardiac tissue without the involvement of an anatomic obstacle. *Circ Res* 1977;41:9-18.

8. Yan GX, Antzelevitch C. Cellular basis for the electrocardiographic J wave. *Circulation* 1996;93:372-379.

9. Toyoshima H, Burgess MJ. Electrotonic interaction during canine ventricular repolarization. *Circ Res* 1978;43:348-356.

10. Gough W, Mehra R, Restivo M, et al. Reentrant ventricular arrhythmias in the late myocardial infarction period in the dog: 13. Correlation of activation and refractory maps. *Circ Res* 1985;57:432-442.

11. Wang Z, Fermini B, Nattel S. Repolarization differences between guinea pig atrial endocardium and epicardium: Evidence of a role of Ito. *Am J Physiol* 1991;260:H1501-H1506.

12. Wang Z, Fermini B, Nattel S. Delayed rectifier outward current and repolarization in human atrial myocytes. *Circ Res* 1993;73:276-285.

13. Surawicz B. Ventricular fibrillation and dispersion of repolarization. *J Cardiovasc Electrophysiol* 1997;8:1009-1012.

14. Ideker RE, Smith WM, Wallace AG, et al. A computerized method for the rapid display of ventricular activation during the intraoperative study of arrhythmias. *Circulation* 1979;59(3):449-458.

15. Witkowski F, Corr P. An automated simultaneous transmural cardiac mapping system. *Am J Physiol* 1984;247:H661-H668.

16. Steinhaus BM. Estimating cardiac transmembrane activation and recovery times from unipolar and bipolar extracellular electrograms: A simulation study. *Circ Res* 1989;64:449-462.

17. Haws C, Lux R. Correlation between in vivo transmembrane action potential durations and activation recovery intervals from electrograms. *Circulation* 1990;81:281-288.

18. Millar CK, Kralios FA, Lux RL. Correlation between refractory periods and activation-recovery intervals from electrograms: Effects of rate and adrenergic interventions. *Circulation* 1985;6:1372-1379.

19. Yuan S, Blomstrom-Lundqvist C, Olsson SB. Monophasic action potentials: Concepts to practical applications. *J Cardiovasc Electrophysiol* 1994;5:287-308.

20. Koller BS, Karasik PE, Solomon AJ, et al. Relation between repolarization and refractoriness during programmed electrical stimulation in the human right ventricle: Implications for ventricular tachycardia induction. *Circulation* 1995;91:2378-2384.

21. Kuo C, Munakata K, Reddy CP, et al. Characteristics and possible mechanisms of ventricular arrhythmia dependent on the dispersion of action potential durations. *Circulation* 1983;67:1356-1357.

22. Franz MR, Swerdlow CD, Liem LB, et al. Cycle length dependence of human action potential duration in vivo. *J Clin Invest* 1988;82:972-979.

23. Behrens S, Li CL, Fabritz CL, et al. Shock-induced dispersion of ventricular repolarization: Implications for the induction of ventricular fibrillation and the upper limit of vulnerability. *J Cardiovasc Electrophysiol* 1997;8:998-1008.

24. Fabritz CL, Kirchhof PF, Behrens S, et al. Myocardial vulnerability to T wave shocks: Relation to shock strength, shock coupling interval, and dispersion of ventricular repolarization. *J Cardiovasc Electrophysiol* 1996;7:231-242.

25. Kirchhof PF, Fabritz CL, Zabel M, et al. The vulnerable period for low and high energy T-wave shocks: Role of dispersion of repolarisation and effect of d-sotalol. *Cardiovasc Res* 1996;31:953-962.

26. Salama G, Morad M. Merocyanine 540 as an optical probe of transmembrane electrical activity in the heart. *Science* 1976;191:485-487.

27. Windisch H, Muller W, Tritthart H. Fluorescence monitoring of rapid changes in membrane potential in heart muscle. *Biophys J* 1985;48:877-884.

28. Loew LM. Design and characterization of electrochromic membrane probes. *J Biochem Biophys Methods* 1982;6:243.

29. Slavik J. measurement of membrane potential. In *Fluorescent Probes in Cellular and Molecular Biology*. Boca Raton: CRC Press; 1994:155-166.

30. Loew LM, Cohen LB, Dix J, et al. A naphthyl analog of the aminostyryl pyridinium class of potentiometric membrane dyes shows consistent sensitivity in a variety of tissue, cell, and model membrane preparations. *J Membr Biol* 1992;130:1-10.

31. Salama G, Lombardi R, Elson J. Maps of optical action potentials and NADH fluorescence in intact working hearts. *Am J Physiol* 1987;252:H384-H394.

32. Pertsov AM, Davidenko JM, Salomonsz R, et al. Spiral waves of excitation underlie reentrant activity in isolated cardiac muscle. *Circ Res* 1993;72:631-650.

33. Rosenbaum DS, Kaplan DT, Kanai A, et al. Repolarization inhomogeneities in ventricular myocardium change dynamically with abrupt cycle length shortening. *Circulation* 1991;84:1333-1345.

34. Dillon SM, Morad MA. A new laser scanning system for measuring action potential propagation in the heart. *Science* 1981;214:453-456.

35. Knisley SB, Blitchington TF, Hill BC, et al. Optical measurements of transmembrane potential changes during electric field stimulation of ventricular cells. *Circ Res* 1993;72:255-270.

36. Girouard SD. *Design and Validation of a High Resolution Cardiac Action Potential Mapping System Using Voltage-Sensitive Dyes* [Master's thesis]. Cleveland, OH: Case Western Reserve University; Department of Biomedical Engineering. 1993.

37. Libbus I. *Design and Validation of a High Resolution Microscopic Action Potential Mapping System Using Voltage-Sensitive Dyes* [Master's thesis].

Cleveland, OH: Case Western Reserve University; Department of Biomedical Engineering. 1997.

38. Girouard SD, Laurita KR, Rosenbaum DS. Unique properties of cardiac action potentials recorded with voltage-sensitive dyes. *J Cardiovasc Electrophysiol* 1996;7:1024-1038.

39. Salama G. Optical measurement of transmembrane potential in heart. In Loew L (ed): *Spectroscopic Probes of Membrane Potential.* CRC Uniscience Publications; 1988:132-199.

40. Akar FG, Yan G, Antzelevitch C, et al. Optical maps reveal reentrant mechanism of torsade de pointes based on topography and electrophysiology of mid-myocardial cells. *Circulation* 1997;96(8):I555. Abstract.

19

Effects of Heart Rate and Antiarrhythmic Drugs on Dispersion of Ventricular Repolarization Measured by Multiple Monophasic Action Potential Recordings

Markus Zabel, MD, Stefan H. Hohnloser, MD and Michael R. Franz, MD, PhD

Introduction

The role of heterogeneity or dispersion of ventricular repolarization (DVR) in the genesis of reentry ventricular arrhythmias has been demonstrated in several studies.[1-4] Moreover, among other electrophysiologic factors, the occurrence of polymorphic torsades de pointes (TdP) as the classic proarrhythmic effect of action potential prolonging drugs has been linked to an increased DVR.[5-8] A number of studies exist that report the influence of antiarrhythmic drugs on QT interval dispersion, a noninvasive electrocardiographic measure.[8-12] Quinidine and sotalol have been reported to increase QT dispersion (QTd),[9,10,12] to exert a

Supported by a Merck International Fellowship in Clinical Pharmacology (M.Z.) and a Department of Veterans Affairs Merit Review Grant (M.R.F.)

From Franz MR (ed): *Monophasic Action Potentials: Bridging Cell and Bedside.* ©Futura Publishing Company, Inc., Armonk, NY, 2000.

neutral effect, or even to decrease it,[10,11] while amiodarone was described to have a neutral effect or to decrease dispersion.[11] While comparisons between various antiarrhythmic drugs with regard to proarrhythmia are important,[13] clinical studies on QTd have been questioned for their usefulness.[14-16] On the other hand, experimental studies on the influence of antiarrhythmic drugs on DVR are scarce. It is therefore the objective of this chapter to characterize the effects of various antiarrhythmic drugs on DVR as studied in an isolated rabbit heart model. Specifically, quinidine as the prototype of class Ia substances, d-sotalol as a pure class III agent, and amiodarone, a drug with a complex electrophysiologic profile,[17] are reviewed. Because bradycardia has been described as an important contributing factor in the genesis of TdP,[13] the influence of heart rate, in particular, is considered.

Rate Dependence of Action Potential Duration and DVR

The rate dependence of the duration of repolarization, ie, action potential duration (APD) or the QT interval from the surface electrocardiogram (ECG), is well established[18,19] and necessitates rate correction of clinical measurements of the QT interval.[20-22] The physiologic basis of rate dependence of DVR is unclear, although rate correction of QTd has been common practice. Zabel et al[23] have assessed rate dependence of APD and DVR in an experimental study. They used a customized Langendorff set up for isolated intact rabbit hearts, which permitted the simultaneous recording of up to 10 monophasic action potentials (MAPs) at various heart rates. Data acquisition and subsequent analysis of the signals was done digitally; DVR was defined as the maximal difference of APD measured at 90% of repolarization (APD_{90}). Dispersion of APD_{90} was very similar over a wide range of heart rates studied (Fig. 1, panel A). Figure 1, panel B shows dispersion of APD_{90} for the entire range of cycle lengths studied. The results show that DVR other than duration of repolarization is not dependent on heart rate. This assumption could be confirmed in a recent clinical study of the influence of heart rate on a number of electrocardiographic variables of DVR at atrial pacing and exercise testing.[24] For clinical measurements of DVR (ie, determination of QTd and related variables of the surface ECG), it should therefore be deducted that a correction for heart rate is unnecessary. An increase of DVR at slow heart rates may well be observed with the additional influence of antiarrhythmic drugs, as described below.

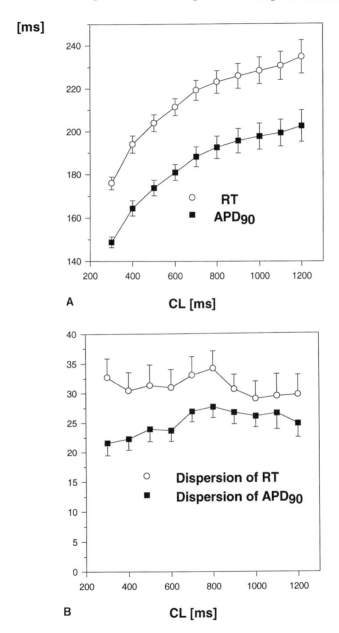

Figure 1. A. Rate dependence of action potential duration. The mean ± SE is plotted for cycle lengths between 300 milliseconds and 1200 milliseconds. **B**. Rate dependence of the dispersion of action potential duration. The mean ± SE is plotted for cycle lengths between 300 milliseconds and 1200 milliseconds. APD_{90} = action potential duration at 90% repolarization; CL = cycle length; RT = repolarization time. From Reference 23, with permission.

Effects of Antiarrhythmic Drugs

Effects on APD

In a second experimental study,[25] the effect of 3 antiarrhythmic drugs on repolarization was evaluated in a total of 55 isolated rabbit hearts. Quinidine and d-sotalol were added to the perfusate in increasing concentrations; amiodarone was prefed to the respective rabbits for 4 weeks. All three drugs—quinidine, d-sotalol, and amiodarone—prolonged APD_{90} as compared to baseline. D-sotalol prolonged APD_{90} in a concentration-dependent and reverse rate-dependent manner (Fig. 2, panel A). This prolongation was most pronounced at long cycle lengths and at the highest concentration of d-sotalol. At long cycle lengths, quinidine also led to a dose-dependent prolongation of APD_{90} (Fig. 2, panel B). Amiodarone prolonged APD_{90} over the entire range of cycle lengths (Fig. 2, panel C).

Effect on DVR

DVR was defined as the difference of maximal and minimal APD_{90} (as described in the above paragraph). D-sotalol did not affect DVR at a concentration of 10^{-6} M (Fig. 3, panel A), as compared to baseline. At 10^{-5}

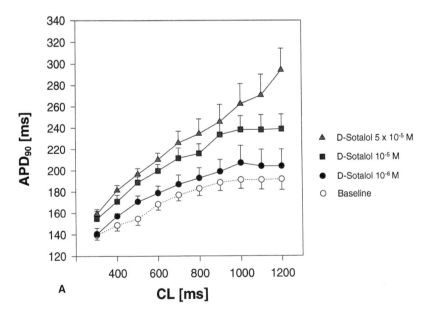

Figure 2. A. Action potential durations ± SEM at cycle lengths between 300 milliseconds and 1200 milliseconds during baseline and during 3 concentrations of d-sotalol. *Continues.*

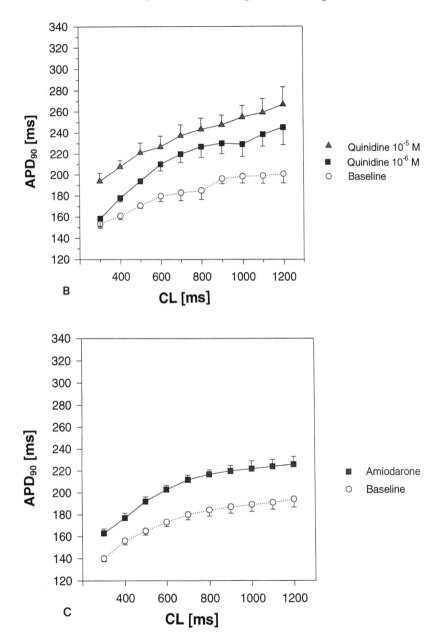

Figure 2 (*continued*). **B**. Action potential durations ± SEM at cycle lengths between 300 milliseconds and 1200 milliseconds during baseline and during 2 concentrations of quinidine. **C**. Action potential durations ± SEM at cycle lengths between 300 milliseconds and 1200 milliseconds in untreated (n=18) compared to amiodarone-treated (n=17) hearts. APD_{90} = action potential duration at 90% repolarization; CL = cycle length. From Reference 25, with permission.

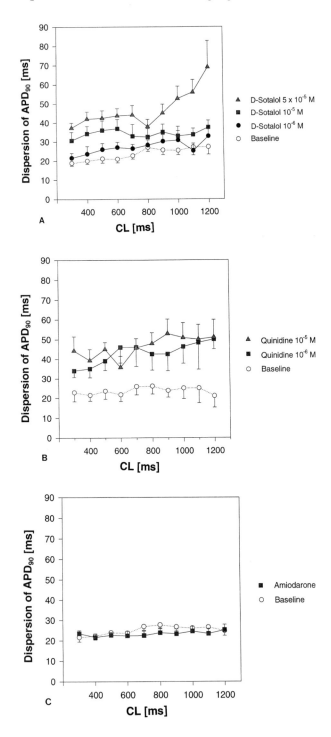

M, an increase in DVR was observed at all cycle lengths. This increase was more pronounced with the high concentration of d-sotalol, particularly at long cycle lengths. DVR increased during administration of both concentrations of quinidine (Fig. 3, panel B). In contrast to d-sotalol, this difference was similar at all cycle lengths tested and with both concentrations of quinidine. Amiodarone did not affect DVR (Fig. 3, panel C).

Implications of Antiarrhythmic Drug Effects on DVR for Proarrhythmia

The characteristic effects of the antiarrhythmic drugs on DVR described in the above paragraph can help explain the different incidence of proarrhythmic effects observed in patients. The majority of cases of drug-induced TdP occur at high dosages of sotalol.[13,26] In accordance with these clinical observations, the experimental data demonstrate the largest increase in DVR with the highest concentration of d-sotalol and at the longest cycle length tested. As demonstrated in previous studies and in the rabbit heart model of TdP described below,[27] an increased DVR[5,7,27,28] as well as the occurrence of early afterdepolarizations (EADs)[5,7,27-31] are considered to be the two major electrophysiologic mechanisms underlying the occurrence of antiarrhythmic drug-induced TdP. In contrast to the results obtained with d-sotalol, the effects of quinidine on DVR were independent of the drug's concentration and were similar at all heart rates. These experimental findings are in agreement with the clinical observations indicating that quinidine-induced TdP appears to be independent of the dosage administered[30] and the reported increased QTd during therapy with quinidine.[9,12] Although amiodarone increased APD to a similar extent as d-sotalol or quinidine, it did not lead to an increase in DVR. This response may be considered an important factor in its low proarrhythmic potential,[13,31] and is in accordance with the findings of two clinical studies which measured a similar effect of amiodarone on QTd.[9,11]

←――

Figure 3. A. Dispersion of ventricular repolarization ± SEM at cycle lengths between 300 milliseconds and 1200 milliseconds during baseline and after addition of 3 concentrations of d-sotalol. **B.** Dispersion of ventricular repolarization ± SEM at cycle lengths between 300 milliseconds and 1200 milliseconds during baseline and after addition of 2 concentrations of quinidine. **C.** Dispersion of ventricular repolarization ± SEM at cycle lengths between 300 milliseconds and 1200 milliseconds in untreated (n=18) compared to amiodarone-treated (n=17) hearts. APD_{90} = action potential duration at 90% repolarization; CL = cycle length. From Reference 25, with permission.

Induction of Proarrhythmia with Increased DVR and Electrolyte Imbalances

Until recently, only an intact rabbit model[32] or an in vivo dog model[33] was available for the study of the mechanisms of drug-induced TdP arrhythmias as suggested above. El-Sherif et al[5] added an in vivo puppy model that mimicked the sodium channel defect of the congenital long QT syndrome. Extending the above experiments with d-sotalol, Zabel et al[27] developed an *isolated* rabbit heart model, giving further insight into the relative role of DVR and EADs in proarrhythmic effects. In addition to the capability of the experimental Langendorff set up to assess DVR by measuring multiple MAPs simultaneously, EADs could be directly quantified in the tracings and the induced arrhythmias could be verified by means of the simultaneous volume-conducted ECG.[34] TdP was induced in the presence of a high concentration of d-sotalol (10^{-4} M), and shortly after lowering of the concentrations of potassium and magnesium in the perfusate (Fig. 4). The presence of bradycardia was also necessary in order to observe polymorphic triggered arrhythmias. Other than in the above described drug study,[25] the additional element of electrolyte imbalance led to the occurrence of triggering EADs. Figure 5 illustrates the changes in APD and DVR observed after initiation of low potassium and magnesium concentrations in the perfusate from one representative experiment. Immediately after the

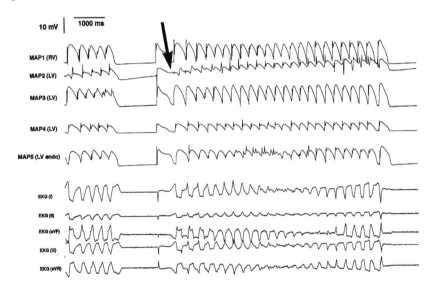

Figure 4. Induction of a 24-beat torsades de pointes. Note the typical undulating pattern of the electrocardiogram. The episode is triggered from an left ventricular endocardial MAP. From Reference 27, with permission.

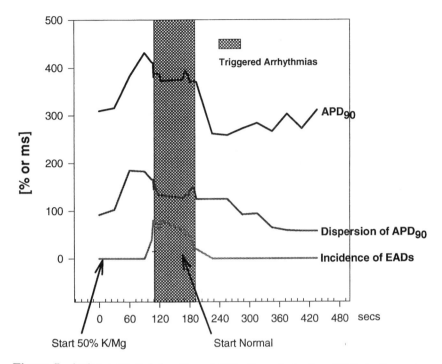

Figure 5. Action potential duration at 90% of repolarization (APD_{90}), dispersion of ventricular repolarization, and incidence of early afterdepolarizations (EADs) before, during, and after 3 minutes of perfusion with a low concentration of potassium and magnesium. The shaded area represents the time window during which triggered arrhythmias occurred. Note that the occurrence of triggered arrhythmias is closely linked to a high incidence of EADs. Adapted from Reference 27, with permission.

change of the perfusate, both APD_{90} and DVR increased sharply. After about 90 seconds, EADs arose in several MAP locations, quickly increased in amplitude and number (Figs. 4 and 5), and gave rise to triggered arrhythmias with bigeminy, couplets, and runs of TdP. Remarkably, all episodes of TdP terminated spontaneously. In addition to providing a simple experimental model to compare antiarrhythmic drugs or other pharmacologic agents for their propensity to develop TdP, the data clearly confirm the influence of DVR in proarrhythmia.

Summary

Heart rate does not influence DVR. Differential effects of antiarrhythmic agents can help explain the different clinical incidence of proarrhythmia. Finally, an increased DVR and occurrence of EADs are important cofactors in a newly developed isolated rabbit heart model of TdP.

References

1. Han J, Moe GK. Nonuniform recovery of excitability in ventricular muscle. *Circ Res* 1964;14:44.

2. Merx W, Yoon MS, Han J. The role of local disparity in conduction and recovery time on ventricular vulnerability to fibrillation. *Am Heart J* 1977;94:603-610.

3. Kuo CS, Munakata K, Reddy CP, Surawicz B. Characteristics and possible mechanism of ventricular arrhythmia dependent on the dispersion of action potential durations. *Circulation* 1983;67:1356-1367.

4. Kuo CS, Reddy CP, Munakata K, Surawicz B. Mechanism of ventricular arrhythmias caused by increased dispersion of repolarization. *Eur Heart J* 1985;6(suppl D):63-70.

5. El-Sherif N, Caref EB, Yin H, Restivo M. The electrophysiologic mechanism of ventricular arrhythmias in the long QT syndrome: Tridimensional mapping of activation and recovery patterns. *Circ Res* 1996;79:474-492.

6. Surawicz B. Electrophysiologic substrate of torsade de pointes: Dispersion of repolarization or early afterdepolarizations? *J Am Coll Cardiol* 1989;14:172-184.

7. Habbab MA, El-Sherif N. Drug-induced torsades de pointes: Role of early afterdepolarizations and dispersion of repolarization. *Am J Med* 1990;89:241-246.

8. Day CP, McComb JM, Matthews J, Campbell RW. Reduction in QT dispersion by sotalol following myocardial infarction. *Eur Heart J* 1991;12:423-427.

9. Hii JT, Wyse DG, Gillis AM, et al. Precordial QT interval dispersion as a marker of torsade de pointes. Disparate effects of class Ia antiarrhythmic drugs and amiodarone. *Circulation* 1992;86:1376-1382.

10. Hohnloser SH, van de Loo A, Kalusche D, et al. Does sotalol-induced alteration of QT dispersion predict effectiveness or proarrhythmic hazards? *Circulation* 1993;88:I397. Abstract.

11. Cui G, Sen L, Sager P, et al. Effects of amiodarone, sematilide, and sotalol on QT dispersion. *Am J Cardiol* 1994;74:896-900.

12. Hohnloser SH, van de Loo A, Baedeker F. Efficacy and proarrhythmic hazards of pharmacologic cardioversion of atrial fibrillation: Prospective comparison of sotalol versus quinidine. *J Am Coll Cardiol* 1995;26:852-858.

13. Hohnloser SH, Singh BN. Proarrhythmia with class III antiarrhythmic drugs: Definition, electrophysiologic mechanisms, incidence, predisposing factors, and clinical implications. *J Cardiovasc Electrophysiol* 1995;6:920-936.

14. Statters DJ, Malik M, Ward DE, Camm AJ. QT dispersion: Problems of methodology and clinical significance. *J Cardiovasc Electrophysiol* 1994;5:672-685.

15. Surawicz B. Will QT dispersion play a role in clinical decision-making? *J Cardiovasc Electrophysiol* 1996;7:777-784.

16. Coumel P, Mason-Blanche P, Badlini F. Dispersion of ventricular repolarization: Reality? Illusion? Significance? *Circulation* 1998;97:2491-2493.

17. Singh BN, Venkatesh N, Nademanee K, et al. The historical development, cellular electrophysiology and pharmacology of amiodarone. *Prog Cardiovasc Dis* 1989;31:249-280.

18. Franz MR, Swerdlow CD, Liem LB, Schaefer J. Cycle length dependence of human action potential duration in vivo. Effects of single extrastimuli, sudden sustained rate acceleration and deceleration, and different steady-state frequencies. *J Clin Invest* 1988;82:972-979.

19. Arnold L, Page J, Attwell D, et al. The dependence on heart rate of the human ventricular action potential duration. *Cardiovasc Res* 1982;16:547-551.

20. Bazett HC. An analysis of the time-relations of electrocardiograms. *Heart* 1920;7:353.
21. Franz MR. Time for yet another QT correction algorithm: Bazett and beyond. *J Am Coll Cardiol* 1994;23:1554-1556.
22. Karjalainen J, Viitasalo M, Mäntäri M, Manninen M. Relation between QT intervals and heart rates from 40 to 120 beats/min in rest electrocardiograms of men and a simple method to adjust QT interval values. *J Am Coll Cardiol* 1994;23:1547-1553.
23. Zabel M, Woosley RL, Franz MR. Is dispersion of ventricular repolarization rate dependent? *PACE* 1997;20:2405-2411.
24. Zabel M, Franz MR, Klingenheben T, et al. Rate-dependence of the QT interval and of QT dispersion: Comparison of atrial pacing and exercise testing. *Circulation* 1997;86:I324. Abstract.
25. Zabel M, Hohnloser SH, Behrens S, et al. Differential effects of d-sotalol, quinidine and amiodarone on dispersion of ventricular repolarization in the isolated rabbit heart. *J Cardiovasc Electrophysiol* 1997;8:1239-1245.
26. Hohnloser SH, Woosley RL. Sotalol. *N Engl J Med* 1994;331:31-38.
27. Zabel M, Hohnloser SH, Behrens S, et al. Electrophysiological features of torsade de pointes: Insights from a new isolated rabbit heart model. *J Cardiovasc Electrophysiol* 1997;8:1148-1158.
28. Surawicz B. Electrophysiologic substrate of torsade de pointes: Dispersion of repolarization or early afterdepolarizations? *J Am Coll Cardiol* 1989;14:172-184.
29. El-Sherif N, Bekheit SS, Henkin R. Quinidine-induced long QTU interval and torsade de pointes: Role of bradycardia-dependent early afterdepolarizations. *J Am Coll Cardiol* 1989;14:252-257.
30. Roden DM, Woosley RL, Primm RK. Incidence and clinical features of the quinidine-associated long QT syndrome: Implications for patient care. *Am Heart J* 1986;111:1088-1093.
31. Hohnloser SH, Klingenheben T, Singh BN. Amiodarone-associated proarrhythmic effects. A review with special reference to torsade de pointes tachycardia. *Ann Intern Med* 1994;7:529-535.
32. Carlsson L, Almgren O, Duker G. QTU-prolongation and torsade de pointes induced by putative class III antiarrhythmic agents in the rabbit: Etiology and interventions. *J Cardiovasc Pharmacol* 1990;16:276-285.
33. Vos MA, Verduyn SC, Gorgels AP, et al. Reproducible induction of early afterdepolarizations and torsade de pointes arrhythmias by d-sotalol and pacing in dogs with chronic atrioventricular block. *Circulation* 1995;91:864-872.
34. Zabel M, Portnoy S, Franz MR. Electrocardiographic indexes of dispersion of ventricular repolarization: An isolated heart validation study. *J Am Coll Cardiol* 1995;25:746-752.

20

Dispersion of Ventricular Repolarization and Arrhythmias:

Basic and Clinical Correlates

Daniel P. Higham, MBBS, MRCP and Professor Ronald W.F. Campbell, MB, ChB, FRCP, FESC[†]

Introduction

Nonuniform changes in repolarization may lead to spatial dispersion of ventricular refractoriness. Animal experiments and computer models have confirmed that such dispersion may be sufficient to generate reentrant ventricular arrhythmias including ventricular fibrillation.[1] Abnormalities of repolarization may also cause triggered activity, which is an arrhythmia mechanism responsible for events in various clinical situations such as the long QT syndrome[2] and drug proarrhythmia.[3] Given the importance of dispersion of repolarization to arrhythmogenesis, characterizing and quantifying this feature should have a major application in patient management.

The QT Interval

In current clinical practice, the only widely practiced assessment of repolarization is that made by measuring the QT interval. Strictly, the

[†]Deceased

From Franz MR (ed): *Monophasic Action Potentials: Bridging Cell and Bedside.* ©Futura Publishing Company, Inc., Armonk, NY, 2000.

QT interval is a measure of ventricular recovery rather than just one of repolarization (Fig. 1). Changes in the QT interval may therefore arise as a result of changes in activation or repolarization or both, and such changes may be either arrhythmogenic or antiarrhythmic.

All normal/abnormal deflections recorded by the electrocardiogram (ECG) depend on the origin and behavior of the underlying ionic currents and their transmission through the extracellular tissue spaces to the body surface. The process of describing the surface ECG complex given the myocardial potentials is the inverse problem of electrocardiography. Several models have been developed to try and solve this problem. They range from Eindhoven's simple dipole theory,[4] multiple dipole theory,[5] solid angle analysis,[6] and volume integral analysis.[7] The more complex of these models are able to accurately derive the QRS complex given the underlying myocardial potential. Modeling ventricular repolarization is, however, a much more difficult problem. The voltage changes experienced are much more complex and occur over longer distances and over a slower time course. The voltage gradients during repolarization are considerably smaller and thus the surface potential changes are also much smaller. Indeed, whether

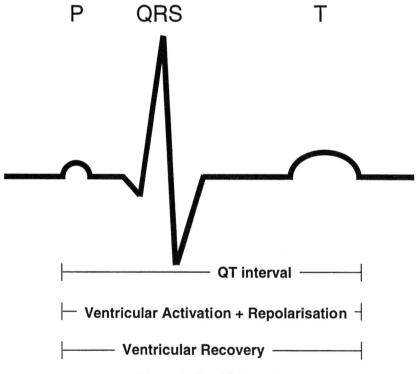

Figure 1. The QT interval.

repolarization occurs due to propagation (like ventricular activation) or is predetermined by regional action potential durations (APDs) is uncertain. Theoretical models leading to accurate explanations of T wave duration and morphology still elude us.

In the use of monophasic action potential (MAP) recordings in both animal experiments and in humans, several basic principles relating to the T wave and thus the QT interval have been established. Burdon-Sanderson and Page[8] demonstrated concordance between MAPs and surface ECG potential recordings. With the application of heat to the apex of the frog heart model they were using, they were able to shorten APD in this region, and by doing so, alter the shape of the T wave. Cowan and coworkers[9] recorded epicardial MAPs from 10 sites in 10 patients undergoing routine cardiac surgery, and demonstrated a marked dispersion of activation time and APD. Similar findings were obtained by Franz et al[10] with use of endocardial recordings. Both studies describe an inverse relationship between activation time and APD that was postulated to account for the concordant shape of the T wave in humans (Fig. 2). The presence of an endocardial-to-epicardial difference in APDs has also been described[10] and is also important in determining T wave shape, with endocardial APDs usually being longer. Thus, T wave shape and duration are determined by the repolarization process, but a complete understanding of the whole process involved has not yet been achieved.

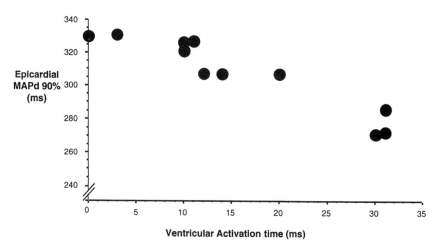

Figure 2. Inverse relationship between ventricular activation time and epicardial MAP. MAPd 90% = monophasic action potential duration at 90% repolarization.

Measurement of the QT Interval

The methodology of estimating the QT interval from the surface ECG is surprisingly poorly developed and is not standardized.[11] QT measurement in a single-lead ECG is relatively straightforward, but the standard 12-lead ECG poses problems. The usual practice is to measure a single arbitrary lead, which may be either a prespecified lead,[12] the lead with the largest T wave, or the lead with the longest QT interval. The situation is further complicated by defining T wave end (tangent or baseline approximation), using rate "correction," T wave morphology, and the presence of U waves. This "single lead" approach to QT has some justification but it does not reveal potentially important information about regional homogeneity.

When each of the 12 leads of the surface ECG are measured, there are small but consistent differences in QT intervals.[13] This phenomenon was first described in 1952 by Lepeschkin and Surawicz,[14] but was largely ignored. The origin of these variations in the QT interval has been investigated. They are not artefactual; this suggests that they may reflect regional changes in ventricular recovery. Proving the latter is a considerable technical challenge and all the current evidence is circumstantial through the correlation of QT variations with clinical arrhythmogenesis. A simple measure of the variation has been proposed—QT dispersion (QTd). QTd is the QT maximum minus the QT minimum, and is considered a measure of the dispersion of underlying ventricular recovery (Fig. 3). Since the first clinical paper that used the concept,[13] there have been scores of reports positively

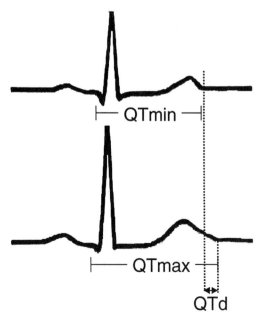

Figure 3. QT dispersion (QTd) is the QT maximum minus the QT minimum, and is considered a measure of the dispersion of underlying ventricular recovery.

associating QTd with either arrhythmia risk or death. Data exist for long QT syndrome,[15] acute-phase myocardial infarction,[16] late myocardial infarction,[17] heart failure,[18] proarrhythmia,[19] and diabetes.[20]

Impressive as such biological evidence is, it is no substitute for direct correlations of regional cardiac ventricular recovery with its expression on the body surface.

This chapter describes experiments correlating epicardial ventricular recovery estimated from epicardial MAPs with the body surface QT interval as recorded by the standard 12-lead ECG. There follows a detailed review of the clinical evidence that QTd predicts arrhythmias in a variety of pathologic situations.

Body Surface QT and Epicardial Ventricular Recovery in Humans

Almost all of the evidence that changes in body surface QT reflect underlying changes in ventricular recovery are circumstantial. Direct evidence in humans is lacking but it is possible to obtain multiple-point recordings of epicardial ventricular recovery. The purpose of this study was to examine the hypothesis underlying QTd by correlating direct measurements of epicardial ventricular recovery in humans with simultaneous recordings of body surface QT interval.

Patients and Methods

Measurements were made in patients who were undergoing routine coronary artery bypass grafting, aortic valve replacement, or arrhythmia surgery. All had given informed consent to the mapping procedures, which had received ethical approval. Fifty patients were considered for the study. One patient refused consent, and in 2 patients, the studies were not performed because their surgery was deferred. Perioperative mapping and ECG studies were thus performed in 47 patients. Because of the complex nature of epicardial MAP recordings, adequate data were obtained in only 22 patients, and in 5 of these, the electrocardiographic data were unsatisfactory for QT analysis. Thus, the data presented below are on 17 patients with direct epicardial MAP recordings and surface QT interval analysis in sinus rhythm.

MAP recordings were made with the use of a hand-held, roving, double-spike spatula electrode (Fig. 4). This technique is technically demanding. The surgeon holds the electrode with firm contact pressure against the epicardial surface, compensating for mechanical movement of the heart. Stable recordings usually develop within seconds and, in good subjects,

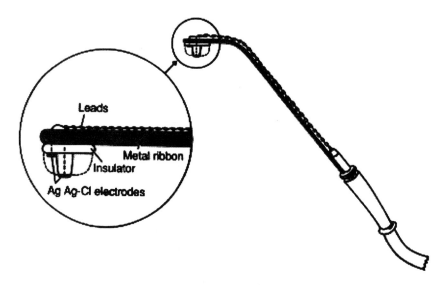

Figure 4. Diagram of the MAP probe.

it is possible to map nearly the entire ventricular surface within 4 minutes.[9] The epicardial MAPs had amplitudes ranging between 15 and 60 mV. To avoid distortion, the electrode must be applied perpendicular to the epicardial surface, the manual spatula handle aiding in this process. Recordings are difficult or impossible to obtain in patients with fatty hearts or in those with considerable areas of epicardial scarring. The skill of the mapping surgeon using the instrument is a key factor in obtaining good quality recordings.

The Signals

The double-spike ring probe permits recording of two MAPs at each myocardial location (Fig. 5). This doubles the chance of obtaining suitable MAPs for analysis. For this study, signals were recorded via a purpose-built bioelectric amplifier with a range of frequency characteristics down to 2 DC. MAPs were recorded using a long time constant (AC) recording (low-frequency cut-off at 0.007 Hz; time constant 22 seconds; high-frequency cut-off at 100 Hertz). Long time constant AC recording was facilitated by a baseline reset facility which rapidly restored the signal range channel. A fixed hook epicardial ventricular reference electrode gave an activation signal. This electrode was usually placed in the anterior wall of the left ventricle. A binary code recording system was developed to allow rapid recording of position and voltage gain, which greatly improved the speed of mapping. The MAP signals were displayed on a real-time color

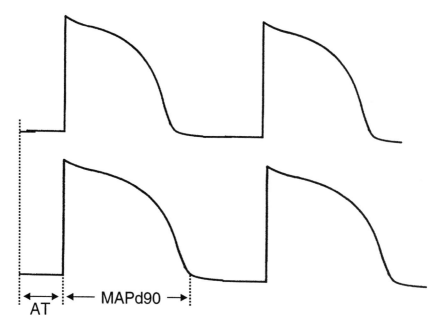

AT MAPd90

Figure 5. With the double-spike ring probe, two MAP recordings are made at each myocardial location.

monitor display to assist the surgeon in optimizing the quality of the recording. Quite fine adjustments of the probe often made great improvements to the signal quality.

MAPs were recorded in this way from the 12 epicardial sites: 1 anterior and 1 posterior right ventricular site and 10 left ventricular sites, as indicated on the standard epicardial map (Fig. 6).

In addition to routine ECG monitoring, each patient had a full 12-lead surface electrode set applied. As saphenous vein harvesting was to be performed in many patients, the right and left leg leads were applied on the respective upper lateral thighs. Leads V_1 and V_2 were more widely separated than normal to allow access for the bone saw to create the median sternotomy. All of the ECG leads were carefully applied and connections were secured under waterproof tape.

A baseline 12-lead ECG was obtained, and then again at specific times and procedural points during the operation. Epicardial mapping was started after 4 minutes of cardiopulmonary bypass to allow a stable state to be reached.[9] The important surface ECG recordings were recorded at the start and at the end of the acquisition of MAP data. During the monophasic recording, the open chest was approximated as closely as possible, but obviously, despite the spatula probe design, it is inevitable that the surface ECG V leads are not as close to the heart as under normal circumstances.

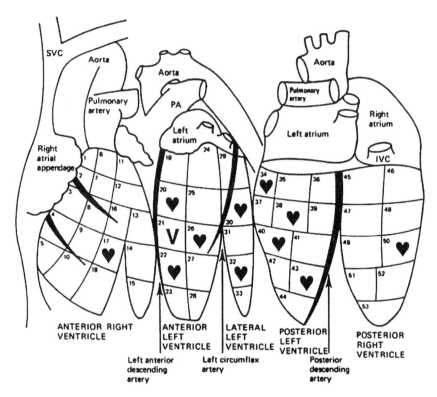

Figure 6. Epicardial MAP illustrating sites of epicardial MAP recording, IVC = inferior vena cava; PA = pulmonary artery; SVC = superior vena cava; V = site of V reference; ♥ = sites of epicardial MAP recording.

ECGs were recorded at 50 mm s^{-1} and at standard gain (10 mV$_2$/cm). QT intervals were measured by use of a single-point manual digitizing system according to procedures that have been previously published.[13] The protocol demanded that MAP signals be recorded quickly when there was hemodynamic and temperature stability. Instability, surgical urgency, and technical problems in obtaining signals accounted for the reduced data available for analysis.

MAP data were recorded on tape and analyzed by use of a commercially available software package for both MAP measurement (monophasic action potential duration at 90% repolarization [MAPD$_{90}$]) and for simple interval measurement to determine activation time. Sections of data of sufficient quality were transferred to disk to facilitate computerized measurements. Reproducibility of measurement for the action potential software was ±1%. Similarly, using cursor measurement, the interval between the activation signal and MAP upstroke indicating the activation time was actually measured to within ±0.5 millisecond. Thus, activation time and repolarization times were measured for each of the epicardial positions allowing calculation of epicardial ventricular recovery time.

Ventricular recovery time dispersion was calculated by subtracting the minimum dispersion value from the maximum dispersion value obtained. For inclusion into the study, all patients had to have at least a minimum of 7 recordings of ventricular recovery time from the 12 sites and 7 analyzable QT intervals from the 12 leads of the surface ECG.

The Findings

Figure 7 shows the plot of the QTd results versus the ventricular recovery time dispersion results. There was a good correlation between QTd and ventricular recovery time dispersion, although, obviously, a wide variation was seen. Mean QTd was 52 ± 18 milliseconds with a mean ventricular recovery time dispersion of 67 ± 22 milliseconds. There was a significant correlation between QTd and ventricular recovery time dispersion using ordinary least squares regression analysis. The correlation coefficient is 0.74; 95% confidence intervals 0.62 to 0.87; $P<0.001$. Table 1 summarizes raw data from each of the patients. Dispersion of activation times and

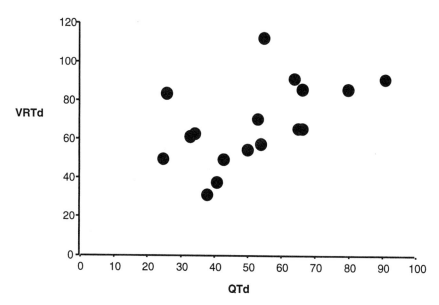

Figure 7. QT dispersion results versus ventricular recovery time dispersion results.

Table 1
Results of Perioperative Epicardial MAP
Mapping Studies in Sinus Rhythm

Patient No.	Activation Time Dispersion	APd$_{90}$ Dispersion	VRT Dispersion	QTd
1	55	40	65	66
2	50	50	70	53
3	110	86	91	64
4	71	103	83	26
5	32	49	49	25
6	38	51	49	43
7	37	81	91	91
8	23	70	57	54
9	21	130	112	55
10	37	85	61	33
11	22	60	65	65
12	36	53	54	50
13	31	59	37	41
14	23	55	63	34
15	36	35	31	38
16	80	97	86	80
17	117	121	86	65

MAPd$_{90}$ = monophasic action potential duration at 90% of repolarization; QTd = QT dispersion; VRT = ventricular recovery time.

MAPD$_{90}$ times are also given. It should be noted that these do not necessarily correspond, given the inverse relationship between MAPD and activation times.

Discussion

This study confirms that QTd correlates reasonably with underlying ventricular recovery time dispersion. Such a finding is important, as alterations in ventricular recovery time may arise by various means such as slowed conduction, dispersion of APDs, and the presence of afterdepolarizations (Fig. 8). These underlying electrophysiologic changes may thus be assessed by a measurement of QTd and perhaps in the clinical situation, may provide a measure of arrhythmia risk. It is not surprising that there is a wide variation among the results. The experimental conditions do not reflect the clinical situation of recording a 12-lead ECG, as the V leads would normally be closer to the heart. Because of the need for rapid assessment of ventricular recovery times, we were limited to 12-point mapping and, as discussed earlier, the data only

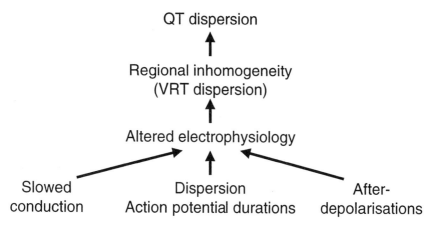

Figure 8. Possible causes of QT dispersion.

Table 2
Factors that Influence Surface QT Dispersion

1. Cardiac electrophysiology:	action potential durations
	conduction time
	afterdepolarizations
	areas of depolarized myocardium (eg, ischemia)
2. Cardiac geometry:	cardiac hypertrophy (symmetrical/ asymmetrical)
	wall motion abnormalities
3. Cardiac innervation:	neurohormonal asymmetry
4. ECG recording:	electrode placement
	tissue impedance
	biological signal processing

measure ventricular recovery time at the epicardial surface and do not take into account the presence of endocardial/epicardial repolarization gradients, which are well known to influence the nature and time course of the T wave. A very close correlation would not be expected. However, the results provide convincing evidence that QTd really does reflect underlying ventricular recovery time dispersion. It should, however, be noted that ventricular recovery time dispersion will not be the sole determinant of the surface QTd. Important factors in the generation of surface QTd are listed in Table 2. These factors should all be considered when assessing this measurement.

QTd: Clinical Correlates of Dispersion of Ventricular Repolarization

Since the concept of QTd was first discussed in 1988, there has been a rapid increase in the literature surrounding the subject. The literature has largely focused on several main categories of patients: those with long QT syndrome, those with hypertrophic cardiomyopathy, those with ischemic heart disease and acute myocardial infarction, those with heart failure, and, finally, clinical situations where drug proarrhythmia is a problem.

Long QT Syndrome

Long QT syndromes are characterized by the presence of a prolonged QT interval with the occurrence of ventricular arrhythmia, usually of the torsades de pointes type, or polymorphic ventricular tachycardia. Long QT syndromes may be congenital, drug-induced, or acquired (idiopathic).[2] The concept of body surface QT variation reflecting dispersion of underlying ventricular recovery is supported by studies in patients with long QT syndromes. Gavrilescu and Luca[21] demonstrated large variations in myocardial recovery using MAPs recorded from the right ventricular endocardium in these patients. Body surface mapping of ECG potentials also confirmed large variations in surface ECG intervals in these patients.[22] Recently, in an animal model of acquired long QT syndrome, Carlsson and coworkers[23] demonstrated that alterations in surface QTd were directly related to changes in underlying MAPs and that increasing dispersion was associated with the appearance of torsades de pointes arrhythmias.

Day and coworkers[15] studied two groups of patients. The first group comprised 10 patients with a history of ventricular arrhythmia and prolonged QT interval (9 congenital, 1 quinidine-related) taken from either published case reports or from their own patient population. The second group consisted of 14 patients who were taking sotalol as part of a randomized, controlled trial following myocardial infarction, all of whom had a corrected QT (QTc) interval of greater than 500 milliseconds. The mean QTc interval was 645 milliseconds in the arrhythmogenic long QT group compared to 572 in the group taking sotalol. The respective QTc dispersion values were 178 ± 18 versus 60 ± 7 milliseconds. The suggestion was made that QTd may improve the prediction of arrhythmogenesis by detecting abnormalities in repolarization. Linker et al[24] reported on 9 patients with congenital long QT syndromes and compared them with age-match controls. Mean QTc intervals were prolonged on affected patients who were not receiving treatment (590±80 versus 430±12 milliseconds), and mean QTc dispersion values were also higher. In patients subsequently taking β-blockers to control their arrhythmias, the QTc value and QTd values were not significantly altered. Linker and coworkers suggested that although the QTd was increased in patients with long QT syndromes, its clinical relevance remained uncertain.[24] Priori and coworkers[25] studied a much larger group of 28 patients with idiopathic long QT syndrome. These patients were divided into 3 categories: those before institution of therapy, those controlled on β-blockers, and those who were not controlled by β-blockade and who had undergone left cardiac sympathetic denervation. They also had a group of 15 healthy controls. Two parameters of interlead QT variability were assessed: QTd, and QT relative dispersion defined as the standard deviation of the QT/QT average × 100. The authors quoted both native and rate-corrective values. The changes in the various parameters between the 4 groups followed the same pattern. Considering QTd, the mean values were 65±16 milliseconds and 73±33 milliseconds in patients taking β-blockers with good arrhythmia control; however, QTc dispersion was significantly higher in the group presenting prior to starting any drugs (140±18 milliseconds) and also in the group requiring left stellate sympathectomy (156-58 milliseconds). QTd and QT relative dispersion were better predictors of responses to therapy than a single QT measurement.

QTd in Patients with Hypertrophic Cardiomyopathy

In 1992, Dritsas and coworkers[26] reported the effect of amiodarone therapy on QTd in patients with hypertrophic cardiomyopathy. Mean QTd levels were significantly lower in patients taking amiodarone (48±10 versus 78±17 milliseconds), whereas amiodarone produced significant QT prolongation (488±21 versus 451±23 milliseconds). These changes were not related to arrhythmic events. Miorelli and coworkers[27] studied the long-term variability of QTd in a group of 3 patients with hypertrophic cardiomyopathy. Late potentials were absent and only 1 patient had documented nonsustained ventricular tachycardia. They measured the maximum QTc interval and QTc dispersion retrospectively and compared them with 10 matched controls. In the control group, QTc dispersion values never exceeded 80 milliseconds (mean value 30±10, 44±8 milliseconds), whereas in 2 of the 3 patients who developed ventricular fibrillation with hypertrophic episodes of cardiomyopathy, QTd increased progressively during the follow-up period and, at the time of the event, all showed a value exceeding 100 milliseconds. In the group studied, sotalol but not amiodarone reduced QTc dispersion values. This study, despite the small number of patients involved, clearly suggests that QTd may have a useful role for predicting clinical arrhythmic events in high-risk patients.

QTd in Ischemic Heart Disease

In 1985, with use of body surface mapping techniques, Mirvis[28] was able to demonstrate significant regional differences in the QT interval in patients following myocardial infarction. Cowan and coworkers[13] confirmed the increased QTd in the surface 12-lead ECG QT intervals in patients with myocardial infarction compared with a group of patients without cardiac disease. Day et al[29] studied the effect of sotalol on QTd following myocardial infarction without arrhythmias. Sotalol reduced QTd in these patients compared to a matched placebo group. Higham et al[16] showed that patients with acute myocardial infarction had higher levels of QTd than patients with unstable angina and that patients who suffered ventricular fibrillation tended to have higher levels still. By analyzing the various components of the QT interval (QT minimum, QT apex, and QT end), they showed that QTd was not just a phenomenon of QT prolongation but that there were shifts in QT apex minimum that suggested that underlying action potential shortening also contributed to the various QT changes seen.

The acute effect of ischemia on electrocardiographic changes can be studied using coronary angioplasty. Tarabey et al[30] presented studies in 18 patients undergoing coronary angioplasty, in whom balloon inflation provoked ST elevation. QTd increased from a mean of 43 ± 20 milliseconds to 61 ± 19 milliseconds, and this was without a significant effect of QT maximum but evidence of a decrease in QT minimum (390 ± 43 milliseconds to 361 ± 43 milliseconds). No significant changes in QT measures were observed in 8 patients who had ST depression and in 8 patients without ST changes. Moreno et al[31] found that the greater the blood flow after thrombolytic therapy for myocardial infarction, the smaller the QTd was on a 12-lead ECG. Kelly et al[32] had suggested that in most patients following coronary angioplasty, QTd is reduced despite the acute changes discussed previously. QTd is increased in patients with previous myocardial infarction and seems to reflect the severity of underlying coronary artery disease. Using a nested case control study, Manttari et al[33] showed that in middle-aged men with normal conventional QT intervals, QT peak dispersion was an independent risk factor for sudden cardiac death but not for fatal myocardial infarction.

In patients with impaired left ventricular function, analysis of repolarization dispersion from the 12-lead surface ECG appears to identify patients with chronic heart failure who are at high risk of sudden cardiac death.[18] In 1994, Barr et al[34] also produced data suggesting that analysis of QTd predicted sudden unexpected death in chronic heart failure.

QTd is a dynamic phenomenon. It alters rapidly during balloon inflation during coronary angioplasty. It changes markedly following successful thrombolysis and it also alters during exercise. Indeed, changes in QTd with exercise appear to improve the accuracy of exercise testing for coronary artery disease in both men and women.[35]

QTd and Prevention of Ventricular Arrhythmias

Pye et al, in 1994, assessed QT interval dispersion on the surface ECG in patients with sustained ventricular arrhythmias.[36] This study excluded patients with recent myocardial infarction or ongoing ischemia, and used a control group of patients with myocardial disease but with no history of arrhythmias. There was a significantly greater mean QTd (77 milliseconds) in patients with arrhythmias compared with the control group (mean 38 milliseconds). The results held for the various groups of patients with ventricular tachycardia whether post myocardial infarction, due to dilated cardiomyopathy, or in patients with ventricular tachycardia and normal hearts. The authors also noticed a significant negative correlation between left ventricular function and QTd in patients with ventricular arrhythmias.

Davey and coworkers[37] studied QTd with chronic heart failure and left ventricular hypertrophy in relation to the autonomic nervous system and Holter tape abnormalities. They found that QTd was increased in patients with left ventricular hypertrophy, and tended to increase in patients with heart failure. These findings were unrelated to the occurrence of autonomic abnormalities or to the incidence of nonsustained ventricular arrhythmias on 24-hour tape. The lack of relationship between QTd and arrhythmic events on the tapes may be related to the arrhythmia type analyzed. Ventricular ectopic beats may arise from a focal myocardial source, and the mechanism of their generation may be unrelated to regional QT changes, perhaps explaining the negative results in this study. Lee et al[38] compared the performance of precordial QTd, the presence of late potentials, and reduced left ventricular ejection fraction for the identification of inducible ventricular tachycardias. QT apex dispersion in 56 patients with inducible ventricular tachycardia (72 ± 55 milliseconds) was greater than that in 106 patients without inducible ventricular tachycardia (55 ± 36 milliseconds). QT apex dispersion partition of more than 68 milliseconds identified inducible ventricular tachycardia with a specificity of 75% and sensitivity of 45%. Late potentials and reduced ejection fraction were superior to QTd alone for identification of inducible ventricular tachycardia, but abnormal QT apex dispersion still remained a significant additional predictor. Using 24-hour Holter monitoring, Puljevic et al[39] showed that increased QTd was associated with ventricular tachycardia and that a level of 80 milliseconds had a sensitivity of 72% and specificity of 86%. Late potentials were also a risk marker for ventricular tachycardia in this study. QTd thus appears to provide extra information with regard to predicting ventricular arrhythmias in patients with cardiac disease.

QTd and Antiarrhythmic Drugs

The effects of some antiarrhythmic drugs such as amiodarone and sotalol on QTd have been discussed in the previous sections of this chapter. Sedgwick and coworkers[40] studied the effect of dofetilide, a new class III antiarrhythmic agent, on the dispersion of right ventricular MAPs recorded from the endocardial wall at the apex and outflow tract. While the APD prolonged with subsequent administration of the drug, there was no increase in dispersion of the APDs between the two sites. Similar findings were noted in the surface QT recordings, with prolongation of the QT interval but no increase in QTd.

In 1992, Hii and coworkers[41] published a paper concerning the role of precordial QTd as a marker for torsades de pointes. They illustrated the disparate effects of class I antiarrhythmic drugs and amiodarone. They concluded that an increased regional QT interval dispersion during class Ia drug therapy was associated with torsades de pointes. Long-term amiodarone therapy in these same patients with a history of torsades de pointes induced by class Ia drugs produced comparable QT interval prolongation but did not increase QT interval dispersion. Measurement of QT interval dispersion rather than single QT values appeared to distinguish between the proarrhythmic and antiarrhythmic actions of drugs in this study.

Conclusions

QTd reflects underlying dispersion of ventricular recovery. It appears to be a useful tool for assessing regional variations and changes in ventricular recovery. Current evidence suggests that QTd increases in various clinical situations, and this appears to be related to the risk of ventricular arrhythmias and sudden death.

References

1. Janse MJ, Wit AL. Electrophysiologic mechanism of ventricular arrhythmias resulting from myocardial ischaemia and infarction. *Physiol Rev* 1989; 69:1049-1069.
2. Jackman WM, Friday KJ, Anderson JL. The long QT syndrome: A critical review, new clinical observations and a unifying hypothesis. *Prog Cardiovasc Dis* 1988;2:115-172.
3. The Sicilian Gambit. A new approach to the classification of antiarrhythmic drugs based on their actions on arrhythmogenic mechanisms. Task Force of the Working Group on Arrhythmias of the European Society of Cardiology. *Circulation* 1991;84(4):1831-1851.
4. Einthoven W, Fahr G, de Waart A. On the direction and manifest size of the variations of potential in the human heart and on the influence of the position of the heart on the form of the electrocardiogram. *Am Heart J* 1950;40(2):163-193.

5. Holt JH, Barnard ACL, Lynn MS, Svendsen P. A study of the human heart as a multiple dipole electrical source: 1. Normal adult male subjects. *Circulation* 1969;40:687-696.

6. Holland RP, Arnsdorf MF. Solid angle theory and the electrocardiogram: Physiologic and quantitative interpretations. *Prog Cardiovasc Dis* 1977;19:431-457.

7. Kootsey JM, Johnson EA. The origin of the T wave. *CRC Crit Rev Bioengineer* 1980;4:233-270.

8. Burdon-Sanderson J, Page FJM. On the time relations of the excitatory process in the ventricle of the heart of the frog. *J Physiol* 1880;2:384-435.

9. Cowan JC, Hilton CJ, Griffiths CJ, et al. Sequence of epicardial repolarisation and configuration of the T wave. *Br Heart J* 1988;60:424-433.

10. Franz MR, Bargheer K, Rafflenbeul W, et al. Monophasic action potential mapping in human subjects with normal electrocardiograms: Direct evidence for the genesis of the T wave. *Circulation* 1987;75:379-386.

11. Campbell RWF, Gardiner P, Amos PA, et al. Measurement of the QT interval. *Eur Heart J* 1985;6(suppl D):81-85.

12. Moller M. QT interval in relation to ventricular arrhythmias and sudden cardiac death in post myocardial infarction patients. *Acta Med Scand* 1981;210:73-77.

13. Cowan JC, Yusoff K, Moore M, et al. Importance of lead selection in QT interval measurement. *Am J Cardiol* 1988;61(1):83-87.

14. Lepeschkin E, Surawicz B. The measurement of the QT interval of the electrocardiogram. *Circulation* 1952;6:378-388.

15. Day CP, McComb JM, Campbell RWF. QT dispersion: An indication of arrhythmia risk in patients with long QT intervals. *Br Heart J* 1990;63:342-344.

16. Higham PD, Furniss SS, Campbell RWF. QT dispersion and components of the QT interval in ischemia and infarction. *Br Heart J* 1995;73(1):32-36.

17. Glancy J, Garratt C, Woods K, Bono D. QT dispersion and mortality after myocardial infarction. *Lancet* 1995;345:945-948.

18. Fu GS, Meissner A, Simon R. Repolarization dispersion and sudden cardiac death in patients with impaired left ventricular function. *Eur Heart J* 1997;18:281-289.

19. Thomas SHL, Ford GA, Higham PD, et al. Effects of terodiline on the QT interval and QT dispersion. *Clin Pharm Therapeut* 1993;53:136.

20. Langen KJ, Ziegler D, Weise F, et al. Evaluation of QT interval length, QT dispersion and myocardial m-iodobenzylguanidine uptake in insulin-dependent diabetic patients with and without autonomic neuropathy. *Clin Sci* 1997;93(4):325-333.

21. Gavrilescu S, Luca C. Right ventricular monophasic action potentials in patients with long QT syndrome. *Br Heart J* 1978;40:1014-1018.

22. De Ambroggi L, Negroni MS, Monza E, et al. Dispersion of ventricular repolarization in the long QT syndrome. *Am J Cardiol* 1991;68:614-620.

23. Carlsson L, Abrahamsson C, Andersson B, et al. Proarrhythmic effects of the class III agent almokalant: Importance of infusion rate, QT dispersion and early afterdepolarizations. *Cardiovasc Res* 1993;27(12):2186-2193.

24. Linker N, Colonna P, Kekwick C, et al. Assessment of QT dispersion in symptomatic patients with congenital long QT syndromes. *Am J Cardiol* 1992; 69(6):634-638.

25. Priori SG, Napolitano C, Diehl L, Schwartz PJ. Dispersion of the QT interval. A marker of therapeutic efficacy in the idiopathic long QT syndrome. *Circulation* 1994;89(4):1681-1689.

26. Dritsas A, Gilligan D, Nihoyannopoulos P, Oakley CM. Amiodarone reduces QT dispersion in patients with hypertrophic cardiomyopathy. *Int J Cardiol* 1992;36(3):345-349.
27. Miorelli M, Buja G, Melacini P, et al. QT interval variability in hypertrophic cardiomyopathy patients with cardiac arrest. *Int J Cardiol* 1994;45(2):121-127.
28. Mirvis DM. Spatial variation of QT intervals in normal persons with acute myocardial infarction. *J Am Coll Cardiol* 1985;5:625-631.
29. Day CP, McComb JM, Matthews J, Campbell RWF. Reduction in QT dispersion by sotalol following myocardial infarction. *Eur Heart J* 1991;12:423-427.
30. Tarabey R, Sukenik D, Molnar J, Somberg JC. Effect of intracoronary balloon inflation at percutaneous transluminal coronary angioplasty on QT dispersion. *Am Heart J* 1998;135(3):519-522.
31. Moreno F, Villanueva T, Karagounis L, Anderson J. Reduction of QT interval dispersion by successful thrombolytic therapy in acute myocardial infarction. TEAM-2 Study Investigators. *Circulation* 1994;90(1):94-100.
32. Kelly RF, Parillo JE, Hollenberg SM. Effect of coronary angioplasty on QT dispersion. *Am Heart J* 1997;134(3):399-405.
33. Manttari M, Oikarinen L, Manninen V, Viitasalo M. QT dispersion as a risk factor for sudden cardiac death and fatal myocardial infarction in a coronary risk population. *Heart* 1997;78(3):268-272.
34. Barr CS, Naas A, Freeman M, et al. QT dispersion and sudden unexpected death in chronic heart failure. *Lancet* 1994;343:327-329.
35. Stoletniy LN, Pai RG. Usefulness of QTc dispersion in interpreting exercise electrocardiograms. *Am Heart J* 1995;130:918-921.
36. Pye M, Quinn AC, Cobbe SM. QT interval dispersion: A non-invasive marker of susceptibility to arrhythmia in patients with sustained ventricular arrhythmias? *Br Heart J* 1994;71(6):511-514.
37. Davey PP, Bateman J, Mulligan IP, et al. QT interval dispersion in chronic heart failure and left ventricular hypertrophy: Relation to autonomic nervous system and Holter tape abnormalities. *Br Heart J* 1994;71(3):268-273.
38. Lee KW, Okin PM, Kligfield P, et al. Precordial QT dispersion and inducible ventricular tachycardia. *Am Heart J* 1997;134(6):1005-1013.
39. Puljevic D, Smalcelj A, Durakovic Z, Goldner V. QT dispersion, daily variations, QT interval adaptation and late potentials as risk markers for ventricular tachycardia. *Eur Heart J* 1997;18(8):1343-1349.
40. Sedgwick ML, Rasmussen HS, Cobbe SM. Effects of the class III antiarrhythmic drug dofetilide on ventricular monophasic action potential duration and QT interval dispersion in stable angina pectoris. *Am J Cardiol* 1992;70(18):1432-1437.
41. Hii JT, Wyse DG, Gillis AM, et al. Precordial QT interval dispersion as a marker of torsade de pointes. Disparate effects of Class Ia antiarrhythmic drugs and amiodarone. *Circulation* 1992;86:1376-1382.

21

Validation of Electrocardiographic Variables of Dispersion of Ventricular Repolarization with Direct Myocardial Repolarization Measurements

Markus Zabel, MD, Paul R. Lichtlen, MD, Axel Haverich, MD and Michael R. Franz, MD, PhD

Introduction

The importance of the dispersion of ventricular repolarization (DVR) in the genesis of ventricular arrhythmias has been shown both experimentally and in clinical electrophysiologic studies.[1-5] In patients, DVR can be measured invasively using endocardial or epicardial catheter mapping by means of the monophasic action potential (MAP) contact electrode method,[6-8] and noninvasively, using extensive multilead body surface potential mapping.[9-12] Neither of these two methods, however, is available or practical for widespread clinical evaluation of DVR. As a result, QT dispersion (QTd) calculated as the range of QT intervals ($QT_{max} - QT_{min}$) has been proposed as a simple noninvasive measurement of DVR available from

From Franz MR (ed): *Monophasic Action Potentials: Bridging Cell and Bedside.* ©Futura Publishing Company, Inc., Armonk, NY, 2000.

the 12-lead surface electrocardiogram (ECG).[13] Since the initial proposal by Campbell and associates,[13] this simple electrocardiographic measurement has been evaluated in numerous studies.[14-28] Currently, it is uncertain whether QTd can be applied as a simple risk marker in patients at increased arrhythmia risk post myocardial infarction[17-20,25,30-32] or with congestive heart failure.[21-24,26,30-32] However, QTd seems to be useful for the assessment of arrhythmia risk in patients with the long QT syndrome[11-13,15] or for evaluation of proarrhythmic effects of action potential prolonging drugs.[13,14] Besides, dynamic changes in response to exercise and/or ischemia have been suggested to provide useful information.[27,28] Recently, QTd measurements have been automatized by use of digital 12-lead ECGs.[29] During the ongoing enormous research efforts on QTd, only one study, in abstract form, was available that correlates QTd with dispersion of recovery time as calculated from MAP recordings taken during cardiac surgery.[33] The number of patients and recordings, however, was low in this study. Thus, for a relatively long period of time, no proper validation of QTd was available. This chapter reviews the two published validation studies[34,35] that correlate QTd and other electrocardiographic variables with direct measurements of DVR.

Experimental Set Up for Evaluation of Electrocardiographic Variables of DVR

To accomplish the objective of correlating potentially useful electrocardiographic variables with the dispersion of action potential duration (APD) and recovery time, a novel isolated heart preparation (Fig. 1) was developed by Zabel et al.[34] Four silver-silver chloride electrode pellets were positioned in a simulated "Einthoven" configuration to the walls of the tissue bath, which had a diameter similar to that of a rabbit thorax. Six additional electrodes were mounted in a circular pattern on the anterior wall of the bath to record unipolar Wilson leads. Six to 8 evenly spread contact MAP electrodes were spring mounted around the centrally placed Langendorff-perfused rabbit heart. Two to 3 electrodes were placed on the right ventricular epicardium, and another 4 to 6 were evenly spread over the left ventricle. In addition to the epicardial MAPs, right ventricular and left ventricular endocardial MAPs were recorded by means of catheters. With use of this set up, a 12-lead volume-conducted ECG and up to 10 MAP signals were recorded simultaneously from the isolated rabbit heart.

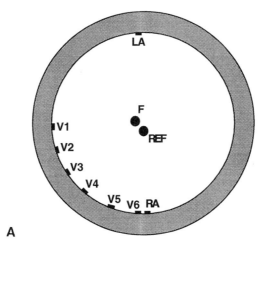

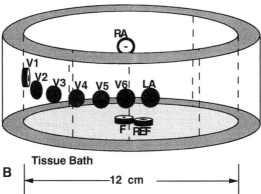

Figure 1. Experimental set up for simultaneous measurements of MAPs and electrocardiograms in an isolated rabbit heart. From Reference 34, with permission.

MAP Mapping
in the Human Heart

With use of contact electrode catheters, Franz et al[6,35] obtained sequential endocardial MAP recordings for evaluation of DVR in the human heart during cardiac catheterization in 11 patients. On average, 8 MAPs from 6 prespecified left ventricular endocardial regions (anteroapical, inferoapical, diaphragmatic, basoseptal, apicoseptal, and posterolateral; Fig. 2) were obtained. In a similar manner, MAPs were recorded by means of a contact electrode probe in 6 patients during cardiac surgery. An average of 6

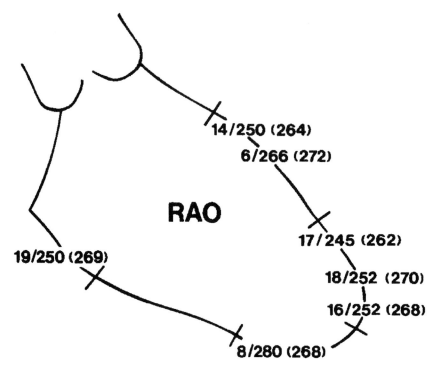

14/250 (264)

6/266 (272)

RAO

17/245 (262)

18/252 (270)

16/252 (268)

19/250 (269)

8/280 (268)

Figure 2. Dispersion of ventricular repolarization measured by means of an endocardial MAP catheter in the human ventricle. Activation times and action potential duration are given for various MAP recording locations. From Reference 6, with permission.

epicardial mapping sites were covered from both ventricles.[6,35] The dispersion of MAP durations at 90% repolarization (APD_{90}) was defined as APD_{90max} − APD_{90min}, whereas dispersion of recovery time (RT = APD_{90} + activation time) was defined as RT_{max} − RT_{min}.

Electrocardiographic Analysis of DVR

In the experimental study,[34] volume-conducted ECGs were recorded digitally, whereas in the human study ECGs were available on paper with a recording speed of 50 mm/s. With use of a new method,[35,36] ECGs were scanned, edited, and converted to a digital file. Subsequently, digital ECGs were submitted to customized software for interactive analysis of all electrocardiographic variables of DVR proposed in the literature. The computer program used customized algorithms to detect important features of the electrocardiographic waveforms such as Q onset, J point, T peak, and T end, and then displayed vertical spikes superimposed on the signal, marking these points for confirmation or manual correction by the observer.

Standard QTD and Related Variables

JT, JTc (JT corrected by the Bazett formula), QT, and corrected QT (QTc) intervals were averaged among all analyzable leads. Rate correction was done by use of the Bazett formula. Conventional QTd, JTd, QTc dispersion, and JTc dispersion were calculated as the maximum minus the minimum interval duration of all analyzable ECG leads. Adjusted QTd[37] and relative QTd involving the standard deviation of QT intervals[15] were also determined. All electrocardiographic variables were recalculated on the basis of the 6 precordial leads only.[14,15]

New Electrocardiographic Variables of DVR

Because the T wave vector is generated from inhomogeneous recovery throughout the heart,[6,38-40] T wave width, measured by the T peak to T end (TPE) interval, and T wave area, representing a summation of T wave vectors, were hypothesized by Zabel et al[34] to reflect DVR. These variables were first tested in the experimental validation study described here[34] and were subsequently evaluated clinically[22,25] as well as in the human validation study.[35] In support of this hypothesis, the consideration of the TPE interval as a measure of transmural DVR was recently described by Antzelevitch et al.[41,42] Their experiments provided evidence that delayed repolarization of M cells residing in the mid myocardium contributes significantly to DVR.[41,42] These findings, however, were derived from a single electrocardiogram lead in an arterially perfused canine wedge preparation. Finally, the ratio of the QT_{peak} to QT_{end} interval was added as a measure of the late repolarization phase.

Experimental Validation Study [34]
(Fig. 3)

Measured from approximately 100 data points at different pacing rates and under additional drug influence, QTd and JTd showed a significant correlation with the dispersion of APD_{90} (r=0.61, $P<0.001$ and r=0.64, $P<0.001$, respectively) and the dispersion of recovery time (r=0.59, $P<0.001$ and r=0.58, $P<0.001$, respectively). T wave area exhibited an excellent correlation with dispersion of APD_{90} and recovery time (r=0.79, $P<0.0001$ and r=0.82, $P<0.0001$, respectively), as did the TPE interval (r=0.81, $P<0.001$

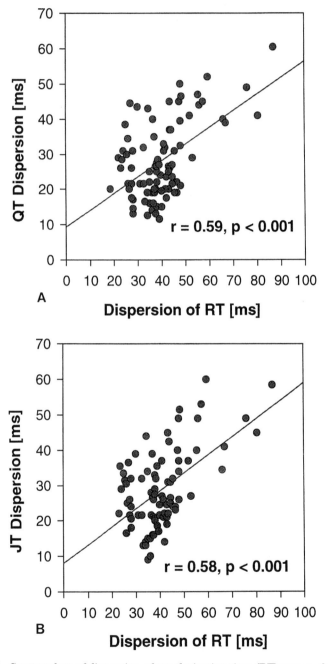

Figure 3. Scatter plots of dispersion of repolarization time (RT) versus electrocardiographic variables from the experimental validation study. **A**. QT dispersion; **B**. JT dispersion. *Continues.*

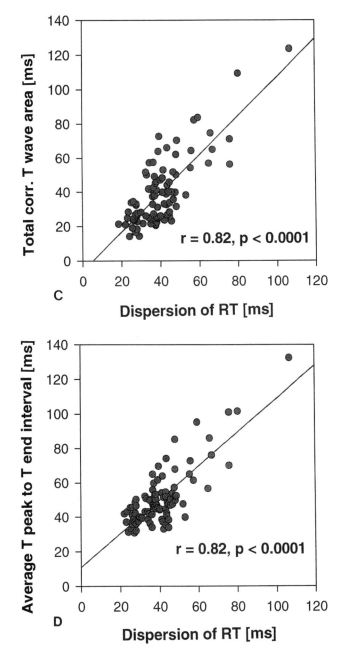

Figure 3 (*continued*). **C**. Average total T wave area; **D**. average TPE interval. From Reference 34, with permission.

and r=0.82, *P*<0.001, respectively). Thus, the TPE interval and the area under the T wave were identified to reflect DVR better than QTd and JTd.

Human Heart Validation Study [35]
(Fig. 4)

MAP recordings matched with 12-lead ECGs were available in 17 patients, 7 of whom had confirmed left ventricular hypertrophy due to aortic valvular disease at echocardiography. QTd exhibited a reasonable correlation with dispersion of recovery time (r=0.67, *P*<0.01), which was remarkably similar to that observed in the experimental study. The coefficients for correlations between myocardial dispersion measurements (dispersion of APD_{90} and dispersion of RT) and all studied electrocardiographic

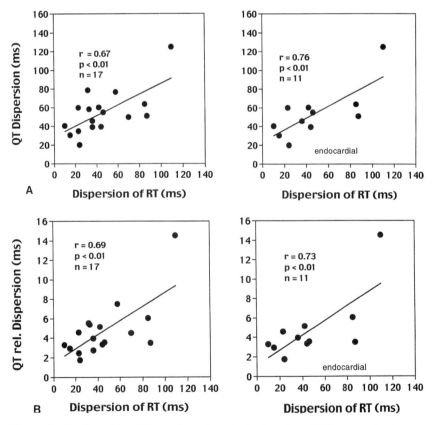

Figure 4. Scatter plots of dispersion of repolarization time (RT) versus electrocardiographic variables from the human validation study. **A**. QT dispersion; **B**. QT relative dispersion. *Continues.*

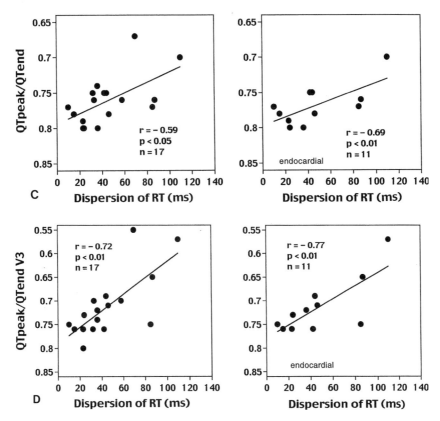

Figure 4 (*continued*). C. QT_{peak}/QT_{end} ratio; **D.** QT_{peak}/QT_{end} ratio in lead V3. From Reference 35, with permission.

variables are shown in Table 1 (panels A and B). Among them the QT_{peak}/QT_{end} ratio in V3 (r=−0.72, P<0.01) and averaged over all analyzable leads (r=−0.59, P<0.01) exhibited one of the best correlations, with dispersion of recovery time that was further improved when endocardial measurements were considered alone. T area measures did not correlate with dispersion of recovery time but discriminated between the presence and absence of left ventricular hypertrophy. Several examples of the correlation scatter plots are shown in Figure 4. Beyond demonstrating a reasonable correlation between electrocardiographic variables of DVR and the direct myocardial MAP measurements, this study allowed a comparison among currently proposed variables of DVR. Many of the studied electrocardiographic variables exhibit a similar and significant correlation with the invasive measurements. Importantly, this is true for the initial standard QTd variable ($QT_{max} − QT_{min}$), which has been widely used by many investigators. Adjusted and relative QTd did not show an improved association with the

Table 1A

Coefficients for Correlations Between
12-Lead ECG Variables and MAP Measurements

Variable	Dispersion of APD_{90} All Recordings n=17	Dispersion of RT All Recordings n=17	Dispersion of APD_{90} Endocardial n=11	Dispersion of RT Endocardial n=11
JTD	0.60*	0.45	0.55	0.60*
JTcD	0.56*	0.42	0.57	0.64*
JTD_{adj}	0.61**	0.46	0.58	0.62*
JTD_{rel}	0.62**	0.57*	0.58	0.64*
QTD	0.69**	0.67**	0.69*	0.76**
QTcD	0.62**	0.58*	0.65*	0.74**
QTD_{adj}	0.69**	0.66**	0.70*	0.76*
QTD_{rel}	0.66**	0.69**	0.65*	0.73*
TPE	0.23	0.41	0.71*	0.63*
TA	−0.25	−0.12	−0.01	−0.04
TA_{late}	−0.27	−0.15	−0.02	−0.08
QT_{peak}/QT_{end}	−0.25	−0.59*	−0.65*	−0.69*

Table 1B

Coefficients for Correlations Between
Precordial ECG Variables and MAP Measurements

Precordial Variable	Dispersion of APD_{90} All Recordings n = 17	Dispersion of RT All Recordings n = 17	Dispersion of APD_{90} Endocardial n = 11	Dispersion of RT Endocardial n = 11
JTD	0.55*	0.43	0.76**	0.71*
JTcD	0.47*	0.35	0.76**	0.76**
JTD_{rel}	0.61**	0.50*	0.67*	0.66*
QTD	0.55*	0.50*	0.69*	0.71*
QTcD	0.46*	0.39	0.65*	0.71*
QTD_{rel}	0.53*	0.54*	0.56	0.62*
TPE	0.26	0.41	0.72*	0.62*
TA	−0.27	−0.17	−0.10	−0.10
TA_{late}	−0.30	−0.20	−0.07	−0.13
QT_{peak}/QT_{end} V3	−0.45	−0.72**	−0.79**	−0.77**

invasive measurements in this study. Importantly, an identical association was found for precordial electrocardiographic variables. This suggests that most of the ventricular heterogeneity in repolarization is found within the 6 unipolar chest leads. Similar to the results of the experimental validation study,[34] variables involving the JT interval correlate better with dispersion of APD_{90}, while those variables involving the QT interval better reflect dispersion of RT. Rate correction of QTd resulted in a decreased correlation with the myocardial measurements in this study. This further supports the hypothesis that DVR is independent of heart rate—as recently demonstrated by Zabel et al experimentally[43] and in patients[44]—and that the practice of rate correction of QTd should be abandoned.

Does the 12-Lead ECG Reflect Local or Global Repolarization?

While the above validation studies prove that DVR (ie, a measure defined by local differences in repolarization) can be assessed from the 12-lead surface ECG, it had long been thought that T waves in the various leads of the surface ECG are a reflection of a common T wave vector defining global repolarization. The study by Mirvis[10] using 150 simultaneous precordial unipolar ECG leads was the first to reveal regional repolarization differences on the body surface. In retrospect, this study was able to give a clear estimate of the expected QTd values in normal subjects and in postmyocardial infarction patients. These were confirmed by Cowan and coworkers,[45] who were the first to calculate interlead differences in the QT interval within the 12-lead surface ECG. These differences provide the basis for the concept of QTd and cannot be explained by different projections of a T wave vector. It can be hypothesized that the T wave reflects a combination of local and global repolarization vector forces. Moreover, it can be expected that more local information from the vicinity of the unipolar electrodes will be carried by the Wilson chest leads while more global repolarization vectors will be represented in the bipolar limb leads. It is therefore conceivable that the unipolar chest leads are most useful for QTd measurements and contain most of the DVR information of the full set of 12 surface ECG leads. Additionally, even the T wave of a single precordial lead seems to convey a large portion of the precordial or even 12-lead information content, as the QT_{peak}/QT_{end} ratio measured from lead V3 exhibited an excellent correlation with DVR as assessed by means of MAP recordings.

Summary

DVR can be assessed from the 12-lead surface ECG as has been validated in an experimental model and in the human heart. Several new electrocardiographic variables have been proposed, including the TPE interval. Several variables exhibit similar accuracy in determination of true myocardial dispersion. Variables involving the terminal part of repolarization such as the QT_{peak}/QT_{end} ratio—even from a single lead—may add to the assessment of DVR from the human heart.

References

1. Han J, Moe GK. Nonuniform recovery of excitability in ventricular muscle. *Circ Res* 1964;14:44.
2. Merx W, Yoon MS, Han J. The role of local disparity in conduction and recovery time on ventricular vulnerability to fibrillation. *Am Heart J* 1977;94:603-610.
3. Kuo CS, Munakata K, Reddy CP, et al. Characteristics and possible mechanism of ventricular arrhythmia dependent on the dispersion of action potential durations. *Circulation* 1983;67:1356-1367.
4. Kuo CS, Reddy CP, Munakata K, et al. Mechanism of ventricular arrhythmias caused by increased dispersion of repolarization. *Eur Heart J* 1985;6(suppl D):63-70.
5. Vassallo JA, Cassidy DM, Kindwall KE, et al. Nonuniform recovery of excitability in the left ventricle. *Circulation* 1988;78:1365-1372.
6. Franz MR, Bargheer K, Rafflenbeul W, et al. Monophasic action potential mapping in human subjects with normal electrocardiograms: Direct evidence for the genesis of the T wave. *Circulation* 1987;75:379-386.
7. Franz MR, Chin MC, Sharkey HR, et al. A new single catheter technique for simultaneous measurement of action potential duration and refractory period in vivo. *J Am Coll Cardiol* 1990;16:878-886.
8. Franz MR. Method and theory of monophasic action potential recording. *Prog Cardiovasc Dis* 1991;33:347-368.
9. Sylven JC, Horacek BM, Spencer CA, et al. QT interval variability on the body surface. *J Electrocardiol* 1984;17:179-188.
10. Mirvis DM. Spatial variation of QT intervals in normal persons and patients with acute myocardial infarction. *J Am Coll Cardiol* 1985;3:625-631.
11. De Ambroggi L, Bertoni T, Locati E, et al. Mapping of body surface potentials in patients with the idiopathic long QT syndrome. *Circulation* 1986;74:1334-1345.
12. De Ambroggi L, Negroni MS, Monza E, et al. Dispersion of ventricular repolarization in the long QT syndrome. *Am J Cardiol* 1991;68:614-620.
13. Day CP, McComb JM, Campbell RW. QT dispersion: An indication of arrhythmia risk in patients with long QT intervals. *Br Heart J* 1990;63:342-344.
14. Hii JTY, Wyse GD, Gillis AM, et al. Precordial QT interval dispersion as a marker of torsade de pointes. *Circulation* 1992;86:1376-1382.
15. Priori SG, Napolitano C, Diehl L, et al. Dispersion of the QT interval: A marker of therapeutic efficacy in the idiopathic long QT syndrome. *Circulation* 1994;89:1681-1689.
16. Barr CS, Naas A, Freeman M, et al. QT dispersion and sudden unexpected death in chronic heart failure. *Lancet* 1994;343:327-329.
17. Zareba W, Moss AJ, le Cessie S. Dispersion of ventricular repolarization and arrhythmic cardiac death in coronary artery disease. *Am J Cardiol* 1994;74:550-553.

18. Moreno FL, Villanueva T, Karagounis LA, et al. Reduction in QT interval dispersion by successful thrombolytic therapy in acute myocardial infarction. TEAM-2 Study Investigators. *Circulation* 1994;90:94-100.
19. Perkiömäki JS, Koistinen MJ, Yli-Mayry S, et al. Dispersion of the QT interval in patients with and without susceptibility to ventricular tachyarrhythmias after previous myocardial infarction. *J Am Coll Cardiol* 1995;26:174-179.
20. Glancy JM, Garratt CJ, Woods KL, et al. QT dispersion and mortality after myocardial infarction. *Lancet* 1995;345:945-948.
21. Fei L, Goldman JH, Prasad K, et al. QT dispersion and RR variations on 12-lead ECGs in patients with congestive heart failure secondary to idiopathic dilated cardiomyopathy. *Eur Heart J* 1996;17:258-263.
22. Zabel M, Ney G, Fischer SR, et al. QRS width in the 12-lead surface ECG but not variables of QT dispersion predict mortality in the CHF-STAT trial. *PACE* 1996;19:589. Abstract.
23. Fu GS, Meissner A, Simon R. Repolarization dispersion and sudden cardiac death in patients with impaired left ventricular function. *Eur Heart J* 1997;18:281-289.
24. Pinsky DJ, Sciacca RR, Steinberg JS. QT dispersion as a marker of risk in patients awaiting heart transplantation. *J Am Coll Cardiol* 1997;29:1576-1584.
25. Zabel M, Klingenheben T, Franz MR, et al. Assessment of QT dispersion for prediction of mortality or arrhythmic events after myocardial infarction: Results of a prospective long-term follow-up study. *Circulation* 1998;97:2543-2550.
26. Zabel M, Franz MR, Klingenheben T, et al. QT dispersion as a marker of risk in patients awaiting heart transplantation? *J Am Coll Cardiol* 1998;31:1442-1443.
27. Sporton SC, Taggart P, Sutton PM, et al. Acute ischemia: A dynamic influence on QT dispersion. *Lancet* 1997;349:306-309.
28. Stoletniy LN, Pai RG. Value of QT dispersion in the interpretation of exercise stress test in women. *Circulation* 1997;96:904-910.
29. Yi G, Prasad K, Elliot P, et al. T wave complexity in patients with hypertrophic cardiomyopathy. *PACE* 1998;21:2382-2386.
30. Statters DJ, Malik M, Ward DE, et al. QT dispersion: Problems of methodology and clinical significance. *J Cardiovasc Electrophysiol* 1994;5:672-685.
31. Surawicz B. Will QT dispersion play a role in clinical decision-making? *J Cardiovasc Electrophysiol* 1996;7:777-784.
32. Coumel P, Mason-Blanche P, Badlini F. Dispersion of ventricular repolarization: Reality? Illusion? Significance? *Circulation* 1998;97:2491-2493.
33. Higham PD, Hilton CJ, Aitcheson JD, et al. Does QT dispersion reflect dispersion of ventricular recovery? *Circulation* 1992;86:I392. Abstract.
34. Zabel M, Portnoy S, Franz MR. Electrocardiographic indexes of dispersion of ventricular repolarization: An isolated heart validation study. *J Am Coll Cardiol* 1995;25:746-752.
35. Zabel M, Lichtlen PR, Haverich A, et al. Comparison of ECG variables of dispersion of ventricular repolarization with direct myocardial repolarization measurements in the human heart. *J Cardiovasc Electrophysiol* 1998;9:1279-1284.
36. Zabel M, Portnoy S, Fletcher RD, et al. A program for digitizing of ECG tracings on paper and accurate interactive measurement of QT intervals and ECG parameters of ventricular repolarization. *J Am Coll Cardiol* 1995;25:374A. Abstract.
37. Day CP, McComb JM, Campbell RWF. QT dispersion in sinus beats and ventricular extrasystoles in normal hearts. *Br Heart J* 1992;67:39-41.

38. Wilson FN, MacLeod AG, Barker PS, et al. The determination and the significance of the areas of the ventricular deflections of the electrocardiogram. *Am Heart J* 1934;10:46.

39. Harumi K, Burgess MJ, Abildskov JA. A theoretic model of the T wave. *Circulation* 1966;34:657-668.

40. Spach MS, Barr RC. Origin of epicardial ST-T wave potentials in the intact dog. *Circ Res* 1976;39:475-487.

41. Antzelevitch C, Nesterenko VV, Shimizu W, et al. Electrophysiological characteristics of the M cell. In Franz MR, Schmitt C, Zrenner B (eds): *Monophasic Action Potentials*. Berlin, Heidelberg: Springer; 1997:212-226.

42. Shimizu W, Antzelevitch C. Sodium channel block with mexiletine is effective in reducing dispersion of repolarization and preventing torsade de pointes in LQT2 and LQT3 models of the long-QT syndrome. *Circulation* 1997;96:2038-2047.

43. Zabel M, Woosley RL, Franz MR. Is dispersion of ventricular repolarization rate dependent? *PACE* 1997;20:2405-2411.

44. Zabel M, Franz MR, Klingenheben T, et al. Rate-dependence of the QT interval and of QT dispersion: Comparison of atrial pacing and exercise testing. *Circulation* 1997;96:I-325. Abstract.

45. Cowan JC, Yusoff K, Moore M, et al. Importance of lead selection in QT interval measurement. *Am J Cardiol* 1988;61:83-87.

22

Mapping of the Spatial Correlation Between the Activation and Repolarization Properties in the Normal Ventricle

Lior Gepstein, MD, Gal Hayam, BSc and Shlomo A. Ben-Haim, MD, DSc

Introduction

Abnormalities of the myocardial activation and repolarization patterns are generally believed to play an important role in the genesis of cardiac arrhythmias. Numerous studies have shown that functional heterogeneity in the activation (slow conduction) or the repolarization (increased dispersion) properties of the myocardial tissue is a major prerequisite for the genesis and maintenance of reentrant arrhythmias.[1-5]

One example of the role of abnormal activation in arrhythmogenesis is the induction of ventricular tachycardia during the chronic stages of healed myocardial infarction. This arrhythmia is generally believed to be reentrant and involves a critical area of slow conduction substrate within the scar.[3] Similarly, several clinical and experimental studies also support the role of augmented dispersion of repolarization in the generation of various cardiac arrhythmias.[4] Examples of experimental models in which

From Franz MR (ed): *Monophasic Action Potentials: Bridging Cell and Bedside.* ©Futura Publishing Company, Inc., Armonk, NY, 2000.

dispersion of repolarization appears to play an important role include the circus-movement tachycardia (leading circle reentry) induced by Allessie et al[5] in isolated segments of rabbit atrial muscle, and the ventricular arrhythmias elicited 3 to 5 days after coronary ligation in dogs.[2] It is generally believed, however, that in many cases both mechanisms are involved and that they tend to be mutually interdependent.[2]

Although endocardial activation patterns have been measured in numerous clinical studies, relatively little information exists regarding the spatial distribution of endocardial repolarization patterns and its role in arrhythmogenesis. Similarly, there are little data in the literature regarding the possible spatial interaction between these two processes in the global heart. Since both processes play an important role in arrhythmogenesis, such interactions may have important clinical implications.

A major hurdle in the assessment of the spatial distribution of the activation and repolarization patterns in the clinical setting has been the inability to accurately associate endocardial spatial and electrophysiologic information. In this chapter we describe the current knowledge of the spatial interactions between activation and repolarization. We also describe recent results from our laboratory in using a new, catheter-based, electroanatomic mapping technique to assess the 3-dimensional (3-D) spatial distribution of endocardial activation, repolarization, and activation-recovery interval (ARI) distribution in the healthy swine heart.[6]

3-D Mapping of Left Ventricular Activation, ARI, and Repolarization Patterns in the Normal Swine Endocardium

The 3-D endocardial activation and repolarization patterns of the left ventricle (LV) were assessed in 13 healthy male pigs during different activation patterns (sinus rhythm and atrial and ventricular pacing).

To enable the regional and global spatial assessment of endocardial activation and repolarization patterns, we used a recently developed, catheter-based, nonfluoroscopic, electroanatomic endocardial mapping technique.[6-8] This new method uses ultralow magnetic fields to accurately determine the location and orientation of a miniature passive magnetic sensor incorporated just proximal to the tip of a 7F deflectable electrophysiologic catheter. By sampling the location of the tip of the roving mapping catheter, simultaneous with the local electrogram recorded from its tip electrode, at a plurality of endocardial sites, a 3-D electroanatomic map can be reconstructed in real time, with the electrophysiologic information color-coded and superimposed on the chamber's geometry (Fig. 1).

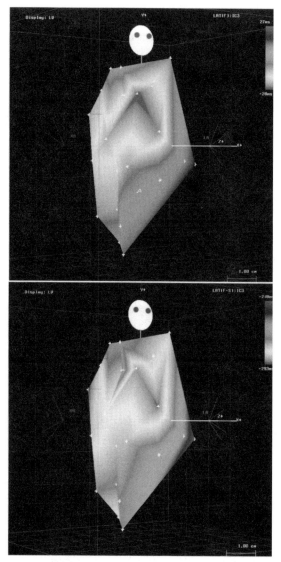

Figure 1. Right anterior oblique view of a 3-dimensional electroanatomic map of the swine left ventricle (LV). **A.** Activation map of the LV during sinus rhythm. The earliest activation site, represented by the red area, is located at the anterosuperior septum. The activation then spread to the rest of the endocardium, with the postero-basal area activated last (blue and purple areas). Yellow and green represent areas with intermediate local activation times (LATs). Total activation time of this ventricle was 47 milliseconds. **B.** Activation-recovery interval (ARI) map of the same ventricle. Colors represent ARI values recorded at each site, with red corresponding to sites with the longest ARIs, blue and purple indicating short ARIs, and yellow and green representing areas with intermediate values. Note the homogenous gradient of ARI resembling the activation sequence, with the longest ARIs (red) located along the septum (earliest activation). See color plate. *Continues.*

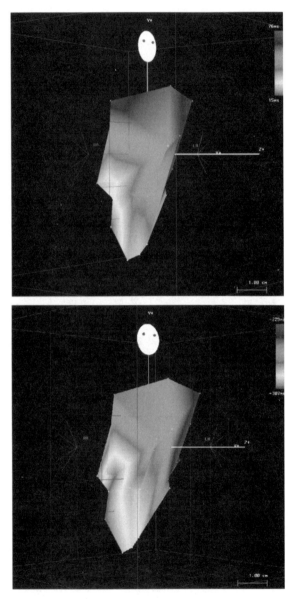

Figure 1 (*continued*). **C**. Activation map of the LV during pacing from the RV inferior septum (cycle length = 350 milliseconds). Total activation time was 61 milliseconds. **D**. ARI map of the same ventricle during pacing. Note again the inverse spatial correlation between ARIs and activation times, with the longest ARIs (red) located at the sites of earliest activation and than shortens gradually as activation proceeds. See color plate.

Activation Patterns

The local activation time (LAT) at each sampled site was determined from the intracardiac unipolar electrogram (filtered at 0.5 to 400 Hz). LAT was defined as the time interval between a fiducial point on the body surface electrocardiogram and the steepest negative intrinsic deflection (dV/dt_{min}) in the local unipolar recording.

Panels A and C of Figure 1 present the typical activation patterns of the swine LV during sinus rhythm (or atrial pacing) and during right ventricular (RV) inferoseptal pacing shown from a right anterior oblique view. The earliest activation site during sinus rhythm (represented in the map as the red area) was noted at the anterosuperior septum, with a second endocardial breakthrough noted more posteriorly. The activation then proceeded to the rest of the ventricle, with relatively fast conduction toward the apex. The latest activation occurred at the posterobasal and posterolateral areas (colored blue and purple in the map). This observed sequence of activation pattern agrees well with the endocardial activation pattern in humans previously described by Durrer et al.[9]

As expected, during RV septal pacing, the earliest LV activation site was noted at the inferior septum and then spread to the rest of the ventricle, with the basal and posterolateral areas activated last (Fig. 1, panel C). An interesting physiologic phenomenon that can also be noted in this figure is the anisotropic properties of the myocardium, with faster conduction velocity along the longitudinal direction.

ARI Patterns

The local repolarization time (LRT) was determined from the timing of the local T wave in the unipolar recording, by use of a method previously described by Wyatt et al[10] and later modified by Millar et al.[11] With use of these methods, LRT was defined as the dV/dt_{max} in the local T wave for negative and biphasic T waves and as the dV/dt_{min} for positive T waves. The ARI at each site was then determined as the time difference between the corresponding LRT and LAT. With use of this method, experimental studies in both humans and animals have shown high correlation between ARI and local action potential duration (APD) measured by transmembrane action potential, monophasic action potential (MAP), and the effective refractory period determined by the extrastimulus technique.[10-12]

Panels B and D of Figure 1 represent typical electroanatomic maps showing the ARI patterns of the LV during sinus rhythm and RV pacing, respectively. Colors represent the values of ARI measured at each site, with red representing areas with long ARIs, blue and purple indicating areas with short ARIs, and green and yellow symbolizing sites with intermediate values. Note that the ARI pattern closely resembled that of the activation (Fig. 1, panels A and C). During sinus rhythm, a homogeneous gradient of ARIs was noted along the LV, with the longest ARIs observed at the septal area (corresponding to the site of earliest activation) and the shortest ARIs observed at the posterobasal region. The range of ARI distribution during sinus rhythm was 63 ± 7 milliseconds (270 ± 16 [mean shortest ARI] to 331 ± 20 milliseconds [mean longest ARI]). Similarly, during RV septal pacing, the ARI maps resembled the corresponding activation maps, with the inferior septum having the longest ARIs, the posterolateral areas characterized by the shortest ARIs, and a gradual decrease in ARI values between them. The range of LV ARI dispersion during ventricular pacing at a cycle length of 350 milliseconds was 65 ± 5 milliseconds (182 ± 8 to 247 ± 12 milliseconds).

Relationship Between Activation Times and ARIs

When examining the activation and ARI maps, one of the most intriguing findings is the close resemblance of the spatial distribution of the two processes. An inverse correlation was noted, such that sites that were activated earlier had longer ARIs than sites that were activated late. This resulted in a homogeneous gradient of ARI shortening as the activation proceeded from the earliest site of activation. Interestingly, this phenomenon was observed independent of the specific depolarization pattern, sinus rhythm, or ventricular pacing.

The inverse correlation between the activation time and ARI was further evaluated when the pooled ARI values from all sampled sites were correlated with their respective LATs in each map. Using linear regression analysis, a significant inverse correlation was noted between LAT and ARI for all rhythms in each of the maps ($r^2=0.76\pm0.03$ and 0.77 ± 0.02 for sinus rhythm and ventricular pacing, respectively). Figure 2 demonstrates the typical relationship between the measured ARI and the corresponding LAT values sampled in one animal. Note the inverse correlation between activation and ARI during both sinus rhythm and ARI, such that progressively later activation times are associated with progressively shorter ARIs.

Repolarization Pattern

The LRT of a given endocardial site is a summation of the measured LAT and the ARI of the relevant site. The tight spatial coupling noted between the activation and ARI patterns, in which sites that are activated early are associated with longer ARIs and sites that are activated late are coupled with shorter ARIs, tends therefore to synchronize repolarization.

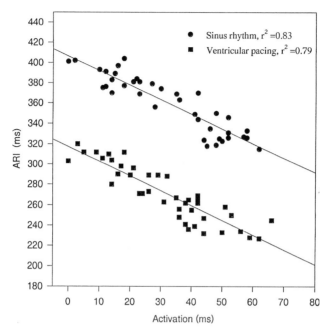

Figure 2. Linear regression analysis of the relationship between activation-recovery interval (ARI) and local activation time values pooled from all sampled sites in one animal during sinus rhythm and right ventricular pacing. A significant inverse correlation was noted in both rhythms indicating that progressively later activation times are associated with progressively shorter ARIs.

Hence, total dispersion of repolarization in the LV was found to be relatively short, averaging less than 40 ms during the different depolarization patterns studied. Furthermore, the observed total dispersion of repolarization was significantly smaller than that of ARI and even than that of activation.

Although in all the repolarization maps, total dispersion was relatively narrow, 3 types of endocardial repolarization patterns were noted. In some maps the repolarization sequence resembled that of activation, in others it was reversed, whereas in some cases the earliest repolarization site was located between the earliest and latest activation sites.

Significance and Possible Mechanisms of the Spatial Coupling Between Activation and ARI

The results reported above present several intriguing findings. The first finding is the observed spatial coupling between the activation and

ARI patterns. The inverse correlation found between activation and APD (estimated by the ARI) results in gradual shortening of the APD as the activation proceeds and, consequentially, in relatively narrow range of the termination of repolarization. The second interesting finding is that the inverse correlation between activation times and ARI was independent of the specific type of depolarization sequence. Hence, marked changes in the spatial distribution of ARI occurred when the activation pattern changed.

The inverse relationship between activation and APD was also noted previously in a number of in vitro and in vivo studies as well as in a number of computer simulations.[13-16] These studies, most of which were conducted in isolated tissue preparations or in a limited number of epicardial sites, also noted the shortening of APD as activation proceeds. Specifically, Zubair et al[13] noted marked effects of the activation sequence on the spatial dispersion of refractory periods at 36 sites within a 1-cm^2 region of the epicardial surface of the canine pulmonary conus. Similarly, Osaka et al[14] examined the influence of the activation sequence on action potential configuration in the epicardial surface of isolated pieces (2.5 cm^2) of canine ventricular myocardium. They found that APD shortened gradually as the recording site was moved further from the stimulation site. In their study, the spatial gradient of APD was found to be steeper in the transverse than in the longitudinal direction.

One possible mechanism proposed to explain the effects of the activation sequence on repolarization is electrotonic interactions. Studies in isolated ventricular muscle and Purkinje fiber preparations have shown that repolarization (anodal) currents applied during repolarization shorten the action potential, and that depolarization (cathodal) currents applied during repolarization prolong the action potential.[17-19] Thus, electrotonic currents flowing from sites that are activated late to neighboring sites activated earlier would tend to increase the APD in the latter sites and decrease the APD in the former sites.

The inverse correlation between activation and APD was also noted by Costard-Jäckle et al,[20] who studied the effect of ectopic pacing on the distribution of ventricular epicardial APDs (measured by MAP recordings) in the isolated Langendorff-perfused rabbit hearts. During both prolonged atrial and ventricular pacing, they noted an inverse relationship between activation and APD (r=0.76, slope = −1.63, and r=0.68, slope = −0.68, during atrial and ventricular pacing, respectively). This resulted in a relatively synchronized epicardial repolarization time. Another important finding in their study was that abrupt changes in the activation sequence perturbed the inverse correlation between the activation and APD patterns. Thus, immediately after changing the activation sequence from atrial to ventricular pacing, the inverse correlation disappeared. Nevertheless, continuation of the ventricular pacing produced slow changes that restored the inverse relationship. Similarly, immediately after switching back to atrial pacing the inverse relationship was lost again but reappeared slowly after 1 hour of pacing.

The latter results may suggest that additional factors other than electrotonic interactions alone may be responsible for the coupling between the sequence of activation and APD. The authors speculated that repeated current flow in the same direction through the intercellular gap junctions might have a modulating effect on the electrotonic interactions between the cells. This process might gradually decrease the gap junction resistance even further, thereby amplifying the electrotonic effects with time.

Clinical Implications

The results presented above may have a number of significant clinical implications. Dispersion of repolarization usually parallels the dispersion of refractoriness. Augmented dispersion of repolarization has been shown in numerous studies to increase the propensity of ventricular arrhythmias both clinically and in experimental models. As discussed earlier, dispersion of repolarization is determined by the summation of regional differences in activation times and APD.

In humans, the mechanism of increased dispersion of repolarization may vary with the disease process. Vassalo et al[21] measured recovery of excitability at multiple LV endocardial sites in 3 groups of patients. In normal subjects, the range of LV recovery times was 52 milliseconds. In patients with previous myocardial infarction and ventricular tachycardia, dispersion of recovery time was 90 milliseconds, mainly due to prolonged activation times. In contrast, the increased dispersion of recovery times (114 milliseconds) in patients with the long QT syndrome was primarily due to increased dispersion of refractory periods.

The tight spatial coupling between the activation and ARI patterns, resulting in an inverse correlation between the two processes, may serve as an important physiologic mechanism in the prevention of ventricular arrhythmias in the normal myocardium. The shortening of APD as the activation proceeds tends to synchronize repolarization both globally and regionally, and may thus serve as an important antiarrhythmic mechanism. As discussed earlier, the tight dependency between the spatial distribution of activation and repolarization may be caused by electrotonic interactions through intercellular gap junctions. One may therefore speculate that in the presence of a pathology that decreases cell-to-cell conductivity, this spatial coupling may be lost, resulting in an increased dispersion of repolarization and in an increased propensity to arrhythmogenesis. Such mechanism may be responsible for the increased propensity for ventricular arrhythmias in patients with LV hypertrophy, especially those with T wave inversion.[22] Interestingly, two human studies[23,24] have found increased dispersion of repolarization in these patients, simultaneous with the disappearance of the inverse relation between activation time and APD. These findings may be related to the variety of cellular and histologic alterations found in LV hypertrophy including marked connective tissue infiltration, changes in fiber orientation, and loss or thickening of cardiac gap junctions.[25] Nevertheless, additional basic investigation as well as clinical studies would have to further test this hypothesis.

The inverse relationship between APD and activation times may also provide insight into the paradox of T wave concordance. In the normal electrocardiogram, despite the fact that on the cellular level depolarization and repolarization produce deflections of opposite polarities, the T wave has the same polarity as the QRS complex. In a study published by Franz et al,[26] MAPs were recorded from 54 LV endocardial sites in 7 patients and 23 epicardial sites in 3 patients. By plotting the APD measured at all sites as a function of the corresponding activation times, they also noted an inverse relationship. Interestingly, the average linear regression slope of this plot in the 10 patients was −1.32. The fact that the correlation between LAT and APD, found at both the endocardial and epicardial surfaces, had a negative slope that was greater than a unity may support the hypothesis that T wave concordance results from opposite directions of the repolarization and depolarization waves, at least in some parts of the myocardium. These results also support the concept of a transmural repolarization gradient in the human myocardium (with the epicardium repolarizing significantly earlier than the endocardium) opposite to that of the depolarization.

Finally, the ability to accurately associate in vivo endocardial spatial and electrophysiologic information may become a valuable clinical and research tool. This may allow a better understanding of the spatial interaction between different electrophysiologic properties of the heart in both health and disease, consequentially improving our understanding of the regional and global mechanisms involved in arrhythmogenesis.

References

1. Han J, Moe GH. Nonuniform recovery of excitability in ventricular muscle. *Circ Res* 1964;14:44-60.
2. Gough WB, Mehra R, Restivo M, et al. Reentrant ventricular arrhythmias in the late myocardial infarction period in the dog: Correlation of activation and refractory maps. *Circ Res* 1985;57:432-442.
3. Callans DJ, Josephson ME. Ventricular tachycardia in the setting of coronary artery disease. In Zipes DP, Jalife J (eds): *Cardiac Electrophysiology: From Cell to Bedside*. 2nd ed. Philadelphia: WB Saunders; 1995:788-811.
4. Kuo CS, Munakata K, Reddy CP, Surawicz B. Characteristics and possible mechanism of ventricular arrhythmia dependent on the dispersion of action potential durations. *Circulation* 1983;67:1356-1367.
5. Allessie MA, Bonke FI, Schopman FJ. Circus movement in rabbit atrial muscle as a mechanism of tachycardia. II. The role of nonuniform recovery of excitabil-

ity in the occurrence of unidirectional block, as studied with multiple microelectrodes. *Circ Res* 1976;39:168-177.

6. Gepstein L, Hayam G, Ben-Haim SA. Activation-repolarization coupling in the normal swine endocardium. *Circulation* 1997;96:4036-4043.

7. Ben-Haim SA, Osadchy D, Schuster I, et al. Novel, non-fluoroscopic, in vivo navigation and mapping technology. *Nat Med* 1996;2:1393-1395.

8. Gepstein L, Hayam G, Ben-Haim SA. A novel method for nonfluoroscopic, catheter-based, electroanatomical mapping of the heart: In vitro and in vivo accuracy results. *Circulation* 1997;95:1611-1622.

9. Durrer D, van Dam RT, Freud GE, et al. Total excitation of the isolated human heart. *Circulation* 1970;41:899-912.

10. Wyatt RF, Burgess MJ, Evans AK, et al. Estimation of ventricular transmembrane action potential duration and repolarization times from unipolar electrograms. *Am J Cardiol* 1981;47:488. Abstract.

11. Millar CK, Kralios FA, Lux RL. Correlation between refractory periods and activation-recovery intervals from electrograms: Effects of rate and adrenergic interventions. *Circulation* 1985;72:1372-1379.

12. Chen P-S, Moser KM, Dembitsky WP, et al. Epicardial activation and repolarization patterns in patients with right ventricular hypertrophy. *Circulation* 1991;83:104-118.

13. Zubair I, Pollard AE, Spitzer KW, Burgess MJ. Effects of activation sequence on the spatial distribution of repolarization properties. *J Electrocardiol* 1994;27:115-127.

14. Osaka T, Kodama I, Tsuboi N, et al. Effects of activation sequence and anisotropic cellular geometry on the repolarization phase of action potential of dog ventricular muscles. *Circulation* 1987;76:226-236.

15. Toyoshima H, Burgess MJ. Electrotonic interaction during canine ventricular repolarization. *Circ Res* 1978;43:348-356.

16. Lesh MD, Pring M, Spear JF. Cellular uncoupling can unmask dispersion of action potential duration in ventricular myocardium: A computer modeling study. *Circ Res* 1989;65:1426-1440.

17. Weidman S. Effect of current flow on the membrane potential of cardiac muscle. *J Physiol (Lond)* 1951;115:227-236.

18. Cranfield PF, Hoffman BF. Propagated repolarization in heart muscle. *J Gen Physiol* 1958;41:633-649.

19. Vassalle M. Analysis of cardiac pacemakers potentials using a "voltage clamp" technique. *Am J Physiol* 1966;210:1335-1341.

20. Costard-Jäckle A, Goetsch B, Antz M, Franz MR. Slow and long-lasting modulation of myocardial repolarization produced by ectopic activation in isolated rabbit hearts: Evidence for cardiac memory. *Circulation* 1989;80:1412-1420.

21. Vassallo JA, Cassidy DM, Kindwall KE, et al. Nonuniform recovery of excitability in the left ventricle. *Circulation* 1988;78:1365-1372.

22. McLenachan JM, Henderson E, Morris KI, et al. Ventricular arrhythmias in patients with hypertensive left ventricular hypertrophy. *N Engl J Med* 1987;317:787-792.

23. Cowan JC, Hilton CJ, Griffiths CJ, et al. Sequence of epicardial repolarisation and configuration of the T wave. *Br Heart J* 1988;60:424-433.

24. Franz MR, Bargheer K, Lichtlen PR, et al. Myocardial repolarization in normal and hypertrophied human left ventricles. In Butrous GS, Schwartz P (eds): *Clinical Aspects of Ventricular Repolarization.* London: Farrand; 1989:219-226.

25. Wendt-Galliteli MF, Jacob R. Time course of electron microscope alterations in the hypertrophied myocardium of Goldblatt rats. *Basic Res Cardiol* 1977;72:209-213.
26. Franz MR, Bargheer K, Rafflenbeul W, et al. Monophasic action potential mapping in human subjects with normal electrocardiograms: Direct evidence for the genesis of the T wave. *Circulation* 1987;75:379-386.

23

Abnormal Relationship Between Activation and Repolarization in Human Left Ventricular Hypertrophy

Michael R. Franz, MD, PhD and Klaus Bargheer, MD

Introduction

Ventricular hypertrophy often is characterized not only by augmented QRS voltage but also by typical repolarization abnormalities (so-called "strain pattern") in the surface electrocardiogram (ECG).[1] Hypotheses advanced to explain these repolarization abnormalities include secondary T wave changes due to changes in ventricular activation, and primary T wave changes due to changes in action potential duration (APD) independent of activation disturbances.[2-4] Results from intracellular action potential recordings in tissue preparations excised from animals with experimentally induced left ventricular hypertrophy remain inconclusive: lengthening of APD,[5,6] shortening of APD,[7] and disparate changes in APD[8] between different areas of the ventricle have all been observed. Also, the clinical relevance of such in vitro data for in vivo T wave changes is unclear because: 1) excised, artificially superfused tissue preparations are no longer exposed to autonomic transmitters; 2) the hemodynamic loading conditions that caused the hypertrophy in the first place are removed; and 3) the effect

From Franz MR (ed): *Monophasic Action Potentials: Bridging Cell and Bedside.*
©Futura Publishing Company, Inc., Armonk, NY, 2000.

of the natural activation sequence on repolarization cannot be determined after the tissue has been dissected from the ventricle. Subendocardial ischemia also has been implicated as a cause of electrocardiographic "strain,"[9-12] but direct evidence for myocardial ischemia in human left ventricular hypertrophy (LVH) is lacking.

With the introduction of the contact electrode technique, monophasic action potential (MAP) recording has become clinically feasible and safe, even in the left ventricle.[13,14] We used this technique to record MAPs from multiple left ventricular endocardial and epicardial sites in 10 patients with typical LVH-associated repolarization abnormalities and compared them with similar recordings in 13 patients with normal left ventricles and normal ECGs. Our objective was to identify electrophysiologic changes in hypertrophied myocardium which may explain LVH-associated T wave abnormalities.

Patient Population

The study population consisted of 23 patients. The mean age was 53 years, with a range from 16 to 70 years. There were 18 men and 5 women. All patients gave written informed consent prior to the study, which had been approved by the Universities" Committees on Human Investigation.

The *comparison* group (group I) consisted of 12 male patients and 1 female patient (age 51 ± 11 years). Of these patients, 8 had coronary artery disease, 1 had mild aortic valve disease, 1 had mild aortic coarctation, 1 had mitral stenosis, and 2 had no structural heart disease. All patients were free from prior myocardial infarction and had normal left ventricles, as assessed by M-mode and 2-dimensional echocardiography or ventriculography; ejection fractions ranged from 55% to 79%. All patients had normal ECGs with normal PR, QRS, and QT intervals, QRS axes between $-10°$ and $+90°$, and normally shaped concordant ST-T waves with T wave axis within 50° of QRS axis. None of the patients received any cardioactive drug regimen at least 5 half-lives before cardiac catheterization or surgery. Data from 10 of these 13 patients have been published previously.[14]

The *LVH* group (group II) consisted of 6 male patients and 4 female patients (age 57 ± 9 years; mean $\pm$ SD) who all had LVH due to longstanding aortic valve disease. Eight patients had aortic stenosis, 2 of those were combined with aortic insufficiency, and 2 patients had aortic insufficiency alone. Patients in this group fulfilled both echocardiographic and electrocardiographic criteria of LVH. Increased wall thickness with (4 patients) and without (6 patients) increased cavity dimensions was present in these 10 patients by M-mode and 2-dimensional echocardiography. All had R or

S wave voltage in the precordial or limb leads meeting at least one of the following voltage criteria suggesting LVH: deepest S wave in V_1 or V_2 added to the largest R wave in V_5 or V_6 greater than 3.5 mV, and R wave in aVL greater than 1.5 mV.[15] In addition to increased voltage, all 10 patients had left ventricular hypertrophy-typical repolarization abnormalities (so-called "strain pattern") in the resting ECG: descending upwardly convex ST segments, asymmetric negative or biphasic T waves with rapid return to baseline or terminal positivity, T wave inversion in V_6 greater than 3 mm and T inversion greater in V_6 than in V_4, or QRS-T wave axis disparity $\geq 180°$ in the frontal plane. Patients with QRS duration greater than 0.12 seconds or obvious left bundle branch block morphology were excluded from the study. Six patients had concomitant coronary artery disease. No patient had a history of prior myocardial infarction. Three patients were on digitalis therapy which was not discontinued.

Endocardial MAP Mapping

Endocardial MAP mapping was performed with the patient in the nonsedated, postabsorptive state during sinus rhythm. Multiple site recordings were obtained in 7 patients from group I and 5 patients from group II, by use of contact electrode catheters manufactured by EP Technologies (San Jose, CA), according to the specifications described earlier.[13] Indications for left cardiac catheterization in group I were suspected coronary artery disease in 5 patients and evaluation of mild aortic valve disease and mild aortic coarctation, respectively, in 2 other patients. Recordings were made sequentially and were distributed as evenly over the endocardial surface as possible, as judged by multiple plane fluoroscopy.[14] If sinus rate varied by more than 5 beats/min, right atrial pacing was performed at the slowest rate that would overdrive the spontaneous rhythm. All MAP signals were recorded with a high-impedance, direct-current coupled, differential preamplifier (EP Technologies, model 1001). The preamplified MAP and 3 standard electrocardiogram leads (usually lead I, aVF, and V_1) were displayed simultaneously on a multichannel recorder and recorded at a paper speed of 100 or 250 mm/s (model 1000, Gould Instruments, Cleveland, OH).

Epicardial MAP Mapping

Epicardial MAP mapping was performed in 5 patients from group I and 5 patients from group II, during open-chest cardiac surgery just prior to initiation of cardiopulmonary bypass. Indications for surgery were coronary artery bypass grafting (4 patients) and mitral regurgitation (1 patient) in group I, and aortic valve replacement in group II. Epicardial MAP recordings were obtained with a special handheld probe.[14] This probe had the exploring electrode mounted on an elastic yet flexible special alloy spatula that was flat enough to fit comfortably inside the epicardial-pericardial space and allowed stable epicardial MAP recordings even from posterior and inferior aspects of the in situ beating human ventricle. Recordings were made during stable sinus rhythm or during right atrial pacing at a constant rate. A detailed map of the left ventricular surface was used to identify the location from which each recording was made. Most recordings were made from the lateral, posterior, and inferior aspects of the left ventricle. These areas were covered by pericardium or lung tissue and were not exposed to the cooling effect of room air. MAP recordings were amplified by the same method as were the endocardial recordings, and 3 electrocardiographic limb leads (I, II, and aVF) were recorded simultaneously, at a paper speed of 100 or 250 milliseconds on a Honeywell VR16 chart recorder.

Data Analysis

To eliminate effects of heart rate on APD in individual patients, only measurements during regular sinus rhythm (± 5 beats/min) or during regular atrial pacing were analyzed. MAP analysis was limited to stable recordings judged on the basis of isoelectric resting potentials, action potential amplitudes exceeding 20 mV, and constant morphology for at least 5 consecutive beats. Accuracy of the measured intervals was within 5 milliseconds, as determined by repeated measurements made by two different observers. At least 3 consecutive MAP recordings were measured at each site, and intervals at a single site were found reproducible with less than 2% variation.

Endocardial and epicardial MAP recordings were analyzed as follows (Fig. 1): AT = delay from the earliest QRS deflection (in any lead) to the rapid upstroke of the MAP; APD = interval from MAP upstroke to 90% repolarization; and total repolarization time (RT) = the sum of AT and APD. Electrical dispersion (a measure of myocardial electrophysiologic nonuniformity) of each of the 3 variables, AT, APD, and RT, was defined as the difference, in milliseconds, between the shortest and longest measurement in a patient's left ventricle, according to the method of Kuo et al.[16] Individual patient data were averaged for the group with normal left ventricles and the group with LVH. It has been suggested that in normal hearts, regional myocardial repolarization is influenced by the time of regional myocardial activation.[14,17-19] We therefore examined the relationship between AT and APD in both patient groups by subjecting all recordings in a given patient to simple linear regression analysis.

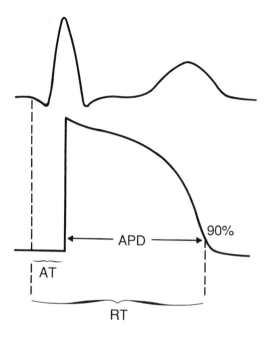

Figure 1. Method of analyzing MAP recordings for activation time (AT), action potential duration at 90% repolarization (APD), and total repolarization time (RT), the sum of AT and action potential duration.

Statistics

Data from group I and II were averaged and compared by unpaired Student t tests. Results from linear regression analysis of APD over AT are reported as slope and r^2 values. Significance of correlation was determined by Pearson's correlation coefficients. For all data, differences with P values of less than 0.05 were considered significant.

Results

MAPs were recorded from 7 to 12 (mean 9.3 ± 1.8) endocardial and 6 to 20 (mean 13.4 ± 3.8) epicardial sites in group I patients, and from 6 to 10 (mean 8.5 ± 1.4) endocardial and 8 to 15 (mean 9.8 ± 2.8) epicardial sites in group II patients. MAP recordings had amplitudes between 20 and 40 mV. There were no qualitative differences in MAP morphology between the two groups, with all recordings having normal configurations, with sharp upstrokes, distinct plateaus, and smooth final repolarization contours.

Activation Time

Endocardial activation time (AT) was similar in group I (18.6 ± 9.6 milliseconds; mean$\pm$SD) and group II (23.3 ± 13.1 milliseconds; NS). Epicardial AT was significantly longer in group II patients (59.6±30.3 milliseconds) than in group I patients (45.4±15.5 milliseconds; $P<0.05$) (Table 1).

Dispersion of APD and RT

Endocardial APD was significantly more disparate in group II patients (73.5±26.9 milliseconds) than in group I patients (39.6±16.8; $P<0.01$), but dispersion of epicardial APD was similar in both groups (31.8±14.5 and 49.3±14.0; NS). Dispersion of RT was significantly greater at both the endocardium and epicardium in group II as compared to group I patients (Table 1). Global data (endocardial and epicardial data lumped) yielded similar results (Table 2). Of particular interest was that in group I patients, RT was significantly less dispersed than APD (29.0±16.0 milliseconds versus 44.1±17.3 milliseconds; $P<0.05$), while in group II patients, the magnitude of dispersion of APD and RT was similar (57.6±34.1 versus 62.5±28.5; NS) (Table 3).

Relationship Between AT and APD

The relationship between AT and APD was examined by plotting of APD as a function of AT. Summary data are shown in Table 4. All but 1

Table 1
MAP Data Separated for Endocardial and Epicardial Recordings

	AT (ms)	Dispersion of APD (ms)	Dispersion of RT (ms)
Group I endo	18.6±9.6	39.6±16.8	25.4±13.7
	NS	P<0.05	P<0.01
Group II endo	23.5±13.1	73.5±26.9	78.5±27.4
Group I epi	45.4±15.4	49.3±14.0	32.6±18.3
	P<0.05	NS	P<0.05
Group II epi	59.6±30.3	31.8±14.5	56.3±20.9

Data are mean ± standard deviation. AT = activation time; APD = action potential duration; RT = repolarization time.

Table 2
MAP Data Based on Whole Left Ventricle Analysis

	AT (ms)	Dispersion of APD (ms)	Dispersion of RT (ms)
Group I	31.7±19.8	44.1±17.3	29.0±16.0
	NS	NS	P<0.001
Group II	41.8±29.7	57.6±34.1	62.5±28.5

Data are mean±standard deviation. Abbreviations same as in Table 1.

Table 3
Comparison of Dispersion of Action Potential Duration and
Repolarization Time in Group I and Group II

	Group I	Group II
APD dispersion (ms)	44.1±17.3	57.6±34.1
	P<0.05	NS
RT dispersion (ms)	29.0±16.0	62.5±28.5

Comparison based on whole left ventricle analysis. Data are mean±standard deviation. Abbreviations same as in Table 1.

Table 4
Linear Regression Analysis of Relationship Between Activation Time
and Action Potential Duration in Group I and Group II Patients

Patient	Slope	r Squared	P Value
Group I			
1	−1.27	0.91	<.0001
2	−1.48	0.57	<.01
3	−1.16	0.76	<.0001
4	−0.83	0.44	<.05
5	−1.24	0.79	<.0001
6	−0.82	0.53	<.005
7	−2.11	0.63	<.0001
8*	−2.00	0.45	NS
9*	−0.90	0.42	<.05
10*	−1.43	0.69	<.005
11*	−0.99	0.66	<.005
12*	−1.01	0.60	<.05
13*	−0.84	0.86	<.001
mean	−1.24	0.64	
±SD	0.44	0.16	
Group II			
14	−1.22	0.10	NS
15	0.22	0.02	NS
16	−0.69	0.41	NS
17	−0.66	0.03	NS
18	0.42	0.09	NS
19*	−0.60	0.17	NS
20*	−0.22	0.11	NS
21*	0.35	0.34	NS
22*	−0.46	0.69	<0.05
23*	0.05	0.24	NS
mean	−0.28	0.22	
±SD	0.53	0.21	

*Monophasic action potential recordings taken from left ventricular epicardium; all others from left ventricular endocardium.

of 13 group I patients demonstrated significant inverse correlation between AT and APD, indicating that progressively longer AT was associated with progressively shorter APD. The average slope of the linear regression lines, derived from the 7 endocardial and 6 epicardial data sets of group I patients was -1.24 ± 0.44, with a significant average correlation coefficient of $r^2 = 0.64 \pm 0.16$. In contrast, group II exhibited no inverse correlation between AT and APD. The mean linear regression slope of APD on AT was -0.28 ± 0.53. Statistically significant correlation was found in only 1 of 10 group II patients, but the slope of this patient's linear regression was lower (-0.45) than in any of the group I patients (Table 3). Representative examples of the correlation between APD and AT for both groups are shown in Figure 2.

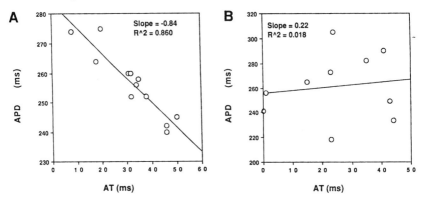

Figure 2. Linear regression analysis for the relationship between activation time (AT) and action potential duration (APD) in a group I patient (**A**) and a group II patient (**B**). Both panels represent endocardial data.

Panel A of Figure 3 demonstrates that the inverse correlation between AT and APD in group I patients has a synchronizing effect on RT; longer ATs were compensated by shorter APDs, which caused RTs to be more uniform than either AT or APD. Panel B of Figure 3 demonstrates that the greater nonuniformity of RT in group II resulted from both greater APD differences and lack of inverse correlation between AT and APD.

Discussion

This human heart study provides direct data on both left ventricular activation and repolarization in patients with LVH and electrocardiographic repolarization abnormalities, and compares these data with those from a group of patients with normal left ventricles and ECGs. Data on human ventricular activation properties have been presented before,[20-22] and our data are essentially consistent with them, including delayed epicardial activation

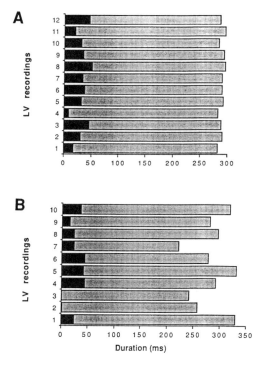

Figure 3. Diagrammatic representation of activation time (AT) (filled bars) and action potential duration (APD) (shaded bars) in a group I patient (**A**) and a group II patient (**B**). Data are the same as in Figure 2 and demonstrate that the inverse correlation between AT and APD in normal myocardium (**A**) synchronizes total repolarization time (represented by the right edge of the horizontal stacked bars). In left ventricular hypertrophy (**B**), despite similar AT differences, APD was more disparate and unrelated to AT, resulting in much greater dispersion of RT.

in LVH.[22] This discussion therefore focuses on differences in repolarization characteristics between normal and hypertrophied human ventricles, and on abnormalities in the relationship between AT and APD in LVH.

Relationship Between AT and APD and Implications for T Wave Morphology

It has been postulated that T wave concordance is due to opposite directions of activation and repolarization waves.[2] We previously reported the first direct evidence for the validity of this hypothesis for the genesis of the normal human T wave,[14] and the extended patient population in this study confirms those data. In addition, the present study identified, in hypertrophied human left ventricles, electrophysiologic abnormalities which may explain the accompanying T wave inversion. While in nonhypertrophied left ventricles APD was inversely related to AT, with a mean linear regression slope of –1.24, such inverse relationship between AT and APD was lacking in patients with LVH. An inverse relation between AT and APD means that, on average, repolarization proceeds in a direction opposite to that of activation, a finding which is consistent with T wave concordance in normal hearts.[14] Conversely, absence of this inverse relation, as found in hypertrophied left ventricles, is compatible with discordant T waves. This hypothesis, for which our data seem to provide direct support, is schematically illustrated in Figure 4.

The electrocardiographic T wave is produced by regional differences in total ventricular RT, which is the sum of AT and APD. Thus, changes in total RT may result from changes in AT (secondary T wave changes), changes in APD (primary T wave changes), or a combination of the two. The increase in epicardial ATs therefore may be responsible, at least in part, for the increased dispersion of epicardial RTs measured in the group with LVH, and the corresponding T wave changes would, according to traditional terminology, be classified as "secondary." However, abnormally increased dispersion of repolarization was observed also at the endocardial surface of the hypertrophied left ventricles where ATs were normal. Fur-

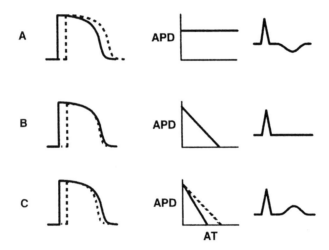

Figure 4. A model to explain T wave polarity on the basis of the relationship between activation time (AT) and action potential duration (APD). **A**. A theoretical relationship is shown, in which each increment in AT is matched precisely by a corresponding decrement in APD. In this case, repolarization would occur simultaneously at all ventricular sites, the linear regression would have a slope of -1.0 and a correlation coefficient of 1.0, and the electrocardiogram (ECG) would exhibit no T wave at all but rather an isoelectric line. **B**. The relationship between AT and action potential duration in subjects with normal T waves. Action potential duration is inversely related to AT, with a slope slightly greater than negative unity (-1.24±0.44; mean ± SD, in our study). This renders the direction of the repolarization wave opposite to that of depolarization, a situation which is consistent with, and which can explain the paradox of, T wave concordance. **C**. The situation encountered in patients with left ventricular hypertrophy. With a correlation coefficient near zero (0.22±0.21), it might be said that ventricular APD is distributed at random, with no significant slope in either positive or negative direction. On average then, repolarization would travel in the same direction as depolarization, and in the ECG would cause a deflection opposite to that of depolarization.

thermore, measurements from both the endocardial and epicardial surfaces of the hypertrophied ventricles had in common the fact that they showed an absence of an inverse correlation between AT and APD, whereas such an inverse relation was present at both the endocardial and epicardial surfaces in all electrocardiographically normal ventricles. These findings indicate an alteration in the regional distribution of APD in the hypertrophied ventricles, and the T wave changes resulting from this alteration would be classified as "primary."

Possible mechanisms underlying the [hypertrophy-induced] T wave changes can only be appreciated if one takes into account a newer concept about the genesis of the ventricular gradient. Rosenbaum et al[23,24] have recently challenged the dogmatic categorization into primary and secondary T wave changes and have advanced the theory that the ventricular gradient is not independent of the activation sequence but rather is created by it. This conclusion was based on a systematic analysis of electrocardiographic records obtained during and after sustained changes in the ventricular activation sequence (as caused by temporary ventricular pacing or intermittent left bundle branch block) which showed that long-lasting alterations in ventricular activation shift ventricular repolarization in such a way that the main repolarization vector is once again oriented in the same direction as the main depolarization vector. Chatterjee et al[25] reported similar results. Because these activation-sequence–dependent T wave changes develop only very slowly, and require an even longer time to dissipate after restoration of the normal activation sequence, Rosenbaum et al[23] ascribed to the myocardium the property of "memory" by which the myocardium "learns" and 'remembers" a sustained period of altered activation sequence. Direct experimental evidence for the cardiac "memory" inferred by Rosenbaum et al has been obtained from direct experimental recordings in isolated rabbit hearts.[26]

One mechanism that has been suggested to cause activation-dependent modulation of APD is electrotonic interaction.[23,26,27] Electrotonic current from the areas to be excited last may retard repolarization of areas excited earlier in the activation sequence, and current from areas to repolarize first may speed repolarization in areas not yet repolarized.[27] Direct evidence for this hypothesis has been obtained in voltage clamp experiments[28] and from action potential recordings in Purkinje fiber-ventricular muscle junctions.[29]

Possible Cellular Mechanisms Underlying the Genesis of the Normal T Wave and Alterations in LVH

If T wave concordance in the normal ECG is due to electrotonic modulation of ventricular repolarization by the sequence of ventricular activation, one must ask why such concordance is lost in patients with advanced LVH and inverted T waves. LVH is associated with a variety of cellular or histologic alterations, including changes in fiber orientation,[30] marked connective tissue infiltration,[8,30] loss or thickening of gap junctions,[31] and increase in basal membrane thickness.[32] It is possible that some or all of these alterations diminish or alter electrotonic interaction in the heart so that APD no longer is influenced by AT. The random distribution of APD in the hypertrophied ventricle, with no apparent negative or positive correlation to AT, may therefore result from a lack of intercellular electrical communication which in normal hearts permits activation to modulate repolarization. This hypothesis is in keeping with experimental evidence for nonuniform electrotonic interaction and increased disparity of APD in hypertrophied cat[8] and rat[33] myocardium, as well as electrical uncoupling un guinea pig left ventricular hypertrophy.[34]

Are Hypertrophy-Related T Wave Changes a Sign of Myocardial Ischemia?

Repolarization abnormalities in patients with LVH are sometimes called "strain pattern."[1,3] This ill-defined term seems to imply some stress-induced form of myocardial ischemia which, if true, would have significant clinical import. This assumption may appear plausible at first sight because: 1) increases in afterload force the ventricle to work harder; 2) the increase in capillary density does not match the increase in muscle mass; 3) the coronary vascular reserve is reduced because of increased coronary vascular resistance[9-12]; and 4) the resulting mismatch between perfusion and metabolic requirements is expected to be greatest at subendocardial muscle layers.[10] However, myocardial ischemia as the underlying cause of LVH-associated repolarization abnormalities has never been verified by direct data. In this study, MAP recordings from hypertrophied left ventricles were qualitatively normal, with sharp upstrokes, distinct plateau phases, and steep final repolarization slopes. In both animal[35-37] and clinical studies,[38,39] MAP recordings have been shown to be highly sensitive markers of ischemia, and are markedly different from those recorded from normal myocardium, distinguishable by an increase in AT, due to slowing of conduction velocity of the cardiac impulse, and loss of plateau duration. Although MAPs were recorded from a limited number of sites, ischemia, if present, should not have gone undetected (especially in endocardial recordings), considering the alleged diffuse nature of ischemia in LVH. Also, endocardial AT did not differ significantly between the two study groups, while endocardial mapping studies in patients with coronary artery disease have reported significantly longer ATs.[40] Delayed epicardial activation in patients with LVH as compared to those without LVH, also reported by others,[22] can be explained by the greater wall thickness and therefore prolonged conduction time from the inner to the outer surface of the hypertrophied ventricle, and needs not be interpreted as evidence of ischemia. In contrast to the implications of "strain," our data and hypothesis are compatible with an altered ventricular gradient and T wave inversion without requiring the assumption of myocardial ischemia.

Study Limitations

The following limitations apply to this clinical study: 1) Dispersion of AT, APD, and RT were measured as the difference between the shortest and longest value in each patient. Although the range of APDs recorded per patient was large, we may have missed the true extremes in a given patient. 2) Our data were not obtained at identical heart rates, and it cannot be excluded that heart rate alters APD and RT nonuniformly over the heart. 3) Local AT was determined as the interval between the onset of QRS and the MAP upstroke. Because of the limited number of electrocardiogram leads recorded, it is possible that we may have missed the very earliest beginning of ventricular activation. However, because all measurements were referenced to the earliest QRS deflection in the same lead, the relationship between AT and APD or RT, respectively, should not be affected. 4) Patients in the comparison group (group I) were not free from heart disease, and several patients with LVH (group II) also had coronary artery disease. None of the patients, however, had a history of prior myocardial infarction, ECGs in group I were normal, and group II patients presented no clinical evidence of ischemia during rest.

Increased Dispersion of Repolarization in LVH and Implications for Arrhythmogenesis

The abnormal relationship between AT and APD in patients with LVH not only provides an attractive alternate explanation for T wave inversion but may be relevant for the greater arrhythmia propensity reported for this group of patients. As illustrated in Figures 3 and 4, an inverse correlation between AT and APD that has a regression slope near unity (-1.24 in our control group) tends to synchronize total ventricular RT. Conversely, lack of an inverse correlation between AT and APD, as found in LVH, allows for a more random distribution of APD and, consequently, greater dispersion of RT. It is well recognized that uniformity of ventricular repolarization is important for protecting the ventricle from reentrant arrhythmias.[16,17,40] Greater dispersion of repolarization in patients with LVH may thus be a factor contributing to the increased arrhythmia susceptibility and the positive predictive value of electrocardiographic LVH for sudden death, both previously reported for this group of patients.[41-47] Under this aspect, it is particularly noteworthy that LVH is associated with an increased risk of arrhythmias and sudden cardiac death only when electrocardiographic voltage criteria of LVH are accompanied by typical repolarization abnormalities.[46,47]

References

1. Marriott HJL. *Practical Electrocardiography*. Baltimore: Williams & Wilkins; 1977:51-61.
2. Wilson FN, MacLeod AG, Barker PS. The T deflection of the electrocardiogram. *Trans Assoc Am Physicians* 1931;46:29-38.
3. Surawicz B. Electrocardiographic diagnosis of chamber enlargement. *J Am Coll Cardiol* 1986;8:711-724. Review.
4. Autenrieth G, Surawicz B, Kuo CS, Arita M. Primary T wave abnormalities caused by uniform and regional shortening of ventricular monophasic action potential in dog. *Circulation* 1975;51:668-676.
5. Keung EC, Aronson RS. Transmembrane action potentials and the electrocardiogram in rats with renal hypertension. *Cardiovasc Res* 1981;15:611-614.
6. Bassett AL, Gelband H. Chronic partial occlusion of the pulmonary artery in cats. Change in ventricular action potential configuration during early hypertrophy. *Circ Res* 1973;32:15-26.
7. Gülch RW, Baumann R, Jacob R. Analysis of myocardial action potential in left ventricular hypertrophy of Goldblatt rats. *Basic Res Cardiol* 1979;74:69-82.
8. Cameron JS, Myerburg RJ, Wong SS, et al. Electrophysiologic consequences of chronic experimentally induced left ventricular pressure overload. *J Am Coll Cardiol* 1983;2:481-487.
9. Dunn FG, Pringle SD. Left ventricular hypertrophy and myocardial ischemia in systemic hypertension. *Am J Cardiol* 1987;60:191-221.
10. Breisch EA, White FC, Nimmo LE, Bloor CM. Cardiac vasculature and flow during pressure-overload hypertrophy. *Am J Physiol* 1986;251:H1031-H1037.
11. Thomas DP, Phillips SIJ, Bove AA. Myocardial morphology and blood flow distribution in chronic volume-overload hypertrophy in dogs. *Basic Res Cardiol* 1984;79:379-388.
12. O'Keefe DD, Hoffman JT, Cheitlin R, et al. Coronary blood flow in experimental canine left ventricular hypertrophy. *Circ Res* 1978;43:43-51.
13. Franz MR. Long-term recording of monophasic action potentials from human endocardium. *Am J Cardiol* 1983;51:1629-1634.
14. Franz MR, Bargheer K, Rafflenbeul W, et al. Monophasic action potential mapping in human subjects with normal electrocardiograms: Direct evidence for the genesis of the T wave. *Circulation* 1987;75:379-386.
15. Scott RC. The electrocardiographic diagnosis of left ventricular hypertrophy. *Am Heart J* 1960;59:155-156.
16. Kuo CS, Munakata K, Reddy CP, Surawicz B. Characteristics and possible mechanism of ventricular arrhythmia dependent on the dispersion of action potential durations. *Circulation* 1983;67:1356-1367.
17. Burgess MJ, Green LS, Millar K, et al. The sequence of normal ventricular recovery. *Am Heart J* 1972;84:660-669.

18. Abildskov JA. The sequence of normal recovery of excitability in the dog heart. *Circulation* 1975;52:442-446.

19. Autenrieth G, Surawicz B, Kuo CS. Sequence of repolarization on the ventricular surface in the dog. *Am Heart J* 1975;89:463-469.

20. Durrer D, Van Dam RT, Freud GE, et al. Total excitation of the isolated human heart. *Circulation* 1970;41:899-912.

21. Cassidy DM, Vassallo JA, Marchlinski FE, et al. Endocardial mapping in humans in sinus rhythm with normal left ventricles: Activation patterns and characteristics of electrograms. *Circulation* 1984;70:37-42.

22. Wiener I, Mindich B, Pitchon R. Epicardial activation of the human ventricle: Effects of left ventricular hypertrophy. *Am J Cardiol* 1982;50:1095-1098.

23. Rosenbaum MB, Blanco HH, Elizari MV, et al. Electrotonic modulation of the T wave and cardiac memory. *Am J Cardiol* 1982;50:213-222.

24. Rosenbaum MB, Sicouri SJ, Davidenko JM, Elizari MV. Heart rate and electrotonic modulation of the T wave: A singular relationship. In Zipes DP, Jalife J (eds): *Cardiac Electrophysiology.* New York, London: Grune & Stratton; 1985:485-488.

25. Chatterjee K, Harris A, Davies G, Leatham A. Electrocardiographic changes subsequent to artificial ventricular depolarization. *Br Heart J* 1969;31:770-779.

26. Costard-Jaeckle A, Franz MR. Slow and long-lasting modulation of myocardial repolarization produced by ectopic activation in isolated rabbit hearts: Evidence for cardiac "memory." *Circulation* 1989;80:1412-1420.

27. Hoffman BF. Electronic modulation of the T-wave. *Am J Cardiol* 1982;50:361-362.

28. Vassalle M. Analysis of cardiac pacemaker potentials using a 'voltage clamp" technique. *Am J Physiol* 1966;210:1335-1341.

29. Sasyniuk BI, Mendez C. A mechanism for reentry in canine ventricular tissue. *Circ Res* 1971;28:3-15.

30. Hatt PY, Jouannot P, Moravec J, Swynghedauw B. Current trends in heart hypertrophy. *Basic Res Cardiol* 1974;69:479-483.

31. Maron BJ, Ferrans VJ, Roberts WC. Ultrastructural features of degenerated cardiac muscle cells in patients with cardiac hypertrophy. *Am J Pathol* 1975;79:387-434.

32. Wendt-Gallitelli MF, Jacob R. Time courses of electron microscopic alterations in the hypertrophied myocardium of Goldblatt rats. *Basic Res Cardiol* 1977;72:209-213.

33. Keung EC, Aronson RS. Non-uniform electrophysiological properties and electrotonic interaction in hypertrophied rat myocardium. *Circ Res* 1981;49:150-158.

34. Cooklin M, Wallis WR, Sheridan DJ, Fry CH. Changes in cell-to-cell electrical coupling associated with left ventricular hypertrophy. *Circ Res* 1997;80:765-771.

35. Franz MR, Flaherty JT, Platia EV, et al. Localization of regional myocardial ischemia by recording of monophasic action potentials. *Circulation* 1984;69:593-604.

36. Kingaby RO, Lab MJ, Cole AW, Plamer TN. Relation between monophasic action potential duration, ST segment elevation, and regional myocardial blood flow after coronary occlusion in the pig. *Cardiovasc Res* 1986;20:740-751.

37. Dill SG, Lab MJ. Changes in monophasic action potential duration during the first hour of regional myocardial ischaemia in the anaesthetized pig. *Cardiovasc Res* 1987;21:908-915.

38. Taggart P, Sutton P, Runnalls M, et al. Use of monophasic action potential recordings during routine coronary-artery bypass surgery as an index of localized myocardial ischaemia. *Lancet* 1986;1:1462-1465.

39. Donaldson RM, Taggart P, Swanton H, et al. Effect of nitroglycerin on the electrical changes of early or subendocardial ischaemia evaluated by monophasic action potential recordings. *Cardiovasc Res* 1984;18:7-13.

40. Vassallo JA, Cassidy DM, Kindwall KE, et al. Nonuniform recovery of excitability in the left ventricle. *Circulation* 1988;78:1365-1372.

41. Olshausen KV, Schwarz F, Apfelbach J, et al. Determinants of the incidence and severity of ventricular arrhythmias in aortic valve disease. *Am J Cardiol* 1983;51:1103-1109.

42. Klein RC. Ventricular arrhythmias in aortic valve disease: Analysis of 102 patients. *Am J Cardiol* 1984;53:1079-1083.

43. Schwartz LS, Goldfischer J, Sprague GJ, Schwartz SP. Syncope and sudden death in aortic stenosis. *Am J Cardiol* 1969;23:647-658.

44. Olshausen KV, Witt T, Schmidt G, Meyer J. Ventricular tachycardia as a cause of sudden death in patients with aortic valve disease. *Am J Cardiol* 1987;59:1214-1215.

45. Messerli FH, Ventura HD, Elizardi DJ, et al. Hypertension and sudden death. Increased ventricular ectopic activity in left ventricular hypertrophy. *Am J Med* 1984;77:18-22.

46. McLenachan JM, Henderson E, Morris KI, Dargie HJ. Ventricular arrhythmias in patients with hypertensive left ventricular hypertrophy. *N Engl J Med* 1987;317:787-792.

47. Messerli FH, Soria F. Ventricular dysrhythmias, left ventricular hypertrophy, and sudden death. *Cardiovasc Drugs Ther* 1994;8(suppl 3):557-563.

Section IV

Evaluation of Antiarrhythmic Drug Effects:
Introduction

The effects of antiarrhythmic drugs are well studied in isolated myocardial tissue preparations. However, these basic data often cannot explain the sometimes unanticipated effects of antiarrhythmic drugs in the clinical laboratory. Such discrepancy between basic and clinical data on antiarrhythmic drug effects and efficacy may be related to a variety of conditions. Among these are the intrinsic differences between an isolated strip of heart tissue perfused by an artificial solution as opposed to an intact in situ human heart that is blood-perfused, exposed to autonomic influences, and modified by multiple diseases which foster arrhythmias.

In this section data are presented, by experts, on the effects of antiarrhythmic drugs on myocardium in the setting of isolated heart tissue and in clinical scenarios. This interesting topic is discussed in terms of use dependence of antiarrhythmic drugs, use dependence-countering effects of adrenergic stimulation, drug-induced postrepolarization refractoriness, and the effects of combining class I and class III drugs.

24

Frequency Dependence of Class I and Class III Antiarrhythmic Agents Explaining Their Antiarrhythmic and Proarrhythmic Properties

Luc Hondeghem MD, PhD

The monophasic action potential (MAP) provides a powerful tool for studying the action of drugs in the whole heart. This chapter describes a novel MAP recording electrode that has been used since 1990 in over 10,000 experiments, and illustrates its use in the study of anti- and proarrhythmic drug actions.

The KCl-MAP Recording Electrode

The MAP is usually recorded between a gently touching electrode and an electrode that firmly contacts the tissue either by pressure or by suction.[1] The firm contact damages the underlying cells, leading to depolarization and unexcitability. As a result, a potential difference develops between the recording electrodes which resembles the action potential. Unfortunately, healing mechanisms electrically isolate the damaged cells and, in the process, the amplitude of the MAP can quickly decline, frequently necessitating the repositioning of the electrodes to a new site. The need for repositioning

From Franz MR (ed): *Monophasic Action Potentials: Bridging Cell and Bedside.*
©Futura Publishing Company, Inc., Armonk, NY, 2000.

is inconvenient for long-term recordings. In addition, to the extent that not all action potentials are identical,[2] it may also introduce errors. This problem can be circumvented by depolarizing a pool of cells with KCl: the depolarized cells are also inactive, but since they are not damaged, stable recordings can be expected for extended periods of time. Although recording between a pool of KCl-depolarized tissue and a silver wire yields the expected MAP, it still has several problems.

Initially, the MAP recordings made with pure isotonic KCL (as described above) still declined so that they became useless in about 1 hour. It was found that addition of 1.8 mM $CaCl_2$ slowed the run-down of the signals. In addition, the quality and stability of the recordings increased with the size of the depolarized pool until it reached a diameter of approximately 1 mm. For larger diameters it became more difficult to obtain a good seal, and leakage of KCl over the epicardium became a problem. Therefore, to minimize the effects of any KCl leakage, the electrode must be angled in such a way that leaked KCl runs away from the heart over the electrode (Fig. 1).

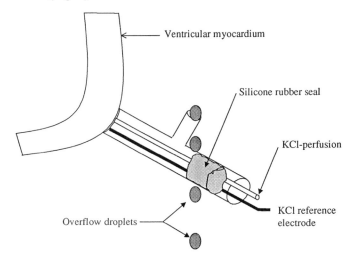

Figure 1. A T-shaped tubing of 1 mm internal diameter is mounted on a 25-cm flexible plastic rod (not shown) and positioned against the ventricular epicardium. The pressure is adjusted to the minimum that does provide a seal between the electrode and the epicardium. The electrode tubing is angled so that any leakage would run away from the heart down the outside of the tube. In the tube are glued with silicone rubber a silver wire (solid black) and a fine capillary polyethylene tubing, both extending to the tip of the electrode. The silver wire is grounded while the capillary is perfused with a salt solution containing 140 mM KCl and 1.8 mM $CaCl_2$ at a rate of approximately 1 mL/min. The perfusate flows from the tip backwards to exit via the open end of the T connector, which is pointed up so that a small hydrostatic pressure of about 1 cm water results at the tip. In order to minimize noise pickup, the electrode solution is passed through a drip chamber positioned close to the heart (not shown).

The signals, however, still declined as a function of time, and occasionally the electrode became very noisy. It was noted that the noise was usually associated with the formation of an air bubble in the tip of the KCl electrode. Remaining run-down of the MAP could have been be due to damage of the cells or to elution of the KCl in the electrode tip. Some improvement in stability resulted after the electrode was mounted on a flexible 25-cm plastic rod. This allowed maintenance of gentle contact with a moving heart, while minimizing damage by pressure.

The most striking improvement resulted when the electrode tip was slowly perfused. This perfusion not only maintains the KCl depolarization, it also flushes away any possible air bubbles. In order to minimize the noise, the KCl is passed through a drip chamber as close as possible to the heart, and the KCl pool in the electrode is used as reference ground. In rare instances where the signals still deteriorate, it is frequently sufficient to briefly increase the KCl flow through the electrode tip. With this arrangement stable MAPs are usually recorded for many hours.[2]

The cells depolarized with isotonic KCl (Fig. 2) have, according to the Nernst equation, a transmembrane potential of 0 mV and can no longer participate in any activity. In contrast, the cells remote from the KCl electrode have, under normal conditions, a negative membrane potential of approximately –85 mV during diastole and a positive membrane potential of approximately +25 mV during the plateau. The change in membrane

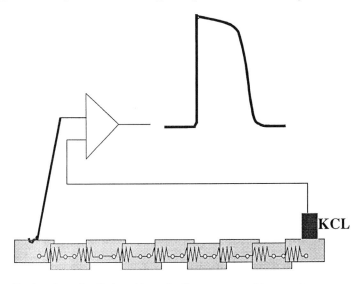

Figure 2. A string of cells is schematically represented by gray boxes, connected by resistors. At the left, the active recording electrode potential is modulated by the local changes in membrane potential. In contrast, the cells at right are permanently depolarized by KCl. The potential difference between the two electrodes is amplified so that a MAP can be recorded.

potential at one electrode but not at the other leads to the MAP (for more details on MAP recordings see chapters 1 through 8).

Modulated Receptor Theory

Ion channels are embedded in a cell membrane across which exists an electrical field that switches with each action potential from about −85 to +25 mV (ie, 110 mV). Since this potential change occurs over a distance of only 10 nm, each action potential induces a change in electrical field in excess of 100,000 V/cm. This strong change of electrical field induces conformational changes in the ion channel proteins that can modify their conductance: the channels are said to open and close. According to Hodgkin and Huxley,[3] sodium channels are closed at rest (R in Fig. 3), but upon depolarization they activate (A in Fig. 3) and transiently become open. Upon maintained depolarization (during the plateau) they inactivate (I in Fig. 3), ie, they close again. Hondeghem and Katzung[4] proposed that, in addition to changing conductance of the channels, these conformational changes can also modulate the affinity for drugs interacting with cardiac channels: rested, activated, and inactivated channels can bind drug to form respectively RD, AD, and ID channels (Fig. 3). Drug-associated channels may also become rested, activated, and inactivated as a function of voltage and time, but the voltage dependence is shifted (eg, to more negative potentials) and the kinetics changed (eg, slowed). In addition, drug-associated channels may have altered conductance (eg, they may not conduct when activated).

For useful sodium channel blockers, the rested state has a much lower affinity than the activated and/or inactivated states; therefore the level of block will be reduced by hyperpolarization (favoring the low-affinity rested state) and by slow heart rates (longer diastolic intervals where the rested state is predominant). Conversely, the effect of a given concentration will be augmented by depolarization and short cycle lengths: the channels spend more time in the activated and inactivated states (high-affinity states).

Similar modulated receptor algorithms have been applied to drug interaction with calcium[5] and potassium channels.[6]

Applications of the KCl-MAP
Electrode to Study Class I Action

The MAP recording consists typically of 4 phases: the upstroke, the plateau, repolarization and diastole. The KCl-MAP electrode has an important advantage for drug study as it can be left in place for the duration of

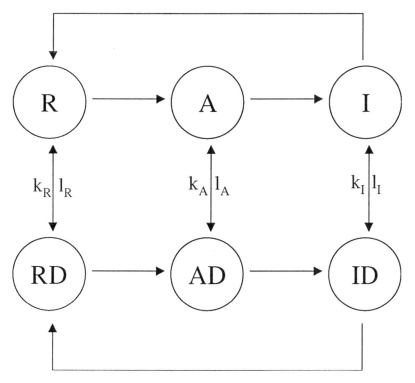

Figure 3. Schematic representation of the modulated receptor theory applied to sodium channels. At negative potentials the channels are rested (R), upon depolarization they activate (A), but during maintained depolarization they inactivate (I). The drugs can bind and unbind to each of these states with characteristic association (k_R, k_A, and k_I) and dissociation (l_R, l_A and l_I) rate constants. Binding of drug leads to RD, AD, and ID states. The drug-associated channels also exhibit voltage-dependent transitions between the states, but these are frequently shifted to more negative potentials. In addition, drug-associated channels may not conduct when activated.

the experiment. The MAP has been used in the past primarily to study class I (slowing of conduction by block of sodium channels) and class III (prolongation of refractoriness by prolongation of the action potential duration [APD]) drug effects.[7] Study of class I action is usually done by studying changes related to the upstrokes.

Conduction Time

Conduction velocity through cardiac tissue can be measured by recording the conduction time between at least 2 electrodes. When only 2 electrodes are used, a change in pathway of activation can seriously distort a drug effect upon conduction. However, when multiple electrodes are used, it is highly unlikely that consistent changes of conduction times would be caused by changes in pathways.

Upstroke Velocity

The maximum upstroke velocity of action potentials is frequently used to estimate drug effects on sodium channels. The upstroke of the MAP can also be differentiated.[8] While sodium channel block can reduce the upstroke of the MAP, the latter is a complex function not only of sodium channel current, but also of conduction and loading conditions. Therefore, although lack of changes in upstroke velocity may suggest that an agent does not have a class I action, slowing of the upstroke is not a reliable measure of the extent of sodium channel block. Only if conduction times and upstroke velocity measurements used at multiple sites consistently yield changes of similar magnitude can one expect that they may reflect a change that is somewhat proportional to the block of sodium channels.

Cardiac Activity Signals

Activation of each cardiac cell or fiber generates a small electrical vector. Since the number of cells/fibers activated per unit time and the direction of activation continuously change, it follows that the heart must generate high-frequency signals. These should be superimposed on the upstroke (where the activations occur) and should normally not exist during the plateau or diastole. When making normal assumptions about resting potential, action potential amplitude, upstroke velocity, APD, number of cardiac cells per unit length, and intracellular connectivity, then impulses compute to propagate through a matrix of cells at velocities near 1 m/s. Most importantly, for the duration of the propagation the cellular matrix emits high-frequency signals (approximately 1 kHz).[9] These cardiac activity signals (CAS) most likely originate from discontinuous propagation across cell and fiber boundaries. Indeed, computations of propagation through uniform conduction media does not yield any CAS-like signals.

When differentiating the action potential between a bandwidth of 250 Hz and 5 kHz (a bandwidth normally filtered away by cardiac electrophysiologists), one can readily see that in synchrony with cardiac activation there occurs a burst of signals that is not present during the plateau (Fig. 4). The duration of the CAS (determined as the time during which the high-frequency signals exceeds the 99% confidence interval of the back-

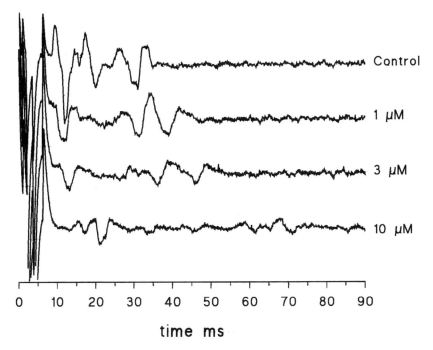

Figure 4. Cardiac activity signals (CAS) obtained from a Langendorff-perfused rabbit heart. The data were sampled at 10 kHz (exp. 6068). The top trace shows that under control, activation signals lasted about 35 milliseconds. Following equilibration with 1 μM quinidine, CAS lasted 42 milliseconds. In 3 μM the duration of the CAS increased to 50 milliseconds and in 10 μM CAS prolonged to exceed 70 milliseconds.

ground noise, see Fig. 4), is the time during which the electrodes sense cardiac activation. Obviously, the more electrodes are placed over the heart, the less the chance that the activation of some remote tissue will not be registered. In more than 10,000 experiments, I have summed the CAS signals from 3 electrodes and found that this can very satisfactorily measure class I drug effects. Use-dependent block of sodium channels results in a beat-by-beat lengthening of the CAS duration and the onset of action is much faster for lidocaine[10] than for quinidine.[11] The use-dependent prolongation of CAS by sodium channel blockers is accentuated by depolarization and ischemia.[12] Upon discontinuation of a stimulation train, the accumulated prolongation of CAS declines exponentially,[12] and the recovery requires many seconds for quinidine[11] but is completed in a few hundred milliseconds for lidocaine.[10] These changes are very similar to those obtained with other techniques.[5]

As conduction is slowed by block of sodium channels (Fig. 4), the CAS duration is not only prolonged, its amplitude is also reduced. As a result, it becomes increasingly difficult to determine the exact point of termination of CAS. For this reason, whenever CAS exceeds 90 milliseconds in the rabbit (a prolongation in excess of 100%), I no longer consider the measurements reliable. During ventricular reentry tachycardia (CAS becomes continuous but regular) and fibrillation (CAS becomes continuous but random), it becomes also not practical to measure conduction with this technique.

Although the CAS shown in Figure 4 come from MAP electrodes on the ventricle, it can also be recorded from electrodes on the atria, between any pair of standard electrodes and from standard pacemaker leads. CAS has even been recorded from precordial leads in human, although in this situation there are considerable signal-to-noise problems.[13]

Applications of the KCl-MAP
Electrode to Study Class III Action

Following the unfavorable results from the CAST trial,[14] the use of class I agents has markedly declined and the popularity of class III agents has increased accordingly.[15] Unfortunately, most of the clinically available agents lengthen APD primarily at slow heart rates, but have much less effect at fast heart rates (reverse use dependence).[16] It is difficult to envision how drugs that prolong the APD at normal heart rates (when not needed) but not during tachycardia could be effective antitachycardia agents. To the contrary, excessive prolongation following long cycle lengths can lead to repolarization disturbances: hesitations of repolarization, early afterdepolarizations (EADs), ectopic beats, torsades de pointes (TdP), and fibrillation. It is hence not unexpected that agents that can be proarrhythmic at normal to slow heart rates, while loosing their antiarrhythmic property during tachycardia, might not be beneficial or even detrimental.[17] Only amiodarone has been shown to maintain its class III action during tachycardia,[18] and it is also the only one that has been reported to save lives.[19] An agent that does not prolong the APD at normal heart rates but use-dependently prolongs it upon tachycardia (until the tachycardia is rendered impossible to sustain), is expected to be highly effective.[2]

In studying class III effects on the MAP in over 10,000 experiments, it has become evident that: 1) class III agents that exhibit reverse use dependence can be proarrhythmic; 2) as class III agents slow repolarization, the likelihood of proarrhythmia increases; and 3) serious proarrhythmia is frequently preceded by temporal and spatial variability of APD. Because of the importance of these 3 aspects, they are discussed in separate sections below.

Prolongation of Plateau versus Prolongation of Repolarization

Although there definitely is a relationship between the extent of prolongation of APD and proarrhythmia,[20] this relationship is not a very tight one: some drugs can trigger EADs for only a minor prolongation of APD while others can yield very long prolongations of the APD before causing any signs of proarrhythmia. For agents that prolong the APD, the greater the ratio of prolongation during repolarization to the prolongation during the plateau, the greater the risk of proarrhythmia. In extremis, agents that shorten the plateau and prolong repolarization (triangulation of the action potential) are champions of proarrhythmia (EADs, TdP, fibrillation). Conversely, agents that lengthen the plateau while shortening the repolarization do not exhibit repolarization disturbances.

Slowing of repolarization results in at least 4 predictable dangers (Fig. 5): 1) When spending too much time in the calcium window current, repolarization can stall or reverse and lead to EADs early during repolarization. This may explain the reversal of class III-induced proarrhythmia by

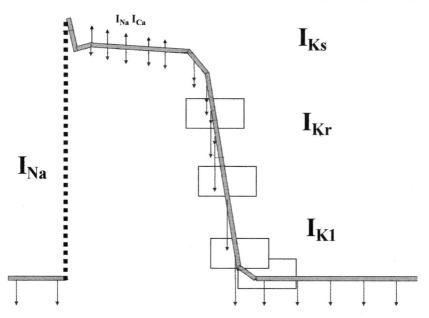

Figure 5. Schematic representation of the action potential. The upstroke is caused by the influx of a large, fast, transient, inward sodium current. During the plateau very little current flows (high impedance): inward sodium and calcium currents slowly decline against slowly increasing outward currents (primarily i_{Kr}, i_{Ks} and i_{K1}). During repolarization the action potential transverses 4 danger windows: calcium window current, sodium window current, reactivation of the sodium channels, and the vulnerable period.

calcium channel blockers.[21] 2) Transition through the sodium window current can similarly promote EADs during late during repolarization and may similarly explain the reversal of proarrhythmia by sodium channel blockers.[22,23] 3) A slow final repolarization prolongs the time of reactivation of the sodium current, which is also proarrhythmic.[24] 4) Insufficient repolarizing outward currents early during diastole facilitate ectopics due to imperfect synchronization of repolarization and facilitation of depolarization by inward current flow. For these reasons, a safe class III effect by block of repolarizing outward currents (i_{Kr}, i_{Ks}, or i_{K1}) may be difficult to achieve.

In contrast, use-dependent prolongation of the APD can also be achieved by activating very small amounts of inward current during the plateau. A more positive plateau may augment the activation of repolarizing outward currents, thus speeding up repolarization. If the activator binds use-dependently and dissociates promptly during normal diastole, then there can be no net prolongation of APD at normal heart rates. However, during tachycardia (more activations yield more binding; while less diastole yields less unbinding), the activator could accumulate and use-dependently prolong the APD until the tachycardia can no longer exist: chemical defibrillator.[25] The profile of a more robust plateau with little lengthening of APD at slow heart rates, faster repolarization, and primarily prolongation of APD upon acceleration of the heart can readily be recognized by the MAP electrode, making it an excellent tool for screening.

Instability of APD: A Predictor of Serious Proarrhythmia

Chemicals that prolong the APD frequently cause repolarization disturbances. Proarrhythmia is commonly recognized in the MAP recordings a few minutes before it actually happens: the APDs become unpredictable from beat to beat (temporal instability) and from site to site (spatial instability). Instabilities past 40% repolarization appear especially dangerous. In panel A of Figure 6, the APD for 10% to 90% repolarization (APD_{10} and APD_{90}, respectively) is plotted for each action potential. Upon the start of a perfusion with sotalol (10 μM), the APD was prolonged within 1 minute. Initially, the prolongation was primarily due to a slowing of repolarization around APD_{30} to APD_{40}. However, after 2 minutes of sotalol perfusion, APD_{40} to APD_{90} was also slowed, and the beat-by-beat APD became unstable. The scatter was sometimes large enough that points of different colors started to mix up. By 10 minutes perfusion with sotalol, repolarization disturbances and EADs became prominent enough to trigger many ectopics. As a result, in the second 10-minute perfusion with sotalol, the computer counted 227 ectopics.

It is important to stress that the instability of APD not only tends to develop earlier than the ectopics, the instability of APD is usually also noted

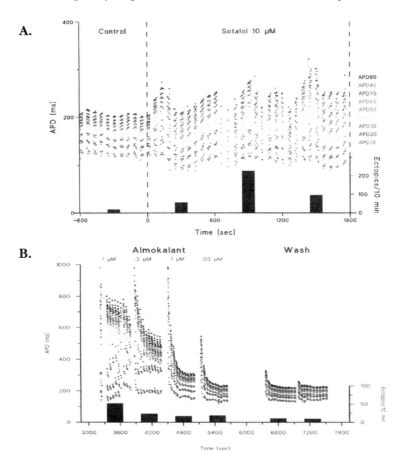

Figure 6. A. The effects of 10-μM sotalol upon the APD_{10} to APD_{90} (exp. 8321). Every minute, a train of 30 action potentials was applied at 1 Hz and the durations of every fourth nonectopic action potential are plotted (when there are many ectopics, fewer points are plotted, eg, from 660 to 780 seconds). Note that sotalol not only lengthens the APD, it also markedly slows repolarization especially between APD_{30} and ADP_{90}. In addition, the stability of the action potential is greatly reduced, especially between 40% and 80% repolarization: scatter of points is much increased, sometimes so markedly that the colors representing different APDs start mixing. **B.** The effects of almokalant (exp. 8537) on APD_{10} to APD_{90}. At 1 μM, the drug elicits numerous arrhythmias while the APD exhibits very marked variability. At 0.3 μM, the arrhythmias decline markedly but the variability remains extensive. Due to overlap of the points, the magnitude is somewhat underestimated. But note example APD_{10} and APD_{20}, and, although more difficult to see, the variability is even more marked as repolarization proceeds (see APD_{90}). At 0.1 μM there is only variability left at APD_{90}. At 0.03 μM the only remaining effect is the reverse use dependence (seen as a marked increase in APD following a long rest period). However, during wash also, this latter effect declines as the APDs approach the control values. Permission for publication of these data kindly provided by Dr. G. Duker from Astra-Hässle. See color plate.

at lower concentrations than the appearance of ectopics. For example, as shown in panel B of Figure 6, instability of APD_{90} started to appear at 0.1 µM almokalant; at 0.3 µM there was much triangulation of the action potential and the instability became very marked from APD_{20} to APD_{90} (and there was even some at APD_{10}); at 1 µM there was also a dramatic increase in arrhythmias.

It should be noted that when the APD becomes unstable, frequently this is associated with spatial nonuniformity; a long APD at one site may coincide with a short APD at another. Spatial and temporal dispersions of APD are well appreciated contributors to reentry.

Reverse Use Dependence[16]

The first action potential following a long rest period is markedly prolonged, but it then use-dependently shortens to reach a steady state value. The sotalol experiment shown in panel A of Figure 6 did not exhibit much reverse use dependence. However, the almokalant perfusion (Fig. 6, panel B) not only resulted in marked instability, it also triggered marked reverse use dependence.

In general (and in order of importance), as instability of the APD increases (temporal dispersion), as APD becomes nonuniform between sites (spatial dispersion), as the reverse use dependence becomes more marked, and as repolarization slows, the greater becomes the likelihood that TdP and fibrillation will ensue.

Finally, it should be noted that upon repolarization (like upon depolarization), the heart generates numerous electrical vectors. The cardiac repolarizing signals have a lower bandwidth and amplitude than CAS, which makes their recording technically more difficult. When the action potentials become unstable and triangulate, the duration of the cardiac repolarizing signals should widen. Widening of cardiac repolarizing signals could provide a powerful warning signal for impending proarrhythmia problems.

Conclusions

Long-term stable MAP recordings can be recorded by the KCl-MAP electrode. CAS signals (during the upstroke) can be used to study class I actions. Class III actions can occur by lengthening of the plateau or repolarization phase. The latter is anticipated to be proarrhythmic by at least 4 mechanisms. Ideally, class III agents should do little to the normal action potential, but upon initiation of a tachycardia they should vigorously lengthen the plateau in a use-dependent fashion until the tachycardia must terminate. Agents that cause reverse use dependence, triangulation of the action potential, or (most importantly) induce instability of APD, are proarrhythmic. The MAP recording electrode is ideally suited to recognize these important electrophysiologic parameters.

References

1. Franz MR. Monophasic action potentials recorded by contact electrode method: Genesis, measurements, and interpretations. In Franz MR (ed): *Monophasic Action Potentials: Bridging Cell and Bedside*. Armonk, NY: Futura Publishing Co., Inc.; 1999:3-17.

2. Liu DW, Gintant GA, Antzelevitch C. Ionic bases for electrophysiological distinctions among epicardial, midmyocardial, and endocardial myocytes from the free wall of the canine left ventricle. *Circ Res* 1993;72:671-687.

3. Hodgkin AL, Huxley AF. A quantitative description of membrane current and its application to conduction and excitation in nerve. *J Physiol* 1952;117:500-544.

4. Hondeghem LM, Katzung BG. Time- and voltage-dependent interactions of antiarrhythmic drugs with cardiac sodium channels. *Biochim Biophys Acta* 1977;472:373-398.

5. Hondeghem LM, Katzung BG. Antiarrhythmic agents: The modulated receptor mechanism of action of sodium and calcium channel-blocking drugs. *Ann Rev Pharmacol Toxicol* 1984;24:387-423.

6. Roden DM, Bennett PB, Snyders DJ, et al. Quinidine delays IK activation in guinea pig ventricular myocytes. *Circ Res* 1988;62:1055-1058.

7. Vaughan Williams EM. Classification of antiarrhythmic agents. In Vaughan Williams EM (ed): *Antiarrhythmic Drugs*. Berlin: Springer-Verlag; 1989:45-67.

8. Koller B, Franz MR. New classification of moricizine and propafenone based on electrophysiologic and electrocardiographic data from isolated rabbit heart. *J Cardiovasc Pharmacol* 1994;24:753-760.

9. Hondeghem K, Aerden M. *Investigation of Cardiac Electrical Activity in the High Frequency Domain* [Electronic Engineering thesis UDC: 615.84 (043)]. Belgium: Department of Applied Sciences, KU Leuven; 1997.

10. Matsubara T, Clarkson CW, Hondeghem LM. Lidocaine blocks open and inactivated cardiac sodium channels. *Naunyn Schmiedebergs Arch Pharmacol* 1987;336:224-231.

11. Snyders DJ, Hondeghem LM. Effects of quinidine on the sodium current of guinea pig ventricular myocytes. Evidence for a drug-associated rested state with altered kinetics. *Circ Res* 1990;66:565-579.

12. Chen CM, Gettes LS, Katzung BG. Effect of lidocaine and quinidine on steady state characteristics and recovery kinetics of (dV/dt)max in guinea pig ventricular myocardium. *Circ Res* 1975;37:20-29.

13. Hondeghem LM. A device and a method for recording and monitoring cardiac activity signals. International Patent Application PCT/BE95/00123.

14. Echt DS, Liebson PR, Mitchell LB, et al, and the CAST Investigators. Mortality and morbidity in patients receiving encainide, flecainide, or placebo. *N Engl J Med* 1991;324:781-788.

15. Singh BN. Choice and chance in drug therapy of cardiac arrhythmias: Technique versus drug-specific responses in evaluation of efficacy. *Am J Cardiol* 1993;72:114F-124F.

16. Hondeghem LM, Snyders DS. Class III antiarrhythmic agents have a lot of potential, but a long way to go: Reduced effectiveness and dangers of reverse use-dependence. *Circulation* 1990;81:686-690.
17. Waldo AL, Camm AJ, de Ruyter H, et al. Effect of d-sotalol on mortality in patients with left ventricular dysfunction after recent and remote myocardial infarction. The SWORD Investigators. Survival With Oral d-Sotalol. *Lancet* 1996;348:7-12.
18. Sager PT, Uppal P, Follmer C, et al. Frequency-dependent electrophysiologic effects of amiodarone in humans. *Circulation* 1993;88:1063-1071.
19. Sim I, McDonald KM, Lavori PW, et al. Quantitative overview of randomized trials of amiodarone to prevent sudden cardiac death. *Circulation* 1997;96:2823-2829.
20. Carlsson L, Almgren O, Duker G. QTU-Prolongation and torsades de pointes induced by putative class III antiarrhythmic agents in the rabbit: Etiology and interventions. *J Cardiovasc Pharmacol* 1990;16:276-285.
21. Roden DM. Early after-depolarizations and torsade de pointes: Implications for the control of cardiac arrhythmias by prolonging repolarization. *Eur Heart J* 1993;14:56-61.
22. Chezalviel-Guilbert F, Davy JM, Poirier JM, Weissenburger J. Mexiletine antagonizes effects of sotalol on QT interval duration and its proarrhythmic effects in a canine model of torsade de pointes. *J Am Coll Cardiol* 1995;26:787-792.
23. Abrahamsson C, Carlsson L, Duker G. Lidocaine and nisoldipine attenuate almokalant-induced dispersion of repolarization and early afterdepolarizations in vitro. *J Cardiovasc Electrophysiol* 1996;7:1074-1081.
24. Starmer CF, Lastra AA, Nesterenko VV, Grant AO. Proarrhythmic response to sodium channel blockade. Theoretical model and numerical experiments. *Circulation* 1991;84:1364-1377.
25. Hondeghem LM. Ideal antiarrhythmic agents: Chemical defibrillators. *J Cardiovasc Electrophysiol* 1991;2:169-177.

25

Effect of d-Sotalol on the Vulnerable Window of Ventricular Fibrillation, and a Definition of the "Area of Vulnerability"

Paulus F. Kirchhof, MD and
C. Larissa Fabritz, MD

Introduction

The deleterious effects of strong electrical stimuli on the electrical activity of the heart[1] have been known for almost 100 years. Investigation of the prerequisites for the induction of these often lethal arrhythmias[2,3] resulted in a description of the vulnerable period of the heart, the only time interval in the cardiac cycle during which short electrical stimuli induce ventricular fibrillation (VF). The development of the automatic cardioverter defibrillator has renewed the interest in myocardial vulnerability to high-energy shocks and has led to studies of the vulnerable period for single T wave shocks. The vulnerability to T wave shocks, which are commonly applied clinically[4,5] to induce VF during implantation of defibrillators or postoperative defibrillation threshold (DFT) testing, has been found to coincide with the ascending[6] and, to some extent, the descending[7] limb of the T wave of the surface electrocardiogram (ECG). This

From Franz MR (ed): *Monophasic Action Potentials: Bridging Cell and Bedside.*
©Futura Publishing Company, Inc., Armonk, NY, 2000.

finding concurs with the old hypothesis[2,3,8,9] that the vulnerability of the heart relates to the late repolarization phase of the action potential. However, this hypothesis has not yet been directly tested.

Previous studies referred to a single vulnerable period, usually determined for an arbitrary stimulus strength.[4,8] According to the strength interval relation,[10,11] a stronger stimulus excites the heart at earlier repolarization states. The interest in vulnerability to T wave shocks has been spurred further by the discovery[5,12,13] that the upper limit of vulnerability (ULV) and DFT correlate closely. A better determination of the optimal ULV coupling interval might abolish discrepancies that have been observed between the ULV and DFT.[4] The existence of a ULV and a lower limit of vulnerability (LLV) as well as a vulnerable period, together, suggests a bimodal function of cardiac vulnerability to T wave shocks.

D-sotalol is an agent whose efficacy against ventricular arrhythmias has been attributed to its action potential prolonging effect[14-19] and a hypothesized reduction in dispersion of repolarization, but recent data[20] have demonstrated proarrhythmic effects of d-sotalol in postinfarction patients.

The aims of the studies presented in this chapter were 1) to determine the vulnerable period for electrical field shocks at two different shock strengths, one slightly above the fibrillation threshold and one close to the ULV; 2) to determine the upper and lower limits of vulnerability with respect to these vulnerable periods, and in relation to the directly measured dispersion of repolarization; 3) to test whether a homogeneous, 2-dimensional "area of vulnerability" exists, defined in time (coupling interval) and shock strength dimensions; 4) to relate the coupling intervals and the durations of the vulnerable periods to the dispersion of 7 simultaneously recorded monophasic action potentials (MAPs) and to the T wave of a volume-conducted ECG; and 5) to investigate the effects of d-sotalol on the dispersion of ventricular repolarization and the associated vulnerable periods.

Methods

Preparation of Isolated Rabbit Hearts

Seven MAPs were recorded simultaneously from isolated, Langendorff-perfused rabbit hearts, as described before,[21-24] with use of Franz Ag/AgCl contact MAP-pacing combination electrodes[25,26] capable of recording and pacing from the same catheter site. MAPs were recorded simultaneously from 5 epicardial sites and 2 left ventricular endocardial sites. The epicardial recordings were located as follows: 1 on the right ventricular free wall, 1 on the right ventricle close to the posterior septum, 2 on the basal and apical left ventricular free wall, and 1 on the left ventricle close to the anterior septum. Usually, MAP amplitudes were greater than 5 mV, with a minimal amplitude of 3.5 mV. Pacing was performed through one of the endocardial MAP catheters using a custom pacing program run on a Macintosh IIfx computer and a stimulus isolator. A volume-conducted ECG[22,24,27] was recorded simultaneously. Of the 3 available Einthoven leads, the lead with the longest monophasic T wave[4] was recorded. An example for a simultaneous recording of 7 MAPs and the tissue bath ECG during steady state pacing is shown in Figure 1.

Field Shock Application

Fibrillation and defibrillation shocks were delivered by an experimental defibrillator via two 5×5 cm rectangular stainless steel plate electrodes placed on opposite walls of the tissue bath. A monophasic shock waveform

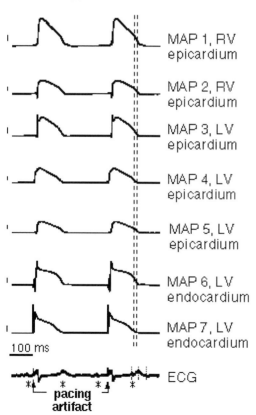

Figure 1. Simultaneous recording of 7 MAPs and lead II of the tissue bath (volume-conducted) electrocardiogram (ECG) during steady state pacing at 600 milliseconds cycle length. The upper 2 MAPs were recorded from the right ventricular epicardium, the middle 3 MAPs from the left ventricular epicardium, and the lower 2 from the left ventricular endocardium. The vertical lines to the left of each recording provide a 1-mV reference calibration for each MAP recording. The dotted lines mark the shortest repolarization time (in MAP 7) and the longest repolarization time (in MAP 1) at the 90% repolarization level. The dispersion of repolarization of the MAP recordings at 90% repolarization is the interval between these lines. Arrows mark artifacts generated by pacing stimuli. * = P waves in the ECG. The 3 dotted lines in the ECG recording mark the mid upslope, peak, and mid downslope of the T wave. Neither the mid upslope nor the peak nor the mid downslope of the T wave coincided with the dispersion of 90% repolarization as measured directly by the 7 MAPs.

truncated after 5 milliseconds was applied. The size of the plate electrodes exceeded the dimensions of the centrally located heart in every direction, thus exposing the whole heart to the shock field. Measurements of the potential gradients in the tissue bath demonstrated a highly uniform shock field in the center of the bath where the heart was positioned.

Protocol

The heart was paced at 600-millisecond basic cycle length from 1 of the 2 endocardial MAP catheters. This cycle length was relatively long, hence close to cycle lengths observed in the human heart, and it guaranteed stable paced rhythms in all hearts without ectopic ventricular activity. Prior to delivery of a shock, the heart was allowed to recover for 3 minutes if the shock did not induce VF, and for 5 minutes if the shock induced VF. Steady state MAP durations were assessed prior to each shock. Experiments showing changes in steady state MAP duration of more than 3% or MAP amplitude of more than 15% in more than 2 MAP recordings were excluded from the analysis.

Determination of the Vulnerable Period and Effect of d-Sotalol

The ULV and the LLV, or fibrillation threshold, were estimated at the peak of the T wave with use of an up-down protocol[28] in 50-V steps. Two voltages were scanned for the vulnerable period, one of them 50 V below the estimated ULV (high shock voltage), the other 50 V above the estimated LLV (low shock voltage). To determine the vulnerable period for each of the two shock strengths, shocks were applied at different coupling intervals in steps of 5 milliseconds. Coupling intervals were defined as the interval from the pacing artifact to the shock artifact, and were verified by off-line analysis. The vulnerable period was scanned to determine the shortest and longest VF-inducing coupling interval. The contingency of the vulnerable period was tested by delivering shocks in coupling interval steps of ≤10 milliseconds throughout the vulnerable period. The borders of the vulnerable period were determined with 5-millisecond accuracy. The duration of the vulnerable period was calculated as the difference between the longest and the shortest coupling interval at which VF was induced. This procedure was repeated for the second shock strength. The order of determination of the two vulnerable periods was changed randomly.

Baseline data were verified by random reproduction of 6 previously delivered shocks. After completion of the baseline protocol, d-sotalol was added to the perfusate at a concentration of 2×10^{-5} mol/L while the heart was continually paced at 600 milliseconds cycle length. MAP durations were analyzed every 5 minutes. The protocol was repeated when ≥45-minute drug loading time had elapsed and MAP prolongation by d-sotalol had reached a constant value (±2.5 milliseconds) at pacing with 600 milliseconds cycle length for at least 5 minutes.

Defining the Area of Vulnerability

In an additional series of 11 experiments, the boundaries of the hypothesized "area of vulnerability" or "vulnerable field" were determined with 10- to 20-V and 5- to 10-millisecond accuracy. Four transition zones from VF to no or nonsustained arrhythmia were determined as illustrated in Figure 2: 1) the longest VF-inducing coupling interval; 2) the shortest VF-inducing coupling interval; 3) LLV; and 4) ULV.

Determination of Longest and Shortest Arrhythmogenic Coupling Intervals

The first shock was applied at the peak of the highest monophasic T wave[4,5] at a shock voltage considered appropriate to induce VF (250 to 300 V). If this shock did not induce VF, coupling interval and shock strength

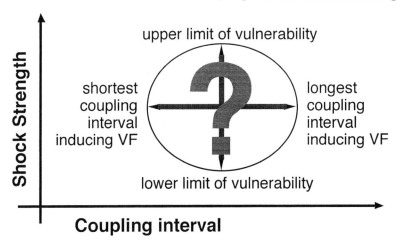

Figure 2. Protocol scheme for determination of an "area" or "field" of vulnerability defined by shock strength (y axis) and coupling interval (x axis). By adapting shock strength and coupling interval interactively in staircase-like steps at the outer limits of the vulnerable field, the borders of vulnerability were determined as 1) the longest ventricular fibrillation (VF)-inducing coupling interval; 2) the shortest VF-inducing coupling interval; 3) the lower limit of vulnerability; and 4) the upper limit of vulnerability.

were adjusted as necessary to induce VF. Once VF was initiated, the shock coupling interval was increased in steps of 20 milliseconds, in order to determine the longest arrhythmogenic coupling interval, until VF was no longer inducible. The last coupling interval (which no longer induced VF) was then decreased by 10 milliseconds. Depending on whether VF was induced, the coupling interval was either decreased or increased by 5 milliseconds for the following shock. The procedure was repeated, targeting the border of vulnerability in staircase-like steps with shock strengths increased and decreased by 30- to 50-V steps until VF was no longer inducible. The same steps were adapted for the determination of the shortest arrhythmogenic coupling intervals approaching refractoriness by decreasing instead of increasing the coupling intervals of the shocks.

LLV and ULV

To determine the LLV, the shortest and longest coupling intervals at the lowest VF-inducing voltage were averaged. At this averaged coupling interval, the lowest VF-inducing shock voltage was determined using a modified up-down method[28] in steps of 10 V. The shock strength that was 10 V below the lowest VF-inducing voltage was then tested at shock coupling intervals 5 and 10 milliseconds shorter and longer than the averaged coupling interval. If VF was again inducible, the modified up-down method was repeated at this new coupling interval. The LLV was determined with an accuracy of 5 and 10 milliseconds and 10 V. The protocol for the LLV determination was adapted from determination of the ULV: the average of the shock coupling intervals of the highest VF-inducing shock voltages was adjusted and the up-down method applied until the ULV was determined with a 5- and 10-millisecond and 10-V accuracy. Shocks at the ULV and LLV were repeated at the end of the protocol to test for reproducibility.

For determination of the DFT, defibrillation shocks were applied after 6 to 12 seconds of sustained VF. The first shock strength was set to 450 V. If defibrillation was effective, shock strength was lowered by 50 V for the next VF episode. If defibrillation failed, a rescue shock was applied, and the defibrillation shock strength was increased by 50 V for the following defibrillation shock. The DFT of each heart was calculated as the mean of the lowest shock strength that defibrillated and the highest shock strength that failed to defibrillate,[29,30] as suggested by other groups.

Direct Analysis of Dispersion of Ventricular Repolarization by Multiple MAP Recordings

MAPs were analyzed for action potential duration (APD) at 90%, 70%, and 50% repolarization[30] as the interval from the fastest MAP upstroke to the respective repolarization level, as described before. Activation time was measured as the time between the pacing artifact and the fastest upstroke of the MAP. Repolarization time was defined as the sum of activation time and APD. Analysis was performed at least once every hour of the protocol during steady state. The dispersion of repolarization was calculated by subtracting the minimal repolarization time from the maximal repolarization time recorded from the 7 MAP electrodes. The computer analysis was randomly verified by manual measurements of APDs at 50%, 70%, and 90% repolarization, and of activation time.

ECG Analysis

Five ECG parameters were analyzed: 1) QRS duration; 2) time from the stimulus-evoked Q wave (pacing artifact in Fig. 1) to the mid upslope of the T wave; 3) time from the Q wave to the peak of the T wave; 4) time from the Q wave to the mid downslope of the T wave; and 5) time from the mid upslope to the mid downslope of the T wave. The mid upslope was defined as the time point when the ascending T wave reached 50% of its maximal amplitude. The mid downslope was defined as the time point when the descending T wave returned to 50% of its maximal amplitude. The periods from the mid upslope to the peak and from the mid upslope to the mid downslope of the T wave were calculated.

Arrhythmia Definitions

Due to its small myocardial mass, the rabbit heart is prone to recover spontaneously from an episode of induced VF. Studies in our laboratory[22,23] and in those of others[31,32] demonstrated that more than 5 extra beats were consistently induced by shocks of coupling intervals and shock energies that induced sustained VF at least once. In addition, the ECG characteristics of the spontaneously terminating episodes that lasted more than 5 extra beats were similar to ECG characteristics during episodes that required external defibrillation. Therefore, VF and nonfibrillating episodes were defined as follows: an episode was regarded as VF if at least 6 full excitations showing cycle lengths of less than 160 milliseconds were induced by a shock in every MAP recording. Induction of 2 to 5 action potentials was regarded as nonsustained arrhythmia, and induction of 0 to 1 action potential as no arrhythmia.

Statistical Analysis

The dispersion of repolarization at baseline and after addition of d-sotalol was compared using the Student paired t test. Coupling intervals of the two vulnerable periods were also compared using the paired *t* test. In order to relate dispersion of repolarization to the vulnerable periods, the shortest and longest repolarization times at 50%, 70%, and 90% and the T wave parameters were compared with the left and right boundaries of the vulnerable periods, the ULV and LLV, using both paired *t* tests and linear regression, where applicable. These correlations enabled a comparison of the dispersion of repolarization and the vulnerable periods in terms of duration and coupling interval referenced to the pacing stimulus. A *P* value less than 0.05 was considered significant.

Results

Vulnerable Period for Low and High Shock Strengths

Shocks that induced VF were clustered within a discrete time interval for each of the two shock strengths, the vulnerable periods. Only shocks delivered within these vulnerable periods induced VF, while shocks delivered outside of the vulnerable periods did not induce VF. Each vulnerable period was bordered by a narrow transition zone (5- to 10-millisecond duration) during which shocks reproducibly induced 2 to 5 extra beats (2.7 ± 0.8 premature ventricular contractions [PVCs]; mean $\pm$ SD; Fig. 3). Shock strengths of the two vulnerable periods were 234 ± 90 V for the low and 294 ± 100 V for the high shock strength (mean $\pm$ SD). The vulnerable period had a duration of 30 ± 14 milliseconds for the low shock strength (range from 15 to 60 milliseconds), and a duration of 34 ± 12 milliseconds for the high shock strength (range from 20 to 50 milliseconds; Table 1). There was no significant difference in the durations of the two vulnerable periods ($P>0.2$). The shortest coupling interval that induced VF (left limit of the vulnerable period) was 16 ± 17 milliseconds shorter for the high shock strength than for the low shock strength, and the longest coupling interval that induced VF (right limit of the vulnerable period) was 8 ± 12 milliseconds shorter for the high shock strength than for the low shock strength ($P<0.005$; Table 1). The vulnerable period was thus shifted leftward to shorter coupling intervals by the higher shock strength.

Dispersion of Repolarization

Dispersion of ventricular repolarization was 31 ± 12 milliseconds at 90% repolarization (range from 20 to 47 milliseconds), 32 ± 11 milliseconds at 70% repolarization (range from 21 to 60 milliseconds), and 38 ± 15 milliseconds at 50% repolarization (range from 22 to 65 milliseconds; $P=NS$; Table 2). Repolarization times ranged from 201 ± 19 milliseconds to 232 ± 17

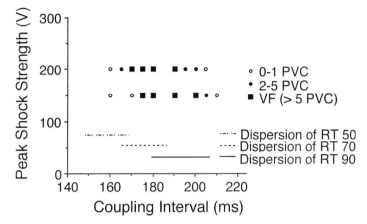

Figure 3. Example of the two vulnerable periods determined in one heart at baseline. Each dot represents a delivered shock and indicates the shock coupling interval (x axis), shock strength (y axis), and type of arrhythmia induced (coded by the dot type). Shocks that induced ventricular fibrillation (VF) are indicated by squares, shocks that induced nonsustained arrhythmias by small closed dots, and shocks that induced no arrhythmia by open dots. The vulnerable periods coincide with the dispersion of repolarization at 70% (vulnerable period for high shock strength) and 90% (vulnerable period for low shock strength). Dispersion of repolarization at 50% (RT 50) does not coincide with either of the two vulnerable periods.

milliseconds at 90% repolarization, from 188 ± 13 milliseconds to 220 ± 19 milliseconds at 70% repolarization, and from 166 ± 6 milliseconds to 203 ± 15 milliseconds at 50% repolarization. All differences between repolarization times at different repolarization levels were significant ($P<0.01$; Table 2).

Effects of d-Sotalol

d-Sotalol shifted both vulnerable periods to longer coupling intervals by an average of 29 ± 15 milliseconds ($P<0.05$) for both the high and the low shock strength. The duration of the vulnerable periods remained unchanged ($P=NS$; Table 1). The shift of the vulnerable period to shorter coupling intervals by the high shock strength as compared to the low shock strength was still significant after infusion of d-sotalol (Table 1).

d-Sotalol prolonged repolarization time of all MAPs at 50%, 70%, and 90% repolarization by 37 milliseconds, 37 milliseconds, and 40 milliseconds, respectively (Table 2). Activation time remained unchanged after addition of d-sotalol; prolongation of repolarization was hence caused by a prolongation of APD. Dispersion of repolarization of the MAPs was not significantly changed by d-sotalol at either of the 3 repolarization levels analyzed (Table 2) at the basic cycle length of 600 milliseconds.

Table 1

Shortest and Longest Coupling Intervals of Shocks
Inducing Ventricular Fibrillation at Baseline and After Addition of D-Sotalol

	Baseline Shortest CI [ms]	Baseline Longest CI [ms]	Baseline Duration [ms]	d-Sotalol Shortest CI [ms]	d-Sotalol Longest CI [ms]	d-Sotalol Duration [ms]
High shock strength	185±13.9	226±27.8	34.2±11.6	214±8.4	250±17	36±12.4
Low shock strength	201±25.6	232±24.7	30±13.5	230±17.6	265±26.5	35±16.5

All durations are given in milliseconds as mean ± standard deviation. CI = coupling interval.

Table 2
Shortest and Longest ATs, RT_{50}, RT_{70}, RT_{90}, and Dispersion of Repolarization During Steady State Pacing at Baseline and After Addition of D-Sotalol

	Baseline Shortest [ms]	Baseline Longest [ms]	Baseline Dispersion [ms]	d-Sotalol Shortest [ms]	d-Sotalol Longest [ms]	d-Sotalol Dispersion [ms]
AT	11.3±6.6	40.8±6.2	—	13.3±13.5	43.9±4.1	—
RT_{50}	166±6.4	203±15.1	38±14.8	193±17	235±21.4	42±18.7
RT_{70}	188±13.4	220±19	32.1±11.4	218±13.9	255±21	36.7±6.8
RT_{90}	201±19.1	232±16.8	31±11.8	240±17.6	277±21	36.7±16

All durations are given in milliseconds as mean ± standard deviation. Steady state pacing has a 600-ms cycle length. AT = activation time; RT_{50} = repolarization time at 50% repolarization; RT_{70} = repolarization time at 70% repolarization; RT_{90} = repolarization time at 90% repolarization.

Correlation of Vulnerable Periods with Dispersion of Repolarization

The left limit of the vulnerable period for the low shock strength coincided with the shortest repolarization time at 90% repolarization, and the left limit of the vulnerable period for the high shock strength coincided with the shortest repolarization time at 70% repolarization. Similarly, the right limit of the vulnerable period for the high shock strength coincided with the longest repolarization time at 70% repolarization, and the right limit of the vulnerable period for the low shock strength coincided with the longest repolarization time at 90% repolarization. The average differences were smaller than 10 milliseconds and not significantly different from zero (Tables 1 and 2). Linear regression analysis between the limits of the two vulnerable periods and the shortest and longest repolarization times at 70% and 90% repolarization using both baseline and d-sotalol data confirmed that 1) the shortest and longest repolarization times at 90% repolarization coincided with the vulnerable period for low shock strengths, and 2) the shortest and longest repolarization times at 70% repolarization coincided with the vulnerable period for high shock strengths (Fig. 4). Figure 5 summarizes these results graphically.

Upper and Lower Limits of Vulnerability

For every shock coupling interval, a discrete highest and lowest shock strength that induced VF could be determined. The ULV was significantly higher than the maximal strength of shocks at any other VF-inducing coupling interval, differing from the second highest VF-inducing shock strength by a mean of 40 ± 27 V ($P < 0.05$). Conversely, the shock strength of the LLV was significantly smaller than the shock strength at any other VF-inducing coupling intervals, differing from the second lowest VF-inducing shock strength by a mean of 39 ± 32 V ($P < 0.05$). The ULV and LLV therefore represented discrete points, in terms of coupling interval and of shock strength. Shocks delivered at the shock strength of the ULV or the LLV, but at 5 to 10 milliseconds shorter or longer coupling intervals, induced significantly less arrhythmias (ULV: 37 ± 36 versus 4 ± 3 PVC; LLV: 31 ± 25 versus 3 ± 2 PVC; $P < 0.001$).

Relation Between the ULV and the DFT

The DFT could be determined in 7 of 11 experiments. It was not significantly different from the ULV. The average difference was $3.5 \pm 10\%$ of the ULV ($P = $ NS; Table 3). The highest deviation of the DFT from the ULV was 20% of the ULV voltage. In all other experiments the differences were ≤10% of the ULV voltage (Table 3).

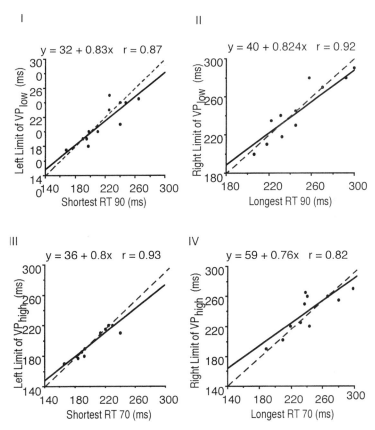

Figure 4. Linear regressions of the left and right limits of the two vulnerable periods with the shortest and longest repolarization times at 70% and 90% repolarization for the combined baseline and d-sotalol data in 7 hearts. The correlations were highly significant ($P<0.001$). Analysis of variance of the correlation coefficients showed that the regression lines were not significantly different from the line of identity ($P>0.2$). **I.** Correlation of the left limit of the vulnerable period for low shock strengths (VP_{low}) with the shortest repolarization time at 90% repolarization (RT 90). **II.** Correlation of the right limit of the vulnerable period for low shock strengths with the longest repolarization time at 90% repolarization. **III.** Correlation of the left limit of the vulnerable period for high shock strengths (VP_{high}) with the shortest repolarization time at 70% repolarization (RT 70). **IV.** Correlation of the right limit of the vulnerable period for high shock strengths with the longest repolarization time at 70% repolarization.

The Area of Vulnerability

When arrhythmic responses to single shocks were plotted as a function of shock coupling intervals and shock strengths, a highly homogenous *field* or area of vulnerability was disclosed, within which all VF-inducing shocks were clustered (Fig. 6). This area of vulnerability was surrounded by a relatively narrow transition zone; shocks applied within close proximity of the vulnerable field, ie, at 10-millisecond shorter or longer coupling intervals, or at 100 to 150 V higher or lower shock strengths, resulted in nonsustained arrhythmias or no arrhythmias. The spread between the shortest and longest arrhythmogenic coupling interval, ie, the maximal width of the vulnerable field, averaged 29 ± 7 milliseconds. The LLV shock strength was 210 ± 39 V, and the ULV shock strength 442 ± 42 V. The difference in shock strength between the ULV and the LLV, ie, the range of VF-inducing shock strengths, was 232 ± 57 V. A vulnerable field, defined by the ULV, LLV, shortest and longest VF-inducing coupling interval, approximated the shape of a rhomboid and comprised $92\pm7\%$ of all shocks inducing

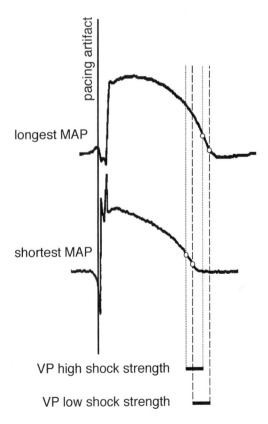

Figure 5. Summary of the correlations between repolarization and the vulnerable periods. Representative for the 7 MAP recordings, the MAPs showing the longest (top recording) and shortest (bottom recording) durations are plotted. The dashed lines mark the repolarization times at 90%, and the dotted lines the repolarization times at 70% repolarization. The dispersion is therefore delineated by the interval between the two dotted lines for 70% repolarization and between the two dashed lines at 90% repolarization. Below, the vulnerable periods are marked by two horizontal lines for the high shock strength (VP high shock strength) and low shock strength (VP low shock strength). The vulnerable periods are determined by dispersion of repolarization at the corresponding repolarization level.

Table 3

Comparison of ULV and DFT in V and Their Differences in Absolute
Values and in Percent of the ULV Voltage

	ULV[V]	DFT[V]	Δ[V]	Δ[%]
1	570	550	−20	−3.5
2	350	375	25	6.7
3	500	450	−50	−10
4	450	540	90	20
5	450	450	0	0
6	450	500	50	11.1
7	410	410	0	0
Average	454.3±69	467.9±65	13.6±46	3.5±10

DFT = defibrillation threshold; ULV = upper limit of vulnerability; V = peak shock voltage;
Δ = difference in absolute value; Δ[%] = difference in percent of ULV voltage.

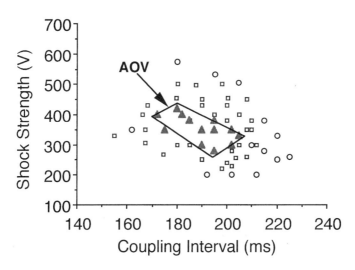

- ○ No Arrhythmia
- ▫ Non Sustained Arrhythmia
- ▲ Ventricular Fibrillation

Figure 6. Example of the 2-dimensional field of vulnerability in one heart. Shock responses are plotted as a function of coupling interval and shock strength. Lines were drawn by eye through the outer boundaries of the vulnerable field, which approximated a rhomboid.

VF, while greater than 95% of the shocks applied outside of the field did not induce VF. An "average" vulnerable field, from a summary of the data from all 11 experiments, is shown in Figure 7. An absolute vulnerable field existed for all experiments between 300 and 350 V and between 190 and 200 milliseconds: within these ranges, nothing but VF was induced.

The Vulnerable Field Rhomboid Has a Leftward Tilt

The shortest average VF-inducing coupling interval occurred at shock strengths 50±67 V higher than the longest average VF-inducing coupling interval ($P<0.01$). Likewise, the average ULV occurred at coupling intervals 7±10 milliseconds shorter than the average LLV ($P<0.05$). This difference corresponded to 24% of the maximal width of the vulnerable field. Both the vertical shift of the left corner of the vulnerable field rhomboid over its right corner and the horizontal shift of the ULV leftward of the LLV

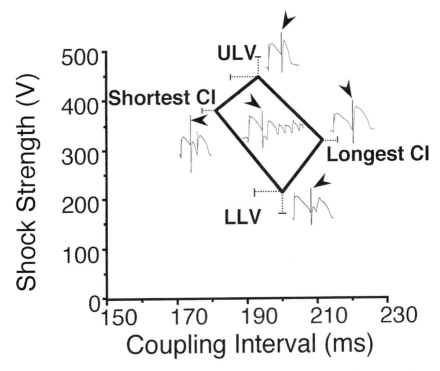

Figure 7. Average vulnerable field or area of vulnerability (AOV). The upper limit of vulnerability (ULV), the lower limit of vulnerability (LLV), and the shortest and longest ventricular fibrillation-inducing coupling intervals are shown in a plot of coupling interval versus shock strength averaged from 11 experiments (mean ± SD). The MAP recordings displayed within and outside this field show typical shock responses in one of the 7 MAPs. Arrows indicate the shock artifact.

allowed an approximation of the vulnerable field by a leftward tilted rhomboid (Fig. 7). VF was induced by $92\pm7\%$ of all shocks applied within the boundaries of this rhomboid, while greater than 95% of the shocks applied outside of this rhomboid did not induce VF. The shift of the vulnerable period to shorter coupling intervals with higher shock strengths is concordant with this leftward tilt of the area of vulnerability.

ECG Data

The ECG data are summarized in Table 4. d-Sotalol prolonged repolarization, as indicated by the prolonged intervals from the pacing artifact to the points on the T wave measured. QRS duration and morphology were not changed by d-sotalol, indicating an essentially unchanged conduction velocity and activation sequence. Both vulnerable periods comprised the peak of the T wave. The mid upslope of the T wave occurred within the vulnerable period for high shock strengths. The vulnerable period for the high shock strength began earlier than the mid upslope of the T wave and ended shortly after the peak of the T wave. The vulnerable period for the low shock strength began before the peak of the T wave, and extended to coupling intervals shortly before the mid downslope of the T wave. The correlation between the right and left limits of the vulnerable periods and the T wave parameters was weak (r=0.6 to 0.72; intercept >50 milliseconds.). The T wave also did not provide a marker for the differentiation between the two vulnerable periods. In the experiments that aimed to determine the area of vulnerability, mean ECG intervals were 167 ± 10 milliseconds from the pacing artifact to the mid upslope of the T wave, 205 ± 9 milliseconds from the pacing artifact to the T wave peak, and 224 ± 9 milliseconds from the pacing artifact to the mid downslope of the T wave. In all hearts, the vulnerable field fell within the interval between the mid upslope and the mid downslope of the T wave. The earliest VF-inducing

Table 4
ECG Intervals at Baseline and After Addition
of D-Sotalol at 600-ms Cycle Length

	Baseline [ms]	D-Sotalol [ms]
QRS Duration	18 ± 30	19 ± 32
Pacing Spike to Mid Upslope of T Wave	174.5 ± 22.5	244 ± 19.8
Pacing Spike to Peak of T Wave	220.1 ± 27.2	280.7 ± 17.5
Pacing Spike to Mid Downslope of T Wave	241 ± 28	302 ± 14.2
Mid Upslope to Peak of T Wave	45.6 ± 8.3	36.2 ± 10.6
Mid Upslope to Mid Downslope of T Wave	76.4 ± 9.8	57.5 ± 11.5

All durations are given in milliseconds as mean $\pm$ standard deviation.

coupling interval and the ULV fell within the interval between the mid upslope and the peak of the T wave in 10 of 11 hearts. The average coupling interval of the LLV was shorter than the peak of the T wave in 6 of 11 hearts, and longer than the peak of the T wave in 5 of 11 hearts. The longest VF-inducing coupling interval occurred between the peak and the mid downslope of the T wave in all hearts.

Discussion

The present investigation of the vulnerability of the myocardium to single shocks yielded several relevant findings: 1) The dispersion of ventricular repolarization, as determined by multiple simultaneous MAP recordings, correlates closely with the vulnerable period to single electrical shocks. 2) Higher shock strengths shift the vulnerable period to the left, ie, to shorter coupling intervals as measured from the pacing artifact to the shocks inducing VF. 3) The vulnerable period for low shock strengths just above the fibrillation threshold is approximated by the shortest and longest repolarization time at the 90% level, while the vulnerable period for high shock strengths just below the ULV is approximated by the shortest and longest repolarization time at the 70% level. The direct assessment of dispersion of ventricular repolarization by multiple MAP recordings was found to be a better predictor of the vulnerable period than the T wave of the surface ECG. 4) In this precisely controlled experimental model, a homogeneous area of vulnerability exists, defined by the shortest and longest coupling interval that induced VF, the LLV, and the ULV. For monophasic shocks, this area of vulnerability resembles a rhomboid tilted toward shorter coupling intervals, ie, to the left. 4) d-Sotalol prolonged MAP durations at multiple sites and shifted the vulnerable period to longer coupling intervals without changing the dispersion of repolarization or its correlation to the vulnerable periods.

Correlation of the Vulnerable Period with Dispersion of Repolarization

A number of studies[3,33,34] have reported an indirect link between the dispersion of repolarization and the susceptibility to arrhythmias. A correlation of the vulnerable period with the dispersion of repolarization has previously been hypothesized[8,9,12] for the induction of VF by a local stimulus. The present study is the first to demonstrate a direct correlation between the vulnerable period for high-energy field shocks and the dispersion of ventricular repolarization measured directly using multiple MAP recordings.

Leftward Shift of the Vulnerable Period with Higher Shock Strengths

Previous studies[3,4,6,35] have referred to one single vulnerable period without regard to possible changes of the vulnerable period caused by different shock strengths. The present study determined the vulnerable period for two different shock strengths: one close to the fibrillation threshold, or LLV, and one close to the ULV. The high shock strength caused a significant leftward shift of the vulnerable period to shorter coupling intervals, but did not affect its duration. Concordant with this leftward shift, the optimum correlation between the boundaries of the vulnerable period and the dispersion of repolarization shifted from the 90% repolarization level for low shock strengths to the 70% repolarization level for high shock strengths. This is in keeping with the strength interval relation[10,11,36] and with studies[37,38] showing that refractoriness, as well as partial and complete excitability of the myocardium, are closely related to its repolarization level.

Mechanism of Vulnerability to Electrical Field Shocks

Epicardial mapping studies[6,39-41] have related the induction of VF by a single shock to reentry of multiple activation wave fronts in different patterns of multiple excitation and propagation. A shock encountering tissue with dispersed repolarization[23,40,42-44] may induce new action potentials in regions with short repolarization times, and prolong action potentials in regions with long repolarization times. Thus, a globally applied field shock[23,40,42-44] can initiate premature action potentials with slow conduction in some areas while finding other areas refractory. This is known[6,39,40] to facilitate reentry of multiple activation wave fronts and induction of VF. The leftward shift of the vulnerable period with higher shock strengths can be explained accordingly: the myocardial responsiveness to higher shock strengths is increased[10,11,36] in every region of the myocardium. Due to this effect, a similar pattern of slow excitation and action potential prolongation[23,42] may be induced by a shock applied at less complete repolarization levels, and thus at shorter shock coupling intervals. See chapter 45 for a more detailed discussion of this mechanism. Shibata et al[6] reported that reentry after induction of VF by T wave shocks occurs in different regions for high-strength shocks than for low-strength shocks. This finding is compatible with the present results, as the shortest MAP at 70% repolarization was sometimes not the shortest MAP at 90% repolarization, due to different repolarization slopes.

Correlation of the Vulnerable Period with T Wave Parameters

The coupling intervals of shocks inducing VF for clinical determination of the DFT and the ULV[4,7,12] are usually determined by analyzing the T wave of the surface ECG. The present data confirm[4,12] the approximate concurrence of the vulnerable period with the mid upslope and the peak of the T wave. However, the T wave was not as strong a predictor of the vulnerable period, as was the dispersion of repolarization measured by multiple MAP recordings. The T wave also did not differentiate between the vulnerable period for high and low shock strengths.

Effects of d-Sotalol

In accordance with previous observations[13,14,16] d-sotalol prolonged APD. Prolongation was seen at all MAP recording sites in this study. This was associated with a shift of both the dispersion of repolarization and the vulnerable periods to longer coupling intervals. The range of dispersion of repolarization and the spread of the vulnerable periods were not affected by d-sotalol, nor was the correlation between the two. Therefore, reduction of QT dispersion by the racemate dl-sotalol in patients[15,45,46] cannot be explained by the present findings in the isolated heart, and may rather be attributed to modification of other factors that influence dispersion in the in situ heart, eg, autonomic influences or response to heart rate changes. Experimental studies[17] showed that d-sotalol does not alter vulnerability, whereas dl-sotalol increases the DFT. In accordance with those results, the present study did not show an alteration of arrhythmia vulnerability by d-sotalol. The premature ending of the SWORD trial,[20,47] due to apparent proarrhythmic effects of d-sotalol, concurs with these results.

The Area or "Field" of Vulnerability

When the vulnerability of the heart to single electrical field shocks is defined 2-dimensionally by shock strength and coupling interval, a homogeneous "area of vulnerability" can be delineated between the right and left limit of the vulnerable periods, the ULV, and the LLV (Fig. 7). In this model, only shocks within this area of vulnerability induced VF.

Homogeneity of the Vulnerable Area

Of shocks applied within the extensions of the vulnerable area, $92 \pm 7\%$ induced VF. This indicates that the vulnerable area is homogeneous within its boundaries and provides a high degree of predictability for arrhythmia induction. An area of optimal VF inducibility has been observed,[6,12] but these studies failed to demonstrate in a systematic fashion this degree of uniformity and the shape of this area. In this controlled steady state model, an absolute area of vulnerability existed (190 to 200 milliseconds; 300 to 350 V), in contrast to other studies[6] in less controlled models, even with the relatively small ranges of dispersion and arrhythmogenic shock strengths in this model.

Characteristics of the ULV and LLV

An LLV for field shocks has been determined in dogs.[12,48] A narrowing of the vulnerable period toward the LLV has been documented[12] before. Since its correlation with the DFT was suggested,[49] the ULV has been studied intensively and has been found to vary[6,50] for different shock coupling intervals, suggesting the possibility of a "maximum ULV." In the present study, a definite, discrete highest and lowest arrhythmogenic shock strength was found for each coupling interval within the vulnerable periods. Only the maximum shock strength of shocks applied at variable shock coupling intervals can be regarded as the true ULV, and only the minimum shock strength at varying coupling intervals as the true LLV. According to this definition and our present data, both the ULV and LLV are defined by discrete shock voltages and coupling intervals.

The correlation between ULV and DFT was excellent in the present study (deviation ≤10% in all hearts except one), with an average difference of 3.5% of the ULV shock strength, supporting the growing evidence that these two shock strengths correlate.

Are ULV and LLV Reproducible and Deterministic?

The ventricular DFT is commonly described[51,52] by a probability function. The same concept of probability has been applied to its correlate, the ULV[7,53] and the LLV.[28] In this isolated, controlled heart model of relatively small mass, conditioned by steady state pacing and subjected to relatively uniform shock fields, the ULV and the LLV were distinct and reproducible. This suggests that both the ULV and the LLV may be deterministic rather than probabilistic variables. Deale et al[54] showed how probabilistic observations of the DFT could be produced by complex deterministic models. In an earlier study, Fabiato et al[48] found fixed values for a 100% success rate in defibrillation and for equivalents of ULV and LLV within the same canine heart, while values between different dogs varied greatly. Probabilistic appearance of the ULV in other studies might therefore be explained by instability of electrophysiologic variables, specifically those that change dispersion of repolarization, rather than by random changes in vulnerability. Defining new factors influencing induction and termination of VF, such as dispersion of repolarization,[23,42] changes in autonomic tone, and shock-substrate interactions, might result in better predicting ULV and LLV, and eventually the ability to predict defibrillation success.

Height and Width of the Vulnerable Field

Compared to other models,[6,12] ULV voltages in the present study were relatively low and the LLV voltages were relatively high, resulting in a relatively small vulnerable field amplitude. This may be due to 1) the small mass of the rabbit heart as compared to other species, combined with extrathoracic shock electrode positions[32,55,56]; 2) the resulting relatively small dispersion of repolarization; and 3) the relatively homogenous shock field.

Methodologic Considerations

A limitation of the isolated rabbit heart model is its tendency to spontaneously convert from induced VF. The definition of VF used in this study follows that of several other groups,[32,57,58] and was confirmed by two observations in this study: 1) the highest number of extra beats induced in the nonsustained arrhythmia group was 3.7 ± 1 PVCs (range from 1 to 5), while the lowest number of extra beats in the VF group was 10.2 ± 7 PVCs (range from 6 to 30), showing a sharp increase (6.4 ± 7 PVCs) in the number of extra beats induced above 5 PVCs, and 2) ECG characteristics were similar between episodes of nonsustained and sustained VF.

While the correlations of repolarization times at 70% with the vulnerable period for high shock strengths and at 90% with the vulnerable period for low shock strengths were excellent in this study (Fig. 4), repolarization times at different repolarization levels will probably yield similar correlations with vulnerable periods for different shock strengths. The somewhat shorter duration of the vulnerable periods in the experiments to determine the area of vulnerability can probably be explained by a less detailed protocol to search for the left and right limits of vulnerability as compared to the effort made to determine upper and lower limits of vulnerability.

The ventricular rabbit heart cell has different channel distributions [59] than the human heart, resulting in a differently shaped[60] electrical restitution curve. In addition, our preparation was deprived of autonomic influences. The results obtained in this study therefore require validation in the human heart prior to clinical application.

VF induction by single shocks probably can be fully understood only when local repolarization patterns and shock field gradients, autonomic influences, and anatomic factors such as tissue anisotropy are measured. We did not measure voltage gradients during the ongoing experiment, but determined them within the bath before the isolated heart was placed inside. There was a highly uniform distribution of voltage gradients in the center of the bath. In most clinical settings, the distribution of the shock field is highly asymmetric. Furthermore, as mentioned above, the preparation used for these studies was deprived of autonomic influences. It is hence possible that the precise and reproducible timing of ULV and LLV like they were seen in this model may differ for clinical settings. Different shock waveforms, eg, biphasic[61] shock forms, can also influence the shape of the area of vulnerability. This effect was not investigated in this study.

Conclusion

This study directly confirms the hypothesized influence of repolarization on the induction of arrhythmias by electrical field shocks, and demonstrates that d-sotalol fails to reduce vulnerability to T wave shocks, concordant with the recently published[20,47] negative result of the SWORD trial.

It is probably the interaction of local shock field gradients, shock polarity, tissue anisotropy, and local repolarization levels that determines the local response to a shock, and whether or not arrhythmias are induced. Even the most sophisticated experimental setups do not provide simultaneous monitoring of all these variables. The upper and lower limits of vulnerability might hence be discrete, reproducible values if all factors that influence vulnerability are kept constant, but this hypothesis remains to be tested. The mechanism of induction of VF by single electrical shocks has still not been fully understood 100 years after its first description.

Acknowledgments The authors wish to thank Drs. Michael R. Franz and Ross Fletcher, VA Medical Center, Washington DC, USA, and Drs. Günter Breithardt and Martin Borggrefe, Westfälische Wilhelms-Universität, Münster, Germany, for their support of this work.

References

1. Prevost JL, Batelli F. Sur quelques effets des décharges electriques sur le coeur des mammifères. *Compte Rendu Acad Sci* 1899;129:651.
2. King B. *The Effect of Electric Shock on Heart Action with Special Reference to Varying Susceptibility in Different Parts of the Cardiac Cycle* [PhD thesis]. New York: Columbia University, Aberdeen Press; 1934.
3. Wiggers CJ, Wegren R. Ventricular fibrillation due to single localized induction in condenser shock supplied during the vulnerable phase of ventricular systole. *Am J Physiol* 1940;128:500-505.

4. Chen PS, Feld GK, Kriett JM, et al. Relation between upper limit of vulnerability and defibrillation threshold in humans. *Circulation* 1993;88:186-192.

5. Hwang C, Swerdlow CD, Kass RM, et al. Upper limit of vulnerability reliably predicts transvenous DFT in humans. *PACE* 1994;17:789.

6. Shibata N, Chen PS, Dixon EG, et al. Influence of shock strength and timing on induction of ventricular arrhythmias in dogs. *Am J Physiol* 1988;255:H891-H901.

7. Walker RG, Idriss SF, Malkin RA, et al. Comparison of methods for determining the upper limit of vulnerability. *Circulation* 1993;88:I-593. Abstract.

8. Burgess MJ. Relation of ventricular repolarization to electrocardiographic T wave-form and arrhythmia vulnerability. *Am J Physiol* 1979;236:402.

9. Zipes DP. Electrophysiological mechanisms involved in ventricular fibrillation. *Circulation* 1975;52:120-130.

10. Davidenko JM, Levi RJ, Maid G, et al. Rate dependence and supernormality in excitability of guinea pig papillary muscle. *Am J Physiol* 1990;259:H290-H299.

11. Michelson EL, Spear JF, Moore EN. Strength-interval relations in a chronic canine model of myocardial infarction. Implications for the interpretation of electrophysiologic studies. *Circulation* 1981;63:1158-1165.

12. Lesigne C, Levy B, Saumont R, et al. An energy-time analysis of ventricular fibrillation and defibrillation thresholds with internal electrodes. *Med Biol Eng* 1976;14:617-622.

13. Kidwell GA, Gonzalez MD. Effects of flecainide and D-sotalol on myocardial conduction and refractoriness: Relation to antiarrhythmic and proarrhythmic drug effects. *J Cardiovasc Pharmacol* 1993;21:621-632.

14. Brachmann J, Beyer T, Schmitt C, et al. Electrophysiologic and antiarrhythmic effects of D-sotalol. *J Cardiovasc Pharmacol* 1992;20:S91-S95.

15. Hohnloser SH, Woosley RL. Sotalol. *N Engl J Med* 1994;331:31-38.

16. Huikuri HV, Yli-Mayry S. Frequency dependent effects of d-sotalol and amiodarone on the action potential duration of the human right ventricle. *PACE* 1992;15:2103-2107.

17. Kwan YW, Solca AM, Gwilt M, et al. Comparative antifibrillatory effects of d- and dl-sotalol in normal and ischaemic ventricular muscle of the cat. *J Cardiovasc Pharmacol* 1990;15:233-238.

18. Roden DM. Usefulness of sotalol for life-threatening ventricular arrhythmias. *Am J Cardiol* 1993;72:51A-55A.

19. Schwartz J, Crocker K, Wynn J, et al. The antiarrhythmic effects of d-sotalol. *Am Heart J* 1987;114:539-544.

20. Waldo AL, Camm AJ, Deruyter H, et al. Effect of d-sotalol on mortality in patients with left ventricular dysfunction after recent and remote myocardial infarction. *Lancet* 1996;348:7-12.

21. Behrens S, Li C, Kirchhof P, et al. Reduced arrhythmogenicity of biphasic versus monophasic T-wave shocks. Implications for defibrillation efficacy. *Circulation* 1996;94:1974-1980.

22. Fabritz CL, Kirchhof PF, Behrens S, et al. Myocardial vulnerability to T wave shocks: Relation to shock strength, shock coupling interval, and dispersion of ventricular repolarization. *J Cardiovasc Electrophysiol* 1996;7:231-242.

23. Kirchhof PF, Fabritz CL, Behrens S, et al. Induction of ventricular fibrillation by T wave field-shocks in the isolated perfused rabbit heart: Role of nonuniform shock responses. *Basic Res Cardiol* 1997;92:35-44.

24. Kirchhof PF, Fabritz CL, Zabel M, et al. The vulnerable period for low and high energy T wave shocks: Role of dispersion of repolarisation and effect of d-sotalol. *J Cardiovasc Res* 1996;31:953-962.

25. Franz MR, Burkhoff D, Spurgeon H, et al. In vitro validation of a new cardiac catheter technique for recording monophasic action potentials. *Eur Heart J* 1986;7:34-41.

26. Franz MR, Chin MC, Sharkey HR, et al. A new single catheter technique for simultaneous measurement of action potential duration and refractory period in vivo. *J Am Coll Cardiol* 1990;16:878-886.

27. Franz MR, Cima R, Wang D, et al. Electrophysiological effects of myocardial stretch and mechanical determinants of stretch-activated arrhythmias [published erratum appears in *Circulation* 1992;86:1663]. *Circulation* 1992; 86:968-978.

28. Cha YM, Peters BB, Birgersdotter-Green U, et al. A reappraisal of ventricular fibrillation threshold testing. *Am J Physiol* 1993;264:H1005-H1010.

29. Daubert JP, Frazier DW, Wolf PD, et al. Response of relatively refractory canine myocardium to monophasic and biphasic shocks. *Circulation* 1991;84:2522-2538.

30. Franz MR, Kirchhof PF, Fabritz CL, et al. Computer analysis of monophasic action potential recordings: Manual validation and clinically pertinent applications. *PACE* 1995;18:1666-1678.

31. Jones DL, Klein GJ, Gulamhusein S, et al. The repetitive ventricular response: Relationship to ventricular fibrillation threshold in dogs. *PACE* 1983;6:1258-1267.

32. MacConaill M. Ventricular fibrillation thresholds in Langendorff perfused rabbit hearts: All or none effect of low potassium concentration. *Cardiovasc Res* 1987;21:463-468.

33. Brugada J, Brugada P, Boersma L, et al. On the mechanisms of ventricular tachycardia acceleration during programmed electrical stimulation. *Circulation* 1991;83:1621-1629.

34. Taggart P, Sutton P, Lab M, et al. Interplay between adrenaline and interbeat interval on ventricular repolarisation in intact heart in vivo. *Cardiovasc Res* 1990;24:884-895.

35. Kolman BS, Verrier RL, Lown B. The effect of vagus nerve stimulation upon vulnerability of the canine ventricle: Role of sympathetic-parasympathetic interactions. *Circulation* 1975;52:578-585.

36. Langberg JJ, Calkins H, Sousa J, et al. Effects of drive train stimulus intensity on ventricular refractoriness in humans. *Circulation* 1991;84:181-187.

37. Franz MR, Costard A. Frequency-dependent effects of quinidine on the relationship between action potential duration and refractoriness in the canine heart in situ. *Circulation* 1988;77:1177-1184.

38. Franz MR, Swerdlow CD, Liem LB, et al. Cycle length dependence of human action potential duration in vivo. Effects of single extrastimuli, sudden sustained rate acceleration and deceleration, and different steady-state frequencies. *J Clin Invest* 1988;82:972-979.

39. Chen PS, Wolf PD, Dixon EG, et al. Mechanism of ventricular vulnerability to single premature stimuli in open-chest dogs. *Circ Res* 1988;62:1191-1209.

40. Frazier DW, Wolf PD, Wharton JM, et al. Stimulus-induced critical point. Mechanism for electrical initiation of reentry in normal canine myocardium. *J Clin Invest* 1989;83:1039-1052.

41. Zhou X, Daubert JP, Wolf PD, et al. Epicardial mapping of ventricular defibrillation with monophasic and biphasic shocks in dogs. *Circ Res* 1993;72:145-160.

42. Behrens S, Li C, Fabritz CL, et al. Shock-induced dispersion of ventricular repolarization: Implications for the induction of ventricular fibrillation and the

upper limit of vulnerability [In Process Citation]. *J Cardiovasc Electrophysiol* 1997;8:998-1008.

43. Dillon SM. Optical recordings in the rabbit heart show that defibrillation strength shocks prolong the duration of depolarization and the refractory period. *Circ Res* 1991;69:842-856.

44. Knisley SB, Smith WM, Ideker RE. Effect of field stimulation on cellular repolarization in rabbit myocardium. Implications for reentry induction. *Circ Res* 1992;70:707-715.

45. Campbell RWF, Furniss SS. Practical considerations in the use of sotalol for ventricular tachycardia and ventricular fibrillation. *Am J Cardiol* 1993;72:80A-85A.

46. Day CP, McComb JM, Matthews J, et al. Reduction in QT dispersion by sotalol following myocardial infarction. *Eur Heart J* 1991;12:423-427.

47. Waldo AL. Effect of d-sotalol on mortality in patients with left ventricular dysfunction after recent and remote myocardial infarction [Erratum]. *Lancet* 1996;348:416.

48. Fabiato A, Coumel P, Gourgon R, et al. Le seuil de réponse synchrone des fibres myocardiqes. Application à la comparaison expérimentale de l'efficacité des différentes choc électriques de défibrillation. *Arch Mal Coeur* 1967;60:527-544.

49. Chen PS, Shibata N, Dixon EG, et al. Comparison of the defibrillation threshold and the upper limit of ventricular vulnerability. *Circulation* 1986;73:1022-1028.

50. Chen PS, Feld GK, Mower MM, et al. Effects of pacing rate and timing of defibrillation shock on the relation between the defibrillation threshold and the upper limit of vulnerability in open chest dogs. *J Am Coll Cardiol* 1991;18:1555-1563.

51. Davy JM, Fain ES, Dorian P, et al. The relationship between successful defibrillation and delivered energy in open-chest dogs: Reappraisal of the "defibrillation threshold" concept. *Am Heart J* 1987;113:77-84.

52. Jones DL, Irish WD, Klein GJ. Defibrillation efficacy. Comparison of defibrillation threshold versus dose-response curve determination. *Circ Res* 1991;69:45-51.

53. Huang J, Kenknight BH, Walcott GP, et al. Effects of transvenous electrode polarity and waveform duration on the relationship between defibrillation threshold and upper limit of vulnerability. *Circulation* 1997;96:1351-1359.

54. Deale OC, Wesley R Jr, Morgan D, et al. Nature of defibrillation: Determinism versus probabilism. *Am J Physiol* 1990;259:H1544-H1550.

55. Guse PA, Walcott GP, Rollins DL, et al. Defibrillation electrode configurations developed from cardiac mapping that combine biphasic shocks with sequential timing. *Am Heart J* 1992;124:1491-1500.

56. Wharton JM, Richard VJ, Murry CE, et al. Electrophysiological effects of monophasic and biphasic stimuli in normal and infarcted dogs. *PACE* 1990;13:1158-1172.

57. Cooper RA, Alferness CA, Smith WM, et al. Internal cardioversion of atrial fibrillation in sheep. *Circulation* 1993;87:1673-1686.

58. Merillat JC, Lakatta EG, Hano O, et al. Role of calcium and the calcium channel in the initiation and maintenance of ventricular fibrillation. *Circ Res* 1990;67:1115-1123.

59. Brown HF, Noble D, Noble SJ, et al. The relationship between the transient inward current (TI) and other components of slow inward current in mammalian cardiac muscle. *Jpn Heart J* 1986;1:127-142.

60. Kurz RW, Ren XL, Franz MR. Dispersion and delay of electrical restitution in the globally ischaemic heart. *Eur Heart J* 1994;15:547-554.
61. Behrens S, Li C, Kirchhof PF, et al. Reduced arrhythmogeneity of biphasic versus monophasic T wave shocks: Implications for defibrillation efficacy. *Circulation* 1996;94:1674-1680.

26

Are Newer Class III Antiarrhythmic Drugs Better?

Experimental and Clinical Data

Claus Schmitt, MD, Juergen Schreieck, MD and Bernhard Zrenner, MD

The Challenge to Develop New Class III Antiarrhythmic Agents

The dilemma of current pharmacologic antiarrhythmic treatment is that only two types of antiarrhythmic agents, β-blockers and amiodarone, now appear to offer arrhythmia mortality reduction by preventing ventricular fibrillation in patients with cardiac disease. Sotalol and amiodarone, two complex class III antiarrhythmic agents, were shown to be effective in reducing symptomatic ventricular tachycardias.[1] The reduction of life-threatening arrhythmias and sudden death in patients at increased risk was shown for amiodarone in large placebo-controlled trials (EMIAT[2] and CAMIAT[3]), and was suggested for sotalol in a large non-placebo–controlled trial (ESVEM[4]). However, several other large controlled trials with both drugs did not find a significant reduction in overall mortality (for sotalol[5]; for amiodarone: EMIAT,[2] CAMIAT,[3] and CHF-STAT[6]). Nevertheless, a recent meta-analysis of 13 randomized controlled trials of prophylactic amiodarone in patients with recent myocardial infarction and congestive heart failure found a small but significant reduction in total mortality of 13% with amiodarone.[7] Since the complex action of sotalol and, especially,

From Franz MR (ed): *Monophasic Action Potentials: Bridging Cell and Bedside.* ©Futura Publishing Company, Inc., Armonk, NY, 2000.

amiodarone is responsible for many adverse effects, the challenge was to develop so-called pure class III antiarrhythmic drugs. These agents, like d-sotalol, ibutilide, and dofetilide, have been designed to achieve selective action potential prolongation. The responsible mechanisms are the inhibition of repolarizing K^+ currents and, for ibutilide, an additional prolongation of the slowly inactivating, inward sodium current.

The following lessons were learned from clinical studies with these so-called pure class III antiarrhythmic drugs. First, these pure class III antiarrhythmics seem to be unsafe. In particular, the SWORD trial[8] demonstrated an excess mortality in postinfarction patients treated with d-sotalol. Second, the rather complex action of amiodarone and sotalol improve efficacy and safety of both drugs.

However, the question arises as to whether selective action potential prolongation per se is an effective and safe mechanism. In light of the recently disappointing results, especially of the SWORD study,[8] the development of many pure class III antiarrhythmic agents (such as E-4031, MS-551, almokalant, MK 499, ambasilide, sematilide, and tedisamil) has been stopped. The only pure class III agents in further clinical development are dofetilide, azimilide, and ibutilide. Ibutilide is the first so-called pure class III antiarrhythmic that was introduced into clinical use for pharmacologic conversion of atrial flutter and fibrillation.[1]

Clinical Studies

Efficacy of Class III Antiarrhythmic Drugs for the Treatment of Ventricular Tachyarrhythmias and for Improving Survival

Although 18 years have passed since Edvardsson et al[9] confirmed the class III effect of sotalol in humans with monophasic action potential (MAP) recordings, there is still a controversial debate about the role of its class III effect in relation to its β-blocking activity.

A recent reevaluation of the ESVEM trial[10] tried to analyze the role of the class III effect of sotalol in comparison to the combined use of β-blockers and class I drugs. It appeared that the reduction in mortality found in the sotalol group, in comparison with class I antiarrhythmics, was similar to the use of other beta-blockers in the presence of class I antiarrhythmic agents. The reduction in mortality and sudden death due to the empirical and prophylactic treatment with β-blockers is well defined. The reevaluation of the ESVEM trial, like many other studies, suggests that sudden death and ventricular tachycardia have different mechanisms and that only the incidence of the latter is reduced by class III antiarrhythmics. This is in line with electrophysiologic studies that demonstrate that suppression of inducible sustained ventricular tachycardias with sotalol does not predict efficacy for the reduction of sudden death.[11] Notably, in a small prospective randomized study, sotalol was not superior to a β-blocker (metoprolol) in preventing the recurrence of spontaneous ventricular arrhythmias or in the suppression of the inducibility of ventricular tachycardias.[12] Moreover, in two small prospective randomized studies, sotalol was not superior or worse than metoprolol for preventing the recurrence of ventricular tachycardias or ventricular fibrillation in patients with an implantable cardioverter defibrillator (ICD).[13,14] Therefore, although sotalol is effective in suppressing ventricular tachycardias, strong evidence is still missing as to whether the class III effect of sotalol is beneficial for this indication. There is only strong evidence that the class III effect of sotalol can be detrimental, demonstrated by the SWORD study and by its potential proarrhythmic response.[15]

Comparison of the efficacy of class III drugs for reduction of ventricular arrhythmias, sudden death, and overall mortality is difficult and limited by the lack of large randomized, controlled trials that directly compare different class III antiarrhythmic drugs. One small comparison trial showed no difference between empirical treatment with sotalol or amiodarone with respect to malignant ventricular arrhythmias.[16] In another small prospective randomized study in patients with inducible ventricular tachycardias, a high dose of amiodarone (1.8 g during 10 days) reduced the inducibility of ventricular tachycardias at a higher rate than a high dose of sotalol (480 mg/day). Inducibility was suppressed in 41% of patients in the amiodarone group versus 24% in the sotalol group.[17] A retrospective analysis of the efficacy of amiodarone versus sotalol had similar outcomes for the suppression of inducible ventricular tachycardias.[18] However, this issue should be considered unsettled, and a definitive answer must await further data.[19]

Dofetilide, a pure class III antiarrhythmic drug that is in clinical evaluation, is a methanesulfonanilide derivative and, like d-sotalol, an I_{Kr} blocker.[20] Dofetilide was recently shown to be as effective as sotalol in the suppression of inducible ventricular tachycardias in patients with coronary artery disease who were suffering from symptomatic ventricular tachyarrhythmias.[20a] In the long-term follow-up, antiarrhythmic efficacy and proarrhythmic events of dofetilide and sotalol were similar; however, the tolerability was better for dofetilide due to more cardiac and noncardiac adverse effects of sotalol not related to the antiarrhythmic effect. The DIAMOND studies[21] are two placebo-controlled survival studies of dofetilide in patients either with congestive heart failure or after acute myocardial infarction within the previous 7 days. The studies, which included a total of 3038 patients, were concluded in 1996. Preliminary results[22] indicate that the overall survival was similar in both studies for the placebo group and the dofetilide group. A similar survival study of patients after myocardial infarction and a reduced left ventricular ejection fraction of 15% to 35%

with another pure class III antiarrhythmic drug, azimilide, was recently initiated (ALIVE).

No definite conclusions can be drawn regarding the relative efficacy between any class III antiarrhythmic drugs, not even between the commonly used sotalol and amiodarone. On the basis of currently available experimental data of the new class III antiarrhythmics dofetilide and azimilide, as well as for newer drugs in development, a significantly improved outcome for long-term overall survival with antiarrhythmic treatment cannot be expected, since the mechanisms of action are similar. Future development must focus primarily on the safety of new antiarrhythmic drugs. A better understanding of the mechanisms for proarrhythmia will be the basis for such a development.

Efficacy of Class III Antiarrhythmic Drugs for the Conversion of Atrial Flutter and Fibrillation

In light of recent results demonstrating that implantable defibrillators are superior to antiarrhythmic agents for increasing overall survival,[23,24] the attention to class III agents has focused more and more on their role in the treatment of supraventricular tachyarrhythmias. In particular, the treatment of the most common arrhythmia, atrial fibrillation, is still a domain of pharmacologic treatment. Table 1 gives an overview of the efficacy of class III antiarrhythmics for acute conversion of atrial fibrillation.

Although significant, only small success rates have been achieved for the acute conversion of atrial fibrillation to sinus rhythm with complex class III agents (amiodarone, sotalol[25]). Relatively high success rates have been demonstrated with ibutilide[26,27] and dofetilide[28,29] in placebo-controlled trials; however, differences in trial design and eligibility hamper comparison of different agents. In particular, the duration of atrial fibrillation predicts the success rate of conversion. For oral sotalol, a conversion rate of 52% was reported for atrial fibrillation with recent onset (<48 hours duration),[30] while longer lasting atrial fibrillation could only be converted at a rate of 20% in non-placebo–controlled studies.[31] However, only a small placebo-controlled study has been performed with sotalol for that purpose, showing no significant conversion of atrial fibrillation for sotalol at doses of 1.5 mg/kg.[32] Randomized trials comparing amiodarone or racemic sotalol with class Ia agents (procainamide, quinidine) for acute pharmacologic conversion of atrial fibrillation found that amiodarone was not better than the class Ia agents, and sotalol had a even lower efficacy rate for cardioversion.[25] In contrast, ibutilide (iv) was shown to be significantly more effective than procainamide in acute conversion of atrial fibrillation.[33] In two large placebo-controlled trials, ibutilide achieved a conversion of atrial flutter

Table 1

Acute Pharmacologic Conversion of Atrial Fibrillation Randomized Controlled Trials

Drug	No. Pts.	Success	Comparison Agent	Comparison Agent Success (%)	Reference	Year
Sotalol (iv)	16	13%	placebo	14%	Sung[32]	1995
Sotalol (po)	25	20%	quinidine (po)	60%	Hohnloser[31]	1995
Sotalol (po)	33	52%	quinidine (po)	86%	Halinen[30]	1995
Amiodarone (iv)	26	92%	placebo	71%	Hou[100]	1995
Amiodarone (iv)	50	68%	placebo	60%	Galve[101]	1996
Amiodarone (iv)	32	34%	placebo	22%	Donovan[102]	1995
			flecainide (iv)	59%		
Amiodarone (iv)	10	70%	procainamide (iv)	71%	Chapman[103]	1993
Amiodarone (iv)	27	44%	quinidine (po)	47%	Kerin[104]	1996
Amiodarone (iv/po)	20	60%	quinidine (po)	55%	Zehender[105]	1992
Amiodarone (iv)	40	90%	placebo	67%	Cotter[38]	1998
Amiodarone (po)	33	48%	placebo	0%	Igoumenidis[106]	1998
Ibutilide (iv)	81	31%	placebo	2%	Stambler[26]	1996
Ibutilide (iv)	45	51%	procainamide (iv)	20%	Volgman[107]	1996
Ibutilide (iv)	130	43%	sotalol (iv)	10%	Harry[108]	1996
Ibutilide (iv)	36	35%	amiodarone (iv)	4%	Bianconi[37]	1995
			placebo	4%		
Ibutilide (iv)	59	32%	procainamide (iv)	5%	Stambler[33]	1997
			placebo	0%		
Dofetilide (po)	71	32%	placebo	1%	Singh[36]	1998
Dofetilide (iv)	50	12%	placebo	0%	Falk[28]	1997
Dofetilide (iv)	53	28%	procainamide (iv)	15%	Green[29]	1997
			placebo	0%		

No. Pts. = number of patients who received the drug; success = rate of successful cardioversion to normal sinus rhythm.

in 63% and 58% of subjects, and of atrial fibrillation in 31% and 40%.[26,27] Ibutilide is somewhat favored for acute pharmacologic conversion of atrial flutter and fibrillation in the United States.[25] However, considering the high rate of proarrhythmia (which ranges from 4.3% to 8.3% and manifests as torsades de pointes tachycardias) related to the intravenous use of ibutilide,[33,34] ibutilide cannot be considered a better class III antiarrhythmic agent. A recent small study with the use of intravenous ibutilide (1 to 2 mg) for conversion of atrial fibrillation reported an excessive high rate of proarrhythmia.[35] Ventricular tachycardias occurred in 36% of patients, and 21% required intervention. Thus, the appropriate use of ibutilide requires strict monitoring and a readily available defibrillator.

In two placebo-controlled studies, the new class III antiarrhythmic dofetilide (iv) also demonstrated a high efficacy rate in acute conversion of sustained atrial flutter (54% and 50%), but significantly less for atrial fibrillation (14.5% and 28%).[28,29] The cases of torsades de pointes tachycardias were 6.6% and 3.2% in these studies. Recently, a double-blind, placebo-controlled multicenter study of oral dofetilide for treatment of chronic atrial fibrillation demonstrated that oral dofetilide had a similar conversion rate of atrial fibrillation (32% with dofetilide 500 μg bid versus 1% with placebo) during a treatment of 3 days to that experienced during the intravenous dofetilide trials, but oral dofetilide was less proarrhythmic (no cases of torsades de pointes or death in 71 patients treated with 500 μg dofetilide bid).[36]

There are preliminary data concerning the superior efficacy of new pure class III antiarrhythmics (ibutilide, dofetilide) compared to complex class III antiarrhythmics in atrial flutter/fibrillation. In a double-blind, randomized study for the conversion of atrial flutter and fibrillation, intravenous treatment with ibutilide (1 or 2 mg) was compared with sotalol (1.5 mg/kg). Either dose of ibutilide was significantly more effective than intravenous sotalol in converting atrial fibrillation or atrial flutter to sinus rhythm. The 2-mg ibutilide dose converted 70% of patients with atrial flutter and 43% of patients with atrial fibrillation, while the conversion rate with intravenous sotalol was only 18% and 10%, respectively.[7] Another comparative trial with intravenous dofetilide versus amiodarone (5 mg/kg) for acute termination of atrial flutter/fibrillation led to an overall conversion rate of 4% for placebo compared with 4% for amiodarone and 35% for dofetilide (8 μg/kg).[37] However, this comparative trial did not include a dose dependence of amiodarone. This is particularly important since placebo-controlled trials have demonstrated significant conversion rates for amiodarone.[25] In the above-mentioned study of Bianconi et al[37] amiodarone was used at a rather low dosage and patient monitoring was too short (3 hours) to achieve the delayed converting effect of intravenous amiodarone, which requires at least 12 hours, as demonstrated by Cotter et al.[38]

A final conclusion about the question of whether newer class III agents are better for acute conversion of atrial flutter/fibrillation is not currently possible. However, in contrast to sotalol and amiodarone, new pure class III antiarrhythmics are superior to class Ia drugs in the conversion of atrial fibrillation. Ibutilide and dofetilide seem to be efficient in the conversion of atrial flutter and less so in atrial fibrillation. A decision of whether these new class III antiarrhythmics are better than complex class III antiarrhythmics, especially with respect to their risk/benefit ratio, must await further randomized trials.

The lower efficacy of newer, so-called pure class III agents in terminating atrial fibrillation in comparison to atrial flutter or atrioventricular reentry tachycardias reflects their inverse rate-dependent efficacy in prolongation of the action potential, effective refractory period, and excitation wavelength. Accordingly, the efficacy of sotalol for treatment of supraventricular arrhythmias correlates with the rate of atrial activity. Sotalol is effective in terminating paroxysmal supraventricular tachycardias (mainly atrioventricular nodal reentry tachycardias) in 67% to 83% of patients,[32,39] less efficient in conversion of atrial flutter, and even less efficient in conversion of persistent atrial fibrillation, as described above. Recently, Villemaire et al[40] demonstrated that sotalol doses that failed to terminate atrial fibrillation in a dog model prevented the induction of atrial fibrillation, since sotalol significantly prolongs the wavelength of excitation at slow rates but not at high rates. Thus, during atrial fibrillation, reverse rate-dependent effects lead to an ineffectiveness of common class III antiarrhythmics in terminating it. The inverse rate-dependent action potential prolongation of various pure class III antiarrhythmics has been demonstrated by recordings of MAPs in humans for sotalol,[41,42] d-sotalol,[43] tedisamil,[44] sematilide,[45] and dofetilide.[46,47]

In contrast to sotalol, dofetilide, and ibutilide, the reverse rate-dependent effect of azimilide diminishes at higher concentrations toward a rate-independent effect, making the drug more effective in terminating atrial fibrillation in a dog model.[48] Clinical studies with azimilide for treatment of atrial tachyarrhythmias are currently under way.

Few data are available for the effects of class III drugs on action potentials in the human atrium. For intravenous ibutilide (0.005 to 0.025 mg/kg), a study recording MAPs in the high right human atrium during atrial flutter found a significant action potential prolongation of 15% and a conversion rate of 56%.[49] A more recent study compared the effect of intravenous ibutilide (0.005 to 0.025 mg/kg) on atrial MAPs in patients with atrial flutter and atrial fibrillation.[33] The comparison revealed a significantly greater increase of the action potential duration in atrial fibrillation than in atrial flutter (52% versus 30%). However, the magnitude of the increase in MAP duration was not correlated significantly with arrhythmia termination. Therefore, for the conversion of atrial flutter/fibrillation, the ability of a class III agent to prolong action potentials at high rates seems to be a crucial mechanism. Ibutilide was shown to be more efficient than sotalol for treatment of atrial flutter in the canine sterile pericarditis model, although ibutilide induced less prolongation of refractoriness than sotalol and did not close the excitable gap.[50] Therefore, a specific action of ibutilide in the area of slow conduction was proposed.

Long-Term Antiarrhythmic Therapy to Maintain Sinus Rhythm

Whether sinus rhythm is restored spontaneously, chemically, or electrically, atrial fibrillation recurs frequently in the absence of long-term antiarrhythmic therapy. The rationale to use racemic sotalol for suppression of the recurrence of atrial fibrillation was supported by trials that showed similar efficacy of randomized treatment with sotalol versus quinidine or propafenone.[51,52] Racemic sotalol was better tolerated than quinidine and, importantly, the proarrhythmic risk was lower for sotalol than for quinidine.[31,51] However, only one small randomized, controlled trial was performed that demonstrated the efficacy of sotalol for this subject.[53] It remains unclear whether the effect of sotalol on the maintenance of sinus rhythm is a class III antiarrhythmic effect or only a β-blocker effect. Evidence for a class III effect of sotalol, even at low doses that did not induce proarrhythmia, was demonstrated by two recent studies, where the occurrence of atrial fibrillation and flutter in the short-term follow-up (5 days) after coronary artery bypass surgery was more suppressed by sotalol than with conventional β-blocker treatment.[54,55] However, in the long-term follow-up after direct current cardioversion of atrial fibrillation, we found no different efficacy of sotalol compared to conventional β-blocker treatment for the maintenance of sinus rhythm.[56] Additionally, a recent meta-analysis of placebo-controlled trials of 43 studies from 1976 to 1996 found no advantage in using sotalol over standard β-blocker therapy for prophylaxis of postcoronary bypass atrial fibrillation.[57]

In conclusion, the class III antiarrhythmic action of sotalol seems to offer no important improvement over the efficacy of β-blockade for prophylaxis of atrial fibrillation. This is in line with the first comparative study of amiodarone and sotalol for suppression of recurrent atrial fibrillation, recently presented by Kochiadakis et al.[58] In this small randomized study (70 patients with refractory atrial fibrillation), significantly more patients maintained sinus rhythm in the amiodarone group than in the sotalol group.

Recently, Singh et al[59] reported excellent results with oral dofetilide for maintaining sinus rhythm in patients with atrial fibrillation and flutter. At 6 months, 70% of the patients treated with dofetilide remained in sinus rhythm compared to 26% of the placebo-treated patients. Notably, no cases of torsades de pointes were seen. Therefore, pure class III antiarrhythmics seem to offer an effective and safe treatment strategy for the maintenance of sinus rhythm in patients with recurrent atrial fibrillation. However, their future role in relation to class Ic and complex class III antiarrhythmics (sotalol, amiodarone) remains to be established.

Safety of New, So-Called Pure Class III Antiarrhythmic Drugs

Different from the proarrhythmogenic risk of class Ia antiarrhythmic drugs such as quinidine, which appear to have an idiosyncratic rather than dose-related proarrhythmic risk,[60] the risk of class III agents seems to be clearly related to their dose.[15] This means that it is clearly related to their repolarization prolonging effect.

From the theoretical point of view, the proarrhythmic potential of potassium channel blockade may be directly linked to its cellular antiarrhythmic mechanism resulting from action potential prolongation. This theory is supported by a computer model for a 2-dimensional array of excitable cells based on the Fitz-Hugh Nagumo model, in which premature extrastimuli can induce stationary spiral wave reentry of excitation corresponding to monomorphic tachycardias. In this model it was shown that, due to action potential prolongation, the core of this stationary spiral wave reentry will become unstable and will also drift in a spiral manner, resulting in a torsade-like electrocardiograph. In tissues with inhomogeneities, spiral waves can fraction and spawn new spirals, resulting in fibrillation and death.[61]

The typical proarrhythmic effect of class III drugs is the occurrence of torsades de pointes tachycardias. The occurrence of monomorphic ventricular tachycardias is less common, but not rare. Racemic sotalol induces torsades de pointes in approximately 3% to 4% of patients exposed to the drug with a strict dose dependence[62]; however, the proarrhythmic effects are dose-dependent. With dosages used in the above-mentioned trials for treatment of atrial fibrillation (≤160 mg/day), the risk was less than 1%, and in commonly used dosages for treatment of ventricular tachycardias it was less than 2%. Similar data concerning the proarrhythmic potential of d-sotalol do not exist; however, the excess mortality observed with d-sotalol in the SWORD trial may be due to the drug's proarrhythmic potential.[8] To date, available data from small trials suggest that ibutilide has a high proarrhythmic risk, ranging from 4% to 36%, when used intravenously.[34,35]

For dofetilide, small trials have reported controversial results for proarrhythmia. Results ranged from a zero incidence of proarrhythmic response for the treatment of patients with atrial fibrillation[59] to a few percent for the treatment of patients with ventricular tachycardias with oral administration of dofetilide.[20a] For the intravenous administration of dofetilide the incidence is reported in the range between 3.2% and 10%.[28,29]

The comparison of the proarrhythmia frequencies of the above-mentioned class III antiarrhythmic is hampered not only by difficulties in comparing different dosage regimens and proarrhythmia/efficacy relationships, but most likely by the presence of different risk factors in the studied patient population. For sotalol, the following variables were found to correlate with the risk of torsades de pointes: baseline arrhythmia, history of congestive heart failure, cardiomegaly, New York Heart Association (NYHA) functional class, baseline prolongation of corrected QT (QTc), and gender. In particular, patients with sustained ventricular tachycardias and females were much more predisposed to proarrhythmia.[63] Only one multicenter randomized study compared class III antiarrhythmics for long-term follow-up (1 year). The proarrhythmic response to dofetilide was not significantly different from that to sotalol in patients with coronary heart disease treated for sustained ventricular arrhythmias.[20a] Additionally, the efficacy of both drugs for the suppression of ventricular tachycardias in an electrophysiologic study and for the long-term follow-up was similar. Other adverse effects were significantly lower in the dofetilide-treated group. The study indicates that currently available pure class III antiarrhythmics may not be safer. In contrast, the DIAMOND study[21] demonstrated in a large randomized population of patients with congestive heart failure that dofetilide is neutral with respect to all-cause mortality compared to placebo. These results are strikingly different from those of the SWORD[8] study with d-sotalol, and may offer a possible release of dofetilide for a limited clinical use.

There is disputing the fact that the lowest incidence of proarrhythmia was seen with amiodarone relative to other agents with class III action.[15] The risk of torsades de pointes appears to be less than 1% despite frequently impressive QT prolongation.[64] This may be related to a reduction in transmural ventricular dispersion of repolarization[65] and the absence of an increase of ventricular dispersion in relation to a comparison of dispersion with d-sotalol or quinidine.[66]

Torsades de pointes is the Achilles' heel of the class III agents, and future studies will be needed to focus on mechanisms underlying the differences among various agents that prolong repolarization. The underlying mechanism for prolongation of action potentials for sotalol, dofetilide, and, in part, for ibutilide,[67] as well as for many other drugs that induce torsades de pointes (histamine H_1-receptor antagonists,[68] erythromycin[69]) is a blockade of I_{Kr}. The hypothesis may be proposed that I_{Kr} blockade itself is responsible for a proarrhythmic response. However, a recent study suggested that torsades de pointes is not necessarily associated with an I_{Kr} block, since disopyramide and procainamide are known to induce torsades de pointes, although they do not block I_{Kr} in therapeutic plasma concentrations.[70] Accordingly, we recently observed early afterdepolarizations not only by selective I_{Kr} blockade but also by selective I_{Ks} blockade in the guinea pig ventricle during β-adrenergic activation.[71] Such early afterdepolarizations may give rise to torsades de pointes tachycardias.

Experimental Studies for Strategies to Improve Properties of Class III Antiarrhythmics

The Unfavorable Inverse Rate Dependence

The value of the prolongation of action potentials at more rapid rates than at slow rates in order to maximize antiarrhythmic efficacy and minimize the risk of torsades de pointes is an important concept for future drug development.

Improvement of the Kinetics of I_{Kr} Blockade

The inverse rate dependence diminishes efficacy at high rates and promotes proarrhythmia at low rates. (Basic mechanisms of rate dependence are discussed in chapter 24.) It was hypothesized that this is related to an I_{Kr} blockade, the underlying mechanism of most pure class III antiarrhythmic agents, such as d-sotalol, dofetilide, E4031, ibutilide, azimilide, sematilide, and others. However, recent studies demonstrated that this is not necessarily related to an I_{Kr} blockade. Rate-dependent accumulation of extracellular potassium reduces the binding of methansulfonanilide, such as dofetilide, to *HERG* channel, responsible for I_{Kr}.[72] Another point to consider is the kinetics of binding to the channel. It was demonstrated that open-channel I_{Kr} blockers such as dofetilide and almokalant have very slow kinetics of recovery from blockade at repolarization.[20,73] Carmeliet[20,73] hypothesized that the rapidly binding and slowly unbinding kinetics of dofetilide and other I_{Kr} blockers are responsible for the reverse rate-dependent action. This hypothesis was recently confirmed for the I_{Kr} blocker MS-551, which has a rapid voltage-dependent binding and unbinding to the I_{Kr} channel (fast kinetics of recovery from blockade at repolarized potentials), resulting in a bell-shaped, rate-dependent action potential prolongation and less action potential prolongation at slow heart rates.[74] Therefore, there is still a perspective for evolving selective I_{Kr} blockers with open-channel block. If they have very rapid recovery from blockade at repolarization, a new generation of I_{Kr} blockers may possess the ability to prolong action potentials in a frequency-dependent manner.

Improvement by I_{Ks} Blockade or Nonselective K⁺ Channel Blockade

The main target of current class III antiarrhythmics, especially the methanesulfonanilides (E4031, d-sotalol, sematilide, dofetilide, MK-499), is the I_{Kr} current. The incomplete recovery from inactivation of the I_{Kr} at high heart rates is a strong limitation of I_{Kr} blockade, since the role of I_{Kr} for repolarization diminishes at high heart rates.[75,76] In contrast, the role of I_{Ks} increases at more rapid heart rates, since the channel may accumulate in its activated state.[75] Therefore, I_{Ks} blockade, as a mechanism for action potential prolongation, may improve the rate dependence of class III antiarrhythmics. Selective I_{Ks} blockers such as chromanol 293B and L-735,821 have become available and have been shown to have rate-independent action potential prolonging effects in ventricular myocytes,[77-79] but have not yet been investigated for their antiarrhythmic potential. We recently demonstrated that a nonselective I_K blocker, ambasilide, reveals a rate-independent action potential prolongation not only in the guinea pig ventricle[71,80] but also in human endomyocardium ventricular tissue (Fig. 1).[81] With measurements of MAPs in the right ventricle of patients undergoing electrophysiologic studies, we could confirm this rate-independent effect of ambasilide for humans (Fig. 1).[82] The comparison of ambasilide with a selective I_{Kr} blocker (dofetilide) and a selective I_{Ks} blocker (chromanol 293B) in the guinea pig demonstrated that a combined I_K blockade may be sufficient to achieve a rate-independent class III antiarrhythmic effect (Fig. 2).[71]

Class III drugs that block I_{Ks} seem to improve the efficacy in the treatment of atrial fibrillation, possibly reflecting an improved action potential prolongation at rapid stimulation frequencies. The high efficacy of azimilide[48] and ambasilide,[83] in contrast to d-sotalol,[83] for the treatment of atrial fibrillation in a canine model for atrial fibrillation, may demonstrate this effect.

I_{Ks} blockade, however, seems to increase the likelihood of delayed afterdepolarizations, especially in the presence of β-adrenergic activation,[71] and the risk of this potential proarrhythmic mechanism remains to be elucidated.

Improvement by Combined I_{Kr} and Calcium Channel Blockade

We have recently shown another perspective for an I_{Kr} blocker by combining dofetilide with a calcium antagonist.[84] In the guinea pig papillary muscle, the reverse rate-dependent effect of dofetilide was abolished with diltiazem (Fig. 3). This effect was achieved with a reduced action potential prolongation of dofetilide at low heart rates and an almost unchanged effect at high heart rates. Therefore, the proarrhythmic effect of the I_{Kr}

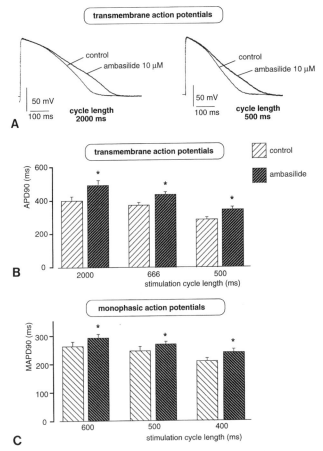

Figure 1. Frequency-independent effect of ambasilide, a pure class III antiarrhythmic agent and nonselective potassium channel blocker, on action potentials of diseased human ventricle in dilated cardiomyopathy or coronary artery disease. **A** and **B**. Transmembrane action potential durations were measured by using intracellular microelectrode techniques in isolated specimens of the left ventricular endomyocardium of human hearts obtained from 10 patients undergoing either heart transplantation or mitral valve replacement. Example of action potentials before drug (control) and after equilibration with 10 μM ambasilide at a stimulation cycle length of 2000 and 500 milliseconds were superimposed in A. Action potential duration at 90% repolarization (APD$_{90}$) before and after 10 μM ambasilide were plotted at different stimulation cycle lengths. Columns are mean values ± SEM; *$P<0.05$, drug versus control. For further details, see Reference 8. **C**. MAPs were measured in the right ventricular apex from 7 patients undergoing electrophysiologic studies after syncope or documented ventricular tachycardias. Stimulation at a cycle length of 600, 500, and 400 milliseconds was performed before and 20 minutes after a intravenous dose of 0.5 to 1.5 mg/kg ambasilide, leading to a plasma level of 6.3±3.3 μM (mean ± SEM). MAP duration at 90% repolarization (MAPD$_{90}$) before and after intravenous ambasilide were plotted at different stimulation cycle lengths. Columns are mean values ± SEM; *$P<0.05$, drug versus control.

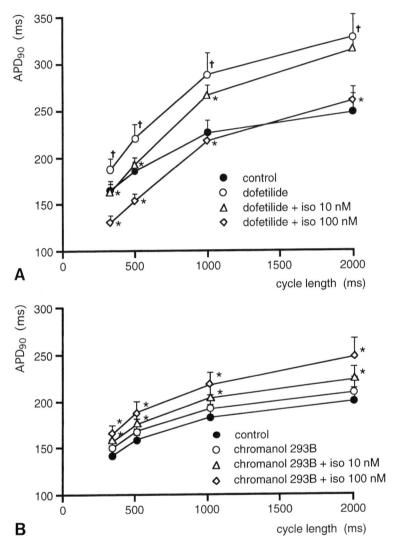

Figure 2. Frequency-dependent effect of two pure class III antiarrhythmics, a selective I_{Kr} blocker, dofetilide (10 nM) (**A**), and a selective I_{Ks} blocker, chromanol 293B (10 μM) (**B**) on action potential duration before and after β-adrenergic stimulation with isoproterenol (iso) in isolated guinea pig papillary muscles (n=10 and n=12, respectively). Transmembrane action potential durations measured at 90% repolarization (APD_{90}) at different stimulation cycle lengths with intracellular microelectrodes were plotted before (control), after equilibration with the class III antiarrhythmic agents, and after exposure to isoproterenol (iso) in concentrations of 10 and 100 nM in the continuous presence of the class III drug. Values are expressed as mean ± SEM. $^{†}P< 0.01$, class III drug versus control; $^{*}P<0.05$, class III drug versus class III drug + isoproterenol. For further details, see Reference 71.

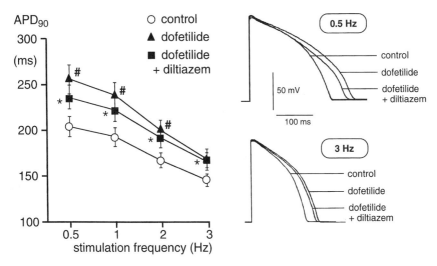

Figure 3. Left: Frequency-dependent effect of a pure class III antiarrhythmic drug, dofetilide (10 nM) with and without the presence of a calcium antagonist (10 μM diltiazem) on action potential duration in 11 isolated guinea pig papillary muscles. Transmembrane action potential durations were measured at 90% repolarization (APD$_{90}$) with intracellular microelectrode techniques before (control), 30 minutes after equilibration with dofetilide, and 30 minutes after exposure to diltiazem in the continuous presence of the dofetilide. Shown are mean values ± SEM. [#]$P<0.01$, dofetilide versus control; [*]$P<0.05$, dofetilide versus dofetilide + diltiazem. Right: Superimposed original action potential recordings at 0.5 and 3 Hz stimulation frequencies. For further details, see Reference 84.

blocker, which should be related to the pronounced action potential prolongation at low heart rates, is reduced without affecting its efficacy at high rates, in terminating tachycardias. Our results may explain the rate-independent or less reversed rate-dependent action potential prolongation of azimilide and amiodarone, two nonselective I_{Kr} blockers that also significantly block inward calcium current.

Improvement by Combined I_{Kr} and Sodium Channel Blockade

The combination of sotalol with a class Ia antiarrhythmic can cause a rate-independent action potential prolongation. This subject is discussed in chapter 28.

Reduced Efficacy of Class III Antiarrhythmic Action During Adrenergic Activation: Improvement by I_{Ks} Blockade

There are several lines of evidence that the antisympathetic actions of sotalol and amiodarone may play a crucial role in mediating a significant component of their beneficial actions. Notably, empirical β-blocker treatment is the most efficient therapy for prophylaxis of torsades de pointes tachycardias in genuine long QT syndrome.

A general disadvantage of I_{Kr} blockers is their reduced efficacy in action potential prolongation in the presence of enhanced adrenergic tonus. This subject is discussed in chapter 27.

Recently, we demonstrated that an I_{Ks} blockade can improve the action potential prolonging effect of a potassium channel blocker in the presence of β-adrenergic stimulation. In a comparative study with a selective I_{Kr} blocker (dofetilide), a nonselective I_K blocker (ambasilide), and a selective I_{Ks} blocker (chromanol 293B), we investigated the effects of β-adrenergic stimulation with isoproterenol in the presence of these different class III agents in guinea pig papillary muscles.[71] The action potential prolonging effect of dofetilide was clearly reduced, the class III effect of ambasilide was less reduced (data here not shown), and, conversely, the class III effect of chromanol 293B was enhanced during β-adrenergic stimulation (Fig. 2). Our data strongly support the hypothesis that I_{Ks} blockade improves the class III antiarrhythmic efficacy during β-adrenergic stimulation. However, in contrast to an I_{Kr} blockade, we observed a considerably high incidence of delayed afterdepolarizations induced by isoproterenol in the presence of an I_{Ks} block with ambasilide or chromanol 293B. Therefore, the important question, whether such an improvement of action potential prolongation during β-adrenergic stimulation by I_{Ks} block is beneficial or detrimental due to proarrhythmia, remains to be elucidated in further studies.

Reduced Efficacy of Class III Action at High K⁺ Levels and Proarrhythmia at Low K⁺ Levels: Improvement by I_{Ks} Blockade

Sotalol and amiodarone were shown to lose their ability to prolong action potential duration in myocardial ischemia.[85,86] Increased extracellular potassium is an important factor in the setting of myocardial ischemia, and has been shown to reduce the efficacy of class III antiarrhythmics. Baskin and Lynch[87] demonstrated that increased extracellular potassium diminishes the class III activity of different methanesulfonanilide I_{Kr} blockers (dofetilide, d-sotalol, E-4031, MK-499). Yang and Roden[70] recently showed for dofetilide that the drug block is strikingly dependent on the extracellular potassium concentration. This phenomenon has substantial clinical implications, as myocardial ischemia as well as rapid stimulation frequencies increase extracellular potassium and thereby reduce efficacy of I_{Kr} blockers in this important situation, for the genesis of arrhythmias. On the other hand, low extracellular potassium in heart failure, which may be aggravated due to diuretic treatment, can cause an increased drug block of I_{Kr}, which may be proarrhythmic due to an excessive action potential prolongation.

We recently demonstrated a way to overcome these general problems of class III antiarrhythmics. In a comparative study of dofetilide and the nonselective K^+ channel blocker, ambasilide, at different extracellular potassium concentrations in the guinea pig papillary muscle, we provided evidence that blocking potassium currents other than I_{Kr}—especially I_{Ks}—achieves a potassium-independent action potential prolongation.[80] Furthermore, we have shown that the adverse reverse rate-dependent effect of dofetilide is pronounced at high potassium concentrations, while the rate-independent effect of ambasilide remains unchanged (Fig. 4). Ambasilide, a nonmethanesulfonanilide potassium channel blocker, is, like dofetilide, an open channel blocker of I_{Kr}.[88,89] Therefore, the most probable mechanism for the advantageous effect of ambasilide in the guinea pig papillary muscle is an I_{Ks} blockade, since other ambasilide-sensitive potassium currents play no role for repolarization in the guinea-pig ventricle.

There are 3 potassium-dependent mechanisms that influence the I_{Kr} current in the presence of dofetilide: first, the potassium-dependent drug-channel interaction; second, the external potassium-dependent activation of the channel, which increases the conductance of the channel in elevated K^{+90}; and third, the potassium gradient, which determines the driving force for the outward current. These characteristics of I_{Kr} channels make a selective I_{Kr} block unlikely to be an ideal class III mechanism in the presence of highly variable external potassium levels in heart disease and during diuretic treatment. In contrast to I_{Kr}, for the I_{Ks} channel, only the third point, the potassium gradient, seems to be significant for the amplitude of the current. This may explain the more stable class III effect of ambasilide at different external potassium levels.

It can, however, be supposed, that an involvement of an I_{Kr} block in a nonselective potassium channel blockade may be an advantageous mechanism, since I_{Kr} increases with high external potassium and thereby contributes to the action potential shortening in myocardial ischemia. Besides ambasilide, azimilide is a nonselective I_K blocker[91] and is likely to open a new perspective for class III antiarrhythmic treatment.

Side-Specific and Event-Specific Class III Antiarrhythmic Action

The general limitation of pharmacologic antiarrhythmic treatment is their inherent proarrhythmic potential. In particular, the induction of ventricular torsades de pointes tachycardias is the major limitation for the treatment of atrial fibrillation with class III agents. A very promising approach and completely new perspective for the treatment of atrial arrhyth-

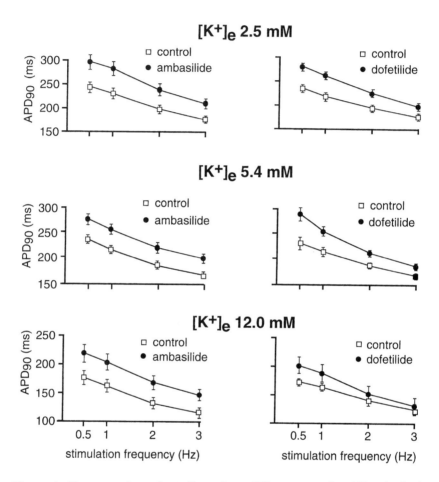

Figure 4. Frequency-dependent effect of two different pure class III antiarrhythmic agents on action potential duration in isolated guinea pig papillary muscles at 3 different extracellular potassium concentrations ($[K^+]_e$). Transmembrane action potential durations were measured at 90% repolarization (APD_{90}) with intracellular microelectrode techniques before (control) and 30 minutes after the addition of either 10 μM ambasilide (right panels), a nonselective I_K blocker (left panel), or 10 nM dofetilide, a selective I_{Kr} blocker (right panels) at different $[K^+]_e$. Shown are mean values ± SEM of at least 10 papillary muscles. For further details, see Reference 80.

mias with class III antiarrhythmics was gained by Wang et al,[92] who characterized the ultrarapid delayed rectifier current (I_{Kur}) in the human atrial myocyte. This current plays an important role for repolarization in the human atrium, but it seems to be functionally absent in the human ventricle.[93,94] Therefore, selective blockade of I_{Kur} may have pronounced class III effects in the human atrium without any effect—especially without any proarrhythmic effect—in the human ventricle. I_{Kur} block may be responsible for the atrial antiarrhythmic effects of quinidine[95] or clofilium.[94] The cloned Kv1.5 channel expressed in cell culture, which is shown to be the molecular equivalent of I_{Kur} in the human atrium,[96] provides a powerful model for screening and development of selective I_{Kur} blockers. Therefore, it seems to be a question of time and effort until a promising new type of class III antiarrhythmic for the treatment of atrial arrhythmias becomes available.

Since I_{Kur} in human atrium is different from canine I_{Kur}, and is absent in most other species, MAP measurements in human atrium will be an important tool for future development of I_{Kur} blockers.

A similar approach would be the development of a selective blocker of the acetylcholine-dependent inward rectifier potassium current ($I_{K ACh}$), which plays a predominant role in the atrium and is less important in Purkinje fibers and absent in ventricular myocytes.[97]

Blockade of ATP-dependent potassium currents ($I_{K ATP}$), as a mechanism for class III antiarrhythmic action, will offer an event-specific antiarrhythmic action. This means that such drugs as glibenclamide prolong repolarization only during ischemia, when $I_{K ATP}$ channels are open, but not during normoxic conditions.[98] Therefore, no proarrhythmic response can be expected in normoxic conditions. Selective $I_{K ATP}$ blockers are currently in clinical evaluation (Hoechst AG, personal communication, 1997). Recently, tedisamil, a nonselective potassium channel blocker, was shown to have antiarrhythmic efficacy in a postinfarcted canine model of ischemic ventricular fibrillation.[99] The authors assumed that this antiarrhythmic effect of tedisamil is due to its known $I_{K ATP}$ blocking action, since they found no electrophysiologic changes during the normoxic state of the heart.

In conclusion, more insights into the basic mechanisms for repolarization, as the results of basic research of potassium channels, in the past decade offer various new targets and exciting perspectives for class III antiarrhythmic therapy. Therefore, the development of new class III antiarrhythmics may open a new era of antiarrhythmic treatment rather than close an old one.

References

1. Singh BN. Controlling cardiac arrhythmias: An overview with a historical perspective. *Am J Cardiol* 1997;80:4G-15G.

 2. Julian DG, Camm AJ, Frangin G, et al, for the European Myocardial Infarct Amiodarone Trial Investigators. Randomized trial of effect of amiodarone on mortality in patients with left-ventricular dysfunction after recent myocardial infarction: EMIAT. *Lancet* 1997;349:667-674.
 3. Cairns JA, Connolly SJ, Roberts R, et al, for the Canadian Amiodarone Myocardial Infarction Arrhythmia Trial Investigators. Randomized trial of outcome after myocardial infarction in patients with frequent or repetitive ventricular premature depolarizations: CAMIAT. *Lancet* 1997;349:675-682.
 4. Manson JW, for the Electrophysiologic Study versus Electrocardiographic Monitoring Investigators. A comparison of seven antiarrhythmic drugs in patients with ventricular tachyarrhythmias. *N Engl J Med* 1993;329:452-458.
 5. Julian DG, Jackson FS, Prescott RJ, et al. Controlled trial of sotalol for one year after myocardial infarction. *Lancet* 1982;1:1142-1147.
 6. Singh SN, Fletcher RD, Singh BN, et al, for the Survival Trial of Antiarrhythmic Therapy in Congestive Heart Failure. Amiodarone in patients with congestive heart failure and asymptomatic ventricular arrhythmias. *N Engl J Med* 1995;333:77-82.
 7. Amiodarone Trials Meta-analysis Investigators. Effect of prophylactic amiodarone on mortality after acute myocardial infarction and in congestive heart failure: Meta-analysis of individual data from 6500 patients in randomised trials. *Lancet* 1997;350:1417-1424.
 8. Waldo AL, Camm AJ, de Ruyter H, et al, for the SWORD Investigators. Effect of d-sotalol on mortality in patients with left ventricular dysfunction after recent and remote myocardial infarction. *Lancet* 1996;348:7-12.
 9. Edvardsson N, Hirsch I, Emanuelsson H, et al. Sotalol-induced delayed ventricular repolarization in man. *Eur Heart J* 1980;1:335-343.
10. Reiffel JA, Hahn E, Hartz V, et al, for the ESVEM Investigators. Sotalol for ventricular tachyarrhythmias: Beta-blocking and class III contributions, and relative efficacy versus class I drugs after prior drug failure. *Am J Cardiol* 1997;79:1048-1053.
11. Haverkamp W, Martinez-Rubio A, Hief C, et al. Efficacy and safety of d,l-sotalol in patients with ventricular tachycardia and in survivors of cardiac arrest. *J Am Coll Cardiol* 1997;30:487-495.
12. Antz M, Cappato R, Kuck KH, et al. Metoprolol versus sotalol in the treatment of sustained ventricular tachycardia. *J Cardiovasc Pharmacol* 1995;26:627-635.
13. Kühlkamp V, Mewis C, Dörnberger V, et al. Efficacy of sotalol and metoprolol in patients with an implanted cardioverter defibrillator. *J Am Coll Cardiol* 1997;29(suppl A):195A. Abstract.
14. Seidl K, Hauer N, Schwick S, et al. Metoprolol is more effective than d,l sotalol for prevention of recurrence of ventricular tachyarrhythmias after implantation of a cardioverter/defibrillator. *J Am Coll Cardiol* 1997;29(suppl A):196A. Abstract.
15. Hohnloser SH, Singh BN. Proarrhythmia with class III antiarrhythmic drugs: Definition, electrophysiologic mechanisms, incidence, predisposing factors and clinical implications. *J Cardiovasc Electrophysiol* 1995;6:920-936.
16. Amiodarone vs Sotalol Study Group: Multicentre randomized trial of sotalol vs amiodarone for chronic malignant ventricular tachyarrhythmias. *Eur Heart J* 1989;10:685-694.
17. Man KC, Williamson BD, Niebauer M, et al. Electrophysiologic effects of sotalol and amiodarone in patients with sustained monomorphic ventricular tachycardia. *Am J Cardiol* 1994;74: 1119-1123.

18. Martinez-Rubio A, Shenasa M, Chen X, et al. Response to sotalol predicts the response to amiodarone during serial drug testing in patients with sustained ventricular tachycardia and coronary artery disease. *Am J Cardiol* 1994;73:357-360.

19. Reiffel JA. Prolonging survival by reducing arrhythmic death: Pharmacologic therapy of ventricular tachycardia and fibrillation. *Am J Cardiol* 1997; 80:45G-55G.

20. Carmeliet E. Voltage- and time dependent block of the delayed K^+ current in cardiac myocytes by dofetilide. *J Pharmacol Exp Ther* 1992;262:809-817.

20a. Boriani G, Lubinski A, Capucci A, et al. A double-blind multicentre crossover study on dofetilide versus sotalol in patients with inducible sustained ventricular tachycardia and coronary artery disease. *Eur Heart J* 1998;19(suppl):111. Abstract.

21. Danish Investigators of Arrhythmia and Mortality On Dofetilide. Dofetilide in patients with left ventricular dysfunction and either heart failure or acute myocardial infarction: Rationale, design, and patient characteristics of the DIAMOND studies. *Clin Cardiol* 1997;20:704-710.

22. Torp-Pedersen C and the Danish Investigations of Arrhythmia and Mortality On Dofetilide (DIAMOND) study group. Dofetilide: A new class III antiarrhythmic drug which is safe in patients with congestive heart failure. *J Am Coll Cardiol* 1998;31(suppl A):160A. Abstract.

23. Böcker D, Haverkamp W, Block M, et al. Comparison of d,l-sotalol and implantable defibrillators for treatment of sustained ventricular tachycardia or fibrillation in patients with coronary artery disease. *Circulation* 1996;94:151-157.

24. AVID—The Antiarrhythmics versus implantable defibrillators (AVID) Investigators. A comparison of antiarrhythmic-drug therapy with implantable defibrillators in patients resuscitated from near fatal ventricular arrhythmias. *N Engl J Med* 1997;337:1576-1583.

25. Ganz LI, Antman EM. Antiarrhythmic drug therapy in the management of atrial fibrillation. *J Cardiovasc Electrophysiol* 1997;8:1175-1189.

26. Stambler BS, Burger AJ, Cassidy DM, et al. Efficacy and safety of repeated intravenous doses of ibutilide for rapid conversion of atrial flutter or fibrillation. *Circulation* 1996;94:1613-1621.

27. Ellenbogen KA, Stambler BS, Wood MA, et al, for the Ibutilide Investigators. Efficacy of intravenous ibutilide for rapid termination of atrial fibrillation and atrial flutter: A dose-response study. *J Am Coll Cardiol* 1996;28:130-136.

28. Falk RH, Pollak A, Singh SN, et al, for the Intravenous Dofetilide Investigators. Intravenous dofetilide, a class III antiarrhythmic agent, for terminating sustained atrial fibrillation or flutter. *J Am Coll Cardiol* 1997;29:385-390.

29. Green MS, Dorian P, Roy D, et al. A randomized, double-blind, placebo-controlled comparison of intravenous dofetilide and procainamide in the acute conversion of atrial fibrillation/flutter. *Circulation* 1997;96(suppl):I-453. Abstract.

30. Halinen MO, Huttunen M, Paakkinen S, et al. Comparison of sotalol with digoxin-quinidine for conversion of acute atrial fibrillation to sinus rhythm (the Sotalol-Digoxin-Quinidine trial). *Am J Cardiol* 1995;26:852-858.

31. Hohnloser SH, van de Loo A, Baedeker F. Efficacy and proarrhythmic hazards of pharmacologic cardioversion of atrial fibrillation: Prospective comparison of sotalol versus quinidine. *J Am Coll Cardiol* 1995;26:852-858.

32. Sung RJ, Tan HL, Karagounis L, et al. Intravenous sotalol for the termination of supraventricular tachycardia and atrial fibrillation and flutter: A multicenter, randomized, double-blind, placebo-controlled study. Sotalol Multicenter Study Group. *Am Heart J* 1995;129:739-748.

33. Stambler BS, Wood MA, Ellenbogen KA, et al. Antiarrhythmic action of intravenous ibutilide compared with procainamide during human atrial flutter and fibrillation. Electrophysiological determinants of enhanced conversion efficacy. *Circulation* 1997;96:4298-4306.

34. Kowey PR, VanderLugt JT, Luderer JR. Safety and risk/benefit analysis of ibutilide for acute conversion of atrial fibrillation/flutter. *Am J Cardiol* 1996;78:46-52.

35. Shenasa H, Nguyen M, Shenasa M. Proarrhythmic effect of ibutilide. *Circulation* 1997;96(suppl I):I383. Abstract.

36. Singh SN, Berk MR, Yellen LG, et al. Oral dofetilide for conversion of patients with chronic atrial fibrillation of atrial flutter to normal sinus rhythm: A multicenter study. *J Am Coll Cardiol* 1998;31(suppl A):369A. Abstract.

37. Bianconi L, Dinelli M, Papalardo A, et al. Comparison of intravenously-administered dofetilide versus amiodarone in the acute termination of atrial fibrillation and flutter: A multi-centered, randomized, double-blind, placebo-controlled study. *Circulation* 1995;92(suppl I):I-774. Abstract.

38. Cotter G, Cotter-Metzkor E, Kaluski E, et al. Acute atrial fibrillation: High dose iv amiodarone facilitates conversion to normal sinus rhythm. When is it necessary? *J Am Coll Cardiol* 1998;31(suppl A):370A. Abstract.

39. Jordaens L, Gorgels A, Stroobandt R, et al. Efficacy and safety of intravenous sotalol for termination of paroxysmal supraventricular tachycardia. *Am J Cardiol* 1991;68:35-40.

40. Villemaire C, Talajic M, Nattel S. Mechanisms by which sotalol prevents atrial fibrillation at doses that fail to terminate the arrhythmias. *Circulation* 1997;96(suppl):I-236. Abstract.

41. Schmitt C, Brachmann J, Karch M, et al. Reverse use-dependent effects of sotalol demonstrated by recording monophasic action potentials of the right ventricle. *Am J Cardiol* 1991;68:1183-1187.

42. Shimizu W, Kurita T, Suyama K, et al. Reverse use dependence of human ventricular repolarization by chronic oral sotalol in monophasic action potential recordings. *Am J Cardiol* 1996;77:1004-1008.

43. Huikuri HV, Yli-Mäyry S. Frequency dependent effects of d-sotalol and amiodarone on the action potential duration of the human right ventricle. *PACE* 1992;15:2103-2107.

44. Bargheer K, Bode F, Klein HU, et al. Prolongation of monophasic action potential duration and the refractory period in the human heart by tedisamil, a new potassium-blocking agent. *Eur Heart J* 1994;15:1409-1414.

45. Sager PT, Nademanee K, Antimisiaris M, et al. Antiarrhythmic effects of selective prolongation of refractoriness. Electrophysiologic actions of sematilide HCl in humans. *Circulation* 1993;88:1072-1082.

46. Sedgwick M, Rasmussen HS, Cobbe SM. Effects of the class III antiarrhythmic drug dofetilide on ventricular monophasic action potential duration and QT interval dispersion in stable angina pectoris. *Am J Cardiol* 1992;70:1432-1437.

47. Sager PT. Frequency-dependent electrophysiologic effects of dofetilide in humans. *Circulation* 1995;92(suppl I):I-774. Abstract.

48. Kanki H, Mitamura H, Sato T, et al. Dose-dependent anti-atrial fibrillation efficacy of azimilide. *Circulation* 1997;96(suppl I):I-383. Abstract.

49. Guo GBF, Ellenbogen KA, Wood MA, et al. Conversion of atrial flutter by ibutilide is associated with increased atrial cycle length variability. *J Am Coll Cardiol* 1996;27:1083-1089.

50. Buchanan LV, LeMay RJ, Walters RR, et al. Antiarrhythmic and electrophysiologic effects of intravenous ibutilide and sotalol in the canine sterile pericarditis model. *J Cardiovasc Electrophysiol* 1996;7:113-119.

51. Juul-Möller S, Edvardsson N, Rehnqvist-Ahlberg N. Sotalol versus quinidine for the maintenance of sinus rhythm after direct current cardioversion of atrial fibrillation. *Circulation* 1990;82:1932-1939.

52. Reimold SC, Cantillon CO, Friedman PL, et al. Propafenone versus sotalol for suppression of recurrent symptomatic atrial fibrillation. *Am J Cardiol* 1994;74:503-505.

53. Singh S, Saini RK, DiMarco J, et al. Efficacy and safety of sotalol in digitalized patients with chronic atrial fibrillation. *Am J Cardiol* 1991;68:1227-1230.

54. Abdulrahman O, Dale HT, Theman TE, et al. Low dose sotalol compared to metoprolol in the prevention of supraventricular arrhythmias alter cardiac surgery. *Circulation* 1997;96(suppl I):I-263. Abstract.

55. Parikka H, Toivonen L, Heikkilä L, et al. Comparison of sotalol and metoprolol in the prevention of atrial fibrillation after coronary bypass surgery. *J Cardiovasc Pharmacol* 1998;31:67-73.

56. Plewan A, Lehmann G, Zrenner B, et al. Maintenance of sinus rhythm after cardioversion of atrial fibrillation: Sotalol vs. Bisoprolol. *Circulation* 1997;96(suppl I):I-264. Abstract.

57. Woodend AK, Nichol G, Carey CY, et al. Sotalol confers no additional benefit over beta-blocker in post-coronary artery bypass atrial fibrillation. *J Am Coll Cardiol* 1998;31(suppl A):383A. Abstract.

58. Kochiadakis GE, Igoumenidis NE, Marketou ME, et al. Class III drugs for suppression of recurrent symptomatic atrial fibrillation. *J Am Coll Cardiol* 1998;31(suppl A):370A. Abstract.

59. Singh SN, Berk MR, Yellen LG, et al. Efficacy and safety of oral dofetilide in maintaining normal sinus in patients with atrial fibrillation/flutter: A multicenter study. *Circulation* 1997;96(suppl I):I-383. Abstract.

60. Roden DM: Torsade de pointes. *Clin Cardiol* 1993;16:683-686.

61. Starmer CF, Romashko DN, Reddy RS, et al. Proarrhythmic response to potassium channel blockade. Numerical studies of polymorphic tachyarrhythmias. *Circulation* 1995;92:595-605.

62. Hohnloser SH. Proarrhythmia with class III antiarrhythmic drugs: Types, risks, and management. *Am J Cardiol* 1997;80:82G-89G.

63. Lehmann MH, Hardy S, Archibald D, et al. Sex differences in risk of torsades de pointes with d,l-sotalol. *Circulation* 1996;94:2534-2541.

64. Hohnloser SH, Klingenheben T, Singh BN. Amiodarone-associated proarrhythmic effects: A review with special reference to torsade de pointes tachycardia. *Ann Intern Med* 1994;121:529-535.

65. Sicouri S, Moro S, Litovsky S, et al. Chronic amiodarone reduces transmural dispersion of repolarization in the canine heart. *J Cardiol Electrophysiol* 1997;8:1269-1279.

66. Zabel M, Hohnloser SH, Behrens S, et al. Differential effects of d-sotalol, quinidine, and amiodarone on dispersion of ventricular repolarization in the isolated rabbit heart. *J Cardiovasc Electrophysiol* 1997;8:1239-1245.

67. Yang T, Snyders DJ, Roden DM. Ibutilide, a methanesulfonanilide antiarrhythmic, is a potent blocker of the rapidly activating delayed rectifier K⁺ current (I_{Kr}) in AT-1 cells. *Circulation* 1995;91:1799-1806.

68. Salata JJ, Jurkiewicz NK, Wallace AA, et al. Cardiac electrophysiological actions of the histamine H1-receptor antagonists astemizole and terfenadine compared with chlorpheniramine and pyrilamine. *Circ Res* 1995;76:110-119.

69. Antzelevitch C, Sun ZQ, Zhang ZQ, et al. Cellular and ionic mechanisms underlying erythromycin-induced long QT intervals and torsade de pointes. *J Am Coll Cardiol* 1996;28:1836-1848.

70. Yang T, Roden DM. Extracellular potassium modulation of drug block of I_{Kr}. Implications for torsade de pointes and reverse use-dependence. *Circulation* 1996;93:407-411.

71. Schreieck J, Wang YG, Gjini V, et al. Differential effect of β-adrenergic stimulation on the frequency-dependent electrophysiologic actions of the new class III antiarrhythmics dofetilide, ambasilide and chromanol 293B. *J Cardiovasc Electrophysiol* 1998;8:1420-1430.

72. Yang T, Snyders D, Roden DM. Discordance between I_{Kr} block and torsades de pointes. *Circulation* 1997;96(suppl):I-554. Abstract.

73. Carmeliet E. Use-dependent block and use-dependent unblock of the delayed rectifier K⁺ current by almokalant in rabbit ventricular myocytes. *Circ Res* 1993;73:857-868.

74. Cheng J, Kamiya K, Kodama I, et al. Differential effects of MS-551 and E-4031 on action potentials and the delayed rectifier K⁺ current in rabbit ventricular myocytes. *Cardiovasc Res* 1996;31:963-974.

75. Sanguinetti MC, Jurkiewicz NK. Two components of cardiac delayed rectifier K⁺ current. Differential sensitivity to block by class III antiarrhythmic agents. *J Gen Physiol* 1990;96:195-215.

76. Sanguinetti MC, Jurkiewicz NK, Scott A, et al. Isoproterenol antagonizes prolongation of refractory period by class III antiarrhythmic agents E-4031 in guinea pig myocytes: Mechanism of action. *Circ Res* 1991;68:77-84.

77. Busch AE, Suessbrich H, Waldegger S, et al. Inhibition of I_{Ks} in guinea pig cardiac myocytes and guinea pig I_{sK} channels by chromanol 293B. *Pflügers Arch* 1996;432:1094-1096.

78. Salata JJ, Jurkiewicz NK, Sanguinetti MC, et al. The novel class III antiarrhythmic agent, L-735,821 is a potent and selective blocker of I_{Ks} in guinea pig ventricular myocytes. *Circulation* 1996;94(suppl I):I-529. Abstract.

79. Bosch RF, Gaspo R, Busch AE, et al. Effects on repolarization of the chromanol 293B, a highly selective blocker of the slow component of the delayed rectifier K⁺ current (I_{Ks}) in human and guinea pig ventricle. *J Am Coll Cardiol* 1997;29(suppl A):512A. Abstract.

80. Gjini V, Korth M, Schreieck J, et al. Differential class III antiarrhythmic effects of ambasilide and dofetilide at different extracellular potassium and pacing frequencies. *J Cardiovasc Pharmacol* 1996;28:314-320.

81. Weyerbrock S, Schreieck J, Karch M, et al. Rate-independent effects of the new class III antiarrhythmic agent ambasilide on transmembrane action potentials in human ventricular endomyocardium. *J Cardiovasc Pharmacol* 1997;30:571-575.

82. Schmitt C, Karch M, Schreieck J, et al. Effect of the new class III antiarrhythmic agent ambasilide on monophasic and transmembrane action potential in human ventricular myocardium. *PACE* 1996;19:692. Abstract.

83. Wang J, Feng J, Nattel S. Class III antiarrhythmic drug action in experimental atrial fibrillation. Differences in reverse use dependence and effectiveness

between d-sotalol and the new antiarrhythmic drug ambasilide. *Circulation* 1994;90:2032-2040.

84. Gjini V, Schreieck J, Korth M, et al. Frequency dependence in the action of the class III antiarrhythmic drug dofetilide is modulated by altering L-type calcium current and digitalis glucoside. *J Cardiovasc Pharmacol* 1998;31:95-100.

85. Cobbe S, Manley S, Alexopoulos D, et al. Interaction of acute myocardial ischemia on the class III antiarrhythmic action of sotalol. *Cardiovasc Res* 1985;19:661-667.

86. Cobbe SM, Manley BS. The influence of ischemia on the electrophysiological properties of amiodarone in chronically treated rabbit hearts. *Eur Heart J* 1987;8:1241-1248.

87. Baskin E, Lynch J. Comparative effects of increased extracellular potassium and pacing frequency on the class III activities of methanesulfonanilide I_{Kr} blocker dofetilide, d-sotalol, E-4031, and MK-499. *J Cardiovasc Pharmacol* 1994;24:199-208.

88. Zhang ZH, Follmer CH, Sarma JSM, et al. Effect of ambasilide, a new class III agent, on plateau currents in isolated guinea pig ventricular myocytes: Block of delayed outward potassium current. *J Pharmacol Exp Ther* 1992;63:40-48.

89. Koidl B, Flaschberger P, Schaffer P, et al. Effects of the class III antiarrhythmic drug ambasilide on outward currents in human atrial myocytes. *Naunyn Schmiedeberg's Arch Pharmacol* 1996;353:226-232.

90. Sanguinetti MC, Jurkiewicz NK. Role of external Ca^{2+} and K^+ in gating of cardiac delayed rectifier K^+ currents. *Pflügers Arch* 1992;420:180-186.

91. Yao JA, Tseng GN. Azimilide (NE-10064) can prolong or shorten action potential duration in canine ventricular myocytes: Dependence on blockade of K, Ca and Na channels. *J Cardiovasc Electrophysiol* 1997;8:184-198.

92. Wang Z, Fermini B, Nattel S. Sustained depolarization-induced outward current in human atrial myocytes. Evidence for a novel delayed rectifier current similar to Kv1.5 cloned channel currents. *Circ Res* 1993;73:1061-1076.

93. Li GR, Feng J, Yue L, et al. Evidence for two components of delayed rectifier K^+ current in human ventricular myocytes. *Circ Res* 1996;78:689-696.

94. Amos GJ, Wettwer E, Metzger F, et al. Differences between outward currents of human atrial and subepicardial ventricular myocytes. *J Physiol* 1996;491:31-50.

95. Wang Z, Fermini B, Nattel S. Effects of flecainide, quinidine and 4-aminopyridine on transient outward and ultrarapid delayed rectifier currents in human atrial myocytes. *J Pharmacol Exp Ther* 1995;272:184-196.

96. Feng J, Wible B, Li GR, et al. Antisense oligodeoxynucleotides directed against Kv1.5 mRNA specifically inhibit ultrarapid delayed rectifier K^+ current in cultured adult human atrial myocytes. *Circ Res* 1997;80:572-579.

97. Pappano AJ, Mubabwa K. Actions of muscarinic agents and adenosine on the heart. In Fozzard HA (ed): *The Heart and the Cardiovascular System*. New York: Raven Press; 1992:1765-1776.

98. Lazdunski M. ATP-sensitive potassium channels: An overview. *J Cardiovasc Pharmacol* 1994;24(suppl):S1-S5.

99. Friedrichs GS, Abreu JN, Driscoll EM, et al. Antifibrillatory efficacy of long-term tedisamil administration in a postinfarcted canine model of ischemic ventricular fibrillation. *J Cardiovasc Pharmacol* 1998;31:56-66.

100. Hou ZY, Chang MS, Chen CY, et al. Acute treatment of recent-onset atrial fibrillation and flutter with a tailored dosing regimen of intravenous amiodarone: A randomized, digoxin-controlled study. *Eur Heart J* 1995;16:521-528.

101. Galve G, Rius T, Ballester R, et al. Intravenous amiodarone in treatment of recent-onset atrial fibrillation: Results of a randomized, controlled study. *J Am Coll Cardiol* 1996;27:1079-1082.
102. Donovan KD, Power BM, Hockings BEF, et al. Intravenous flecainide versus amiodarone for recent-onset atrial fibrillation. *Am J Cardiol* 1995;75:693-697.
103. Chapman MJ, Moran JL, O'Fathartaigh MS, et al. Management of atrial tachyarrhythmias in the critically ill: A comparison of intravenous procainamide and amiodarone. *Intensive Care Med* 1993;19:48-52.
104. Kerin NZ, Faitel K, Naini M. The efficacy of intravenous amiodarone for the conversion of chronic atrial fibrillation: Amiodarone vs quinidine for conversion of atrial fibrillation. *Arch Intern Med* 1996;156:49-53.
105. Zehender M, Hohnloser S, Müller B, et al. Effects of amiodarone versus quinidine and verapamil in patients with chronic atrial fibrillation: Results of a comparative study and a 2-year follow-up. *J Am Coll Cardiol* 1992;19:1054-1059.
106. Igoumenidis NE, Kochiadakis GE, Marketou ME, et al. Amiodarone in the treatment of chronic atrial fibrillation: Results of a randomised, controlled study. *J Am Coll Cardiol* 1998;31(suppl A):183A. Abstract.
107. Volgman AS, Stambler BS, Kappagoda C, et al. Comparison of intravenous ibutilide versus procainamide for the rapid termination of atrial fibrillation or flutter. *PACE* 1996;19:608.
108. Harry JD, Perry KT, Grauwels D, et al. A multinational study comparing the safety and efficacy of intravenous ibutilide fumarate with the safety and efficacy of intravenous dl-sotalol in termination of atrial flutter and atrial fibrillation. Technical Report on file with FDA.

27

Frequency Dependence of Class III Antiarrhythmic Drugs and Reversal by Sympathetic Stimulation

Philip T. Sager, MD and
Alaa Eldin Shalaby, MD

Introduction

There has been a major shift in antiarrhythmic drug development from class I agents to class III drugs that work primarily by prolonging repolarization. Most of these agents manifest their electrophysiologic actions by blocking at least one component of the delayed rectifier potassium current (I_K), although many agents also inhibit other repolarizing currents. Such class III drug-induced increases in the action potential duration (APD) result in prolongation of the wavelength of a reentrant circuit, hopefully leading to tachycardia termination or prevention of initiation. APD prolongation may also result in an inability of reentrant circuits to sustain, by altering the dynamics of the "pivot points."[1] However, as described by Dr. Hondgehem in chapter 24, one significant concern regarding the use of class III antiarrhythmic agents to prevent or terminate arrhythmias is that many agents, when administered to isolated myocytes, prolong the APD to a greater extent during bradycardia than during tachycardia, and such reverse frequency dependence may result in the agent having little or no

Supported in part from a Grant-in-Aid (G1117) from the Greater Los Angeles Chapter of the American Heart Association.
From Franz MR (ed): *Monophasic Action Potentials: Bridging Cell and Bedside.* ©Futura Publishing Company, Inc., Armonk, NY, 2000.

ability to prolong repolarization during the short cycle lengths commonly associated with clinical arrhythmias.[2,3] Conversely, as a result of bradycardia, the agents may cause excessive prolongation of the ventricular APD and QT intervals, heightening the risk of torsades de pointes. The issue is complex because other factors (eg, autonomic influences, ischemia) may affect drug-induced prolongation of repolarization as well as the frequency-dependent response.[4]

The findings of reverse frequency-dependent effects on repolarization have been most completely described in single-cell measurements of action potentials, and the degree to which the properties of clinically evaluated class III agents (eg, sematilide, dofetilide, d,l-sotalol, amiodarone, etc) in isolated tissues correlate with in vivo actions in humans is unclear. Experiments in isolated cells are inherently different from in vivo human determinations, due to species differences in the ionic currents responsible for the cardiac action potential, the loss of the effects of cell-to-cell coupling,[5] experiments performed at nonphysiologic temperatures and milieu (eg, tissue bath versus in vivo conditions), etc. For these reasons it is important to determine the frequency dependence of antiarrhythmic drugs in vivo in humans and not to simply extrapolate the single-cell or animal data to the human condition.

Monophasic action potential (MAP) recordings[6-8] permit the accurate measurement of human atrial and ventricular repolarization, and recent advances in catheter design by Franz and colleagues[9] of a contact silver-silver chloride electrode with a second pair of distal pacing electrodes allows the determination of repolarization and refractoriness at the same cardiac site. These technological advances permit the careful study of the electrophysiologic effects of pharmacologic agents on repolarization and refractoriness and allow drug-induced prolongation of refractoriness to be further delineated as being secondary to prolongation of APD or to other mechanisms such as a delay in recovery of sodium channels during phase 3 of the action potential.[10-12]

This chapter focuses on the in vivo data in humans, examining the frequency-dependent effects of class III antiarrhythmic agents on ventricular electrophysiology and the modulation of drug-induced prolongation of the APD during β-adrenergic sympathetic stimulation.

Frequency-Dependent Ventricular Electrophysiologic Effects of Class III Agents in Humans

Sematilide

Sematilide is a pure class III antiarrhythmic agent developed by Berlex Laboratories (Richmond, CA) that was shown during voltage clamp studies in isolated Purkinje fibers to prolong the APD by blocking I_K (most likely by specifically blocking the delayed rectifier potassium current [I_{Kr}]) without other cardiac actions or effects on the autonomic nervous system.[13-16] We recently examined the frequency-dependent actions of oral sematilide in a cohort of 10 patients undergoing evaluation of malignant ventricular arrhythmias.[15] The right ventricular MAP was recorded from the right ventricle during the patient's baseline drug-free electrophysiologic study. After steady state pacing (cycle lengths of 600, 500, 400, 350, and 300 milliseconds) for at least 150 beats, MAPs were recorded and the APD at 90% repolarization (APD_{90}) was determined. The right ventricular effective refractory period (RVERP) was also measured at the same ventricular site. The QRS duration was determined during steady state ventricular pacing as a measure of ventricular conduction. The patients were then given oral sematilide (mean dose 133 ± 29 mg every 8 hours) and the electrophysiologic measurements were repeated after steady state dosing. The catheter position was rigorously determined during the first electrophysiologic study and the catheter was placed in a similar position during the follow-up examination.

As shown in Figure 1, sematilide significantly prolonged the APD_{90}, and these effects were greater at a cycle length of 600 milliseconds compared to more rapid pacing, demonstrating that sematilide-induced APD prolongation was reverse frequency-dependent ($P<0.02$). When the data were analyzed using the diastolic interval, there was a significant correlation for both the absolute magnitude of sematilide-induced APD_{90} prolongation as

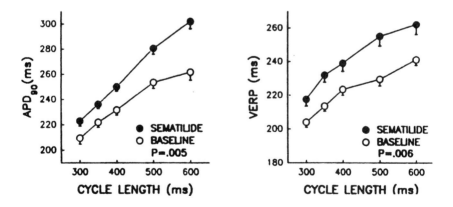

Figure 1. Graphs showing the frequency-dependent effects of sematilide on the action potential duration (APD_{90}) and the right ventricular refractory period (RVERP). Sematilide significantly increased the APD_{90} and the RVERP to a greater extent and for longer as compared to shorter paced cycle lengths ($P<0.05$, repeated measures ANOVA). Modified from Reference 15, with permission from the American Heart Association and the authors.

well as the percent increase in the APD_{90} as compared to the diastolic interval, indicating less prolongation of the APD_{90} during shorter as compared to longer diastolic intervals. The prolongation of the RVERP during sematilide administration paralleled the changes in the APD_{90} and, by use of repeated measures analysis of variance (ANOVA), sematilide-induced prolongation of the RVERP was also shown to be reverse frequency-dependent ($P<0.05$). Sematilide was without any effects on the QRS duration, thus showing a lack of effect on ventricular conduction. It did not alter the $RVERP/APD_{90}$ ratio, indicating that drug-induced increases in refractoriness were solely secondary to increases in repolarization.

In summary, these studies indicate that sematilide increases the APD and these increases in APD_{90} are responsible for the increases in the RVERP. Both repolarization and refractoriness were shown to have reverse frequency dependence and there were no effects on ventricular conduction. While the mechanisms for reverse frequency dependence were not evaluated in the current study, Jurkiewicz and Sanguinetti[17] have demonstrated, using voltage clamp techniques in isolated cells, that the pure class III I_{Kr} blocker dofetilide has reverse frequency dependence in their model and that the mechanism of this phenomenon is that during rapid pacing, due to the short diastolic intervals, I_{Ks} does not have sufficient time to deactivate completely, and thus build-up of I_{Ks} current partially offsets the rate-independent block of I_{Kr} by dofetilide, resulting in enhanced shortening of the APD during rapid pacing. Other possible mechanisms for sematilide-induced reverse frequency dependence include extracellular potassium accumulation at short cycle lengths in the intracellular clefts and subsequent augmentation of the conductance of repolarizing potassium currents, as well as a modulation of the inward calcium current during rapid heart rates.[18,19]

Dofetilide

Dofetilide is a methanesulfonanilide class III agent[17,20,21] that has been demonstrated to be a pure blocker of I_{Kr} and to be devoid of other electrophysiologic or antiadrenergic effects. As discussed above, dofetilide in isolated cell preparations has been shown to demonstrate reverse frequency dependence.[20] Using a methodology similar to that described above for sematilide, Sager[22] determined the effects of dofetilide (0.25 to 0.75 μg orally every 8 hours) on the monophasic APD. Dofetilide significantly prolonged the APD at all paced cycle lengths (Fig. 2) and there was significant reverse frequency dependence with a greater prolongation of the APD_{90} at longer as compared to shorter paced cycle lengths ($P<0.05$ by ANOVA). The changes in APD_{90} were paralleled by similar changes in the

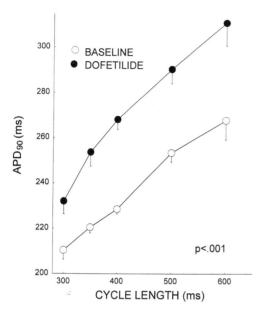

Figure 2. Graph showing the frequency-dependent effects of dofetilide on the action potential duration (APD_{90}). Dofetilide significantly increased the APD_{90} in a reverse frequency-dependent manner ($P<0.05$). Modified from Reference 22, with permission from the American Heart Association and the author.

refractory period and there were no significant changes in the paced QRS duration or the $RVERP/APD_{90}$ ratio.

Two additional studies have examined the effects of intravenous dofetilide on cardiac repolarization. Sedgwick et al[23] administered intravenous dofetilide and measured drug-induced increases in the human MAP between paced cycle lengths at 500 and 800 milliseconds. This study failed to show any frequency dependence of dofetilide over the range of pacing cycle lengths examined. Yuan et al[24] administered intravenous dofetilide to 10 patients and examined the APD_{90} at paced cycle lengths of 500 and 600 milliseconds. They failed to observe a drug-induced difference in APD_{90} prolongation at these two cycle lengths. These two studies differ from the above study of oral dofetilide in that pacing was not performed at the rapid cycle lengths frequently necessary to show reverse frequency dependence (these latter studies used a minimum cycle length of 500 milliseconds as the shortest paced cycle lengths). Thus, it is not surprising that reverse frequency dependence was not observed in these latter studies of intravenous dofetilide, since rapid pacing was not examined.

d,l-Sotalol

The frequency-dependent effects of d,l-sotalol have been determined[25] by use of the methodology discussed above. Seventeen patients were examined at baseline and then during chronic oral d,l-sotalol therapy (362 ± 21 mg/day). In contrast to sematilide or dofetilide, d,l-sotalol significantly prolonged the APD_{90} without frequency-dependent effects (Fig. 3). Interestingly, mild but significant reverse frequency-dependent effects of sotalol on the RVERP were observed. Similar to the above data with dofetilide and sematilide, sotalol had no effect on QRS duration or the $RVERP/APD_{90}$ ratio. Possible explanations for sotalol's lack of frequency-dependent effect on repolarization, as compared to sematilide and dofetilide, are that sotalol blocks multiple ionic channels (I_{Kr}, I_{to}, I_{K1}) and that β-blockade may affect frequency dependence.

In contrast to the above findings, Schmitt et al[26] examined the effects of intravenous d,l-sotalol on the APD_{90} in humans (Fig. 4) and did observe a reverse frequency-dependent effect on this parameter. The different results from these two studies may be related to the fact that the above study measured MAPs after steady state pacing for 200 beats, while Schmitt et al[26] measured the MAPs after only 20 beats, a period that might not have permitted the full accommodation of the action potentials to rapid pacing. In addition, there may be a difference between the effects of intravenous and oral d,l-sotalol and, if β-blockade has an effect on the frequency relationship, this may also vary with oral as compared to intravenous administration. Another intriguing explanation for the different results of the above studies is that the type of underlying heart disease may affect the frequency relationship. Indeed, Schmitt et al[4] have demonstrated in dogs that d,l-sotalol exerts reverse frequency-dependent prolongation of

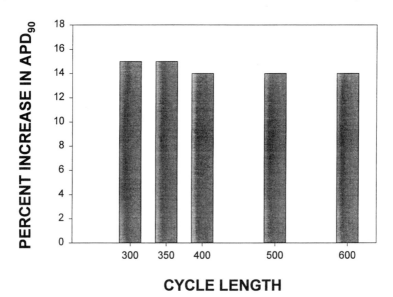

CYCLE LENGTH

Figure 3. Plot showing the frequency-dependent effects of d,l-sotalol on the percent increase in repolarization (APD_{90}). d,l-Sotalol prolonged the APD_{90} without frequency-dependent effects. Modified from Reference 25, with permission.

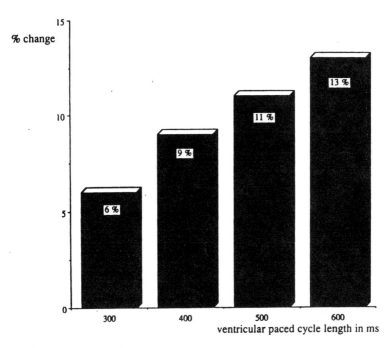

Figure 4. Plot showing the percent increase in the monophasic action potential duration at 90% repolarization (APD_{90}) during d,l-sotalol administration in humans over paced cycle lengths of 300 to 600 milliseconds. Modified from Reference 4, with permission from the *American Journal of Cardiology* and the authors.

repolarization in normal myocardium but that the drug's effects are frequency-independent in chronically infarcted myocardium. Thus, differences in the type of underlying heart disease of the patients could possibly be responsible for the disparate observations. A similar difference in the frequency-dependent effects of quinidine on Purkinje fiber repolarization in normal and infarcted dogs has also been reported.[27] Lastly, Shimizu et al[28] have also evaluated the frequency-dependent effects of d,l-sotalol. In this study, instead of measuring APDs in the same patients before and after d,l-sotalol administration, they took the baseline drug-free measurements in a separate group of patients with different forms of heart disease (concealed accessory pathway in controls versus sustained ventricular arrhythmias in d,l-sotalol patients). Given that the baseline and drug determinations were made in different patients, it is difficult to draw firm conclusions from this study.

d-Sotalol

The frequency-dependent effects of intravenous d-sotalol on human ventricular repolarization have been studied in 6 patients.[29] Over the range of tested cycle lengths (350 to 700 milliseconds), d-sotalol-induced increases in the APD_{90} appeared to be attenuated during rapid pacing.

Amiodarone

Sager et al[30] examined the effects of an 11-day loading regimen of amiodarone (1621 ± 162 mg/day) on human MAPs. The APD_{90} was increased by 10% to 13% compared to baseline, and these increases were independent of the paced cycle lengths (Fig. 5). When the RVERP was examined, there was a mild reverse frequency-dependent effect on this parameter ($P = 0.04$ by ANOVA). However, when the percent increase in the RVERP was determined, there was no significant frequency-dependent effect on this parameter. In addition, the absolute increase in the RVERP at the shortest paced cycle length (300 milliseconds) remained significantly increased by 33 milliseconds (17%; $P < 0.001$). As expected, and in contrast to the data examining d,l-sotalol,[25] dofetilide,[22] and sematilide,[15] when the paced QRS duration was evaluated, there was a significant frequency-dependent effect with a much greater prolongation of this parameter at shorter paced cycle lengths, as compared to longer cycle lengths (Fig. 5), consistent with use-dependent blockade of sodium channels. At the shortest paced cycle length, the QRS duration was prolonged by 28% as compared to baseline values. When the ratio of the $RVERP/APD_{90}$ was examined, this parameter was significantly increased during amiodarone therapy, indicating that the prolongation of the RVERP was secondary to prolongation of repolarization, as well as to time-dependent processes (most likely a delay in recovery of sodium channels during phase 3 of the APD).

In another series of experiments, Huikuri and Yli-Mayry[29] examined the effects of amiodarone on repolarization at baseline and after at least 3 months of oral amiodarone therapy. Over a range of pacing cycle lengths of 700 to 350 milliseconds, amiodarone prolonged the APD by 10% to 13% without frequency-dependent effects. These latter two studies in humans are consistent with the lack of a frequency-dependent effect on repolarization by amiodarone demonstrated in dogs by Anderson et al.[31] The frequency-independent action of amiodarone on repolarization may be related to its nonselective blockade of outward repolarizing potassium currents. The absence of a frequency-dependent effect may explain, in part, amiodarone's potent antiarrhythmic actions and low incidence of proarrhythmia: its ability to prevent arrhythmias by prolonging the APD is preserved during tachycardia and it does not further increase the APD during bradycardia, limiting bradycardia-induced torsades de pointes. In addition, when the RVERP is prolonged to a greater extent than the APD, early afterdepolarizations may fall within the refractory period and thus not propagate.

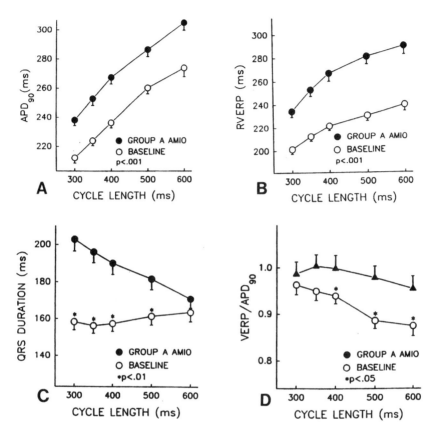

Figure 5. Graphs showing the frequency-dependent effects of amiodarone on electrophysiologic parameters. **A**. The frequency-dependent effect on the action potential duration at 90% repolarization (APD_{90}) demonstrating prolongation of this parameter without frequency-dependent effects. **B**. The frequency-dependent effects of amiodarone on the right ventricular effective refractory period (RVERP) demonstrating a mild reverse frequency-dependent effect (there was no significant percent increase in the RVERP as a function of paced cycle length). **C**. The effects of amiodarone on the QRS duration demonstrating significant frequency-dependent prolongation of this parameter during rapid pacing. **D**. The significant increase in the RVERP/APD_{90} ratio during amiodarone therapy ($P < 0.05$). Reproduced from Reference 30, with permission of the American Heart Association and the authors.

Other Class III Agents

As previously discussed, one likely explanation for the reverse frequency dependence of class III agents is that at rapid rates I_{Ks} has insufficient time to deactivate and there is build-up of I_{Ks} current with resulting shortening of the APD.[17] If this is an important mechanisms in humans, then it would be expected that a drug that blocked I_{Ks} would be devoid of frequency-dependent effects. Ambasilide is an investigational agent that blocks both I_{Ks} and I_{Kr}, and in animal studies was devoid of frequency-dependent effects.[32] Schmitt et al[33] examined MAPs in 7 patients during ambasilide treatment and demonstrated a frequency-independent increase in the APDs. Similar results were obtained in transmembrane recordings from isolated human heart tissue obtained from cardiac transplant recipients. Thus, block of I_{Ks} may result in a more favorable frequency relationship than that of pure I_{Kr} blockade.

Tedisamil is an experimental class III agent that blocks the transient outward current and possibly also I_{Kr}. Its frequency relationship has been examined in humans by use of MAP recordings, and these studies have demonstrated a reverse frequency-dependent prolongation of left ventricular repolarization.[34]

Modulation of Class III Drug-Induced Prolongation of Repolarization by Sympathetic Stimulation

Attention has been increasingly focused on the role the autonomic nervous system appears to play in the development of clinical arrhythmias. For example, β-blockers decrease arrhythmia mortality after myocardial infarction (MI),[35,36] increases in sympathetic activity as measured by norepinephrine spillover have been observed in patients with clinical sustained ventricular arrhythmias,[37] and the ventricular fibrillation threshold in dogs can be significantly reduced during sympathetic nerve stimulation.[38] Sympathetic stimulation by administration of β-adrenergic catecholamines has been shown to significantly attenuate the electrophysiologic actions of class I agents on refractoriness.[23,25,39-42] An important question regarding the use of class III antiarrhythmic agents is to what extent these agents' ability to prolong repolarization are altered during sympathetic stimulation. If the drugs are of clinical benefit by prolonging the APD and these effects are nullified during sympathetic stimulation, this may significantly limit their clinical efficacy.

Beta-adrenergic catecholamines modulate numerous currents in cardiac myocytes, can shorten repolarization by increasing I_{ks},[43] the chloride current (I_{Cl}),[44] and the sodium-potassium pump current,[45] and may improve ventricular conduction by increasing the fast inward sodium current (I_{Na}). In addition, beta stimulation also increases the slow inward calcium current (I_{Ca})[46] and the pacemaker current (I_F). The increase in I_{Ks} may be particularly important. Since many class III antiarrhythmic drugs block the rapidly activating component of I_{Kr}, it is possible that catecholamine-induced increases in I_{Ks} might overwhelm the effects of class III agents to prolong the APD. Indeed, in a recent study, Sanguinetti et al[43] demonstrated that the pure I_{Kr} blocker E-4031 (Fig. 6) increased the refractory period of isolated guinea pig papillary muscles by 50%, but that pretreatment with isoproterenol resulted in a significant decrease from baseline refractory period values despite E-4031 coadministration (these effects of isoproterenol were blocked by timolol). The negation of the effects of E-4031 were secondary to significant increases by isoproterenol of I_{Ks} and the chloride current, with no significant effect on I_{Kr}, which remained significantly inhibited during E-4031 administration. Similarly, the drug-induced prolongation of the ventricular monophasic APD in anesthetized dogs during d-sotalol administration (which exerts its electrophysiologic effects largely through blocking I_{Kr}) was markedly reduced during left stellate ganglion stimulation.[47]

The effects of β-adrenergic stimulation during isoproterenol infusion on the drug-induced prolongation of repolarization of sematilide, amiodarone, and d,l-sotalol have been examined in humans. In a series of experiments, Sager et al[25,48] examined patients undergoing drug-free electrophysiologic study, repeat electrophysiologic study during steady state oral drug dosing (in the case of amiodarone, drug testing was performed after 10.5 days of amiodarone loading), and during concomitant isoproterenol admin-

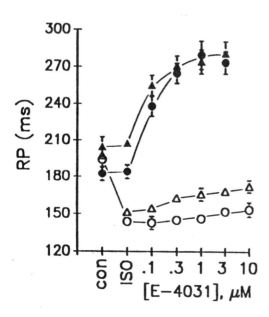

● E−4031 alone
▲ ISO + Timolol + E−4031
○ ISO alone
△ ISO + E−4031

Figure 6. Graphs showing the effects of E-4031 alone, isoproterenol (Iso) plus E-4031, isoproterenol plus timolol plus E-4031, and isoproterenol alone, on the refractory period of isolated guinea pig papillary muscles as a function of E-4031 concentration. E-4031 significantly increased the refractory period and these effects of E-4031 were totally abolished during concomitant isoproterenol administration ($P<0.05$). The effects of isoproterenol on E-4031–induced refractory period prolongation were fully reversed after timolol administration ($P<0.05$). From Reference 43, with permission of the American Heart Association and the authors.

istration (a fixed dose of 35 ng/kg/minute after a 12-minute equilibration period). Electrophysiologic determinations were performed after steady state pacing for 200 beats at paced cycle lengths ranging from 300 to 500 milliseconds (or 600 milliseconds depending on the sinus rate), and MAPs were measured from the right ventricular outflow tract.

Sematilide

Sematilide-induced increases in the APD_{90}[48] were fully reversed during isoproterenol infusion to values similar to those obtained at baseline (Fig. 7; P = ns, sematilide/isoproterenol versus baseline; $P<0.001$, sematilide versus sematilide/isoproterenol). In contrast, when the effects of isoproterenol on the RVERP were investigated, it was found that isoproterenol administration resulted in a significant reduction in the sematilide-induced increases in the RVERP to values significantly shorter than baseline drug-free values ($P<0.001$, sematilide versus sematilide/isoproterenol; $P<0.05$, baseline versus sematilide/isoproterenol). Thus, isoproterenol had a significantly greater effect on the reduction of the RVERP than on the APD_{90}; this was confirmed when the $RVERP/APD_{90}$ was examined and it was found that the normal increase of this ratio observed at short cycle lengths was negated following isoproterenol administration to patients receiving sematilide ($P<0.02$, sematilide versus sematilide/isoproterenol).

The effect of sematilide and sematilide plus isoproterenol on the sustained ventricular tachycardia (VT) cycle length was examined in morphologically similar monomorphic VTs (Fig. 8). While there was a nonsignificant trend for sematilide to increase the sustained VT cycle length, the administration of isoproterenol to patients receiving sematilide resulted in a significant shortening of the sustained VT cycle length compared to sematilide alone ($P=0.006$), and the cycle length tended to be decreased to values below baseline ($P<0.06$). In summary, these data demonstrate that isoproterenol fully reversed the effects of sematilide-induced prolongation of the APD_{90} and reduced the RVERP to values significantly below those obtained at baseline, and also shortened the sustained VT cycle length. These finding suggest that the electrophysiologic actions of a pure I_{Kr}-blocking agent in humans may be readily reversed during periods of increased sympathetic stimulation.

Amiodarone

The effects of isoproterenol on amiodarone-induced changes in cardiac electrophysiology were examined in 22 patients.[48] In contrast to the data obtained with sematilide, amiodarone-induced increases in the APD_{90}

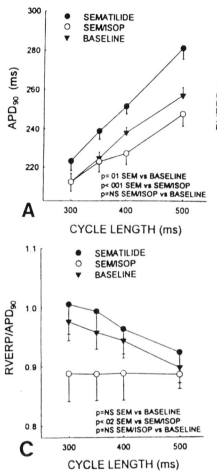

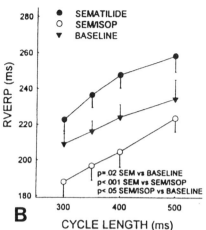

Figure 7. Graphs showing the frequency-dependent effects of sematilide and sematilide plus isoproterenol on electrophysiologic parameters. **A.** The effects on the APD_{90}. Sematilide-induced APD_{90} prolongation was fully reversed by isoproterenol. **B.** The effects on the right ventricular effective refractory period (RVERP). Sematilide-induced RVERP prolongation was reversed by isoproterenol to values significantly below baseline ($P<0.05$). **C.** The effects on the ratio of the right ventricular refractory period and action potential duration ($RVERP/APD_{90}$). During isoproterenol administration to patients receiving sematilide, the $RVERP/APD_{90}$ ratio was significantly reduced ($P=0.02$). Reproduced from Reference 48, with permission from the American Heart Association and the authors.

(Fig. 9) were attenuated but not reversed during isoproterenol infusion and the APD_{90} remained significantly prolonged by 4% to 8% at each paced cycle length compared to baseline values ($P=0.005$). Similar to the effects seen with sematilide, isoproterenol also reduced amiodarone-induced prolongation of repolarization to a significantly greater degree during slower pacing, as compared to more rapid pacing ($P<0.02$). The effects of isoproterenol on refractoriness was consistent with the effects on repolarization, and the RVERP remained significantly prolonged compared to baseline values, by 6% to 8% ($P=0.01$).

When the effects on the paced QRS duration were examined (Fig. 8), it was found that isoproterenol significantly reduced the paced QRS

SEMATILIDE

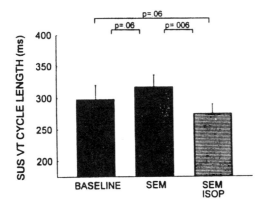

AMIODARONE

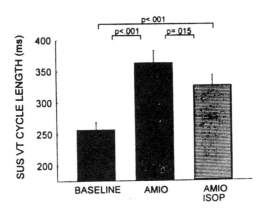

Figure 8. Graph showing the effects of sematilide or amiodarone before or during isoproterenol (ISOP) administration on sustained ventricular tachycardia (SUS VT) cycle length. Top: baseline, sematilide, and sematilide plus isoproterenol. Bottom: baseline, amiodarone, and amiodarone plus isoproterenol. During isoproterenol administration to patients receiving sematilide, the SUS VT cycle length was significantly reduced (P=0.006) compared with sematilide alone, and nonsignificantly reduced (P=0.06) compared with baseline drug-free values. Whereas isoproterenol administration to patients receiving amiodarone significantly reduced (P=0.015) the SUS VT cycle length, the SUS VT cycle length remained significantly prolonged (P<0.001) compared with baseline drug-free values. Modified from Reference 48, with permission of the American Heart Association and the authors.

duration. This reduction in QRS duration was relatively fixed at each paced cycle length (4% to 6% reduction; P=0.005), consistent with an improvement in ventricular conduction, possibly secondary to a relatively fixed increase in the rapid inward sodium current.[49,50] Overall, isoproterenol had no significant effects on the RVERP/APD$_{90}$ ratio. When the effects on morphologically similar VTs were examined, amiodarone alone resulted in a significant prolongation of the induced sustained VT cycle length from 257 ± 12 milliseconds to 363 ± 19 milliseconds (P<0.001). The administration of isoproterenol resulted in a significant reduction in sustained VT cycle length to a mean of 329 milliseconds, but these values remained significantly prolonged compared to baseline drug-free values (P<0.001).

Amiodarone's partial resistance to reversal of its electrophysiologic effects during catecholamine infusion may be secondary to multiple fac-

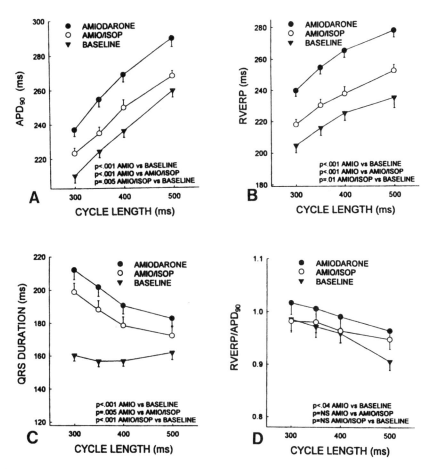

Figure 9. Graphs showing the frequency-dependent effects of amiodarone and amiodarone plus isoproterenol on electrophysiologic parameters. **A.** Amiodarone-induced prolongation of the APD_{90} was attenuated by isoproterenol but remained significantly prolonged compared to baseline values. **B.** Amiodarone-induced prolongation of the right ventricular effective refractory period (RVERP) was attenuated by isoproterenol but remained significantly prolonged compared to baseline values. **C.** The effects on the conduction as determined by the QRS duration. Isoproterenol administration during amiodarone significantly decreased the QRS duration by a fixed amount of 4% to 6% independent of the paced cycle length. **D.** The effects of amiodarone on the RVERP and action potential duration ratio ($RVERP/APD_{90}$). Amiodarone significantly increased the $RVERP/APD_{90}$ ratio compared with baseline values, and isoproterenol had no significant effect on this parameter. Modified from Reference 48, with permission of the American Heart Association and the authors.

tors. Amiodarone is a nonselective blocker of repolarizing potassium currents and some resistance may be offered by partial inhibition of I_{Ks}. It has been suggested that the drug's noncompetitive antiadrenergic effects play the major role in the drug's resistance to reversal during sympathetic stimulation.[48] This would be consistent with the fact that when myocytes are exposed to E-4031 and isoproterenol,[43] E-4031--induced effective refractory period prolongation is fully reversed by catecholamines[51] but these actions are blocked by timolol. The greater reduction in repolarization by isoproterenol at slower pacing, as compared to more rapid pacing, is interesting. Isoproterenol shortens the APD in part by increasing I_{Ks} during rapid pacing[43] secondary to its slow deactivation kinetics. This may limit further increases in this current by isoproterenol during rapid pacing, with less relative shortening of the APD.

d,l-Sotalol

The effects of isoproterenol infusion on d,l-sotalol--induced changes in ventricular electrophysiology were examined in 17 patients.[25] Oral d,l-sotalol significantly prolonged the APD_{90}, and these effects were mildly reduced during isoproterenol administration by 2% to 4% ($P=0.02$ compared to sotalol alone by ANOVA [Fig. 10]). d,l-Sotalol administration resulted in increases in the RVERP of 8% to 17%, but isoproterenol failed to exert

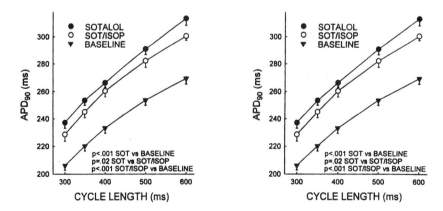

Figure 10. Graphs showing that frequency-dependent effects of d,l-sotalol and d,l-sotalol plus isoproterenol (ISOP) on repolarization (APD_{90}; left panel) and the right ventricular effective refractory period (RVERP; right panel). d,l-Sotalol prolonged the APD_{90} without frequency-dependent effects and the drug's effects on repolarization were only mildly attenuated by isoproterenol. d,l-Sotalol's effects on the RVERP demonstrated reverse frequency dependence and overall isoproterenol's effects on the d,l-sotalol-induced RVERP prolongation were not significant. Modified from Reference 25, with permission.

a significant effect on the RVERP, nonsignificantly reducing this parameter during sotalol therapy by 0% to 3%. Isoproterenol had no effect on the QRS duration of patients receiving sotalol or on the RVERP/APD$_{90}$ ratio. When morphologically similar induced sustained VTs were examined, d,l-sotalol modestly increased the sustained VT cycle length from 272 ± 14 milliseconds to 304 ± 10 milliseconds ($P<0.05$) and isoproterenol had no effect on the sustained VT cycle length (308 ± 12 milliseconds), which remained significantly prolonged compared to baseline values ($P<0.05$). Thus, d,l-sotalol was more resistant than amiodarone or the pure class III agent sematilide to reversal of its electrophysiologic effects.

Groh et al[52] examined the reversal of sotalol's ability to prolong the effective refractory period of guinea pig myocytes and demonstrated that d,l-sotalol was significantly more resistant to reversal than d-sotalol. When whole cell current recordings were examined, d,l-sotalol demonstrated significantly greater blockade of I_{Cl} and I_{Ks} than d-sotalol, whose blockade of I_{Kr} was overwhelmed by increases in the other repolarizing currents during catecholamine infusion.

Summary

The use of MAP recordings in humans has permitted accurate determination of repolarization, including frequency-dependent effects of class III agents. The data show that pure I_{Kr} blockers exerted reverse frequency-dependent effects on repolarization in humans while the effects of amiodarone and ambasilide were frequency-independent. The data on d,l-sotalol is inconsistent. Clearly, in addition to frequency dependence, other factors play an important role in a drug's efficacy, since dofetilide has been shown to have a favorable antiarrhythmic profile.[21,53] Even small increases in the APD during tachycardias may be antiarrhythmic by closing the excitable gap, causing oscillations in refractoriness and conduction,[54-56] or altering the dynamics of "pivot points."[1] Reverse frequency dependence may result in an agent being more efficacious in the prevention of arrhythmia initiation (when the heart rate is initially slow) than in arrhythmia termination (when the heart rate is rapid and when the drug's effects are minimized).[57] Determinants of repolarization are useful to delineate the mechanisms responsible for prolongation of refractoriness by antiarrhythmic agents. Amiodarone-induced prolongation of the ERP was shown to be secondary to APD-prolongation–dependent and –independent processes,[30] and isoproterenol-induced shortening of the RVERP in patients receiving sematilide was demonstrated to be secondary to processes other than APD shortening.[48]

The different class III agents have divergent proclivities for their electrophysiologic actions to be modulated by sympathetic stimulation: d,l-sotalol was highly resistant and amiodarone's effects were partially attenuated, while sematilide's effects were fully reversed during sympathetic stimulation. These findings may have important ramifications on the utility of class III agents to prevent clinical arrhythmias, and they suggest the usefulness of concomitant antiadrenergic maneuvers or of the development of drugs that block currents augmented by β-adrenergic sympathetic stimulation (eg, I_{Ks}, I_{Cl}). While there is a need for more clinical studies to evaluate the benefits of combining antiadrenergic actions to class III drug effects, it is relevant that patients who received the greatest benefit from amiodarone in the EMIAT[58] and CAMIAT[59] post-MI studies were receiving concomitant β-blocker therapy. Interestingly, in a canine model of post-MI ischemic dogs who developed ventricular fibrillation during increased sympathetic activity, d,l-sotalol but not d-sotalol, was effective prophylactic therapy against arrhythmia development.[60,61]

Conclusion

The frequency-dependent effects on repolarization differ significantly among the different class III agents in humans. β-Adrenergic stimulation significantly modulates the electrophysiologic actions of antiarrhythmic agents, and pure I_{Kr} blockers are highly sensitive to reversal of their prolonging effects on repolarization and refractoriness during catecholamine administration. The role of the autonomic nervous system in modulating class III drug effects appears to be clinically important.

Acknowledgment The authors are thankful to Elizabeth Corey for her assistance in the preparation of this manuscript.

References

1. Girouard SD, Pastore JM, Laurita KR, et al. Optical mapping in a new guinea pig model of ventricular tachycardia reveals mechanisms for multiple wavelengths in a single reentrant circuit. *Circulation* 1996;93:603-613.
2. Hondeghem LM, Snyders DJ. Class III antiarrhythmic agents have a lot of potential but a long way to go. Reduced effectiveness and dangers of reverse use dependence. *Circulation* 1990;81:686-690.
3. Nattel S, Zeng FD. Frequency-dependent effects of antiarrhythmic drugs on action potential duration and refractoriness of canine cardiac Purkinje fibers. *J Pharmacol Exp Ther* 1984;229:283-291.
4. Schmitt C, Beyer T, Karch M, et al. Sotalol exhibits reverse use-dependent action on monophasic action potentials in normal but not in infarcted canine ventricular myocardium. *J Cardiovasc Pharmacol* 1992;19:487-492.
5. Laurita KR, Girouard SD, Rudy Y, Rosenbaum DS. Role of passive electrical properties during action potential restitution in intact heart. *Am J Physiol* 1997;273:H1205-H1214.

6. Franz MR, Burkhoff D, Spurgeon H, et al. In vitro validation of a new cardiac catheter technique for recording monophasic action potentials. *Eur Heart J* 1986;7:34-41.

7. Franz MR, Swerdlow CD, Liem LB, Schaefer J. Cycle length dependence of human action potential duration in vivo. Effects of single extrastimuli, sudden sustained rate acceleration and deceleration, and different steady-state frequencies. *J Clin Invest* 1988;82:972-979.

8. Franz MR. Method and theory of monophasic action potential recording. *Prog Cardiovasc Dis* 1991;33:347-368.

9. Franz MR, Chin MC, Sharkey HR, et al. A new single catheter technique for simultaneous measurement of action potential duration and refractory period in vivo. *J Am Coll Cardiol* 1990;16:878-886.

10. Franz MR, Burkhoff D, Yue DT, Sagawa K. Mechanically induced action potential changes and arrhythmia in isolated and in situ canine hearts. *Cardiovasc Res* 1989;23:213-223.

11. Koller BS, Karasik PE, Solomon AJ, Franz MR. Relation between repolarization and refractoriness during programmed electrical stimulation in the human right ventricle. Implications for ventricular tachycardia induction. *Circulation* 1995;91:2378-2384.

12. Lee RJ, Liem LB, Cohen TJ, Franz MR: Relation between repolarization and refractoriness in the human ventricle: Cycle length dependence and effect of procainamide. *J Am Coll Cardiol* 1992;19:614-618.

13. Lynch JJJ, Baskin EP, Nutt EM, et al. Comparison of binding to rapidly activating delayed rectifier K+ channel, I_{Kr}, and effects on myocardial refractoriness for class III antiarrhythmic agents. *J Cardiovasc Pharmacol* 1995;25:336-340.

14. Sager PT, Singh BN. Electrophysiological and pharmacodynamic profile of sematilide HCL. In Singh BN, Wellens HJJ, Hiraoka M (eds): *Electropharmacological Control of Cardiac Arrhythmias.* Mt. Kisco, NY: Futura Publishing Co., Inc.; 1994:525-534.

15. Sager PT, Nademanee K, Antimisiaris M, et al. Antiarrhythmic effects of selective prolongation of refractoriness. Electrophysiologic actions of sematilide HCl in humans. *Circulation* 1993;88:1072-1082.

16. Lee KS, Tsai TD, Lee EW. Membrane activity of class III antiarrhythmic compounds: A comparison between ibutilide, d-sotalol, E-4031, sematilide and dofetilide. *Eur J Pharmacol* 1993;234:43-53.

17. Jurkiewicz NK, Sanguinetti MC. Rate-dependent prolongation of cardiac action potentials by a methanesulfonanilide class III antiarrhythmic agent. Specific block of rapidly activating delayed rectifier K+ current by dofetilide. *Circ Res* 1993;72:75-83.

18. Gjini V, Schreieck J, Korth M, et al. Frequency dependence in the action of the class III antiarrhythmic drug dofetilide is modulated by altering L-type calcium current and digitalis glucoside. *J Cardiovasc Pharmacol* 1998;31:95-100.

19. Li GR, Nattel S. Properties of human atrial I_{Ca} at physiological temperatures and relevance to action potential. *Am J Physiol* 1997;272:H227-H235.

20. Kiehn J, Wible B, Ficker E, et al. Cloned human inward rectifier K+ channel as a target for class III methanesulfonanilides. *Circ Res* 1995;77:1151-1155.

21. Sager PT. New antiarrhythmic agents. *Electrophys Board Rev* In Press.

22. Sager PT. The frequency-dependent effects of dofetilide in humans. *Circulation* 1995;92:II774. Abstract.

23. Sedgwick ML, Rasmussen HS, Cobb SM. Effects of the class III antiarrhythmic drug dofetilide on ventricular monophasic action potential duration and QT interval dispersion in stable angina pectoris. *Am J Cardiol* 1992;70:1432-1437.

24. Yuan S, Wohlfart B, Rasmussen HS, et al. Effect of dofetilide on cardiac repolarization in patients with ventricular tachycardia. A study using simultaneous monophasic action potential recordings from two sites in the right ventricle. *Eur Heart J* 1994;15:514-522.

25. Sager PT, Behboodikhah M. Frequency-dependent electrophysiologic effects of d,l-sotalol and quinidine and modulation by beta-adrenergic stimulation. *J Cardiovasc Electrophysiol* 1996;7:102-112.

26. Schmitt C, Brachmann J, Karch M, et al. Reverse use-dependent effects of sotalol demonstrated by recording monophasic action potentials of the right ventricle. *Am J Cardiol* 1991;68:1183-1187.

27. Montero M, Beyer T, Schmitt C, et al. Differential effects of quinidine on transmembrane action potentials of normal and infarcted canine Purkinje fibers. *J Cardiovasc Pharmacol* 1992;20:304-310.

28. Shimizu W, Kurita T, Suyama K, et al. Reverse use dependence of human ventricular repolarization by chronic oral sotalol in monophasic action potential recordings. *Am J Cardiol* 1996;77:1004-1008.

29. Huikuri HV, Yli-Mayry S. Frequency dependent effects of d-sotalol and amiodarone on the action potential duration of the human right ventricle. *PACE* 1992;15:2103-2107.

30. Sager PT, Uppal P, Follmer C, et al. Frequency-dependent electrophysiologic effects of amiodarone in humans. *Circulation* 1993;88:1063-1071.

31. Anderson KP, Walker R, Dustman T, et al. Rate-related electrophysiologic effects of long-term administration of amiodarone on canine ventricular myocardium in vivo. *Circulation* 1989;79:948-958.

32. Weyerbrock S, Schreieck J, Karch M, et al. Rate-independent effects of the new class III antiarrhythmic agent ambasilide on transmembrane action potentials in human ventricular endomyocardium. *J Cardiovasc Pharmacol* 1997;30:571-575.

33. Schmitt C, Karch M, Schreieck J, et al. Effects of the new class III antiarrhythmic agent ambasilide on monophasic and transmembrane action potential in human ventricular myocardium. *PACE* 1996;19:692. Abstract.

34. Bargheer K, Bode F, Klein HU, et al. Prolongation of monophasic action potential duration and the refractory period in the human heart by tedisamil, a new potassium-blocking agent. *Eur Heart J* 1994;15:1409-1414.

35. Olsson G, Rehnqvist N, Sjogren A, et al. Long-term treatment with metoprolol after myocardial infarction: Effect on 3 year mortality and morbidity. *J Am Coll Cardiol* 1985;5:1428-1437.

36. Yusuf S, Wittes J, Friedman L. Overview of results of randomized clinical trials in heart disease. I. Treatments following myocardial infarction. *JAMA* 1988;260:2088-2093.

37. Meredith IT, Broughton A, Jennings GL, Esler MD. Evidence of a selective increase in cardiac sympathetic activity in patients with sustained ventricular arrhythmias. *N Engl J Med* 1991;325:618-624.

38. Parker GW, Michael LH, Hartley CJ, et al. Central β-adrenergic mechanisms may modulate ischemic ventricular fibrillation in pigs. *Circ Res* 1990;66:259-270.

39. Markel ML, Miles WM, Luck JC, et al. Differential effects of isoproterenol on sustained ventricular tachycardia before and during procainamide and quinidine antiarrhythmic drug therapy. *Circulation* 1993;87:783-792.

40. Morady F, Kou WH, Kadish AH, et al. Effects of epinephrine in patients with an accessory atrioventricular connection treated with quinidine. *Am J Cardiol* 1988;62:580-584.

41. Calkins H, Sousa J, el-Atassi R, et al. Reversal of antiarrhythmic drug effects by epinephrine: Quinidine versus amiodarone [see comments]. *J Am Coll Cardiol* 1992;19:347-352.

42. Jazayeri MR, Van Wyhe G, Avitall B, et al. Isoproterenol reversal of antiarrhythmic effects in patients with inducible sustained ventricular tachyarrhythmias. *J Am Coll Cardiol* 1989;14:705-714.

43. Sanguinetti MC, Jurkiewicz NK, Scott A, Siegl PK. Isoproterenol antagonizes prolongation of refractory period by the class III antiarrhythmic agent E-4031 in guinea pig myocytes. Mechanism of action. *Circ Res* 1991;68:77-84.

44. Harvey RD, Hume JR. Autonomic regulation of a chloride current in heart. *Science* 1989;244:983-985.

45. Boyett NR, Fedida D. Changes in the electrical activity of dog Purkinje fibers at high heart rates. *J Physiol (Lond)* 1984;350:361-391.

46. Reuter H. Calcium channel modulation by neurotransmitter, enzymes and drugs. *Nature* 1983;301:569-574.

47. Vanoli E, Priori SG, Nakagawa H, et al. Sympathetic activation, ventricular repolarization and I_{kr} blockade: Implications for the antifibrillatory efficacy of potassium channel blocking agents. *J Am Coll Cardiol* 1995;25:1609-1614.

48. Sager PT, Follmer C, Uppal P, et al. The effects of beta-adrenergic stimulation on the frequency-dependent electrophysiologic actions of amiodarone and sematilide. *Circulation* 1994;90:1811-1819.

49. Matsuda JJ, Lee H, Shibata EF. Enhancement of rabbit cardiac sodium channels by beta-adrenergic stimulation. *Circ Res* 1992;70:199-207.

50. Lee HC, Matsuda JJ, Reynertson SI, et al. Reversal of lidocaine effects on sodium currents by isoproterenol in rabbit hearts and heart cells. *J Clin Invest* 1993;91:693-701.

51. Manolis AS, Estes NAM III. Reversal of electrophysiologic effects of flecainide on the accessory pathway by isoproterenol in the Wolff-Parkinson-White syndrome. *Am J Cardiol* 1989;64(3):194-198.

52. Groh WJ, Gibson KJ, McAnulty JH, Maylie JG. Beta-adrenergic blocking property of dl-sotalol maintains class III efficacy in guinea pig ventricular muscle after isoproterenol. *Circulation* 1995;91:262-264.

53. Singh S, Berk M, Yellen L, et al. Efficacy and safety of oral dofetilide in maintaining normal sinus in patients with atrial fibrillation/flutter: A multicenter study. *Circulation* 1997;(suppl 70th Scientific Sessions)96:2145. Abstract.

54. Frame LH, Rhee EK. Spontaneous termination of reentry after one cycle or short nonsustained runs. Role of oscillations and excess dispersion of refractoriness. *Circ Res* 1991;68:493-502.

55. Frame LH, Simson MB. Oscillations of conduction, action potential duration, and refractoriness. A mechanism for spontaneous termination of reentrant tachycardias. *Circulation* 1988;78:1277-1287.

56. Guo GB, Ellenbogen KA, Wood MA, Stambler BS. Conversion of atrial flutter by ibutilide is associated with increased atrial cycle length variability. *J Am Coll Cardiol* 1996;27:1083-1089.

57. Villemaire C, Talajic M, Nattel S. Mechanisms by which sotalol prevents atrial fibrillation at doses that fail to terminate the arrhythmia. *Circulation* 1997;96(suppl):I236. Abstract.

58. Julian DG, Camm AJ, Frangin G, et al. Randomised trial of effect of amiodarone on mortality in patients with left-ventricular dysfunction after recent myocardial infarction: EMIAT. European Myocardial Infarct Amiodarone Trial Investigators. *Lancet* 1997;349:667-674.
59. Cairns JA, Connolly SJ, Roberts R, Gent M. Randomised trial of outcome after myocardial infarction in patients with frequent or repetitive ventricular premature depolarisations: CAMIAT. Canadian Amiodarone Myocardial Infarction Arrhythmia Trial Investigators. *Lancet* 1997;349:675-682.
60. Vanoli E, Hull SSJ, Adamson PB, et al. K$^+$ channel blockade in the prevention of ventricular fibrillation in dogs with acute ischemia and enhanced sympathetic activity. *J Cardiovasc Pharmacol* 1995;26:847-854.
61. Schwartz PJ, Billman GE, Stone HL. Autonomic mechanisms in ventricular fibrillation induced by myocardial ischemia during exercise in dogs with healed myocardial infarction. An experimental preparation for sudden cardiac death. *Circulation* 1984;69:790-800.

28

Modification of the Ventricular Tachyarrhythmia Substrate by Combined Class Ia and Class III Drug Treatment:

Role of Use Dependency

S. Douglas Lee MD, Paul Dorian MD, MSc and David M. Newman MD, FACC

The focus of pharmacologic management of ventricular tachyarrhythmias evolved from modification of conduction to modification of repolarization in an attempt to alter the electrical substrate and thus the clinical course of patients prone to sudden cardiac death. Progress in the pharmacologic management of ventricular tachycardia (VT) was made with the availability of drugs that prolong repolarization, such as sotalol[1] and particularly amiodarone, which, like sotalol, prolongs repolarization and possesses antiadrenergic properties and also has class I antiarrhythmic effects. The success of amiodarone has resulted in the common clinical practice of empirical amiodarone administration for the pharmacotherapy of ventricular tachyarrhythmias. Randomized clinical trials of device therapy versus pharmacotherapy have consistently used amiodarone as the drug of choice in prospective comparisons.[2-4] The success of amiodarone in the prevention of sudden death suggests that a combination of multiple

From Franz MR (ed): *Monophasic Action Potentials: Bridging Cell and Bedside.*
©Futura Publishing Company, Inc., Armonk, NY, 2000.

antiarrhythmic mechanisms may act synergistically to improve the chances of success of pharmacologic suppression of VT. The hypothesis may thus be raised that antiarrhythmic effectiveness may also be obtained by combining antiarrhythmic drugs with complementary mechanisms of effect to alter the ventricular tachyarrhythmia substrate.

Mechanisms that may help to explain the beneficial effect of amiodarone or other types of pharmacotherapy have expanded beyond traditional views of prolongation of refractoriness or repolarization to involve concepts which account for the effect of rate- or cycle-length–dependent phenomena on drug action. These mechanisms can be studied with electrophysiologic testing, particularly with the insights provided by monophasic action potential (MAP) recordings. It must be recognized that even these mechanistic insights in the intact human heart are limited to the tissue that can be sampled, and excluded are insights relating to the relationship between heterogeneity of myocardial cellular elements and dysrhythmias[5,6] or the contribution of passive membrane properties to treatment effect.[7,8]

The traditional clinical application of invasive electrophysiologic testing has been to dichotomize the results based on VT inducibility. Using this approach, invasive studies have not been found to be superior to noninvasive tests in predicting clinical outcome (based on VT recurrence).[1] However, interpreting the results of electrophysiologic testing in a manner that emphasizes the continuous nature of the physiologic data may provide greater clinical utility to the test and offer mechanistic insights in the search for rational drug use. Inducibility as an endpoint requires an arbitrary definition of what constitutes a "positive" as opposed to a "negative" test. It may be more appropriate to approach inducibility in a continuous fashion, and indeed supportive data suggest that fewer ventricular responses induced portends a better outcome.[9]

Despite its limitations, the presence or absence of inducibility of VT at electrophysiologic testing remains the standard criterion for predicting the likelihood of success of a particular drug therapy in preventing VT recurrence. Among patients with spontaneous sustained VT and inducible sustained VT at drug-free electrophysiologic study, the inability to induce sustained VT in the presence of an antiarrhythmic drug indicates a low likelihood (<15% per year) of a spontaneous recurrence[10-12]; however, the overall chance of drug success at electrophysiologic study is only 10% to 40%. The likelihood of success of drug therapy varies with factors such as the particular drug employed, the patient, and the number of agents previously tested.[13] Continued ability to induce VT despite antiarrhythmic monotherapy appears to confer a poor prognosis, with an up to 80% risk of arrhythmia recurrence at 1 year.[12] However, the prognostic significance of continued inducibility depends on the drugs tested. Amiodarone, for example, may be associated with low recurrence rates despite high rates of inducibility; recurrence of VT may also be well tolerated, depending on the rate of VT induced.[14]

The generally disappointing results concerning electropharmacologic testing that emerged after the ESVEM trial has led to the current strategy of empirical device or drug therapy for patients with VT. Beyond inducibility, however, prospective studies have demonstrated that amiodarone-induced slowing of induced VT (associated with increased blood pressure, improved hemodynamic tolerance, slowing of cycle length, and prolongation of effective refractory period [ERP]) adequately predicted survival even if VT occurred.[15] Smaller series have highlighted the importance of changes in ERP in predicting drug efficacy.[16] An increase in ERP can be generated by either class III effect or via postrepolarization refractoriness by potent sodium channel blockade.[17] Postrepolarization refractoriness, however, may at the same time promote reentrant proarrhythmia by increasing conduction slowing.[18] Class Ia agents at low doses possess elements of both mechanisms.

Electropharmacologic studies of VT have demonstrated the importance of prolongation of refractoriness in predicting a favorable response to drug therapy.[16,19] Drugs that prolong cardiac refractoriness by delaying repolarization, such as sotalol or amiodarone, have been shown to be superior to sodium channel blocking agents (which primarily slow cardiac conduction) for management of recurrent VT or sudden death.[20,21] Both class I and class III drugs increase refractoriness. An increase in the ventricular ERP (VERP) during antiarrhythmic drug therapy correlates with an increase in VT cycle length.[22,23] Thus, prolonging VERP slows the rate of VT and, with certain drugs (eg, amiodarone), refractoriness is the best indicator of VT cycle length on treatment.[22] Slowing of VT may be an important facet of antiarrhythmic drug therapy, making the arrhythmia more likely to be tolerated hemodynamically.[10,15,24] Its importance has been underplayed due in part to the ambiguity surrounding assessment of hemodynamic tolerance.

Class Ia Antiarrhythmic Agents and Refractoriness

Class Ia drugs include quinidine, procainamide, and disopyramide, and are grouped together according to widely accepted classification schemes because they depress phase 0 of the action potential, slow conduction, and prolong repolarization.[25] Sodium channel blockers prolong refractoriness by shifting the voltage-dependent recovery of sodium channels to a more negative point in the action potential and thereby prolonging time-dependent recovery of excitability.[26-29] Therefore, even when repolarization is complete and membrane voltage has reached its previous baseline negative potential, sodium channels may still not be sufficiently recovered to allow a new action potential, a phenomenon termed *postrepolarization refractoriness*.[30] This is reflected by prolongation of refractoriness relative to repolarization and is quantified by the ratio of ERP to action potential duration (ERP/APD).[31] In addition to prolonging refractoriness by blocking sodium channels, class Ia drugs also prolong APD by directly inhibiting the delayed rectifier potassium current (I_K) by the parent drug or its metabolites.[32,33]

At the receptor level, these drugs bind to a receptor site at the inner pore of the delayed rectifier potassium channel when in the open state.[34,35] The net flow of current may be even more complex because quinidine blocks multiple potassium currents other than I_K in vitro, including the transient outward potassium current (I_{to}) and I_{K1}.[36] The relative extent of refractoriness prolongation or "class III" effect of "class I" drugs decreases as heart rate increases. At slow rates, it is proposed that there are a greater number of potassium channel receptors than sodium channel receptors occupied.[36,37] However, at faster rates the converse applies and thus there are proportionately fewer potassium channels than sodium channels occupied.[38,39] The mechanism of this effect is not known, but increased affinity of the drug to its receptor when the heart rate is low may occur because of decreased accumulation of potassium in the extracellular space.[38,39] Therefore, "class III" effects are more marked at long cycle lengths, whereas sodium channel blockade leading to conduction slowing and "class I" effect occurs to a greater degree at shorter cycle lengths.[31,32,37,40]

Despite a moderate degree of efficacy in patients with sustained ventricular arrhythmias,[41] monotherapy with a class Ia agent is not ideal because of the risk of proarrhythmia which may be as high at 8% per year.[42,43] Clinical trials comparing multiple class I versus class III agents favor the latter, with a decreased likelihood of developing recurrent ventricular arrhythmias during use of sotalol[1,20,44,45] or amiodarone.[21,46,47] These results may be a reflection of the detrimental effects of excessive conduction delay in diseased or abnormal tissue that is observed with sodium channel blockers.[30] Furthermore, animal studies reveal that sodium channel blockade in the context of concomitant myocardial ischemia results in a significantly increased risk of ventricular fibrillation,[17] again reinforcing the case against monotherapy with a class I agent.

Class III Antiarrhythmic Agents and the Concept of Reverse Use Dependence

The electrophysiologic effect of class III drugs is to prolong the action potential. This effect results from a relative reduction in outwardly directed currents or an increase in inwardly directed currents. Prolongation of the action potential is achieved for most class III drugs by blockade of the delayed rectifier outward potassium current (primarily I_{Kr}, the rapid component of this current), which has classically been described as drug-sensitive. Sotalol prolongs APD by blocking the rapid component of the outward potassium current but does not affect the slow component of this current (I_{Ks}). Indeed, most currently available class III effects are mediated through I_{Kr} blockade, and the theoretical possibility exists of even greater prolongation of repolarization if other outward currents can be inhibited.[37]

Multicenter randomized trials have shown sotalol to be more effective in suppressing VT than class I agents alone.[20,45] However, class III effects mediated via I_{Kr} blockade demonstrate what has been termed *reverse use dependence*, a progressive loss of antiarrhythmic effect at rapid cycle lengths.[37] Sotalol is an example of a drug that exhibits reverse use dependence in APD prolongation,[48-52] resulting in an attenuation of the increase in ERP over control as cycle lengths decrease (Fig. 1). Similar to d,l-sotalol, d-sotalol exhibits reverse use dependence in prolongation of ventricular APD.[53] Other drugs in this class for which reverse use dependence has been demonstrated include sematilide,[54,55] dofetilide,[56] E-4031, and UK 66,914.[57] The class III effects of quinidine[27,58,59] and procainamide[37] are also subject to this effect.

A drug or a combination of drugs that prolongs ventricular refractoriness and whose effects are preserved at high cardiac stimulation frequen-

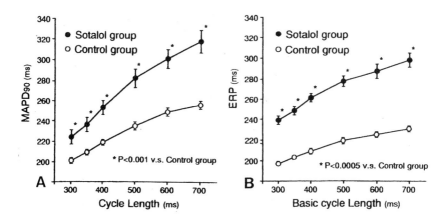

Figure 1. Reverse use dependence observed with sotalol monotherapy. **A.** Increases in the action potential duration that are observed at slow cycle lengths are progressively attenuated at faster rates. **B.** There is also reverse use dependence in refractoriness prolongation, since the primary determinant of refractoriness is prolongation of repolarization. Adapted from *American Journal of Cardiology* 76:1004-1008, 1996, with permission from Excerpta Medica Inc.

cies may be useful for preventing induced and spontaneous VT.[37] In addition to increased drug efficacy, there would theoretically be decreased proarrhythmia if repolarization were not excessively prolonged at slow heart rates.[60-63] The relative lack of reverse use dependence may underscore efficacy of amiodarone, a compound that inherently possesses significant class Ia and class III effects.[23]

It has been speculated that a factor responsible for some of the rate-related loss of drug-induced APD prolongation may the relatively greater contribution of I_{Ks}, a slowly activating outward potassium current, to repolarization at rapid rates.[64] The proposed mechanism involves the incomplete deactivation of I_{Ks} during short diastolic intervals, resulting in a greater net repolarizing current at faster versus slower rates.

Interactions between drug effect and autonomic state may also alter potassium currents and promote reverse use dependence. Clinically, pure I_{Kr} blockade without β-blockade can be harmful, particularly post myocardial infarction and in left ventricular dysfunction, as was demonstrated by the adverse effects of d-sotalol in the SWORD study.[65,66] Other pure I_{Kr} blockers such as sematilide and E-4031 undergo reversal of APD-prolonging effects with the addition of β-adrenergic stimulation,[54,67] which, in voltage clamped guinea pig myocytes, has been shown to be due to a selective β-adrenergic augmentation of I_{Ks} repolarizing current.[67] Adrenergic stimulation can also shorten the APD by increasing rate, I_{to}, the chloride current (I_{Cl}), and the sodium-potassium pump current ($I_{Na-K\ pump}$).[68-73] In patients receiving class III antiarrhythmic therapy, drug-mediated APD prolongation and refractoriness are attenuated by isoproterenol in the electrophysiology laboratory.[74]

As a result, β-blockade may be of additive benefit combined with all antiarrhythmic drugs, particularly in states with high adrenergic tone such as sustained VT. The utility of racemic sotalol and the most recent substudy analysis of CAMIAT and EMIAT support this view with marked additive benefits of amiodarone and β-blockers.[75-78] The class III effects of quinidine on repolarization and refractoriness are reversed with isoproterenol administration.[79] In contrast, at equivalent doses of isoproterenol, the effects of d,l-sotalol on repolarization and VT cycle length are preserved because of its β-adrenergic–blocking property.[79] Prolongation of repolarization observed with d-sotalol is also significantly attenuated or completely reversed by β-adrenergic stimulation.[80] The mechanism of this effect in humans is not clear, but in animal models there is enhanced activity of I_{Ks} by β-adrenergic stimulation which, at the plateau phase of the action potential, is quantitatively similar to I_{Kr}.[64]

Amiodarone, which has multiple mechanisms of action but primarily prolongs repolarization,[81] prolongs the action potential uniformly at different cycle lengths (Fig. 2).[23,53] There is some reverse use dependence of amiodarone on the VERP, and thus amiodarone-induced increase in refrac-

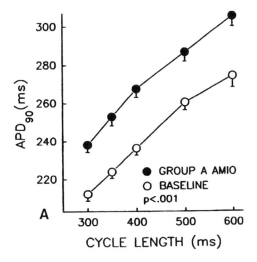

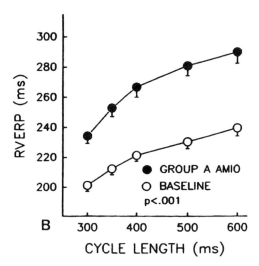

Figure 2. A. Use-dependent prolongation of the action potential is observed with amiodarone monotherapy with a constant incremental increase in action potential duration at 90% repolarization (APD_{90}) at all cycle lengths tested. Dissociation of frequency-dependent effects on ventricular effective refractory period (VERP) are observed when compared with APD_{90} illustrated by the significantly longer prolongation of VERP at longer cycle lengths. **B.** The attenuation of the VERP prolongation of amiodarone may reflect incomplete recovery of sodium channel blockade by the end of repolarization. Adapted from Reference 23.

toriness is reduced at shorter cycle lengths (Fig. 2). Amiodarone also exerts use-dependent sodium channel blockade, and thus the QRS duration is significantly more prolonged at faster cycle lengths after both short- and long-term courses of therapy.[23,82] This effect is consistent with the use-dependent conduction slowing seen with other sodium channel blockers.[83] Prolongation of VERP by amiodarone is thus not fully due to APD prolongation and exhibits time-dependent effects, which may result from incomplete recovery of sodium channel blockade after repolarization.[23]

Mechanistic Models for Antiarrhythmic Drug Combinations

The concepts of increasing wavelength and decreasing the excitable gap to prevent arrhythmias help to conceptualize the problem and to provide some rational basis for antiarrhythmia drug combinations. A rational basis for the use of antiarrhythmic drugs in reentrant arrhythmias requires an understanding of the *wavelength* and the *excitable gap* hypotheses. The wavelength is the spatial representation of the circulating wave of excitation which is expressed mathematically as the product of the functional refractory period (FRP) and the conduction velocity (CV).[84] The wavelength concept was proposed as a predictive tool for determining the effect of drugs on arrhythmias.[85] A tachyarrhythmia would not exist if the wavelength exceeded the length of the reentrant circuit. Therefore, an increase in wavelength would be conducive to termination of reentry, whereas a decrease in wavelength would facilitate reentry.[86] When the wavelength (λ) reaches a critical threshold ($\lambda_{critical}$), it can support a reentrant rhythm.[87]

Sotalol was thus felt to be an ideal antiarrhythmic drug because it increases FRP by prolonging repolarization without decreasing CV, and therefore causes wavelength prolongation.[87] In addition, voltage clamp studies suggest that sotalol may increase CV at fast cycle lengths and it is hypothesized that this is due to reduction in potassium conductance at diastolic potentials.[88] In contrast, class I drugs used as monotherapy may increase FRP but also decrease CV in a use-dependent manner, and therefore do not consistently prolong λ, and may possibly traverse the $\lambda_{critical}$ threshold, promoting reentry.

The excitable gap adds another dimension to the model. An extrastimulus may depolarize tissue with heterogeneous recovery of excitability, leading to block in a region of a potential reentrant circuit. If the area of block has recovered excitability in less time than required for the wave front to conduct around the reentrant circuit, it conducts impulses in the direction opposite to the initiating extrastimulus and permits conduction to proceed around the reentrant circuit. Excitability in this area of "unidirectional block" is primarily determined by refractoriness, and factors that tend to decrease refractoriness facilitate the sustenance of reentry arrhythmias.[89] Furthermore, if conduction is prolonged to a relatively greater extent than refractoriness, the time required for the wave front to propagate around the reentrant circuit will increase, allowing the area of unidirectional block greater time to recover excitability. The excitable gap is widened and reentry is facilitated. In contrast, when refractoriness is prolonged to a relatively greater extent than the time period required for the wave front to return to the area of unidirectional block, the excitable gap may be abolished and circus movement cannot be established.

The limitation of such models is that they may be just two of many important interplaying mechanisms and, as is true for all fixed substrate models, they are limited by the dynamic effects of autonomic tone and ischemia, both of which will act as related and independent arrhythmogenic modalities.[90]

Interest in the combination of antiarrhythmic drugs has been prompted by the lack of efficacy of monotherapies and the toxicity resulting from high doses of individual agents.[91-94] Furthermore, for most drugs used as monotherapy, persistently inducible VT, even if VT slowing is achieved, is associated with a high rate of VT recurrence and sudden death.[95,96] Combinations that have been investigated include drugs of Vaughan Williams classes Ia and Ib,[92] classes I and II,[93,97,98] and classes I and III.[94]

Since β-blockers blunt the effects of catecholamines, which may reverse most drug effects on sodium or I_K blockade, it is not surprising that β-adrenergic antagonists used in combination with class I drugs decrease the incidence of VT and couplets on ambulatory electrocardiographic monitoring and on exercise testing.[99] When metoprolol is added to class I drugs, noninducibility is increased significantly compared with monotherapy class I regimens, with success rates ranging from 30% to greater than 60% when invasive electrophysiologic study is used as a study endpoint.[97,100] A trend toward further increasing the VERP was observed with combination therapy.[101] This has led to studies that used β-adrenergic antagonists as monotherapy in one of the treatment arms in patients who survived VT or ventricular fibrillation.[102]

Sotalol has been studied in combination with class Ib agents (eg, mexiletine, tocainide) for ventricular arrhythmias in patients who failed two or more drugs, including amiodarone monotherapy. The combination was shown to suppress both premature ventricular contractions and inducible sustained VT at electrophysiologic testing and thus was proposed as a possible treatment for drug-refractory ventricular arrhythmias.[103] Amiodarone has also been used in combination with class I drugs, and whereas one study found that sustained VT induction was suppressed when amiodarone alone was ineffective,[104] the majority have not found an impact on inducibility.[103,105,106] Addition of class I agents slows conduction in an additive manner[93,107,108] and potentiates the increase in VERP observed with amiodarone monotherapy.[105] Class Ia (eg, quinidine) and Ic (eg, flecainide, encainide) drugs prolong VT cycle length and decrease the rate of induced VT, making the rhythm more hemodynamically stable when added to amiodarone, despite the lack of impact on inducibility.[103,105,106] Prolongation of conduction was shown to be greatest with encainide, followed by flecainide, with the smallest increment observed with mexiletine. One might predict that a disproportionate prolongation of conduction such that conduction delay is relatively more prominent than refractoriness would widen the excitable gap and predispose to reentrant arrhythmias. This was indeed observed in the patients receiving amiodarone and encainide, which resulted in clinical evidence of proarrhythmia.[103]

Rationale for Sotalol and Class Ia Combination Therapy

Multiple classes of effect, particularly prolongation of repolarization, β-adrenergic blockade, and modest prolongation of conduction, are likely to be effective as has been observed with amiodarone. As previously mentioned, sotalol, like amiodarone, prolongs ventricular refractoriness. Based on experimental[94] and clinical[16,89,109,110] evidence, a regimen consisting of sotalol, which prolongs ventricular repolarization and has β-blocking properties,[81,88,111,112] and quinidine or procainamide, which prolong refractoriness and slow cardiac conduction modestly,[32,81] may be expected to be useful. As observed with amiodarone, it was hypothesized that the combination of sotalol and quinidine or procainamide would also minimize reverse use dependence on refractoriness, characteristic of sotalol alone.[113] Mexiletine and quinidine in combination exhibit an increase in the VERP of a third extrastimulus when triple extrastimuli are applied at close coupling intervals, and may explain the increased clinical benefit of this combination.[92] The clinical and electrophysiologic results of treatment with sotalol and class Ia drug combinations are described in the subsequent parts of this chapter.

Efficacy of the Sotalol and Class Ia Drug Combination

The clinical efficacy of the sotalol and class Ia drug combination was studied in 50 patients with spontaneous sustained VT or ventricular fibrillation who had inducible sustained monomorphic VT.[113] All of these patients had previously been treated with one or more antiarrhythmic drug that failed to suppress inducible VT. Low-dose sotalol (205 ± 84 mg/day; mean $\pm$ standard deviation) plus quinidine (1278 ± 479 mg/day) or procainamide (2393 ± 1423 mg/day) was administered, and on restudy with electrophysiologic testing, 46% of patients were rendered noninducible.[113] VT was inducible but modified in 37% of patients, with modification defined as VT that met all of the following criteria: 1) had an induced VT cycle length ≥ 50 milliseconds longer than baseline cycle length; 2) pacing termination of VT was possible; and 3) was well tolerated with mild or no symptoms, presyncope, or loss of consciousness. Thus, 83% of the original cohort were prospectively followed on the drug combination as long-term therapy. After an average duration of follow-up of approximately 2 years, there were no incidences of sudden death in this treatment group. Actuarial recurrence rates of nonfatal sustained VT were 6% (at 1 year), 6% (at 2 years), and 11% (at 3 years). In patients with VT that was not suppressed or modified at repeat electrophysiologic testing, and in patients not able to tolerate the combination drug therapy, actuarial recurrence rates were 9% (at 1 year), 14% (at 2 years), and 32% (at 3 years). There were no instances of symptomatic proarrhythmia or unexplained syncope, and ambulatory electrocardiographic monitoring did not reveal an increase in the frequency of nonsustained VT or any instances of torsades de pointes. This absence of observed risk of torsades de pointes may have been due to the low doses of sotalol and quinidine/procainamide used in the study that minimized the potential for toxicity of each individual drug.[113]

Simultaneous assessment of postrepolarization refractoriness and the MAP during programmed electrical stimulation afforded insight into the mechanisms that may possibly have resulted in successful clinical prevention of recurrent arrhythmia.[114] The combination of sotalol and a class Ia agent exhibited many of the electrophysiologic effects that would have been expected from the individual drugs as monotherapy. Thus, the combination exhibited prolongation of APD at 90% repolarization (APD_{90}), which was prolonged by 10% (drive cycle 600 milliseconds) and by 13% (drive cycle 400 milliseconds) on therapy. Postrepolarization refractoriness, an attribute of class I antiarrhythmic drug monotherapy, was observed and the ERP/APD ratio increased significantly during therapy consisting of sotalol and class Ia agent. Ventricular refractoriness was markedly prolonged, reflecting the combined effects of prolonged repolarization and postrepolarization refractoriness. Prolongation of right ventricular ERP was marked on combination therapy and was increased to a greater extent than would be expected from monotherapy with either class of drug at similar dosages. Changes in refractoriness that were observed in the right ventricle during drug therapy correlated well with the post-treatment VT cycle length in both modified and nonmodified VT groups. Similarly, functional refractoriness was also prolonged to a significant degree, with increases of 15% (drive cycle 600 milliseconds) and 16% (drive cycle 400 milliseconds) (Fig. 3). These effects occurred with only a modest effect on conduction delay as might be predicted from the low doses of procainamide or quinidine used. The increase in refractoriness was more marked than the moderate increase in conduction time, therefore decreasing the excitable gap.

Beyond the observations that may have been predicted from the electropharmacologic effects of the individual monotherapies, rate-dependent effects were also observed. Repolarization as assessed by APD shortens as the preceding diastolic interval shortens. A similar effect is observed

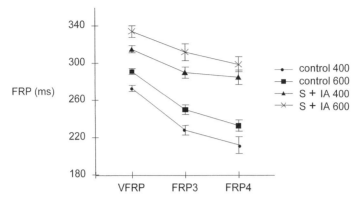

Figure 3. Ventricular functional refractory period (VFRP) and shortest intervals for subsequent extrastimuli (ie, FRP3, FRP4) on no antiarrhythmic drug regimen at cycle lengths of 400 milliseconds (control 400) and 600 milliseconds (control 600); and during therapy with sotalol and a class Ia agent at cycle lengths of 400 milliseconds (S + 1A 400) and 600 milliseconds (S + 1A 600). In the control group, progressive shortening of functional refractoriness with repetitive extrastimuli is observed and is attenuated with combination drug therapy. Reprinted with permission from the American College of Cardiology (*Journal of the American College of Cardiology*, 1997;29:100-105).

with APD-prolonging therapy with class III antiarrhythmic drugs, and a loss of drug effect is how reverse use dependence may be manifested. The combination of sotalol and a class Ia agent attenuates the loss of APD prolongation, and thus at faster rates there is incrementally greater prolongation of repolarization. Postrepolarization refractoriness (ERP-APD$_{90}$ > 0) was observed on therapy, and repetitive extrastimulation with rapidly delivered extrastimuli did not diminish this potentially beneficial effect. In contrast, programmed electrical stimulation in patients not receiving drug therapy, by use of repetitive extrastimulation, shortens successive APDs and diminishes the prolongation of the ERP/APD ratio. As a result of this, capture occurs at progressively less complete levels of cardiac repolarization.[115] This electrophysiologic phenomenon correlates with a high incidence of VT induction and it has been postulated that this may be a mechanism for VT induction in the electrophysiology laboratory by closely coupled extrastimuli.

The absolute difference in refractory periods between treatment and pretreatment cohorts also demonstrates an increased difference with successive extrastimuli (Fig. 4). The absolute prolongation of refractoriness represents drug effect, and the effect is such that with more extrastimuli there is more absolute prolongation of functional refractoriness. If one defines drug effect as the change in electrophysiologic measures from control values, the greater effect on refractory periods for subsequent extrastimuli versus the first extrastimulus represents positive rate depen-

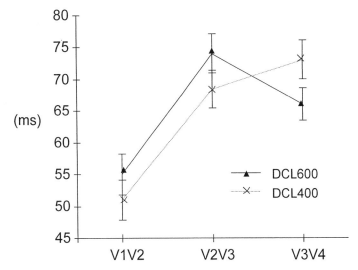

Figure 4. Absolute increase (in milliseconds) in functional refractory period after delivery of single (V1V2), double (V2V3), and triple (V3V4) extrastimuli in patients receiving sotalol plus a class I antiarrhythmic agent versus control at drive cycle lengths of 600 milliseconds (DCL600) and 400 milliseconds (DCL400). There is greater prolongation of function refractoriness for successive beats as the coupling interval shortens, implying greater drug effect at faster rates. Reproduced from Reference 114.

dence of drug effect. This effect, which is observed with the drug combination, occurs on the background of shortening of APD and refractoriness normally seen with successive extrastimuli. The absolute difference increases as extrastimuli become more closely coupled, suggesting that there is greater drug efficacy at faster rates (Fig. 4). Reverse use dependence is a progressive loss of antiarrhythmic effect at faster rates. The term *use dependence* implies that there is persistent drug effect despite a shorter cycle length. Use-dependent effects on repolarization may be further divided into two subcategories where the absolute indexes of drug effect increase progressively with faster rates (*forward use dependence*) or where there is a fixed increase in absolute indexes regardless of cycle length (*fixed use dependence*). One could envision that forward use dependence would be an ideal property of an antiarrhythmic drug for the treatment of tachyarrhythmias and would be better than a drug where there is a fixed absolute increase regardless of rate. During electrophysiologic study with closely coupled extrastimuli there is a decrease in functional refractoriness as more extrastimuli are delivered. When antiarrhythmic therapy is instituted, the absolute prolongation of refractoriness on drug treatment can be compared with the baseline study and it is expected that as the absolute prolongation increases there would be greater likelihood of noninducibility and greater drug effectiveness.

Conclusion

A useful property of an antiarrhythmic regimen may be its multiple classes of antiarrhythmic effect. Adrenergic blockade combined with potassium and modest sodium channel block may be particularly effective; this combination of effects can be achieved by monotherapy with amiodarone or combination therapy with sotalol and agents with class Ia action. Based on electrophysiologic mechanisms, the combination of sotalol and class Ia agents emulates the beneficial properties of amiodarone.

Invasive electrophysiologic testing can lend insight into the mechanism of antiarrhythmic drug effect and may provide potential reasons for the effectiveness of certain antiarrhythmic drugs or drug combinations. Assessment of repolarization in vivo by the use of the MAP catheter contributes to our knowledge of the potential mechanisms of antiarrhythmic drug effectiveness in the context of monotherapy and in the electropharmacodynamic interactions of antiarrhythmic drug combinations. The combination of sotalol and class Ia agents is an example that illustrates the benefits of drug mechanisms which involve: 1) prolonging refractoriness and repolarization; 2) postrepolarization refractoriness; 3) modest prolongation of conduction delay; and 4) nonspecific antiadrenergic and thereby anti-ischemic effects. The drug combination attenuates the rate-dependent shortening of APD and cycle-length--dependent shortening of refractoriness, thus altering reverse use dependence, which is observed with sotalol monotherapy. Furthermore, the peeling back of refractoriness is attenuated on the drug combination. These rate-dependent parameters which can be evaluated during invasive electrophysiologic evaluation warrant further study, and routine assessment of such parameters may help to guide therapy and refine the interpretation and predictive value of electrophysiologic testing in electropharmacologic drug trials and prognostic studies.

References

1. Mason J. A comparison of seven antiarrhythmic drugs in patients with ventricular tachyarrhythmias. *N Engl J Med* 1993;329:452-458.
2. The Antiarrhythmics versus Implantable Defibrillators (AVID) investigators. A comparison of antiarrhythmic drug therapy with implantable defibrillators in patients resuscitated from near fatal ventricular arrhythmias. *N Engl J Med* 1997;337:1576-1583.
3. Moss AJ, Hall WJ, Cannon DS, et al. Improved survival with an implanted defibrillator in patients with coronary artery disease at high risk for ventricular arrhythmia. *N Engl J Med* 1996;335:1933-1940.
4. Connolly SJ, Gent M, Roberts RS, et al. Canadian Implantable Defibrillator Study (CIDS). Study design and organization. CIDS co-investigators. *Am J Cardiol* 1993;72:103F-108F.
5. Sicouri S, Antzelevitch C. Drug-induced afterdepolarizations and triggered activity occur in a discrete subpopulation of ventricular muscle cells (M cells)

in the canine heart: Quinidine and digitalis. *J Cardiovasc Electrophysiol* 1993;4:48-58.

6. Liu DW, Antzelevitch C. Characteristics of the delayed rectifier current (IKr and IKs) in canine ventricular epicardial, midmyocardial, and endocardial myocytes. A weaker IKs contributes to the longer action potential of the M cell. *Circ Res* 1995;76:351-365.

7. Arnsdorff MF, Sawicki GJ. Flecainide and the electrophysiologic matrix: The effects of flecainide acetate on the determinants of cardiac excitability in sheep Purkinje fibers. *J Cardiovasc Electrophysiol* 1996;7:1172-1182.

8. Arnsdorff MF. Cardiac excitability, the electrophysiologic matrix and electrically induced ventricular arrhythmias: Order and reproducibility in seeming electrophysiologic chaos. *J Am Coll Cardiol* 1991;17:139-142.

9. Mitchell LB, Sheldon RS, Gillis AM, et al. Definition of predicted effective antiarrhythmic drug therapy for ventricular tachyarrhythmias by the electrophysiologic study approach: Randomized comparison of patient response criteria. *J Am Coll Cardiol* 1997;30:1346-1353.

10. Waller TJ, Kay HR, Spielman SR, et al. Reduction in sudden death and total mortality by antiarrhythmic therapy evaluated by electrophysiologic drug testing: Criteria of efficacy in patients with sustained ventricular tachyarrhythmia. *J Am Coll Cardiol* 1987;10:83-89.

11. Mitchell LB, Duff HJ, Manyari DE, et al. A randomized clinical trial of the noninvasive and invasive approaches to drug therapy of ventricular tachycardia. *N Engl J Med* 1987;317:1681-1687.

12. Swerdlow CD, Winkle RA, Mason JW. Determinants of survival in patients with ventricular tachyarrhythmias. *N Engl J Med* 1983;308:1436-1442.

13. Spielman SR, Schwartz JS, McCarthy DM, et al. Predictors of the success or failure of medical therapy in patients with chronic recurrent sustained ventricular tachycardia: A discriminant analysis. *J Am Coll Cardiol* 1983;1:401-408.

14. Ferrick KJ, Singh S, Roth JA, et al. Prediction of electrophysiologic study results in patients treated with amiodarone. *Am Heart J* 1995;129:496-501.

15. Horowitz LN, Greenspan AM, Spielman SR, et al. Usefulness of electrophysiologic testing in evaluation of amiodarone therapy for sustained ventricular tachyarrhythmias associated with coronary heart disease. *Am J Cardiol* 1985;55:367-371.

16. Gillis AM, Wyse DG, Duff HJ, Mitchell LB. Drug response at electropharmacologic study in patients with ventricular tachyarrhythmias: The importance of ventricular refractoriness. *J Am Coll Cardiol* 1991;17:914-920.

17. Nattel S, Pedersen DH, Zipes DP. Alterations in regional myocardial distribution and arrhythmogenic effects of aprindine produced by coronary artery occlusion in the dog. *Cardiovasc Res* 1981;15:80-85.

18. Echt DS, Leibson PR, Mitchell LB, et al. Mortality and morbidity in patients receiving encainide, flecainide, or placebo. The cardiac arrhythmia suppression trial (CAST). *N Engl J Med* 1991;324:781-788.

19. Mitchell LB, Wyse DG, Duff HJ. Programmed electrical stimulation studies for ventricular tachycardia induction in humans: I. The role of ventricular functional refractoriness in tachycardia induction. *J Am Coll Cardiol* 1986;8:567-575.

20. Klein RC, and the ESVEM Investigators. Comparative efficacy of sotalol and class I antiarrhythmic agents in patients with ventricular tachycardia or fibrillation: Results of the electrophysiology study versus electrocardiographic monitoring (ESVEM) trial. *Eur Heart J* 1993;14(suppl H):78-84.

21. CASCADE Investigators. Randomized antiarrhythmic drug therapy in survivors of cardiac arrest (the CASCADE study). *Am J Cardiol* 1993;72:280-287.

22. Chiamvimonvat N, Gillis AM, Mitchell LB, et al. Determinants of prolongation of ventricular tachycardia cycle length by amiodarone. *PACE* 1991;14:618.

23. Sager PT, Uppal P, Follmer C, et al. Frequency-dependent electrophysiologic effects of amiodarone in humans. *Circulation* 1993;88:1063-1071.

24. Kadish AH, Buxton AE, Waxman HL, et al. Usefulness of electrophysiologic study to determine the clinical tolerance of arrhythmia recurrences during amiodarone therapy. *J Am Coll Cardiol* 1987;10:90-96.

25. Task Force of the Working Group on Arrhythmias of the European Society of Cardiology. The Sicilian gambit: A new approach to the classification of antiarrhythmic drugs based on their actions on arrhythmogenic mechanisms. *Circulation* 1991;84:1831-1851.

26. Nattel S, Zeng FD. Frequency-dependent effects of antiarrhythmic drugs on action potential duration and refractoriness of canine cardiac Purkinje fibers. *J Pharmacol Exp Ther* 1984;229:283-291.

27. Nademanee K, Stevenson WG, Weiss JN, et al. Frequency-dependent effects of quinidine on the ventricular action potential and QRS duration in humans. *Circulation* 1990;81:790-796.

28. Campbell TJ. Kinetics of onset of rate-dependent effects of class I antiarrhythmic drugs are important in determining their effects on refractoriness in guinea-pig ventricle, and provide a theoretical basis for their subclassification. *Cardiovasc Res* 1983;17:344-352.

29. Davidenko JM, Antzelevich C. Electrophysiological mechanisms underlying rate-dependent changes of refractoriness in normal and segmentally depressed canine Purkinje fibers: The characteristics of postrepolarization refractoriness. *Circ Res* 1986;58:257-268.

30. Roden DM. Ionic mechanisms for prolongation of refractoriness and their proarrhythmic and antiarrhythmic correlates. *Am J Cardiol* 1996;78(suppl 4A):12-16.

31. Lee RJ, Liem LB, Cohen TJ, Franz MR. Relation between repolarization and refractoriness in the human ventricle: Cycle length dependence and effect of procainamide. *J Am Coll Cardiol* 1992;19:614-618.

32. Salata JJ, Wasserstrom A. Effects of quinidine on action potentials and ionic currents in isolated canine ventricular myocytes. *Circ Res* 1988;62:324-337.

33. Roden DM, Bennett PB, Snyders DJ, et al. Quinidine delays I_k activation in guinea pig ventricular myocytes. *Circ Res* 1988;62:1055-1058.

34. Snyders DJ, Knoth KM, Roberds SL, Tamkun MM. Time-, voltage-, and state-dependent block by quinidine of a cloned human cardiac potassium channel. *Mol Pharmacol* 1992;41:322-330.

35. Yeola SW, Rich TC, Uebele VN, et al. Molecular analysis of a binding site for quinidine in human cardiac delayed rectifier K^+ channel: Role of S6 in antiarrhythmic drug binding. *Circ Res* 1996;78:1105-1114.

36. Colatsky TJ, Follmer CH, Starmer F. Channel specificity in antiarrhythmic drug action: Mechanism of potassium channel block and its role in suppressing and aggravating cardiac arrhythmias. *Circulation* 1990;82:2235-2242.

37. Hondeghem LM, Snyders DJ. Class III antiarrhythmic agents have a lot of potential but a long way to go: Reduced effectiveness and dangers of reverse use dependence. *Circulation* 1990;81:686-690.

38. Hohnloser SH, Woosley RL. Sotalol. *N Engl J Med* 1994:331:31-38.

39. Yang T, Roden DM. Extracellular potassium modulation of drug block of I_{kr}: Implications for torsade de pointes and reverse use-dependence. *Circulation* 1996;93:407-411.
40. Roden DM, Hoffman BF. Action potential prolongation and induction of abnormal automaticity by low quinidine concentrations in canine Purkinje fibers. Relation to potassium and cycle length. *Circ Res* 1985;56:857-867.
41. Grace AA, Camm AJ. Quinidine. *N Engl J Med* 1998;338:35-45.
42. Roden DM. Risks and benefits of antiarrhythmic therapy. *N Engl J Med* 1994;331:785-791.
43. Roden DM, Woosley RL, Primm PK. Incidence and clinical features of the quinidine-associated long QT syndrome: Implications for patient care. *Am Heart J* 1986;111:1088-1093.
44. Mason JW, Marcus FI, Bigger JT, et al. A summary and assessment of the findings and conclusions of the ESVEM trial. *Prog Cardiovasc Dis* 1996; 38:347-358.
45. Singh BN, Kehoe R, Woosley RL, et al, for the Sotalol Multicenter Study Group. Multicenter trial of sotalol compared with procainamide in the suppression of inducible ventricular tachycardia: A double-blind randomized parallel evaluation. *Am Heart J* 1995;129:87-97.
46. Moosvi AR, Goldstein S, VanderBrug-Medendorp S, et al. Effect of empiric antiarrhythmic therapy in resuscitated out-of-hospital cardiac arrest victims with coronary artery disease. *Am J Cardiol* 1990;65:1192-1197.
47. Steinbeck G, Greene HL. Management of patients with life-threatening sustained ventricular tachyarrhythmias—the role of guided antiarrhythmic drug therapy. *Prog Cardiovasc Dis* 1996;38:419-428.
48. Schmitt C, Brachmann J, Karch M, et al. Reverse use-dependent effects of sotalol demonstrated by recording monophasic action potentials of the right ventricle. *Am J Cardiol* 1991;68:1183-1187.
49. Sadanaga T, Ogawa S, Okada Y, et al. Clinical efficacy of the use-dependent QRS prolongation and the reverse use-dependent QT prolongation of class I and class II antiarrhythmic agents and their value in predicting efficacy. *Am Heart J* 1993;126:114-121.
50. Hayward RP, Taggart P. Effect of sotalol on human atrial action potential duration and refractoriness: Cycle length dependency of class III activity. *Cardiovasc Res* 1986;20:100-107.
51. Strauss HC, Bigger JT, Hoffman BF. Electrophysiological and β-receptor blocking effects of MJ1999 on dog and rabbit cardiac tissue. *Circulation* 1970;25:661-678.
52. Shimizu W, Kurita T, Suyama K, et al. Reverse use dependence of human ventricular repolarization by chronic oral sotalol in monophasic action potential recordings. *Am J Cardiol* 1996;77:1004-1008.
53. Huikuri HV, Yli-Mayry S. Frequency dependent effects of d-sotalol and amiodarone on the action potential duration of the human right ventricle. *PACE* 1992;15:2103-2107.
54. Sager PT, Follmer C, Uppal P, et al. The effects of β-adrenergic stimulation on the frequency-dependent electrophysiologic actions of amiodarone and sematilide in humans. *Circulation* 1994;90:1811-1819.
55. Sager PT, Nademanee K, Antimisiaris M, et al. Antiarrhythmic effects of selective prolongation of refractoriness. *Circulation* 1993;88:1072-1082.
56. Tande PM, Bjornstad H, Yang T, Refsum H. Rate-dependent class III antiarrhythmic action, negative chronotropy, and positive inotropy of a novel I_k blocking

drug, UK-68,798: Potent in guinea pig but no effect in rat myocardium. *J Cardio-vasc Pharmacol* 1990;16:401-410.

57. Jurkiewicz NK, Sanguinetti MC. Rate-dependent prolongation of cardiac action potentials by a methanesulfonanilide class III antiarrhythmic agent: Specific block of rapidly activating delayed rectifier K^+ current by dofetilide. *Circ Res* 1993;72:75-83.

58. Jackman WM, Friday KJ, Anderson JL, et al. The long QT syndromes: A critical review, new clinical observations and a unifying hypothesis. *Prog Cardiovasc Dis* 1988;31:115-172.

59. Langenfeld H, Kohler C, Weirich J, et al. Reverse use dependence of antiarrhythmic class Ia, Ib and Ic: Effects of drugs on the action potential duration? *PACE* 1992;15:2097-2102.

60. Singh BN, Vaughan Williams EM. A third class of antiarrhythmic action: Effects on atrial and ventricular intracellular potentials, and other pharmacologic actions on cardiac muscle, of MJ 1999 and AH 3474. *Br J Pharmacol* 1970;29:675-687.

61. Herre JM, Sauve MJ, Malone P, Scheinman M. Long-term results of amiodarone therapy in patients with recurrent sustained ventricular tachycardia or ventricular fibrillation. *J Am Coll Cardiol* 1989;12:442-449.

62. Lazzara R. Amiodarone and torsade de pointes. *Ann Intern Med* 1989; 111:549-551.

63. Mattioni TA, Zheutlin TA, Sarmiento JJ, et al. Amiodarone in patients with previous drug-mediated torsade de pointes. *Ann Intern Med* 1989;111:574-580.

64. Sanguinetti MC, Jurkiewicz NK. Two components of cardiac delayed rectifier K^+ current. Differential sensitivity to block by class III antiarrhythmic agents. *J Gen Physiol* 1990;96:195-215.

65. Waldo AL, Camm AJ, deRuyter H, et al. Survival with oral d-sotalol in patients with left ventricular dysfunction after myocardial infarction. Rationale, design, and methods (the SWORD trial). *Am J Cardiol* 1995;75:1023-1027.

66. Waldo AL, Camm AJ, deRuyter H, et al. Effect of d-sotalol on mortality in patients with left ventricular dysfunction after recent and remote myocardial infarction. The SWORD investigators. Survival with oral d-sotalol. *Lancet* 1996;348:7-12.

67. Sanguinetti MC, Jurkiewicz NK, Scott A, et al. Isoproterenol antagonizes prolongation of refractory period by the class III antiarrhythmic agent E-4031 in guinea pig myocytes. Mechanism of action. *Circ Res* 1991;68:77-84.

68. Tovar OH, Jones JL. Epinephrine facilitates cardiac fibrillation by shortening action potential refractoriness. *J Mol Cell Cardiol* 1997;29:1447-1455.

69. Hoffman BF, Singer D. Appraisal of the effects of catecholamines on cardiac electrical activity. *Ann N Y Acad Sci* 1967;193:914-924.

70. Giles W, Nakajima T, Ono K, et al. Modulation of the delayed rectifier K^+ current by isoprenaline in bull-frog atrial myocytes. *J Physiol (Lond)* 1989;415:233-249.

71. Nakayama T, Fozzard HA. Adrenergic modulation of the transient outward current in isolated canine Purkinje cells. *Circ Res* 1988;62:162-172.

72. Harvey RD, Hume JR. Autonomic regulation of delayed rectifier K^+ current in mammalian heart involves G proteins. *Am J Physiol* 1989;257:H818-H823.

73. Boyett NR, Fedida D. Changes in the electrical activity of dog Purkinje fibers at high heart rates. *J Physiol (Lond)* 1984;350:361-391.

74. Newman D, Dorian P, Feder-Elituv R. Isoproterenol antagonizes drug-induced prolongation of action potential duration in humans. *Can J Physiol Pharmacol* 1993;71:755-760.

75. Cairns JA, Connolly SJ, Roberts RS, and the CAMIAT investigators. Randomised trial of outcome after myocardial infarction in patients with frequent or repetitive ventricular premature depolarisations: CAMIAT. *Lancet* 1997;349:675-682.
76. Julian DG, Camm AJ, Frangin G, and the EMIAT investigators. Randomised trial of effect of amiodarone on mortality in patients with left ventricular dysfunction after recent myocardial infarction: EMIAT. *Lancet* 1997;349:667-674.
77. Dorian P, Newman D, Connolly S, et al. Beta blockade may be necessary for amiodarone to exert its antiarrhythmic benefit—results from CAMIAT. *PACE* 1997;20:1144.
78. Kennedy HL. Beta-blocker prevention of proarrhythmia and proischemia: Clues from CAST, CAMIAT, and EMIAT. *Am J Cardiol* 1997;80:1208-1211.
79. Sager PT, Behboodikhah M. Frequency-dependent electrophysiologic effects of d,l-sotalol and quinidine and modulation by beta-adrenergic stimulation. *J Cardiovasc Electrophysiol* 1996;7:102-112.
80. Vanoli E, Priori SG, Nakagawa H, et al. Sympathetic activation, ventricular repolarization and I_{kr} blockade: Implications for the antifibrillatory efficacy of potassium channel blocking agents. *J Am Coll Cardiol* 1995;25:1609-1614.
81. Nattel S. Antiarrhythmic drug classifications: A critical appraisal of their history, present status, and clinical relevance. *Drugs* 1991;41:672-701.
82. Chiamvimonvat N, Mitchell LB, Gillis AM, et al. Use-dependent electrophysiologic effects of amiodarone in coronary artery disease and inducible ventricular tachycardia. *Am J Cardiol* 1992;70:598-604.
83. Villemaire C, Savard P, Talajic M, Nattel S. A quantitative analysis of use-dependent ventricular conduction slowing by procainamide in anesthetized dogs. *Circulation* 1992;85:2255-2266.
84. Rensma PL, Allessie MA, Lammers WJEP, et al. Length of excitation wave and susceptibility to reentrant atrial arrhythmias in normal conscious dogs. *Circ Res* 1988;62:395-410.
85. Smeets JLRM, Allessie MA, Lammers WJEP, et al. The wavelength of the cardiac impulse and reentrant arrhythmias in isolated rabbit atrium. The role of heart rate, autonomic transmitters, temperature and potassium. *Circ Res* 1986;58:96-108.
86. Frame LH, Simson MB. Oscillations of conduction, action potential duration, and refractoriness. A mechanism for spontaneous termination of reentrant tachycardias. *Circulation* 1988;78:1277-1287.
87. Hill BC, Hunt AJ, Courtney KR. Reentrant tachycardia in a thin layer of ventricular subepicardium: Effects of d-sotalol and lidocaine. *J Cardiovasc Pharmacol* 1990;16:871-880.
88. Carmeliet E. Electrophysiologic and voltage clamp analysis of the effects of sotalol on isolated cardiac muscle and Purkinje fibers. *J Pharmacol Exp Ther* 1985;232:817-825.
89. Furukawa T, Rozanski JJ, Moroe K, et al. Efficacy of procainamide on ventricular tachycardia: Relation to prolongation of refractoriness and slowing of conduction. *Am Heart J* 1989;118:702-708.
90. Bigger JT, and the Coronary Artery Bypass Graft Patch Trial Investigators. Prophylactic use of implanted cardiac defibrillators in patients at high risk for ventricular arrhythmias after coronary artery bypass graft surgery. *N Engl J Med* 1997;337:1569-1575.
91. Greenspan AM, Spielman SR, Horowitz LN. Combination antiarrhythmic drug therapy for ventricular tachyarrhythmias. *PACE* 1986;9:565-576.

92. Duff HJ, Mitchell LB, Manyari D, Wyse DG. Mexiletine-quinidine combination: Electrophysiologic correlates of a favorable antiarrhythmic interaction in humans. *J Am Coll Cardiol* 1987;10:1149-1156.

93. Deedwania PL, Olukotun AY, Kupersmith J, et al. Beta blockers in combination with class I antiarrhythmic agents. *Am J Cardiol* 1987;60:21B-28B.

94. Marchlinski FE, Buxton AE, Kindwall KE, et al. Comparison of individual and combined effects of procainamide and amiodarone in patients with sustained ventricular tachyarrhythmias. *Circulation* 1988;78:583-591.

95. Mason JW, Winkle RA. Accuracy of the ventricular tachycardia induction study for predicting long-term efficacy and inefficacy of antiarrhythmic drugs. *N Engl J Med* 1980;303:1073-1077.

96. Gonzalez R, Scheinman MM, Herre JM, et al. Usefulness of sotalol for drug-refractory malignant ventricular arrhythmias. *J Am Coll Cardiol* 1988; 12:1568-1572.

97. Friehling TD, Lipshutz H, Marinchak RA, et al. Effectiveness of propranolol added to a type I antiarrhythmic agent for sustained ventricular tachycardia secondary to coronary artery disease. *Am J Cardiol* 1990;65:1328-1333.

98. Bonavita GJ, Pires LA, Wagshal AB, et al. Usefulness of oral quinidine-mexiletine combination therapy for sustained ventricular tachyarrhythmias as assessed by programmed electrical stimulation when quinidine monotherapy has failed. *Am Heart J* 1994;127:847-851.

99. Hirsowitz G, Podrid PJ, Lampert S, et al. The role of beta blocking agents as adjunct therapy to membrane stabilizing drugs in malignant ventricular arrhythmia. *Am Heart J* 1986;111:852-860.

100. Brodsky MA, Allen BJ, Bessen M, et al. Beta-blocker therapy in patients with ventricular tachyarrhythmias in the setting of left ventricular dysfunction. *Am Heart J* 1988;115:799-808.

101. Brodsky MA, Chough SP, Allen BJ, et al. Adjuvant metoprolol improves efficacy of class I antiarrhythmic drugs in patients with inducible sustained monomorphic ventricular tachycardia. *Am Heart J* 1992;124:629-635.

102. Siebels J, Kuck KH. Implantable cardioverter defibrillator compared with antiarrhythmic drug treatment in cardiac arrest survivors (the cardiac arrest study Hamburg). *Am Heart J* 1994;127:1139-1144.

103. Luderitz B, Mletzko R, Jung W, Manz M. Combination of antiarrhythmic drugs. *J Cardiovasc Pharmacol* 1991;17(suppl 6):S48-S52.

104. Bellocci F, Santarelli P, Montenero A, et al. Value of electrophysiologic testing of amiodarone alone or in combination with class I antiarrhythmic drugs for ventricular tachycardia. *Circulation* 1985;72(suppl II):II274.

105. Toivonen L, Kadish A, Morady F. A prospective comparison of class IA, B and C antiarrhythmic agents in combination with amiodarone in patients with inducible, sustained ventricular tachycardia. *Circulation* 1991;84:101-108.

106. Jung W, Mletzko R, Manz M, et al. Efficacy and safety of combination therapy with amiodarone and type I agents for treatment of inducible ventricular tachycardia. *PACE* 1993;16:778-788.

107. Marchlinski FE, Buxton AE, Josephson ME, Schmitt C. Predicting ventricular tachycardia cycle length after procainamide by assessing cycle length-dependent changes in paced QRS duration. *Circulation* 1989;79:39-46.

108. Waxman HL, Groh WC, Marchlinski FE, et al. Amiodarone for control of sustained ventricular tachyarrhythmia: Clinical and electrophysiologic effect in 51 patients. *Am J Cardiol* 1982;50:1066-1074.

109. Kus T, Costi P, Dubuc M, Shenasa M. Prolongation of ventricular refractoriness by class Ia antiarrhythmic drugs in the prevention of ventricular tachycardia induction. *Am Heart J* 1990;120:855-863.
110. Kus T, Dubuc M, Lambert C, Shenasa M. Efficacy of propafenone in preventing ventricular tachycardia: Inverse correlation with rate-related prolongation of conduction time. *J Am Coll Cardiol* 1990;16:1229-1237.
111. Nademanee K, Feld G, Hendrickson J, et al. Electrophysiologic and antiarrhythmic effects of sotalol in patients with life-threatening ventricular tachyarrhythmias. *Circulation* 1985;72:555-564.
112. Kuchar DL, Garan H, Venditti FJ, et al. Usefulness of sotalol in suppressing ventricular tachycardia or ventricular fibrillation in patients with healed myocardial infarcts. *Am J Cardiol* 1989;64:33-36.
113. Dorian P, Newman D, Berman N, et al. Sotalol and type IA drugs in combination prevent recurrence of sustained ventricular tachycardia. *J Am Coll Cardiol* 1993;22:106-113.
114. Lee SD, Newman D, Ham M, Dorian P. Electrophysiologic mechanisms of antiarrhythmic efficacy of a sotalol and class Ia drug combination: Elimination of reverse use dependence. *J Am Coll Cardiol* 1997;29:100-105.
115. Koller BS, Karasik PE, Solomon AJ, Franz MR. Relation between repolarization and refractoriness during programmed electrical stimulation in the human right ventricle: Implications for ventricular tachycardia induction. *Circulation* 1995;91:2378-2384.

29

Postrepolarization Refractoriness:

Could it Be Why Antiarrhythmic Drugs Work?

Paulus F. Kirchhof, MD, C. Larissa Fabritz, MD and Michael R. Franz, MD, PhD

Introduction

While negative data on the efficacy of antiarrhythmic drugs to prevent sudden cardiac death in high-risk populations is accumulating,[1-11] the mechanisms by which antiarrhythmic drugs suppress tachyarrhythmias or exert proarrhythmic effects are still not well understood. The CAST trials[1,3,4,6] have rebutted the "suppression hypothesis" by demonstrating that sodium channel blocking drugs, especially those drugs with slow binding kinetics (flecainide, encainide), have proarrhythmic effects despite their ability to reduce ectopic ventricular activity. The quest for electrophysiologic measures of antiarrhythmic efficacy has since been expanded to include invasive electrophysiologic studies and serial drug testing[7,12,13] and assessment of dispersion of repolarization,[14,15] and has recently focused on prolongation of action potential duration (APD) and subsequent prolongation of refractoriness as possible antiarrhythmic factors,[11] so far without delineating a measurement that clearly relates to antiarrhythmic efficacy.

From Franz MR (ed): *Monophasic Action Potentials: Bridging Cell and Bedside.* ©Futura Publishing Company, Inc., Armonk, NY, 2000.

Published investigations of epicardial activation mapping[16,17] have suggested that the proarrhythmic effect of sodium channel blocking drugs is mediated by conduction slowing, which shortens the excitation wavelength or creates unidirectional block, thereby providing conditions for reentry, especially in structurally altered hearts. Drugs with sodium channel blocking activity are known to delay the time-dependent recovery of excitability, thereby, in a rate-dependent manner, prolonging refractoriness beyond repolarization[18-20] of the action potential to its resting state. Although the ionic mechanisms of this drug-induced postrepolarization refractoriness (PRR) are not yet well defined, PRR may produce an antiarrhythmic effect, based on the hypothesis that PRR could shield the myocardium against very premature excitation with its associated conduction slowing and wavelength shortening.[18,20,21] As the major mechanism of tachyarrhythmia induction during premature extrastimulation[21-23] is most likely wavelength shortening by premature excitation, PRR could especially prevent tachyarrhythmia induction by programmed ventricular stimulation.

In the study described in this chapter, we compared the effects of two sodium channel blocking drugs[24-30]—procainamide, which has relatively fast dissociation kinetics and is known to prolong the action potential, and propafenone, which has slow dissociation kinetics and divergent APD effects—on APD, conduction time (CT), and PRR during regular pacing, repetitive extrastimulation, and high-frequency burst pacing. These data were correlated with the incidence and type of tachyarrhythmias that were induced.

Methods and Results

Eleven Langendorff-perfused rabbit hearts were studied through use of 6 to 7 simultaneous right and left ventricular endocardial and epicardial monophasic action potential (MAP) recordings[31-34] and a volume-conducted electrocardiogram (ECG), as previously described.[34,35] Repetitive extrastimulation (S2-S5) and burst pacing were performed through one of the endocardial MAP catheters. In 3 experiments, burst stimuli were also applied through a bipolar hook electrode consisting of two platinum wires which were inserted into the left ventricular free wall with an interelectrode distance of 2 to 3 mm and positioned in close proximity (<3 mm) to one of the epicardial MAP electrodes.

Hearts were paced at a 400-millisecond basic cycle length and twice diastolic threshold, with the following arrhythmogenic interventions applied during baseline and after addition of procainamide or propafenone to the perfusate: 1) Repetitive extrastimulation (S2-S5) was performed at twice, 3 times, and 5 times diastolic threshold. Effective refractory periods

(ERPs) were determined by using a protocol consisting of 40 S1 stimuli and extrastimuli introduced in 5-millisecond decrements, starting at 200 milliseconds. Each extrastimulus was set at a coupling interval of ERP + 5 milliseconds, and the next extrastimulus (S3-S5) was applied. 2) High-frequency burst pacing was used because it probes myocardial excitability in a more continuous fashion than intermittent extrastimulation and uncovers the rate-dependent relationship between repolarization and refractoriness with greater resolution and sensitivity. Burst pacing at 2 to 10 times diastolic threshold was applied for 10 seconds via one of the left ventricular MAP catheters (n=11) or through a hook electrode mounted in the apex (n=3) at burst cycle lengths of 10 to 40 milliseconds. Propafenone or procainamide was added to the perfusate, and the entire protocol was repeated after the electrophysiologic drug effect, as assessed by MAPs, had reached a steady state.[36,37]

CT and APD at 90% repolarization (APD_{90}), measured as defined in previous publications[28,34] and elsewhere in this book, were measured during steady state pacing and for each extrastimulus (S2-S5) at the shortest coupling interval (ERP + 5 milliseconds). PRR was defined as the difference between the ERP and the preceding APD_{90} at the pacing site for S2-S5, respectively. During burst stimulation, PRR was measured as the difference between APD_{90} and the following activation.

Steady State Pacing

At baseline, average APD_{90} was 171 ± 11 milliseconds at a 400-millisecond basic pacing cycle length. Procainamide and propafenone prolonged APD_{90} significantly: by 12% and 14%, respectively. CT between the MAP upstroke at the pacing site and that of the 6 other MAP recordings ranged from 5 to 55 milliseconds with an average of 13 ± 8 milliseconds. Procainamide prolonged average CT by an average of 11 ± 11 milliseconds ($85 \pm 85\%$), and propafenone prolonged average CT by an average of 21 ± 11 milliseconds ($161 \pm 85\%$; $P<0.05$ for procainamide versus propafenone).

Repetitive Extrastimulation

Effective Refractory Period

At baseline, repetitive premature extrastimulation caused a progressive decrease in ERPs from 168 ± 21 milliseconds (S2) to 133 ± 21 milliseconds (S5; see Table 1 and Fig. 1). Procainamide did not significantly change ERPs during repetitive extrastimulation, whereas propafenone lengthened ERPs from 209 ± 28 milliseconds at S2 to 187 ± 8 milliseconds at S5 (Table

Table 1

Effective Refractory Periods During Premature Extrastimulation (S2-S5)
at Baseline, with Procainamide, and with Propafenone

Stimulus Number	S2 [ms]	S3 [ms]	S4 [ms]	S5 [ms]
Baseline	168±20	156±19	138±21	133±20
Procainamide	142±18	138±18	133±18	125±14
Propafenone	209±28	206±21	199±15	187±8

All values are given in milliseconds as mean ± standard deviation.

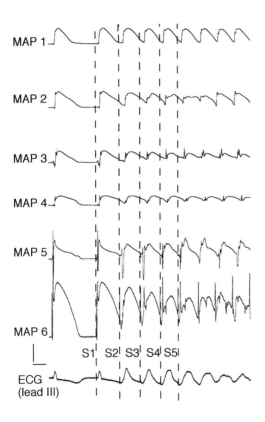

Figure 1. Recording of 6 MAPs and lead 3 of the tissue bath electrocardiogram (ECG) during multiple premature extrastimulation (S2-S5) at baseline. The time of stimulus application is marked by vertical dashed lines. MAPs 1 and 2 are recorded from the right ventricular epicardium, MAPs 3 and 4 from the left ventricular epicardium, and MAPs 5 and 6 from the left ventricular endocardium. The horizontal calibration bar indicates 100 milliseconds, the vertical calibration bar 1 mV (for the ECG), 2 mV (for MAP 6), and 5 mV (for MAPs 1 through 5). Pacing was performed from MAP catheter number 6 until the "tightest" extrastimulus sequence still resulting in capture (ERP + 5 milliseconds) was achieved. The consecutive extrastimuli captured the myocardium at less and less repolarized potentials (progressive "encroachment" of repetitive extrastimuli), initiating ventricular fibrillation. From Kirchhof P, et al. *Circulation* 1998;97:2567-2574.

1). The progressive decrease in ERP observed during multiple extrastimulation at baseline and with procainamide was less pronounced with propafenone.

Conduction Time

Baseline CT between the pacing site and the other MAP recording sites increased progressively for S2 and S3, and remained at an elevated plateau value for S4 and S5 (Table 2). With procainamide, average and maximal CT increased slightly at steady state pacing, without additional conduction-delaying effects during multiple extrastimulation (Fig. 2). Propafenone prolonged average CT at steady state pacing by an average of 21 milliseconds. In addition to this effect during steady state pacing, propafenone progressively prolonged CT during multiple extrastimulation in a use-dependent fashion: average CT increased up to 400% at S5, and similar effects were observed on maximal CT (Fig. 2). Neither the site of maximal CT nor the order of activation between the 7 MAP recordings was modified by procainamide or propafenone.

Postrepolarization Refractoriness

At baseline, ERPs for S2 stimuli were nearly equal to the basic APD_{90}. During repetitive extrastimulation, ERPs shortened not only in absolute terms but also relative to the concomitant APD_{90}. This allowed the subsequent extrastimulus to elicit a new propagated response earlier in the repolarization phase (Fig. 1). The last of the series of repetitive extrastimuli (S5) was able to elicit a new response 10 ± 10 milliseconds before the 90% repolarization level was reached ($P < 0.05$; Table 2). Procainamide and propafenone prolonged ERP during repetitive extrastimulation relative to their concomitant APD_{90}, to an extent that the earliest capture by an extrastimulus occurred *after* 90% repolarization, hence inducing PRR. While procainamide-induced PRR remained constant from S2-S4, propafen-

Table 2
Conduction Times and Postrepolarization Refractoriness During Premature Extrastimulation (S2-S5) at Baseline

Stimulus Number	S1 [ms]	S2 [ms]	S3 [ms]	S4 [ms]	S5 [ms]
Mean CT	13.1±8	16.3±10	19.6±10	18.6±10	18.3±9
Maximal CT	22.1±13	28.2±17	33.8±18	32.2±17	32.6±16
PRR		2±11	−8±11	−7±8	−7±7

All values are given in milliseconds as mean ± standard deviation. CT = conduction time; PRR = postrepolarization refractoriness.

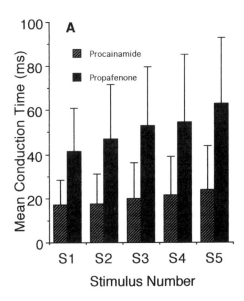

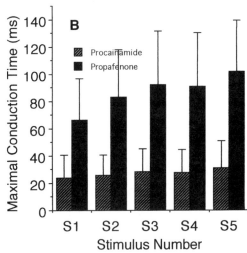

Figure 2. Effects of procainamide and propafenone on conduction times (CT) during premature extrastimulation (S2-S5) at coupling intervals of ERP + 5 milliseconds. The effect of drug on CT, calculated as the CT difference between baseline and drug (y axis) is plotted versus the number of the extrastimulus (S2-S5, x axis). **A.** Changes in mean CT caused by procainamide (striped columns) and propafenone (filled columns). **B.** Changes in maximal CT (symbols as in panel A). From Kirchhof P, et al. *Circulation* 1998;97:2567-2574.

one progressively prolonged PRR in a use-dependent fashion, increasing from S2-S4 (Fig. 3).

Burst Stimulation

At baseline, 65% of all burst stimuli induced ventricular fibrillation (VF). The probability of VF induction increased with increasing stimulus strength and was highest for intermediate burst cycle lengths (20 to 30

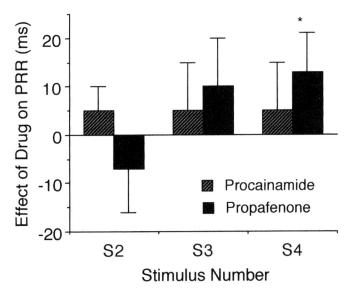

Figure 3. Changes in postrepolarization refractoriness (PRR) induced by procainamide (striped columns) and propafenone (filled columns) during multiple premature extrastimulation. Drug-induced changes in PRR, measured as PRR during drug minus PRR at baseline (y axis), are plotted versus the stimulus number (S2-S4, x axis). Both drugs slightly increased the duration of PRR. Propafenone increased PRR progressively, reaching significant prolongation at S4 ($P<0.05$, see *). At S5, arrhythmia induction rate was too high to yield sufficient data with propafenone. From Kirchhof P, et al. *Circulation* 1998;97:2567-2574.

milliseconds; Table 3). Procainamide decreased the inducibility of VF to 14% of the burst stimuli applied in this study ($P<0.05$ versus baseline). Propafenone did not reduce the incidence of arrhythmia inducibility per se, with 63% of all bursts inducing significant arrhythmias (P = NS versus baseline), but changed the type of the induced arrhythmia from VF (Fig. 4, panel A) to a slow monomorphic ventricular tachycardia (VT) (Fig. 4, panel B). Burst stimulation induced a slow monomorphic VT with propafenone in 57%, and VF in only 6% of the bursts applied. Activation sequence of the multiple MAP recordings and QRS morphology in the tissue bath ECG were constant during tachycardias induced with propafenone (Fig. 4, panel B), consistent with monomorphic tachycardia.

PRR and Arrhythmia Inducibility

At baseline, the average take-off point of premature action potentials was 3 ± 5 milliseconds after repolarization to 90%, ie, PRR of 3 milliseconds. PRR during burst stimulation was only observed with low stimulus strengths and burst frequencies. Reexcitation occurred earlier (at less

Table 3

Probability of Arrhythmia Induction During Burst Stimulation in Percent
Using Different Stimulus Strengths from 2 to 10 Times Diastolic Threshold and Different
Burst Cycle Lengths (Burst Interval) at Baseline, with Procainamide, and with Propafenone

Stimulus Strength	*Twice Threshold*				*3 Times Threshold*				*5–10 Times Threshold*			
Burst interval (ms)	10	20	30	40	10	20	30	40	10	20	30	40
Baseline	0	37.5	37.5	0	50	87.5	86	40	66	100	100	100
Procainamide	0	0	0	0	0	0	0	0	0	100	100	100
Propafenone	0	20	50	33.3	24	50	80	75	100	100	100	100

All values are given in percent of all bursts applied.

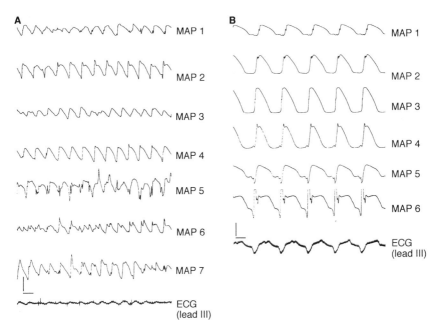

Figure 4. Recordings of 6 MAPs and lead 3 of the tissue bath electrocardiogram (ECG) during ventricular fibrillation (**A**) and monomorphic tachycardia (**B**). In both panels, the arrangement of the recordings is similar: The upper 2 recordings show MAPs from the right ventricular epicardium, the middle 3 from the left ventricular epicardium, and the lowest from the left ventricular endocardium. The bottom-most trace shows lead 3 of the tissue bath ECG. The calibration bars indicate 5 mV for the MAP and 1 mV for the ECG recordings (vertical), and 100 milliseconds (horizontal). **A.** Recording of a typical episode of ventricular fibrillation with procainamide. The activation sequence changes rapidly, almost with every beat. Reactivation occurs early during repolarization, exhibiting periods of low-amplitude MAP signals in several recordings. The tissue bath ECG shows undulations around the baseline. **B.** Recording of a typical episode of monomorphic ventricular tachycardia with propafenone. The activation sequence remains constant during the recording. In every MAP recording, a long diastolic interval of approximately 120 milliseconds is observed. From Kirchhof P, et al. *Circulation* 1998;97:2567-2574.

repolarized "take-off" potentials) during burst stimulation that induced VF than during bursts that did not induce arrhythmias (Fig. 5).

PRR was increased by administration of both procainamide and propafenone, with propafenone producing greater PRR than procainamide (procainamide: 8 ± 9 milliseconds, propafenone: 34 ± 17 milliseconds). Similar to baseline data, bursts that induced VF showed significantly less PRR than other bursts that did not induce arrhythmias with procainamide (Fig. 5). In contrast to those at baseline and with procainamide, bursts that induced arrhythmias (mostly monomorphic VT) with propafenone were not associated with less PRR than were bursts with different frequencies

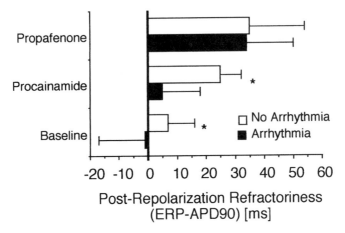

Figure 5. Association of postrepolarization refractoriness (PRR) and induction of arrhythmias at baseline and with procainamide, but not with propafenone, during burst stimulation. PRR, expressed in milliseconds as the interval between action potential duration at 90% repolarization (APD$_{90}$) and the following activation (x axis), is plotted separately for shocks that induce arrhythmias and those that do not induce arrhythmias. From Kirchhof P, et al. *Circulation* 1998;97:2567-2574.

and/or stimulus strengths that did not induce arrhythmias (Fig. 5). PRR was associated with protection against induction of VF with procainamide, but not protection against monomorphic VT with propafenone, during repetitive extrastimulation and burst stimulation. The differential electrophysiologic effects of procainamide and propafenone are summarized and compared in Table 4.

Table 4
Summary of Electrophysiologic Effects
of Procainamide and Propafenone

	Procainamide	*Propafenone*
Action potential duration	+12%	+14%
Postrepolarization refractoriness	+8–15 ms	+10–30 ms
Mean condition time at S5	+94%	+400%
Inducibility of arrhythmias	70% less VF	monomorphic ventricular tachycardia instead of VF
Mean change in wave length	−20% (NS)	−80%

VF = ventricular fibrillation.

Discussion

The present data suggest that PRR might relate to prevention of VF by antiarrhythmic drugs. This hypothesis is supported by the following main findings: 1) Both procainamide and propafenone caused PRR. With either drug, PRR was associated with protection against VF. Propafenone produced greater PRR, and almost completely abolished induction of VF. 2) Use-dependent conduction slowing (caused primarily by propafenone) increased the inducibility of slow monomorphic VT, even in the presence of marked PRR. PRR protects against induction of VF but not monomorphic VT, possibly by preventing microreentry but not macroreentry.

Electrophysiologic Effects Observed in this Study

The effects of procainamide and propafenone on steady state APD concur with those reported in previous publications[20,28,37-39] that showed action potential prolongation with procainamide, and action potential shortening at long cycle lengths and prolongation at short cycle lengths with propafenone. Propafenone prolonged APD_{90} and ERP during repetitive extrastimulation in a use-dependent fashion, possibly attributable to the use-dependent accumulation of propafenone[40] with higher probability of channels in the open state. Probably as a result of higher open-channel probabilities due to subthreshold stimulation,[41] PRR was even more pronounced during burst stimulation.

Procainamide has fast dissociation kinetics[37] and therefore does not exhibit cumulative, use-dependent conduction slowing with multiple premature extrastimulation. In contrast, propafenone has slow dissociation kinetics[38,39,42] and is therefore prone to cumulative sodium channel block with higher probabilities of open sodium channels. This effect can explain both the slower CTs during 400-millisecond pacing and the additional conduction slowing effect of propafenone, but not of procainamide, during multiple premature extrastimulation.

Postrepolarization Refractoriness

During baseline, repetitive extrastimulation caused the ERP to shorten by a greater extent than the concomitant APD_{90}. This shift to capture during earlier repolarization levels with repetitive extrastimulation has been observed previously in the human heart, and has been termed *facilitated excitability* or *progressive encroachment*[20,21,43] of capturing extrastimuli. Encroachment of repetitive extrastimuli, or burst stimuli, onto the repolarization phase of the preceding action potential was associated with tachyarrhythmia induction (Fig. 5). In contrast, drug-induced suppression of excitability during the final repolarization phase (relative refractoriness) eliminated these very premature and arrhythmogenic responses (Figs. 3 and 5). Protracting voltage-dependent and time-dependent recovery of sodium channels until a state of more complete sodium channel availability has been reached could hence be an antiarrhythmic mechanism of sodium channel blocking drugs. Consistent with a more recovered sodium channel availability, CT was shorter at S2 than at S5, the latter of which encroached more onto the repolarization phase (Table 2).

Complete repolarization at the time of reactivation will also prevent excitation during the vulnerable period[34,44] in the late repolarization phase, caused by partial excitability due to dispersion of refractoriness, and thereby preclude arrhythmia induction[33,45,46] via microreentry. By preventing microreentry, PRR could suppress the induction of polymorphic ventricular arrhythmias by burst stimulation or by premature extrastimulation. This explanation is supported by the association between drug-induced PRR and protection against induction of VF, while absence of PRR and presence of facilitated excitability has been associated with induction of tachyar-rhythmias (Fig. 5).

Conduction Slowing Promotes Monomorphic VT

Monomorphic tachycardia is inducible via macroreentry (ie, within a functionally or anatomically preformed reentry circuit). In this setting, reentry can occur due to shortening of activation wavelength below the physical length of a preformed reentry circuit.[47-49] Conduction slowing and action potential shortening both shorten activation wavelength. Given little or no change in APD, a fourfold increase in CT as observed with propafen-one in this study decreases activation wave length fourfold (Table 4), and possibly below the perimeter of the heart, a setting that allows for macroreentry around the circumference of the whole heart in this model. This mechanism may explain the induction of monomorphic tachycardia with propafenone, but not with procainamide. As microreentry occurs within very short intervals[45] at the stimulation site, suppression of microre-entry was probably achieved by PRR intervals of 10 to 30 milliseconds, while this short-term stabilization of excitation at the stimulation site could not prevent macroreentry. In the present study, proarrhythmic effects were caused by usual concentrations of propafenone in the intact, structurally normal heart. Whether propafenone can be used safely in structurally normal hearts, as has been suggested after the CAST trial,[50] is hence ques-tionable.

Study Limitations

The present study was performed in the intact, isolated rabbit heart. The relation between activation wavelength and heart size in the rabbit is different from that in the human, and some electrophysiologic membrane characteristics of the rabbit myocardium[51,52] differ from those of the human heart. Also, in this isolated heart model, no effort was made to model abnormal electrophysiologic and pharmacologic characteristics seen in idiopathic or ischemic myocardial disease. While the present model could demonstrate protective effects of both procainamide and propafenone against the inducibility of VF as well as proarrhythmic effects of propafenone for monomorphic tachycardia, and associate them with effects on PRR and conduction slowing, these class I drug effects need further verification in the clinical setting.

While the analysis of MAP morphology, of activation sequences among the multiple MAP recordings, and of tissue bath ECG morphology provided a reliable distinction between VT and VF (Fig. 4), exact reentry circuits could not be visualized in this study. Whether prevention of VF by propafenone was caused by PRR or by conduction slowing alone, and how propafenone induced monomorphic VT in this model, could not be directly demonstrated in this study.

In the presence of slowly dissociating sodium channel blockers such as propafenone, electrical stimulation may artificially increase PRR and its antiarrhythmic effects due to subthreshold channel activation.[41] Suppression of arrhythmias other than those induced by electrical stimulation may depend on mechanisms other than those described in this study. The present data show that PRR has antiarrhythmic properties during programmed ventricular stimulation. Whether PRR also prevents clinical arrhythmias, or whether PRR is a stimulation-specific antiarrhythmic mechanism that could explain the discrepancy between electrophysiologically inducible and clinically occurring arrhythmias, has yet to be determined.

Conclusions

The results of this experimental study suggest that an important mechanism by which antiarrhythmic drugs with sodium channel blocking properties suppress induction of tachyarrhythmias the production of use-dependent PRR. The results of this study further suggest that, in the case of propafenone, the antiarrhythmic effects of PRR may be offset by the proarrhythmic effects of progressive conduction slowing, which sets the stage for slow monomorphic VT, even in the structurally normal heart. Sodium channel blockers with slow dissociation kinetics are known to cause slow and often incessant monomorphic VT in patients. The ideal antiarrhythmic drug remains to be designed. This study suggests that such an "ideal" drug should produce PRR in a use-dependent fashion, with little or no effect on conduction and propagation of activation wave fronts, to prevent induction of polymorphic ventricular tachyarrhythmias. How PRR can be achieved independently of conduction slowing may be subject of further research involving new antiarrhythmic agents and MAPs.

References

1. Akhtar M, Breithardt G, Camm AJ, et al. CAST and beyond. Implications of the Cardiac Arrhythmia Suppression Trial. Task Force of the Working Group on Arrhythmias of the European Society of Cardiology. *Circulation* 1990;81:1123-1127.
2. Capucci A, Boriani G. Propafenone in the treatment of cardiac arrhythmias. A risk-benefit appraisal. *Drug Saf* 1995;12:55-72.
3. Echt DS, Liebson PR, Mitchell LB, et al. Mortality and morbidity in patients receiving encainide, flecainide, or placebo: The Cardiac Arrhythmia Suppression Trial. *N Engl J Med* 1991;324:781-788.
4. Falk RH, Fogel RI. Flecainide. *J Cardiovasc Electrophysiol* 1994;5:964-981.
5. The Antiarrhythmics versus Implantable Defibrillators (AVID) Investigators. A comparison of antiarrhythmic-drug therapy with implantable defibrillators in patients resuscitated from near-fatal ventricular arrhythmias. *N Engl J Med* 1997;337:1576-1583.
6. Investigators TCASTI. Effect of the antiarrhythmic agent moricizine on survival after myocardial infarction. *N Engl J Med* 1992;327:227-235.
7. Mason JW. A comparison of seven antiarrhythmic drugs in patients with ventricular tachyarrhythmias. Electrophysiologic Study versus Electrocardiographic Monitoring Investigators [see comments]. *N Engl J Med* 1993;329:452-458.
8. Moss AJ, Hall WJ, Cannom DS, et al. Improved survival with an implantable defibrillator in patients with coronary artery disease at high risk for ventricular arrhythmias. *N Engl J Med* 1996;335:1933-1940.
9. Siebels J, Cappato R, Rüppel R, et al. ICD versus drugs in cardiac arrest survivors: Preliminary results of the Cardiac Arrest Study Hamburg. *PACE* 1993;16:552-558.
10. Waldo AL. Effect of d-sotalol on mortality in patients with left ventricular dysfunction after recent and remote myocardial infarction [Erratum]. *Lancet* 1996;348:416.
11. Waldo AL, Camm AJ, Deruyter H, et al. Effect of d-sotalol on mortality in patients with left ventricular dysfunction after recent and remote myocardial infarction. *Lancet* 1996;348:7-12.
12. Borggrefe M, Trampisch HJ, Breithardt G. Reappraisal of criteria for assessing drug efficacy in patients with ventricular tachyarrhythmias: Complete versus partial suppression of inducible arrhythmias. *J Am Coll Cardiol* 1988;12:140-149.
13. Mason JW. A comparison of electrophysiologic testing with Holter monitoring to predict antiarrhythmic drug efficacy for ventricular tachyarrhythmias. *N Engl J Med* 1993;329:445-451.
14. Dillon SM. Synchronized repolarization after defibrillation shocks. A possible component of the defibrillation process demonstrated by optical recordings in rabbit heart. *Circulation* 1992;85:1865-1878.
15. Hohnloser SH, Woosley RL. Sotalol. *N Engl J Med* 1994;331:31-38.
16. Coromilas J, Saltman AE, Waldecker B, et al. Electrophysiological effects of flecainide on anisotropic conduction and reentry in infarcted canine hearts. *Circulation* 1995;91:2245-2263.

17. Restivo M, Yin H, Caref EB, et al. Reentrant arrhythmias in the subacute infarction period. The proarrhythmic effect of flecainide acetate on functional reentrant circuits. *Circulation* 1995;91:1236-1246.

18. Costard JA, Franz MR. Frequency-dependent antiarrhythmic drug effects on postrepolarization refractoriness and ventricular conduction time in canine ventricular myocardium in vivo. *J Pharmacol Exp Ther* 1989;251:39-46.

19. Hondeghem LM, Snyders DJ. Class III antiarrhythmic agents have a lot of potential but a long way to go. Reduced effectiveness and dangers of reverse use dependence. *Circulation* 1990;81:686-690.

20. Lee RJ, Liem LB, Cohen TJ, et al. Relation between repolarization and refractoriness in the human ventricle: Cycle length dependence and effect of procainamide. *J Am Coll Cardiol* 1992;19:614-618.

21. Koller BS, Karasik PE, Soloman AJ, et al. The relationship between repolarization and refractoriness during programmed electrical stimulation in the human right ventricle: Implications for ventricular tachycardia induction. *Circulation* 1995;91:2378-2384.

22. Mason JR, Winkle RA. Accuracy of ventricular tachycardia induction study for predicting long-term efficacy and inefficiency of antiarrhythmic drugs. *N Engl J Med* 1980;303:1073-1077.

23. Wilber DJ, Garan H, Finkelstein D, et al. Out-of-hospital cardiac arrest: Use of electrophysiologic testing in the prediction of long-term outcome. *N Engl J Med* 1988;318:19-24.

24. Task Force of the Working Group on Arrhythmias of the European Society of Cardiology. The Sicilian Gambit. A new approach to the classification of antiarrhythmic drugs based on their actions on arrhythmogenic mechanisms. *Circulation* 1991;84:1831-1851.

25. Connolly SJ, Kates RE, Lebsack CS, et al. Clinical pharmacology of propafenone. *Circulation* 1983;68:589-596.

26. Edvardsson N, Hirsch I, Olsson SB. Acute effects of lignocaine, procainamide, metoprolol, digoxin and atropine on human myocardial refractoriness. *Cardiovasc Res* 1984;18:463-470.

27. Edvardsson N, Hirsch I, Olsson SB. Effects of lidocaine, procainamide, metoprolol, digoxin and atropine on the conduction of premature ventricular beats in man. *Eur Heart J* 1985;6:57-66.

28. Koller B, Franz MR. New classification of moricizine and propafenone based on electrophysiologic and electrocardiographic data from isolated rabbit heart. *J Cardiovasc Pharmacol* 1994;24:753-760.

29. Rosen MR. The classification of antiarrhythmic drugs: How do we educate the scientist and the clinician. In Breithardt G, Borggrefe M, Camm J, Shenasa M (eds): *Antiarrhythmic Drugs*. Berlin, Heidelberg, New York: Springer Verlag; 1995:393-404.

30. Zipes DP, Prystowsky EN, Heger JJ. Electrophysiology and pharmacology of aprindine, encainide, and propafenone. *Ann N Y Acad Sci* 1984;432:201-209.

31. Fabritz CL, Kirchhof PF, Behrens S, et al. Myocardial vulnerability to T wave shocks: Relation to shock strength, shock coupling interval, and dispersion of ventricular repolarization. *J Cardiovasc Electrophysiol* 1996;7:231-242.

32. Franz MR, Chin MC, Sharkey HR, et al. A new single catheter technique for simultaneous measurement of action potential duration and refractory period in vivo. *J Am Coll Cardiol* 1990;16:878-886.

33. Kirchhof PF, Fabritz CL, Behrens S, et al. Induction of ventricular fibrillation by T wave field-shocks in the isolated perfused rabbit heart: Role of nonuniform shock responses. *Basic Res Cardiol* 1997;92:35-44.
34. Kirchhof PF, Fabritz CL, Zabel M, et al. The vulnerable period for low and high energy T wave shocks: Role of dispersion of repolarisation and effect of d-sotalol. *Cardiovasc Res* 1996;31:953-962.
35. Franz MR, Cima R, Wang D, et al. Electrophysiological effects of myocardial stretch and mechanical determinants of stretch-activated arrhythmias [published erratum appears in *Circulation* 1992;86:1663]. *Circulation* 1992; 86:968-978.
36. Eggenreich U, Fleischmann PH, Stark G, et al. Effects of propafenone on the median frequency of ventricular fibrillation in Langendorff perfused guinea-pig hearts. *Cardiovasc Res* 1996;31:926-931.
37. Villemaire C, Nattel S. Modulation of procainamide's effect on cardiac conduction in dogs by extracellular potassium concentration. A quantitative analysis. *Circulation* 1994;89:2870-2878.
38. Tamargo J. Propafenone slows conduction and produces a nonuniform recovery of excitability between Purkinje and ventricular muscle fibers. *J Cardiovasc Pharmacol* 1993;22:203-207.
39. Varro A, Elharrar V, Surawicz B. Frequency-dependent effects of several class I antiarrhythmic drugs on Vmax of action potential upstroke in canine cardiac Purkinje fibers. *J Cardiovasc Pharmacol* 1985;7:482-492.
40. Stark G, Dhein S, Bachernegg M, et al. Frequency-dependent effects of propafenone decrease with duration of ventricular tachycardia in isolated guinea pig hearts. *Eur J Pharmacol* 1994;252:283-289.
41. Shenasa M, Fromer M, Borggrefe M, et al. Subthreshold electrical stimulation for termination and prevention of reentrant tachycardias. *J Electrocardiol* 1992;24:25-31.
42. Winslow E, Campbell JK. Comparative frequency-dependent effects of three class Ic agents, Org 7797, flecainide, and propafenone, on ventricular action potential duration. *J Cardiovasc Pharmacol* 1991;18:911-917.
43. Davidenko JM, Antzelevitch C. Electrophysiological mechanisms underlying rate-dependent changes of refractoriness in normal and segmentally depressed canine Purkinje fibers. The characteristics of post-repolarization refractoriness. *Circ Res* 1986;58:257-268.
44. Wiggers CJ, Wegren R. Ventricular fibrillation due to single localized induction in condenser shock supplied during the vulnerable phase of ventricular systole. *Am J Physiol* 1940;128:500-505.
45. Frazier DW, Wolf PD, Wharton JM, et al. Stimulus-induced critical point. Mechanism for electrical initiation of reentry in normal canine myocardium. *J Clin Invest* 1989;83:1039-1052.
46. Habbab MA, El-Sherif N. Recordings from the slow zone of reentry during burst pacing versus programmed premature stimulation for initiation of reentrant ventricular tachycardia in patients with coronary artery disease. *Am J Cardiol* 1992;70:211-217.
47. Boersma L, Brugada J, Kirchhof C, et al. Mapping of reset of anatomic and functional reentry in anisotropic rabbit ventricular myocardium. *Circulation* 1994;89:852-862.
48. Brugada J, Boersma L, Kirchhof C, et al. Proarrhythmic effects of flecainide. Experimental evidence for increased susceptibility to reentrant arrhythmias. *Circulation* 1991;84:1808-1818.

49. El-Sherif N, Gough WB, Restivo M. Reentrant ventricular arrhythmias in the late myocardial infarction period: Mechanism by which a short-long-short cardiac sequence facilitates the induction of reentry. *Circulation* 1991;83:268-278.
50. Heusch A, Kramer HH, Krogmann ON, et al. Clinical experience with propafenone for cardiac arrhythmias in the young. *Eur Heart J* 1994;15:1050-1056.
51. Brown HF, Noble D, Noble SJ, et al. The relationship between the transient inward current (TI) and other components of slow inward current in mammalian cardiac muscle. *Jpn Heart J* 1986;1:127-142.
52. Kurz RW, Ren XL, Franz MR. Dispersion and delay of electrical restitution in the globally ischaemic heart. *Eur Heart J* 1994;15:547-554.

30

Mechanism of Atrial Flutter Conversion by Class III Antiarrhythmic Drugs

Guilherme Fenelon, MD,
Kenneth A. Ellenbogen, MD,
Mark A. Wood, MD
and Bruce S. Stambler, MD

Atrial flutter is a rapid, regular atrial tachyarrhythmia that occurs in paroxysmal or chronic persistent forms. Atrial flutter is often classified into two major types on the basis of the surface electrocardiogram (ECG): classic or type I atrial flutter, in which the atrial rate may be from 200 to 340 beats/min, and type II atrial flutter with atrial rates greater than 340 beats/min. Whereas less is known about the mechanisms implicated in type II flutter, it is generally accepted that type I flutter is caused by macroreentry within the right atrium.[1] Clinical studies using intracavitary mapping demonstrated that during typical atrial flutter the intra-atrial septum is activated in the inferior-to-superior direction and the free wall is activated superiorly to inferiorly. Most importantly, a critical portion of the reentrant circuit is an area of slow conduction in a narrow isthmus of tissue in the posteroinferior right atrium between the inferior vena cava and the tricuspid annulus.[1] Surgical[2] or catheter[3] ablation of this isthmus of slow conduction has resulted in successful termination and prevention of recurrences of atrial flutter.

From Franz MR (ed): *Monophasic Action Potentials: Bridging Cell and Bedside.*
©Futura Publishing Company, Inc., Armonk, NY, 2000.

Most of our understanding of the mechanisms of atrial flutter termination by antiarrhythmic drugs has emerged from experimental models of atrial flutter.[1] Surprisingly, very limited knowledge exists about the mechanisms of atrial flutter termination by pharmacologic agents in the clinical setting. This undoubtedly relates to the relatively disappointing efficacy of antiarrhythmic drug therapy alone with most class I agents, amiodarone, or d,l-sotalol for arrhythmia termination in patients with atrial flutter. Recently, however, pure class III drugs that selectively prolong repolarization and refractoriness, either alone[4-6] or as an adjunct to atrial overdrive pacing,[7] have been reported effective in terminating atrial flutter in patients. These recent clinical findings confirm prior data in a variety of experimental models that arrhythmias due to reentry can be terminated and suppressed by agents that predominately prolong myocardial refractoriness. However, because none of these animal models has a clear-cut clinical counterpart, it is uncertain whether the experimental data on the mechanisms of atrial flutter termination by antiarrhythmic drugs can be extrapolated to the clinical setting. Furthermore, in contrast to the experience in clinical practice, many drugs with a variety of actions have remarkably high success rates for terminating and controlling atrial flutter in experimental flutter models. As a result, clinical predictions of whether specific electrophysiologic properties of antiarrhythmic drugs will have antiarrhythmic or proarrhythmic effects remain far from ideal, and conversion of atrial flutter with antiarrhythmic agents has been largely empiric. To properly predict clinical effects of antiarrhythmic drugs on atrial flutter, it is important to identify specific electrophysiologic characteristics of the arrhythmia that make a drug with particular electrophysiologic properties antiarrhythmic.

This chapter reviews the current knowledge on the mechanisms of type I atrial flutter termination by antiarrhythmic drugs, with emphasis on class III agents. Type II atrial flutter and atrial flutter related to congenital heart disease and/or cardiac surgery are not discussed.

Mechanisms and Vulnerable Parameters of Atrial Flutter

Components of Reentrant Circuits

An area of unidirectional block is a critical requirement for the establishment of most reentrant circuits such as type I atrial flutter. For both initiation and maintenance of reentry, a circuit must also have adequate boundaries that prevent short circuiting of the impulse. Finally, an additional condition necessary for reentry is that the time for recirculation of the impulse to its site of origin must be longer than the refractory period of the proximal segment of the circuit. In other words, the anatomic length of the circuit should be equal to or longer than the distance traveled by the depolarization wave during the refractory period. The latter is defined as the wavelength, and equals the product of refractory period and conduction velocity. Shorter wavelengths, resulting either from short refractory periods, slow conduction velocities, or both, are more likely to set up reentrant circuits in a given tissue mass than longer wavelengths.[8] The difference in area between the wavelength and the anatomic length of the circuit defines the excitable gap, or that segment of the reentrant circuit that is excitable while the reentrant impulse is traveling around the circuit. The gap may be fully or partially excitable depending on the degree of recovery of excitability of the tissue ahead of the advancing wave front. When the wavelength exceeds the anatomic length of the circuit, the excitable gap closes and reentry ceases.

Excitable Gap in Atrial Flutter

Although some studies suggest that the excitable gap in human atrial flutter is partially excitable, most evidence indicates that atrial flutter has a fully excitable gap.[9-11] The tachycardia cycle length of an excitable gap reentrant circuit is directly proportional to conduction velocity. Action potential duration (APD) and refractoriness are direct determinants of cycle length only if the excitable gap is partially rather than fully excitable. In a reentrant circuit in which the wave front circulates through partially refractory tissue, shortening of APD will increase the excitable gap, accelerate conduction velocity, and decrease tachycardia cycle length. Conversely, in a reentrant circuit with a fully excitable gap, shortening of APD will not result in changes in conduction velocity or in tachycardia cycle length.

We used monophasic action potential (MAP) recordings and pharmacologic agents with differential effects on APD and conduction velocity as tools to determine whether the excitable gap in the atrial flutter reentrant circuit in humans is fully or partially excitable.[10] MAPs were recorded from the right atrium in 41 patients during type I atrial flutter. The MAP catheter was positioned in an area of the right atrium where a stable MAP recording was obtained, usually against the free wall or appendage, and not necessarily from the area of slow conduction. The APD during atrial flutter was measured from the atrial MAP recording and the atrial flutter cycle length was used as index of conduction velocity during atrial flutter. Adenosine (17 ± 3 mg) shortened APD from 166 ± 22 to 149 ± 26 milliseconds (-17 ± 16 milliseconds; $P<0.001$) but did not change atrial flutter cycle length (236 ± 27 to 236 ± 29 milliseconds). Isoproterenol (0.03 µg/kg body weight per minute) decreased both APD (-10 ± 9 milliseconds; $P<0.05$) and flutter cycle length (-7 ± 4 milliseconds; $P<0.05$). Procainamide (15 mg/kg, then 2 mg/min) prolonged APD (40 ± 18 milliseconds, $P<0.001$) and flutter cycle length (61 ± 20 milliseconds, $P<0.001$). The pharmacologically induced changes in flutter cycle length were not correlated with changes in APD. Procainamide's prolongation of APD was reversed by adenosine (-40 ± 24 milliseconds; $P<0.001$) without significantly affecting the flutter cycle length (-4 ± 6 milliseconds; $P=NS$) (Fig. 1). These results suggest that atrial flutter cycle length is determined primarily by conduction velocity and does not depend directly on APD; or, in other words, that the atrial flutter reentrant circuit has a fully excitable gap.

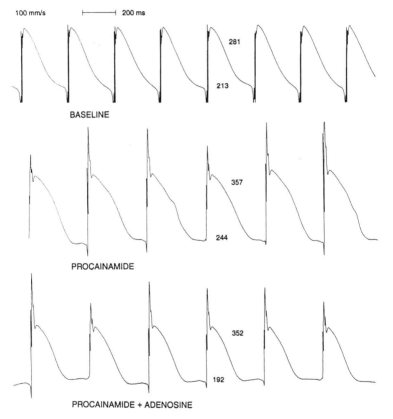

Figure 1. MAPs during atrial flutter at baseline, during procainamide, and during adenosine in the presence of procainamide. The atrial cycle lengths and action potential durations (APDs) are above and below the tracings, respectively. Adenosine reversed the procainamide-induced increase in APD (-52 milliseconds) without significantly altering the increase in cycle length (-5 milliseconds). From Reference 10, with permission.

Vulnerable Parameters of Atrial Flutter

The electrophysiologic parameter(s) of the arrhythmia whose modification has an antiarrhythmic effect has been defined as a vulnerable parameter.[12] In atrial flutter, the major vulnerable parameters involve the refractory period and wavelength, the excitable gap, the anatomic pathway and its boundaries, and the area of slow conduction in the corridor between the inferior vena cava, tricuspid annulus, and coronary sinus.[1] The etiology of slow conduction in the posteroinferior right atrium during type I flutter has yet to be determined, but anisotropy has been implicated in its development.[3,13] The presence of a fully excitable gap in this region indicates that slow conduction within the isthmus is not caused by incomplete recovery from refractoriness. We recently showed that slow conduction during atrial flutter is related to normal MAPs,[13] supporting the concept that functional properties rather than structural abnormalities contribute to the development of slow conduction during atrial flutter. It is clear from surgical and catheter ablation studies that creation of a line of conduction block in the isthmus between the inferior vena cava and either the tricuspid annulus or coronary sinus successfully abolishes atrial flutter and prevents its recurrence.[2,3] Conduction block in the area of slow conduction also occurs in spontaneous, drug-induced, and rapid atrial pacing-induced flutter termination.[1] However, the specific mechanisms that result in conduction block in these situations are not as readily identifiable as in the case of the line of block produced with radiofrequency energy. Several hypotheses have been put forth to explain these mechanisms.

Mechanisms of Atrial Flutter Termination

Spontaneous Tachycardia Termination

The mechanisms that lead a stable, sustained reentrant tachycardia such as atrial flutter to suddenly spontaneously terminate are not well understood but may be related to increases in cycle length variability.[14,15] A premature stimulus or an abrupt change in heart rate may provoke oscillation in conduction velocity and refractoriness at certain sites in a reentrant circuit. The degree of oscillation at a given site of the reentrant circuit forms the basis of beat-to-beat cycle length variability and may be important to maintain stability of a reentrant tachycardia. A reentrant tachycardia becomes stable and sustains itself if the oscillation dampens, and will terminate if the oscillation becomes progressively greater (Figs. 2 and 3).

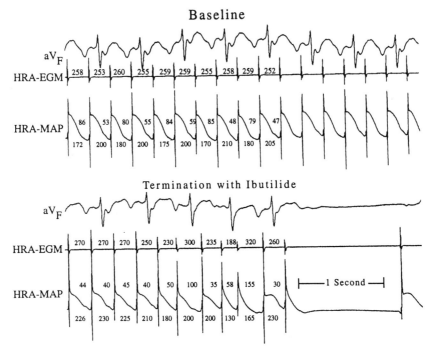

Figure 2. Surface lead aVF, bipolar electrogram (EGM), and MAP recorded from high right atrium (HRA) in a patient at baseline and just before conversion of atrial flutter at 35 minutes after the beginning of ibutilide infusion. Numbers above the electrocardiographic tracing are atrial flutter cycle length, and those above and below the MAP tracings are the diastolic interval and MAP duration, respectively. Mean cycle length for 10 consecutive beats was 257 milliseconds at baseline and 259 milliseconds just before conversion. The beat-to-beat variability in cycle length and diastolic interval were 1 and 2.4 at baseline and 14 and 64 just before conversion, respectively. From Reference 33, with permission.

Experimental studies in atrial flutter have shown an association between spontaneous arrhythmia termination and beat-to-beat cycle length oscillation. In the canine atrial tricuspid ring preparation, conduction velocity and refractoriness vary from site to site in the reentrant circuit, and depend on the duration of the preceding diastolic interval.[14] In this model, a critical event for termination of the arrhythmia is an exceptionally long diastolic interval preceding the next to last cycle that accelerates local conduction and prolongs APD and refractoriness at the site. Similarly, in the canine sterile pericarditis model, spontaneous termination is preceded by a consistent oscillatory pattern occurring over the last two beats: a long cycle followed by a much shorter cycle.[15] In the canine model of atrial flutter created by an anatomic barrier,[16,17] oscillation of cycle length, in addition to resulting from changes in conduction velocity, may also occur

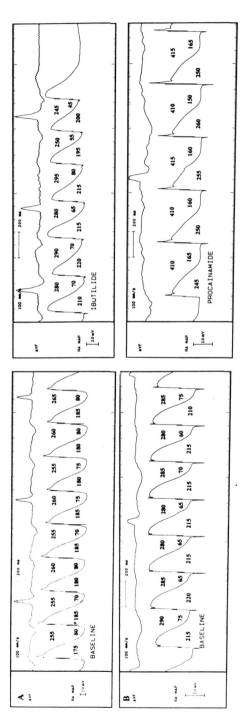

Figure 3. Surface electrocardiogram (lead aVF) and right atrial MAP (RA MAP) recordings during atrial flutter from two patients (A and B) at baseline (left) and during ibutilide or procainamide (right). The atrial cycle length (CL), MAP duration (MAPD), and diastolic interval (DI) are shown above (top number), below, and above (bottom number) the action potential recording, respectively. In patient A, ibutilide (top right) increased mean atrial CL (Δ18 milliseconds) and MAPD (Δ27 milliseconds), decreased DI (Δ-9 milliseconds), increased MAPD/CL (Δ0.05), and terminated atrial flutter after an increase in beat-to-beat atrial CL, MAPD, and DI variability. In patient B, procainamide (bottom right) increased mean atrial CL (Δ125 milliseconds), MAPD (Δ25 milliseconds) and DI (Δ100 milliseconds), decreased MAPD/CL (Δ-0.17), and atrial flutter persisted. From Stambler BS, Wood MA, Ellenbogen KA. Antiarrhythmic actions of intravenous ibutilide compared with procainamide during human atrial flutter and fibrillation. Electrophysiological determinants of enhanced conversion efficacy. *Circulation* 1997;96:4298-4306, with permission of the American Heart Association.

as a result of a change in the pathway length or a disturbance of the pathway by a competing focus. Finally, oscillations in refractoriness with a nearly constant beat-to-beat cycle length can also result in termination of tachyarrhythmias.[14] Local variation in the conduction time may be exactly compensated by changes elsewhere in the circuit so that the cycle length may be nearly constant if not recorded from within the circuit. Although in clinical studies the presence of small beat-to-beat variations in atrial flutter cycle length have been observed,[18,19] the role of cycle length oscillations on the spontaneous termination of the arrhythmia has not been systematically analyzed.

The mechanisms responsible for these interval oscillations have not been fully explained. Previous clinical and experimental studies have demonstrated that these variations are not randomly distributed but occur on a beat-to-beat basis in association with the QRS complex.[18,19] We used time and frequency analysis techniques to investigate the beat-to-beat variation of atrial flutter cycle length.[20] Modulation of the frequency peaks in the power spectra was evaluated by examination of their response to physiologic and pharmacologic interventions. The results suggest that atrial flutter is modulated on a beat-to-beat basis by a complex interplay between the ventricular contraction and the respiratory rate (Fig. 4), possibly mediated via changes in atrial pressure and/or volume and by the autonomic nervous system. Changes in each of these control mechanisms can be detected by alterations in specific bands of the power spectrum. Thus, alterations in the mechanisms that mediate atrial flutter cycle length variability may contribute to spontaneous tachycardia termination.

Drug-Induced Termination of Atrial Flutter

The excitable gap in atrial flutter is considered a vulnerable parameter that is susceptible to antiarrhythmic drugs.[1] It is postulated that class III drugs that are capable of prolonging repolarization without affecting conduction velocity will terminate flutter by increasing the wavelength until the excitable gap closes and reentry is extinguished.[12,21] By prolonging the refractory period, the reentrant impulse initially will be forced to travel in partially refractory tissue, and slowing of tachycardia will occur. With further refractoriness prolongation, the impulse will encroach on absolute refractory tissue, conduction will no longer be possible, and the tachycardia will terminate. The hypothesis that prolongation of refractoriness is critically important to the termination of reentry by antiarrhythmic drugs has been confirmed by a number of experimental studies. However a number of studies have also suggested that antiarrhythmic drugs may terminate reentry by a variety of other diverse mechanisms. The mechanisms impli-

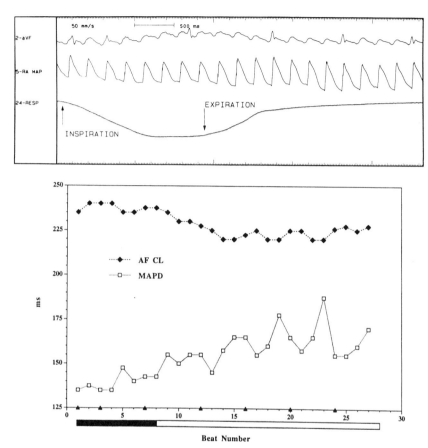

Figure 4. Top: surface electrocardiogram (lead aVF) and right atrial MAP (RA MAP) recorded during atrial flutter along with respiratory activity (RESP). Arrows indicate onset of inspiration and expiration. Bottom: beat-to-beat atrial flutter cycle lengths (AF CL) (filled diamonds) and MAP durations (MAPD) (open squares) obtained from the tracings on top. Filled triangles on the abscissa indicate timing of QRS complexes; filled rectangle below abscissa indicates inspiration; open rectangle below abscissa indicates expiration. During inspiration, atrial flutter cycle lengths are longer and MAPs are shorter than during expiration. From Stambler BS and Ellenbogen KA. Elucidating the mechanisms of atrial flutter cycle length variability using power spectral analysis techniques. *Circulation* 1996;94:2515-2525, with permission of the American Heart Association.

cated in pharmacologic conversion of experimental and clinical atrial flutter are summarized in Table 1.

Experimental Studies

In various models of atrial flutter, the arrhythmia can be consistently interrupted with use of drugs with diverse effects on conduction velocity

Table 1
Mechanisms Leading to Drug-Induced Conduction
Block in the Area of Slow Conduction

	Experimental Flutter	Human Flutter
Beat-to-beat atrial cycle length variability	yes	yes
Failure of safety factor for conduction	yes	unknown
Failure of lateral boundaries (short circuit)*	yes	unknown
Reflection of the reentrant impulse*	yes	unknown

*May be facilitated by, as well as result in atrial cycle length variability.

and refractoriness. Drugs that predominantly decrease conduction velocity (class I agents) such as procainamide,[22] moricizine,[23] disopyramide,[16,24] propafenone,[16,24] flecainide[16,24] or SC-40230[16] terminate atrial flutter by increasing cycle length and preferentially suppressing conduction in the area of slow conduction. The same was unexpectedly observed with the cardiac glycoside ouabain.[1] The class III drugs E-4301,[24] d-sotalol,[16] and dofetilide[25] interrupt atrial flutter by decreasing the excitable gap through a greater prolongation of refractoriness and a lesser slowing of conduction. Conversely, another class III drug (N-acetylprocainamide)[22] terminates atrial flutter without decreasing the excitable gap. In all studies, class III drug-induced prolongation of the wavelength was never sufficient to close the measured excitable gap of the reentrant circuit. Importantly, however, the excitable gap was not determined simultaneously from multiple sites within the circuit or at the moment of tachycardia termination in these studies.

Whether class I and class III agents terminate atrial flutter through different mechanisms is not entirely clear from these studies. Depending on the model, the following modes of arrhythmia termination were observed with both class I and class III drugs: 1) failure of the safety factor for conduction localized to a critical site of slow conduction[23]; 2) failure of a lateral boundary, resulting in short circuiting of the impulse that resets and extinguishes the original circuit[17]; and 3) reflection of the reentrant impulse within the primary path resulting in elimination of the excitable gap.[26] Antiarrhythmic drugs may also have effects on atrial tissue outside of the reentrant circuit that can result in flutter termination. For example, the class III drug d-sotalol may promote ectopic beats outside the reentrant circuit during atrial flutter, which can destabilize the circuit.[17] It is important to note that regardless of the mechanism involved, most episodes of atrial flutter termination have been preceded by beat-to-beat cycle length oscillations. Therefore, it is tempting to speculate that in animal models of atrial flutter, agents with class I (depressing conduction) or class III (prolonging refractoriness and the wavelength) effects induce perturbations of the slow conduction zone that ultimately lead to termination of the arrhythmia.

Clinical Studies

In contrast with experimental atrial flutter, class I and class III drugs do not exhibit the same efficacy in converting human type I atrial flutter. Class Ia and Ic agents have efficacy rates of only 0% to 30% for acute termination of atrial flutter and, in general, these drugs usually only slow the flutter rate without interrupting the arrhythmia.[1,27] Similarly, not all class III drugs are equally effective in terminating atrial flutter. Amiodarone and d,l-sotalol have not been shown to be successful in restoring sinus rhythm in patients with atrial flutter or atrial fibrillation.[21,28] To date, the only drugs that have been proven effective in terminating atrial flutter are selective class III agents such as ibutilide or dofetilide.[4-7,21] In a randomized, double-blind, placebo-controlled trial involving 266 patients with atrial flutter or atrial fibrillation, intravenous ibutilide (1.0+0.5 mg or 1.0+1.0 mg) successfully converted the atrial arrhythmia in 47% of patients, compared with 2% after placebo.[5] Among patients with atrial flutter, the conversion efficacy of ibutilide was 63% (50 of 80 patients), which, interestingly, was significantly higher than the 31% success rate with ibutilide in atrial fibrillation (25 of 81 patients). In a randomized trial of 127 patients,[29] ibutilide (1.0+1.0 mg) was superior to intravenous procainamide (1200 mg) in converting atrial flutter (76% versus 12%) or atrial fibrillation (51% versus 20%; $P<0.005$). Furthermore, in a randomized trial of 319 patients, ibutilide (2.0 mg) was more effective than intravenous d,l-sotalol (1.5 mg/kg) in acute conversion of atrial flutter (70% versus 19%) or atrial fibrillation (44% versus 11%; $P<0.05$). Finally, in another study, both ibutilide and procainamide were equally effective (87% versus 88%) in enhancing termination of atrial flutter by atrial overdrive pacing (Fig. 5).[7] Antiarrhythmic drug-induced changes in tachycardia cycle length and MAP duration (MAPD) were not found to be useful predictors of the ability of rapid pacing to terminate atrial flutter.

The electrophysiologic basis for the striking superiority of ibutilide compared with class I and other nonselective class III drugs in the acute conversion of human atrial flutter has not been fully explained. Ibutilide prolongs APD and refractoriness without directly affecting conduction velocity, and does so without exhibiting reverse use dependence.[21,30] This means that prolongation of refractoriness and APD are not affected by heart rate, with similar increases at slow (bradycardia) and fast (tachycardia) heart rates. The electrophysiologic effects of ibutilide have been attributed to activation of a slow inward plateau current carried by Na^+, and to blockade of the rapidly activating delayed rectifier K^+ current (I_{Kr}).[31] The

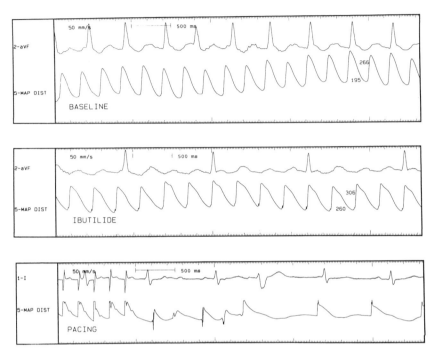

Figure 5. Surface lead aVF, and MAP recorded from the high right atrium (HRA) in a patient at baseline (top), after ibutilide infusion (middle), and immediately before pacing-induced conversion of atrial flutter (bottom). The atrial flutter cycle lengths and MAP durations are shown above and below the tracings, respectively. Note that ibutilide prolonged the atrial flutter cycle length by 39 milliseconds and MAP duration by 65 milliseconds. The last 5 beats of an atrial overdrive pacing train are shown at bottom left. Following infusion of ibutilide, pacing resulted in termination of atrial flutter with several beats of transient atrial fibrillation before resumption of sinus rhythm. From Reference 7, with permission.

efficacy of ibutilide in terminating experimental atrial flutter has also been reported; however, detailed analysis of the mechanisms resulting in arrhythmia conversion was not performed.[32]

Insights into the mechanisms responsible for acute conversion of human atrial flutter by ibutilide and its enhanced efficacy compared with the class Ia drug procainamide were provided by recent studies from our group.[27,33] The antiarrhythmic effects of ibutilide compared with procainamide were evaluated in 89 patients with atrial flutter, by use of right atrial MAP recordings (Figs. 3 and 6).[27] The MAPD and atrial cycle length were used as indexes of repolarization and conduction times, respectively. The diastolic interval was defined as atrial cycle length minus MAPD and was used as an estimate of the excitable gap during reentry. The fraction of the atrial flutter cycle length occupied by the action potential, ie, the ratio

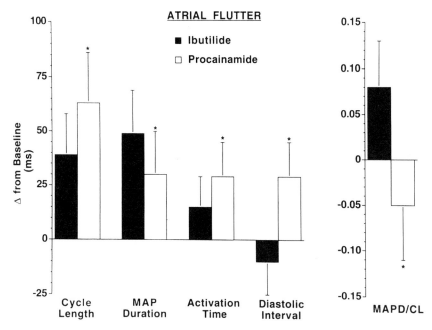

Figure 6. Comparison of the electrophysiologic effects of ibutilide with procainamide during atrial flutter. MAPD = atrial MAP duration; CL = atrial cycle length; *P<0.05 versus ibutilide. Adapted from Stambler BS, Wood MA, Ellenbogen KA. Antiarrhythmic actions of intravenous ibutilide compared with procainamide during human atrial flutter and fibrillation. Electrophysiological determinants of enhanced conversion efficacy. *Circulation* 1997;96:4298-4306, with permission of the American Heart Association.

MAPD/CL (cycle length) was used as a measure of relative drug-induced changes in repolarization to conduction velocity. Theoretically, in a reentrant circuit with a fixed path length, wavelength is proportional to refractory period divided by cycle length. Hence, the MAPD/CL ratio was used as an index of drug-induced changes in wavelength.

As expected, ibutilide was superior to procainamide in converting atrial flutter (29 of 45 patients or 64% versus 0 of 33 patients). Ibutilide and procainamide produced electrophysiologic effects consistent with class III and class Ia antiarrhythmic drug action, respectively (Fig. 6). Ibutilide prolonged MAPD more than cycle length (30% versus 16%), whereas procainamide increased atrial cycle length more than MAPD (26% versus 18%). These effects resulted in a 13% mean increase in MAPD/CL by ibutilide, whereas procainamide decreased this index by 6%. Conversion efficacy was correlated with prolongation of the MAPD/CL and not with changes in MAPD (refractoriness) or CL (conduction velocity) alone. Similar findings were noted with dofetilide (class III) and quinidine (class Ia) in experimental atrial flutter.[25] The former increased wavelength by 11%, whereas the latter reduced the wavelength by 2%.

Corroborating our previous observations,[33] termination of atrial flutter with ibutilide was associated with an increase in beat-to-beat variability in atrial cycle length, MAPD, and diastolic interval (Figs. 2 and 3). These oscillations did not occur in atrial flutter that was not terminated by ibutilide or procainamide, further suggesting that oscillatory termination is an important mechanism by which ibutilide produces flutter termination. As in experimental studies,[1] it seems unlikely that action potential prolongation by ibutilide was sufficient to close the excitable gap and extinguish the circuit. The size of the excitable gap, however, can vary throughout the circuit. A local excitable gap might have been eliminated or reduced by the relatively greater increases in atrial MAPD than cycle length produced by ibutilide. This could result in cycle length oscillations and arrhythmia termination. Detailed recordings from the critical area of slow conduction would help to corroborate these conclusions as well as the precise mechanisms by which ibutilide promotes cycle length oscillations and arrhythmia conversion. Preliminary data suggest that ibutilide prolonged refractoriness and decreased the excitable gap near the entrance to the isthmus of the flutter circuit between the inferior vena cava and tricuspid annulus.[34] Ibutilide shifted the reset response curve determined at this region rightward with a steeper slope and loss of the flat portion. This suggests that ibutilide eliminated the fully excitable gap in this portion of the circuit, forcing impulses to propagate in partially excitable tissue and enhancing interval-dependent conduction delay. Comparison of the effects of ibutilide in other areas of atrium and the reentrant circuit would help determine whether the area of slow conduction responds in some unique manner to class III antiarrhythmic drugs.

Determinants of Ibutilide's Clinical Effects

To properly interpret the superior atrial flutter conversion efficacy of ibutilide in relation to other class III drugs that also have effects on atrial repolarization and refractoriness (eg, d,l-sotalol or amiodarone), some aspects of the clinical effects of antiarrhythmic drugs should be noted. Cardiac arrhythmias result from complex interactions between the components of Coumel's Triangle: namely, substrate, triggers (most commonly extrasystoles), and modulating factors (autonomic nervous system, electrolytes, ischemia, etc.). Therefore, the clinical effectiveness of an antiarrhythmic agent will be determined by the equally complex interactions between the drug and the Coumel's Triangle (Table 2). In order to envision

Table 2

Factors that Modulate Clinical Efficacy of Antiarrhythmic Drugs

Arrhythmia-Related	*Drug-Reated*
Substrate	Heart rate (use and reverse-use
mechanism(s) of the arrhythmia	dependence)
(reentry, automaticity)	Neurohormonal status
heart disease	Electrophysiological actions
(normal heart, structural diseases)	(class I, II, III, or IV)
Triggers	Resting membrane potential
extrasystoles	(voltage dependence)
Modulating factors	Ionic channels
autonomic nervous system	functional state
electrolytes	(open, inactivated, resting)
ischemia	cardiac tissue
	(atrial, ventricular, Purkinje)
	functional and structural
	abnormalities
	($\downarrow$ density)
	Membrane ionic pumps and receptors

From reference 21, with permission.

the clinical effects of class III agents, all of the complexities of arrhythmias and of drugs must be taken into account.

The nature and specific electrophysiologic characteristics of an atrial arrhythmia are important for determining the antiarrhythmic efficacy of a drug with particular electrophysiologic properties. As previously noted, the efficacy of ibutilide and other class III drugs differs significantly in atrial flutter compared with atrial fibrillation.[5] Thus, it is not appropriate, as is often done in some clinical studies, to group both atrial arrhythmias together and not separate success rates according to the arrhythmia category. Furthermore, even when considering a particular type of arrhythmia, the specific electrophysiologic properties of a drug may only be antiarrhythmic if a susceptible substrate is present. In this regard, Fei and Frame[35] showed, in an experimental model of atrial reentry in a fixed circuit, that the properties of the reentrant circuit determine antiarrhythmic drug efficacy for tachycardia termination. The initial size of the excitable gap in the circuit and the presence of an area of the circuit that is susceptible to fixed conduction block were both major determinants of the efficacy of d-sotalol for tachycardia termination and the mechanism by which d-sotalol terminated reentry. Only when the initial excitable gap was short could d-sotalol terminate reentry by prolongation of refractory period and closure of the excitable gap. In contrast, d-sotalol could terminate reentry by producing fixed bidirectional conduction block in an area of slow conduction, regardless of the initial reentry cycle length or duration of the excitable gap. In preparations that developed fixed conduction block during d-sotalol, conduction was slower and more rate-dependent before drug administration at critical sites than in the areas of slowest conduction in preparations that did not develop fixed block. Likewise, we have shown in patients with atrial fibrillation that the baseline atrial fibrillation cycle length and MAPD are important determinants of the efficacy of ibutilide for arrhythmia termination.[27] Efficacy was significantly enhanced by a longer mean atrial fibrillation cycle length (64% for cycle length ≥160 milliseconds versus 0% for cycle length <160 milliseconds; $P<0.001$) or MAPD (57% for MAPD ≥125 milliseconds versus 0% for MAPD <125 milliseconds; $P=0.002$). Longer fibrillation cycle lengths may indicate a reduced complexity of atrial fibrillation circuits or a smaller number of reentrant wavelets, and appear to be an important marker of the efficacy of ibutilide for arrhythmia termination.

It is also important to recognize that class III agents are not all alike.[21] While certain class III compounds have almost exclusively class III effects (d-sotalol, ibutilide), others have significant additional actions of at least one other class such as amiodarone (class I, sodium channel blocker; class II, antiadrenergic; and class IV, calcium channel blocker) and d,l-sotalol (class II effects). Considering, for example, that chronic β-blockade has been shown to modify the frequency content of beat-to-beat variability in atrial flutter cycle length and that sympathetic stimulation can modulate and even reverse class III drug effects on APD, these adjunctive actions may take on much greater importance.[20] Furthermore, class III drugs, such as sotalol, with significant reverse use dependence may have reduced efficacy in terminating atrial tachyarrhythmias, due to their diminished potency in prolonging atrial refractoriness and APD at the rapid rates present during atrial flutter.[21] Finally, class III drugs may exert their electrophysiologic actions by blocking one or more of the outward K+ currents (transient outward current, I_{to}; inward rectifier current, I_{K1}; rapid and slow delayed rectifier currents, I_{Ks} and I_{Kr}) and/or by activating slow inward Na+ current. Thus, a great deal of diversity in cellular ionic action exists among the class III agents. Although this has not yet been demonstrated to be important clinically, these differences may translate into important differences in antiarrhythmic or proarrhythmic effects during interactions with the arrhythmia substrate. This may be particularly relevant if ionic channel alterations are present, as may occur in disease states such as congestive heart failure. Some or all of these diverse electrophysiologic actions are also undoubtedly dependent on the drug's pharmacokinetic properties, dose, and concentration. For example, in isolated guinea pig ventricular myocytes, ibutilide's prolongation of APD exhibits a bell-shaped dose-response curve, indicating that ibutilide has multiple ionic channel activities.[36] Although not observed in humans, at higher concentrations in guinea pig ventricular myocytes, ibutilide can shorten APD by activating an outward K+ current.[37] Therefore, attributing antiarrhythmic effects of class III agents to a single 'class effect" has obvious limitations. Each drug must be considered on an individual basis in each clinical scenario. Ongoing clinical and experimental investigations with ibutilide and other selective class III drugs (azimilide, dofetilide, tedisamil) may further elucidate the mechanisms of class III antiarrhythmic drug action in converting atrial arrhythmias.

Conclusions

Pharmacologic conversion of type I atrial flutter is a complex phenomenon involving mechanisms that are not well understood. Beat-to-beat oscillation in cycle length can be promoted by several mechanisms and is an important marker preceding spontaneous and drug-induced termination of atrial flutter. It seems clear that there are important differences in the antiarrhythmic drug responses of atrial flutter in humans compared with animal models, stressing the limitations of extrapolating data from experimental to the clinical setting. This is illustrated by the disparity between the experimental and clinical converting efficacy of class I and some class III drugs. The recent clinical findings of the enhanced efficacy of selective class III agents, compared with class Ia or Ic agents, in terminating atrial flutter along with MAP recordings in patients with atrial flutter support the concept that termination of atrial flutter is promoted by the relatively greater prolongation of APD and refractoriness than slowing of conduction and tachycardia rate that is induced by selective class III antiarrhythmic drug action. Additional experimental and clinical studies with ibutilide and other selective class III agents that appear efficacious in terminating atrial flutter will help to identify the critical mechanisms involved in termination of this atrial arrhythmia. Specifically, the interaction of antiarrhythmic drugs with the area of slow conduction in the posteroinferior right atrium deserves further study.

References

1. Members of the Sicilian Gambit. Atrial fibrillation and flutter: Mechanisms. In Members of the Sicilian Gambit (eds): *Antiarrhythmic Therapy: A Pathophysiological Approach.* Armonk, NY: Futura Publishing Company, Inc.; 1994:161-179.
2. Klein G, Guiraudon G, Sharma A, et al. Demonstration of macroreentry and feasibility of operative therapy in the common type of atrial flutter. *Am J Cardiol* 1986;57:587-591.
3. Lesh M, Van Hare G, Epstein L, et al. Radiofrequency catheter ablation of atrial arrhythmias. Results and mechanisms. *Circulation* 1994;89:1074-1089.
4. Ellenbogen KA, Stambler BS, Wood MA, et al. Efficacy of intravenous ibutilide for rapid termination of atrial fibrillation and flutter: A dose response study. *J Am Coll Cardiol* 1996;28:130-136.

5. Stambler BS, Wood MA, Ellenbogen K, et al. Efficacy and safety of repeated intravenous doses of ibutilide for rapid conversion of atrial flutter or fibrillation. *Circulation* 1996;94:1613-1621.

6. Falk RH, Pollak A, Singh SN, Friedrich T, for the Intravenous Dofetilide Investigators. Intravenous dofetilide, a class III antiarrhythmic agent, for the termination of sustained atrial fibrillation or flutter. *J Am Coll Cardiol* 1997;29:385-390.

7. Stambler BS, Wood MA, Ellenbogen K. Comparative efficacy of intravenous ibutilide versus procainamide for enhancing termination of atrial flutter by atrial overdrive pacing. *Am J Cardiol* 1996;77:960-966.

8. Rensma P, Allessie M, Lammers W, et al. The length of the excitation wave as an index for the susceptibility to reentrant atrial arrhythmias. *Circ Res* 1988;62:395-408.

9. Josephson ME. Atrial flutter and fibrillation. In *Clinical Cardiac Electrophysiology*. Philadelphia: Lea & Febiger; 1993:275-310.

10. Stambler BS, Wood MA, Ellenbogen KA. Pharmacologic alterations in human type I atrial flutter cycle length and monophasic action potential duration. Evidence of a fully excitable gap in the reentrant circuit. *J Am Coll Cardiol* 1996;27:453-461.

11. Callans DJ, Schwartzman D, Gottlieb CD, et al. Characterization of the excitable gap in human type I atrial flutter. *J Am Coll Cardiol* 1997;30:1793-1801.

12. Task Force of Working Group on Arrhythmias: The Sicilian Gambit: A new approach to the classification of antiarrhythmic drugs, based on their actions on arrhythmogenic mechanisms. *Circulation* 1991;84:1831-1851.

13. Fenelon G, Brugada P. Unipolar waveforms and monophasic action potentials in the characterization of slow conduction in human atrial flutter. *PACE* 1998;21:2580-2587.

14. Frame LH, Simson MB. Oscillations of conduction, action potential duration and refractoriness: A mechanism for spontaneous termination of reentrant tachycardias. *Circulation* 1988;78:1277-1287.

15. Ortiz J, Igarashi M, Gonzalez H, et al. Mechanism of spontaneous termination of stable atrial flutter in the canine sterile pericarditis model. *Circulation* 1993;88:1866-1877.

16. Spinelli W, Hoffman BF. Mechanism of termination of reentrant atrial arrhythmias by class I and class III antiarrhythmic agents. *Circ Res* 1989;65:1565-1579.

17. Boyden PA, Graziano JN. Activation mapping of reentry around an anatomic barrier in the canine atrium: Observations during the action of the class III agent, d-sotalol. *J Cardiovasc Electrophysiol* 1993;4:266-279.

18. Waxman MB, Kirsh JA, Cameron DA, et al. The mechanism of flutter interval alternans. *PACE* 1990;13:138-143.

19. Lammers WJEP, Ravelli F, Disertori M, et al. Variations in human atrial flutter cycle length induced by ventricular beats: Evidence of a reentrant circuit with a partially excitable gap. *J Cardiovasc Electrophysiol* 1991;2:375-387.

20. Stambler BS, Ellenbogen KA. Elucidating the mechanisms of atrial flutter cycle length variability using power spectral analysis techniques. *Circulation* 1996;94:2515-2525.

21. Fenelon G, Stambler BS. Class III antiarrhythmic drugs. An update on electrophysiology, pharmacology, and clinical indications. *Cardiol Clin* 1997;1:137-158.

22. Wu KM, Hoffman BF. Effect of procainamide and N-acetylprocainamide on atrial flutter. Studies in vivo and in vitro. *Circulation* 1987;76:1397-1408.

23. Ortiz J, Nozaki A, Shimizu A, et al. Mechanism of interruption of atrial flutter by moricizine. Electrophysiologic and multiplexing studies in the canine sterile pericarditis model of atrial flutter. *Circulation* 1994;89:2860-2869.

24. Inoue H, Yamashita T, Nozaki A, et al. Effects of antiarrhythmic drugs on canine atrial flutter due to reentry: Role of prolongation of refractory period and depression of conduction to excitable gap. *J Am Coll Cardiol* 1991;18:1098-1104.

25. Cha Y, Wales A, Wolf P, et al. Electrophysiologic effects of the new class III antiarrhythmic drug dofetilide compared to the class IA antiarrhythmic drug quinidine in experimental canine atrial flutter: Role of dispersion of refractoriness in antiarrhythmic efficacy. *J Cardiovasc Electrophysiol* 1996;7:809-827.

26. Pinto JMB, Graziano JN, Boyden PA. Endocardial mapping of reentry around an anatomical barrier in the canine right atrium: Observations during the action of the class IC agent flecainide. *J Cardiovasc Electrophysiol* 1993;4:672-685.

27. Stambler BS, Wood MA, Ellenbogen KA. Antiarrhythmic actions of intravenous ibutilide compared with procainamide during human atrial flutter and fibrillation. Electrophysiological determinants of enhanced conversion efficacy. *Circulation* 1997;96:4298-4306.

28. Sung RJ, Tan HL, Karagounis L, et al. Intravenous sotalol for the termination of supraventricular tachycardia and atrial fibrillation and flutter: A multicenter, randomized, double-blind, placebo-controlled study. *Am Heart J* 1995; 129:739-746.

29. Volgman AS, Carberry PA, Stambler BS, et al. Comparison of intravenous ibutilide versus procainamide for the rapid termination of atrial fibrillation or flutter. *J Am Coll Cardiol* 1998;31:1414-1419.

30. Buchanan LV, Lemay RJ, Gibson JK. Comparison of the antiarrhythmic agents d,l-sotalol HCl and ibutilide fumarate for atrial reverse use dependence and antiarrhythmic effects. *PACE* 1996;19:687. Abstract.

31. Yang T, Snyders DJ, Roden DM. Ibutilide, a methanesulfonanilide antiarrhythmic, is a potent blocker of the rapidly-activating delayed rectifier K^+ current (IKR) in AT 1 cells. *Circulation* 1995;91:1799-1806.

32. Buchanan LV, LeMay RJ, Walters RR, et al. Antiarrhythmic and electrophysiologic effects of intravenous ibutilide and sotalol in the canine sterile pericarditis model. *J Cardiovasc Electrophysiol* 1996;7:113-119.

33. Guo GB-F, Ellenbogen KA, Wood MA, Stambler BS. Conversion of atrial flutter by ibutilide is associated with increased atrial cycle length variability. *J Am Coll Cardiol* 1996;27:1083-1089.

34. Cheng J, Karch MR, Scheinman MM. Electrophysiologic effects of ibutilide in patients with typical atrial flutter. *PACE* 1997;20:1059. Abstract.

35. Fei H, Frame LH. d-Sotalol terminates reentry by two mechanisms with different dependence on the duration of the excitable gap. *J Pharmacol Exp Ther* 1996;277:174-185.

36. Lee KS. Ibutilide, a new compound with potent class III antiarrhythmic activity, activates a slow inward Na^+ current in guinea pig ventricular cells. *J Pharmacol Exp Ther* 1992;262:99-108.

37. Lee KS, Tsai TD, Lee EW. Membrane activity of class III antiarrhythmic compounds: A comparison between ibutilide, d-sotalol, E-4031, sematilide and dofetilide. *Eur J Pharmacol* 1993;234:43-53.

Section V

Torsades de Pointes and Other Triggered Ventricular Arrhythmias:
Introduction

Early and delayed afterdepolarizations (EADs and DADs, respectively) are important triggers of arrhythmias, specifically of the polymorphous ventricular tachycardia and torsades de pointes type. The surface electrocardiogram provides only indirect clues about the existence of such EADs, and cannot identify DADs. Monophasic action potential (MAP) recordings have played a pivotal role in verifying the existence of these slow potentials in the intact experimental heart and clinical setting. This section presents compelling evidence that MAP recordings can detect such specific arrhythmia triggers and also provide direct insight into the mechanism of torsades de pointes arrhythmias.

31

New Theories on the Genesis of Early and Delayed Afterdepolarizations

Bela Szabo, MD, PhD,
Warren M. Jackman, MD, FACC and
Ralph Lazzara, MD, FACC

Early afterdepolarizations (EADs) have been defined as transient retardations in the repolarization of the action potential with or without an upturn in the membrane potential (Em).[1] They are generated in individual cardiac cells in the absence of cell-to-cell interaction or external triggering. EADs are easily recognized in the action potential when they generate an upstroke, but their recognition can be obscured by a great variability in the shape and size of the action potential in various species, cell types, heart rates, and other conditions. EAD that exhibits an upstroke is considered to be a significant arrhythmogenic factor because of its capability to trigger extra action potential. For this practical reason, EADs are frequently described by the upstroke component.[2]

The other component of EADs, the slowing in the repolarization that precedes the upstroke, is less conspicuous and is better recognized in phase plane plots (PPPs)[3-6] than in the action potential (Fig. 1). The PPP is the derivative of the action potential represented as a function of the Em. The PPP as a quantitative description of the net membrane current during the action potential was proposed by Jenerick.[7] Later PPP was used to describe EADs quantitatively.[3,5,6,8]

From Franz MR (ed): *Monophasic Action Potentials: Bridging Cell and Bedside.*
©Futura Publishing Company, Inc., Armonk, NY, 2000.

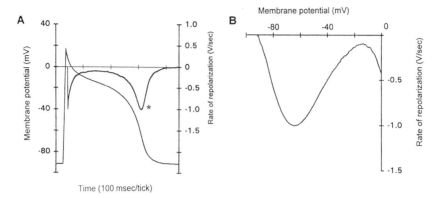

Figure 1. Action potentials in a cardiac ventricular Purkinje fiber under control conditions. **A**. Action potential and the rate of repolarization in time domain (*). **B**. Rate of repolarization in membrane potential domain (the repolarization in phase plane plot is truncated at 0 mV). Modified from Reference 5.

A slowing in the repolarization during EAD appears as a transient decrease in the rate of repolarization in the PPP, and the upstroke appears as a reversal in the direction of change in the rate. The part of the EAD that appears as a slowing in the rate of repolarization has been denoted as *EAD proper* (Fig. 2). The other part of the EAD, in which the direction of change is reversed, has been denoted as the *triggered component of EAD* (Fig. 3).[5] These denominations express the view that it is the EAD proper that is directly related to the underlying pathologic process in EAD, whereas the triggered component is secondary to the effect of EAD proper. The triggered component of EAD can be abolished by inhibitors of I_{Na} or I_{CaL} without abolishing EAD proper, demonstrating a difference in their ionic basis and that the upstroke in EAD is caused by a regenerative current of I_{Na} and/or I_{Ca}.[9,10] The ionic current of EAD cannot be determined directly when action potential is recorded. However, indirect evidence suggests that more than one mechanism exists for EAD generation. It is possible that EADs occurring at the plateau level ("plateau EADs" or "early EADs") and during phase 3 of the action potential ("phase 3 EADs" or "late EADs") are generated by separate mechanisms.[5,11,12]

It has been proposed that plateau EADs are generated by the "L-type Ca^{++} window current mechanism."[13-17] The window current, originally described by Hodgkin and Huxley[18] for Na^+ channels, flows at a range of Em when a fraction of both activation and inactivation gates of Na^+ and L-type Ca^{++} channels are open. This range, ie, a window in the Em, for I_{CaL}, is near -15 mV (Fig. 4).[15] The window current in the L-type Ca^{++} channel ($I_{Ca,w}$) requires a relatively long residence of the Em in the window range for activation; therefore, it is minimal in the normal repolarization of the action potential. However, if the duration of the action potential is length-

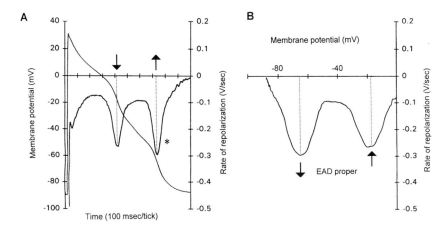

Figure 2. Analysis of early afterdepolarization (EAD) generation in a cardiac Purkinje fiber during Cs⁺ (3.6 mM) treatment. **A.** Action potential and rate of repolarization in time domain (*). **B.** Rate of repolarization in membrane potential domain (the repolarization in phase plane plot is truncated at 0 mV). EAD without an upstroke (EAD proper) appears as a transient decrease in the rate of repolarization. It starts and ends 400 milliseconds and 700 milliseconds, respectively, after the upstroke in the action potential (arrow in A). In the membrane potential domain, EAD starts and ends at -18mV and -65mV, respectively (arrow in B). Modified from Reference 5.

ened at the plateau, there may be sufficient time for an activation of $I_{Ca.w.}$[16] Under experimental conditions the duration of the action potential may be increased at the plateau level by drugs that reduce the inactivation of I_{Na} (eg, by sea anemone toxin, ATXII),[8,19] drugs that increase the amplitude and duration of I_{CaL} (BAY-K8644),[16,20] or drugs that reduce the delayed rectifier K⁺ current (I_K).[13] The plateau EAD starts with a slowly depolarizing phase, a "conditioning phase" probably caused by a gradual activation of $I_{Ca.w.}$[20,21] This phase is followed by a relatively faster upstroke that may be caused by a regenerative I_{CaL} activated by the conditioning phase.

The relative participation of various sarcolemmal currents in the slowing of the repolarization, lengthening of the plateau, and activation of $I_{Ca.w}$ and a regenerative I_{CaL} has been modeled mathematically by use of the Em-dependent kinetic parameters of various currents involved in the ventricular action potential of the guinea pig.[21,22] Experimentally, plateau EADs have been observed in Purkinje fibers and in M cells of the ventricular mid myocardium of the dog.[23] The action potential in the M cells resembles that in Purkinje fibers in that the duration of the plateau is greatly lengthened at reduced rates.[24,25] Slow rates are an important factor in the generation of plateau EADs because of the relatively slow activation of $I_{Ca.w.}$ At normal rates the relatively short systole does not permit $I_{Ca.w}$ to be activated.[21,22]

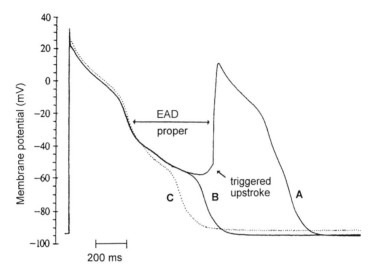

Figure 3. The two components of early afterdepolarization (EAD): EAD proper and triggered upstroke in EAD (**A**) in a Cs+ (3.6 mM) treated cardiac Purkinje fiber. The triggering of the rapid upstroke in EAD occurs at membrane potential of -50 mV (oblique arrow in trace A). Traces **B** and **C**: in the 10th second and 20th second in 3.6 mM $[Ca^{++}]_o$, respectively. EAD proper is inhibited when $[Ca^{++}]_o$ is increased from 1.8 mM to 3.6 mM. A moderate inhibition in EAD proper abolishes the upstroke in EAD completely (trace B). Modified from Reference 5.

The duration of the action potential in the heart is highly sensitive to I_{CaL} inactivation.[26,27] A simulation of Ca^{++}-dependent inactivation of I_{CaL} by Luo and Rudy[22] suggested that a sufficiently fast decrease of the intracellular Ca^{++} transient makes possible the recovery of I_{CaL} during the action potential plateau through the recovery of the Ca^{++}-dependent inactivation gate. The recovery of I_{CaL} may result in the depolarization of the sarcolemma and may generate early EADs. However, Ca^{++} binding to the EF hand,[26,28] which has been shown to be the Ca^{++}-binding motif in the L-type Ca^{++} channel, is little if at all influenced by rapid changes in global cytosolic calcium ($[Ca^{++}]_i$), such as in the myofilament space during Ca^{++} transient[29,31] Simulations of $[Ca^{++}]$ transient in the myofilament (or myoplasmic) space and in the restricted subspace at the internal orificium of L-type Ca^{++} channels show entirely different Ca^{++} kinetics (eg, see Fig. 5 in Reference 26), and the transition of the inactivated channel from "Ca^{++} mode" to the "normal mode" appears to be slow when the sarcolemma is depolarized.[32,33] Therefore, more investigations are required to determine whether the reactivation of I_{CaL} from Ca^{++}-dependent inactivation depends on repolarization[34] and can be a mechanism of early EADs. Late EADs are not generated by $I_{Ca.w}$ but by a Ca^{++}-activated transient inward current.[5] The evidence for this stems from the following observations. Late EADs have been observed

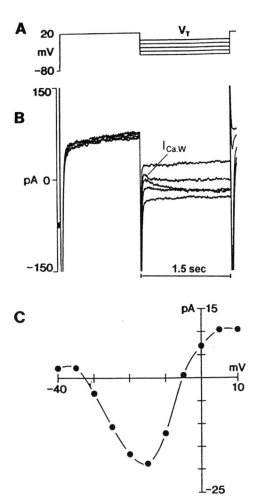

Figure 4. Recovery of L-type Ca++ current in a single canine Purkinje cell. **A.** The voltage clamp protocol. L-type Ca++ current was activated with a voltage clamp step from −80 mV to +20 mV for 1.5 seconds. V_T = repolarizing steps (1.5 seconds) to voltages within the overlapping area of the activation-inactivation curves of L-type Ca++ current (between 0 mV and -40 mV). **B.** Current tracings observed in response to voltage protocols shown in A. Peak current during the first step is off scale. $I_{Ca.w}$ = L-type Ca++ window current. **C.** The current-voltage plot for the L-type Ca++ window current. Modified from Reference 15.

in Purkinje fibers during a "moderate" inhibition of K+ currents that does not generate early EADs but reduces the rate of phase 3 repolarization.[5,35,36] Under these conditions, late EADs are generated after relatively long periods of treatment and after the occurrence of an intracellular accumulation of Ca++. Studies of the mechanism of late EADs have demonstrated that both intracellular Ca++ loading and a lengthening in the duration of the action potential are necessary conditions for a generation of late EAD (Fig. 5). In vitro the generation of late EAD is augmented by Ca++ loading regardless of whether it is produced by increasing [Ca++]o, by reducing [Na+]o, by treatment with β-adrenergic agonists, or by reversing the Na+:Ca++ exchange under conditions of voltage clamp. Ca++ may also accumulate due to a lengthening in the duration of the action potential and in the absence of other effects.[37]

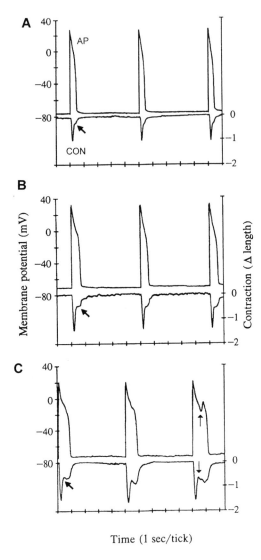

Figure 5. The effect of Ca^{++} loading and K^+ current inhibition in the action potential (AP) and contraction (CON), and early afterdepolarization (EAD) generation in canine ventricular myocytes. **A.** Action potential and contraction at the end of 10 minutes" treatment in high $[Ca^{++}]_o$ (3.6 mM), to load myocytes with Ca^{++}. **B** and **C.** Ten- and 15-minute treatment with Cs^+ (3.6 mM), respectively, following Ca^{++} loading in the same myocyte as in A ($[Ca^{++}]_o$ was 1.8 mM during Cs^+ treatment). Note the increasing amplitude in the contraction and generation of aftercontraction (oblique arrow) indicating that Ca^{++} accumulation continues during Cs^+ treatment in the myocyte. EAD first occurred in the 15th minute of Cs^+ treatment. EAD accompanied the aftercontraction, the onset of EAD being later as compared to the onset of aftercontraction (vertical arrow in C). All of the EADs were preceded by aftercontraction, but some of the aftercontractions appeared without an EAD (eg, first cycle in C).

The accumulation of Ca^{++} in the presence of K^+ current inhibitors may be due to the dependence of Ca^{++} extrusion from the cells on the Em (ie, on the repolarization of the action potential). When the repolarization of the action potential is delayed, there is a delay in the extrusion of Ca^{++}, favoring an intracellular sequestration of Ca^{++} in the sarcoplasmic reticulum (SR). The bias for the sequestration of Ca^{++} in the SR is fostered, in the presence of K^+ current inhibition, by β-adrenergic agonists that enhance Ca^{++} uptake in the SR (Fig. 6).

There are multiple Ca^{++}-dependent phenomena that may be activated when $[Ca^{++}]_i$ is increased. Studies of the role of intracellular Ca^{++} in late

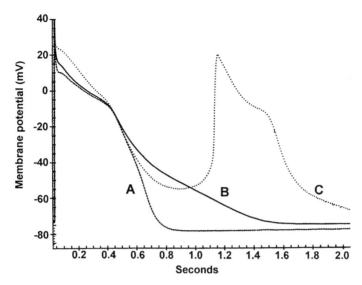

Figure 6. The enhancement of late early afterdepolarizations (EADs) in the ventricular myocardium by epinephrine. **A.** Cs^+ (3.6 mM) does not generate EADs in the ventricular myocardium free of Purkinje fibers in vitro. **C.** The combination of Cs^+ (3.6 mM) with epinephrine (100 nM) treatment generated late EAD. **B.** Increasing $[Ca^{++}]_o$ from 1.8 to 3.6 mM inhibited EAD.

EADs have demonstrated that late EADs occur in conjunction with a rapid rise in $[Ca^{++}]_i$.[5,38-41] The rise in $[Ca^{++}]_i$ during late EADs is inhibited by ryanodine, an inhibitor of Ca^{++} release channels in the SR.[40] The inhibitory effect of ryanodine identifies the SR as a source of Ca^{++} release.

It can be assumed that Ca^{++} ions entering the cells via I_{CaL} during EAD may trigger a Ca^{++} release in the SR. However, a second Ca^{++} release is not observed when I_{CaL} is activated during an early EAD.[21,41] Entry of Ca^{++} through L-type channels when I_{CaL} is reactivated may cause a slight increase in $[Ca^{++}]_i$ during early EAD, but Ca^{++} is largely absorbed by intracellular Ca^{++} binding. During early EAD, I_{CaL} is the only current that becomes more inward during the EAD depolarizing phase. The $Na^+:Ca^{++}$ exchange current (I_{NCX}) becomes less inward because of a binding of intracellular Ca^{++} to sites other than the $Na^+:Ca^{++}$ exchanger and because of the depolarization caused by I_{CaL}.[21]

Late EADs are generated in cardiac cells in which Ca^{++} sequestration is increased in the SR. In the loaded SR, a second Ca^{++} release is possible during an action potential without a reactivation of I_{CaL}. A second Ca^{++} release in the SR may release significantly more Ca^{++} into the filament space as compared to a reactivation of I_{CaL}. This can be judged from the size of the intracellular after-Ca^{++} transient indicated by fura-2, an intracellular Ca^{++} indicator (Fig. 7), and by generation of an aftercontraction (Fig. 5). The amplitude of after-Ca^{++} transient and aftercontraction may be

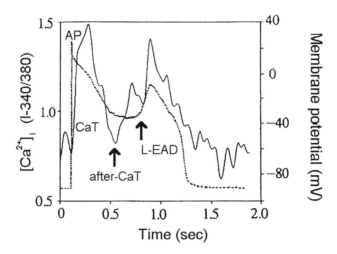

Figure 7. The relationship among the action potential (AP), late early afterdepolarization (L-EAD), intracellular Ca^{++} transient (CaT), and after-Ca^{++} transient (after-CaT) in a canine ventricular myocyte treated in high [Ca^{++}]$_o$ (3.6 mM) and Cs$^+$ (3.6 mM) for 30 minutes and stimulated 0.3 Hz. [Ca^{++}]$_i$ was determined with fura 2 and expressed in terms of Ca^{++}-dependent fluorescence ratio at 340:380 nm. Note the earlier onset in after-CaT relative to the upstroke in L-EAD (arrows).

as high as that of the Ca^{++} transient and contraction in a normal cell that is not loaded with Ca^{++}.

Multiple lines of evidence indicate that after-Ca^{++} transient and after-contraction are spontaneous (ie, they are not triggered by I$_{CaL}$ during late EAD): 1) The onset of after-Ca^{++} transient and aftercontraction precedes the onset of the depolarizing phase of late EAD (Figs. 5 and 7).[41] 2) Late EADs may be abolished without abolishing aftercontraction.[41] 3) After-Ca^{++} transient and aftercontraction may occur during phase 3 repolarization when the Em is negative to the activation range of I$_{CaL}$. 4) During the after-Ca^{++} transient and aftercontraction, the cellular Ca^{++} load decreases, whereas a reactivation of I$_{CaL}$ should have an opposite effect, ie, increasing [Ca^{++}]$_i$. Ca^{++} unloading during an after-Ca^{++} transient and aftercontraction is demonstrated by a decrease in the amplitude of the Ca^{++} transient and contraction during the subsequent cycle that follows a late EAD. Cellular unloading of Ca^{++} may also decrease late EADs during subsequent cycles (Fig. 8).

The mathematical modeling[21] of early EAD excluded the role of I$_{NCX}$ in the depolarizing phase of EAD. Although I$_{NCX}$ is inward throughout most of repolarization, it decreases when another current depolarizes the Em (ie, I$_{CaL}$). However, I$_{NCX}$ increases continuously in the absence of phase 2 EAD due to the increasingly negative Em throughout phase 3 repolarization. When Ca^{++} is released from the SR, these ions may bind to the myofila-

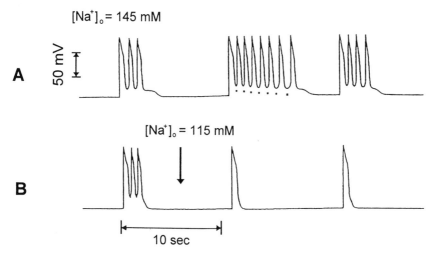

Figure 8. A. Triggering by late early afterdepolarization (EAD). The first action potential is stimulated in each burst and it is followed by two or more triggered action potentials. During a burst of triggered action potentials, late EAD is generated at a progressively more negative membrane potential level and with an increasing coupling interval leading to a self termination of late EAD and triggering. In the second burst of triggered action potential, dots show the trend of change in membrane potential and coupling time of late EAD **B.** Late EAD and triggering is inhibited by reducing $[Na^+]_o$ from 145 mM to 115 mM (30 mM Na^+ replaced by Li^+ = arrow).

ments and to the Na^+:Ca^{++} exchanger. Ca^{++} ions binding to the myofilaments cause the aftercontraction, and those binding to the exchanger stimulate their own extrusion and generate a transient inward current (I_{ti}).

The evidence for the role of I_{NCX} and I_{ti} caused by I_{NCX} in late EAD has been provided by the observation that late EADs: 1) are enhanced by a Ca^{++} loading of cardiac myocytes; 2) occur during a spontaneous Ca^{++} release in the SR; 3) occur after the onset of after-Ca^{++} transient and aftercontraction; 4) may be generated at Em levels at which I_{CaL} is inactivated (Fig. 9); 5) are inhibited by increasing $[Ca^{++}]_o$, which inhibits I_{NCX} (Fig. 3) but increases I_{CaL}; 6) are inhibited by decreasing $[Na^+]_o$ (Fig. 8), which decreases I_{NCX} but does not affect I_{CaL}; 7) cause cellular unloading of Ca^{++}, which promotes self termination in contrast to the effect of I_{CaL}, which increases the cellular load of Ca^{++}; and 8) are suppressed by inhibitors of I_{NCX}.

During spontaneous Ca^{++} release in Ca^{++}-loaded cardiac cells during diastole, an I_{ti} has been observed that is generated by I_{NCX}.[42] I_{ti} was originally observed under conditions when delayed afterdepolarizations (DADs) are generated. The conditions that generate DADs (fast rates, β-adrenergic agonists, cardioactive steroids) cause a shortening in the duration of the action potential: a second (after-) Ca^{++} transient occurs after repolarization is com-

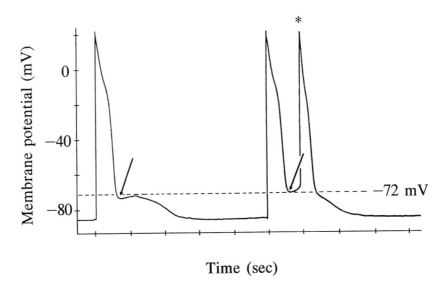

Time (sec)

Figure 9. Late early afterdepolarizations (EADs) in a canine Purkinje fiber. Late EADs (arrows) with and without triggering occurred at a membrane potential of approximately −72 mV after 20 minutes of Cs^+ (3.6 mM) treatment. The first and the second action potentials were stimulated and the third (*) was triggered by late EAD (arrow).

plete. However, under the conditions of Ca^{++} loading at slow rates and a relatively long action potential, a second (after-) Ca^{++} transient may occur and generate an I_{ti} during the repolarization of the action potential. These latter conditions can be mimicked by simulating an action potential of long duration in Ca^{++}-loaded myocytes under conditions of a voltage clamp. Under these conditions, I_{ti} appears over a broad range of Em similar to that of late EADs (Fig. 10). When the voltage clamp is released, EADs appear in the action potential, exhibiting similar Em-dependent and time-dependent parameters as seen in I_{ti}. Since I_{ti} appears in a broad range of Em and interval of time during a long action potential, ie, I_{ti} follows the kinetics of the after-Ca^{++} transient, it is distinguishable from $I_{Ca,w}$, which has a strict and narrow Em dependence and requires a long duration in the window.[15] Because I_{ti} is generated during extrusion of cellular Ca^{++}, which causes Ca^{++} unloading of the cardiac cell, there may be a large beat-to-beat variance in Ca^{++} loading, in spontaneous Ca^{++} release, I_{ti}, and late EADs.

The time of spontaneous Ca^{++} release during the action potential may depend on the magnitude of Ca^{++} loading. A relatively greater Ca^{++} loading may result in a relatively earlier release of Ca^{++} and a relatively earlier generation of late EADs. A late spontaneous Ca^{++} release may generate DADs if repolarization is complete.[43-45] It is not known whether differences exist in the mechanism of DADs when generated at fast or slow rates.

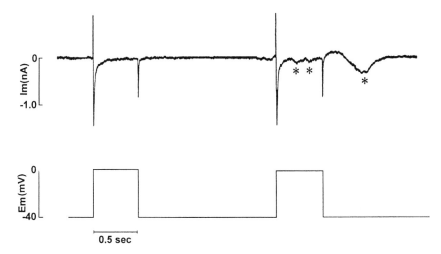

Figure 10. Transient inward current (* in upper trace) in a canine ventricular myocyte. Depolarizing steps of 0.5 seconds from –40 mV holding level to 0 mV were repeated approximately 15 times at 0.2 Hz (lower trace), until transient inward current appeared (*). Voltage clamp was performed with discontinuous clamp using an AXOCLAMP 2A, and microelectrode of 15 MΩ filled with 3 M KCl.

EAD proper may be generated with or without a rapid upstroke in late EAD. Examples are shown in Figures 9 and 11, in which the progression of late EAD generation is shown in Purkinje fibers during Cs$^+$ treatment. EAD proper was generated in the Purkinje fibers at Em levels more negative than -40 mV, at which I_{CaL} is inactivated. A progression of EAD proper resulted in triggering all-or-nothing action potential from an Em level of -72 mV, as shown in Figure 9 and a relatively rapid upstroke from -40 mV, as shown in panel D of Figure 11. A rapid upstroke from the relatively more negative Em level may be caused by I_{Na} and from the less negative Em level by I_{CaL}, both activated by the initial depolarization of EAD proper. Although I_{CaL} may be activated in both early and late EAD, there is a difference in the mechanism of the activation of this current. In early EAD the activating mechanism may be $I_{Ca,w}$, whereas in late EAD it may be a spontaneous Ca^{++} release in the SR and I_{NCX}.

Late EADs have a relatively greater propensity for generation in Purkinje fibers compared to myocytes of the ventricular myocardium. The explanation for this difference may be that ventricular myocytes have a relatively stronger repolarizing current and a faster phase 3 repolarization compared to Purkinje fibers. However, a rapid upstroke in the late EAD generated in Purkinje fibers can produce triggering in the connected myocardium in which no EAD is generated by the same treatment that generates EAD in Purkinje fibers (Fig. 11, panels D and E). Although late EADs are not generated in the ventricular myocardium in vitro if not loaded with

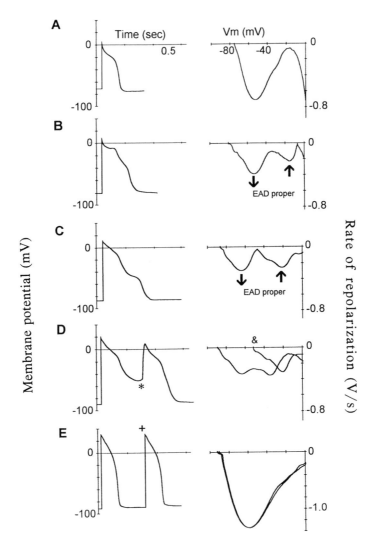

Figure 11. Representative changes in the action potential in a Purkinje fiber and connected ventricular myocardium of guinea pig during exposures to low $[Na^+]_o$ and to Cs^+, low $[K^+]_o$, and slow rates. Action potentials were recorded (left-hand panels) and rate of repolarization calculated (right-hand panels) in a Purkinje network (A through D) and papillary muscle of the right ventricle (E) during subsequent treatments as follows: **A**: in the 10th minute of low $[Na^+]_o$ treatment (Li^+ substitution); **B**: 2 minutes in Cs^+ and low $[K^+]_o$; **C**: 19 minutes in Cs^+ and low $[K^+]_o$; **D**: 37 minutes in Cs^+ and low $[K^+]_o$ in a Purkinje fiber; and **E**: 37 minutes in Cs^+ and low $[K^+]_o$ in the papillary muscle. Only the Purkinje fiber was stimulated (at 0.2 Hz). Plus sign (+) indicates that the second action potential in the papillary muscle was triggered by EAD in the Purkinje fiber (*). Ampersand (&) indicates that the curve is truncated at positive values and the derivative for the triggered upstroke is not shown.

Ca^{++}, they may be generated in vivo in the presence of circulating catecholamines. The enhancing effect of epinephrine in late EAD generation is shown in Figure 6 in a ventricular tissue preparation in which late EAD was not generated in the presence of Cs^+ (3.6 mM) alone, but only after epinephrine had been added to the superfusing solution. Epinephrine increases I_{CaL}, and by this effect it may enhance the generation of early EAD. However, in the experiment shown in the figure, the enhancement of late EAD was not directly caused by I_{CaL}, because EAD was generated at an Em level at which I_{CaL} is inactivated, and it was inhibited by high $[Ca^{++}]_o$, which does not inhibit, but increases, I_{CaL}. It is possible that late EAD generation is augmented by catecholamines in vivo because relatively low doses of Cs^+ have generated EADs not only in Purkinje fibers but also in epicardial and endocardial layers of the ventricular wall.[45,46]

Late EADs and triggering have been observed in MAPs recorded in clinical and experimental settings in vivo. The presence of catecholamines in vivo may enhance the generation of late EAD and triggering when repolarizing K^+ currents are inhibited with drugs or due to abnormal genetic encoding of ionic channels. Catecholamines may enhance late EAD by increasing Ca^{++} uptake in cardiac cells,[47-49] increasing the sequestration and release of this ion in the SR,[50] and increasing the activity of I_{NCX} in the sarcolemma.[49] K^+ current inhibitors increase the duration of the action potential and inhibit the extrusion of Ca^{++} from the cells by reducing the activity of the $Na^+:Ca^{++}$ exchanger during the prolonged depolarization. These effects acting together may result Ca^{++} loading, spontaneous Ca^{++} release, and late EADs.[51]

Adrenergic actions have been known for a long time to generate arrhythmias by first generating EADs. The arrhythmogenic effect of adrenergic activity is enhanced under conditions in which repolarizing K^+ currents are inhibited, such as long QT syndromes. Although β-adrenergic effects increase I_{CaL} and increase both early and late EADs, MAP recordings in vivo have demonstrated late EADs (Fig. 12).

With use of a novel experimental model[52] that enabled the performance of comprehensive electrophysiologic studies in a small mammalian heart in vivo, the effects of perturbations that affect the action potential duration were compared with respect to plateau EADs, late EADs, and DADs. These studies[53] were aimed at elucidating the differential mechanism of the 3 types of afterdepolarizations in guinea pig hearts in vivo. In this study plateau EADs, late EADs, and DADs were induced by Bay K8644, CsCl, and digoxin, respectively. Plateau EADs were abolished with pinacidil, a K^+_{ATP} channel opener that reduces the duration of the plateau. Verapamil abolished late EADs and DADs, probably by reducing the intracellular load of Ca^{++}. In contrast, pinacidil was less effective in inhibiting late EADs than plateau EADs. These data were interpreted to suggest that the mechanism of plateau EADs is different from that of late EADs and DADs, and

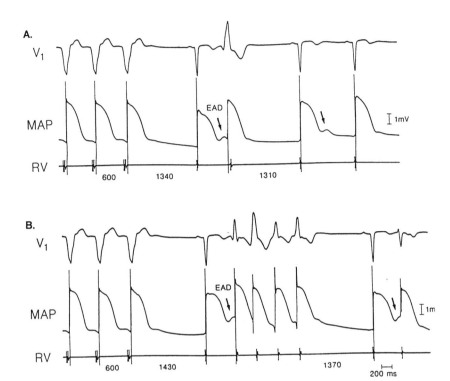

Figure 12. Late early afterdepolarization (EADs) on MAP in an idiopathic, nonfamilial long QT syndrome patient. Upper trace: Electrocardiograph lead V; middle trace: MAP recorded from the right ventricular outflow tract; bottom trace: bipolar electrogram (RV) from the right ventricular apex. Late EADs (arrows) increase when a relatively faster rate is followed by a pause. A relatively longer pause of 1430 milliseconds results in a late EAD followed by a 4-beat episode of ventricular tachycardia. The duration of the action potential at the plateau level is relatively short. From Reference 10.

that late EADs and DADs can share similar mechanisms under conditions of Ca^{++} overload.

Clinical Considerations

Catheter recordings of MAPs (injury potentials) from human hearts have provided convincing evidence that EADs are generated in both the acquired and congenital long QT syndromes and that they provide a triggering mechanism for ventricular ectopy and torsades de pointes.[10,54-63] In the long QT syndromes, adrenergic stimulation through emotion or exertion was recognized very early as a prime provocation of symptoms, arrhythmias, and sudden death.[64,65] β-Adrenergic receptor blockade has been accepted as the standard therapy to prevent arrhythmias in the congenital long QT syndromes, although repolarization and the QT interval often remain prolonged.[66]

Adrenergic stimulation has multiple complex actions on the myocardium and on ion currents. In the congenital long QT syndromes, the ionic mechanisms for prolongation of repolarization are genetically determined abnormalities of ion channels that result in enhancement of noninactivated I_{Na}, reduction of I_{Kr}, or reduction of I_{Ks}.[12] The production of prolonged repolarizations by these abnormal ion currents would not be expected to be significantly worsened by adrenergic stimulation. However, the ionic mechanisms that are activated by prolonged repolarization and that affect Ca^{++} transport to induce EADs would be expected to be strongly affected by adrenergic stimulation. Adrenergic stimulation enhances Ca^{++} entry into the cell via I_{CaL} and augments Ca^{++} uptake by the SR, promoting cellular Ca^{++} loading. By these actions, adrenergic stimulation would be predicted to enhance EADs that are directly dependent on I_{CaL} and EADs that depend on I_{NCX} activated by spontaneous Ca^{++} release from Ca^{++}-loaded SR.

In both the congenital and the acquired long QT syndromes, Ca^{++} channel blockers have been shown in isolated case reports to be effective therapy.[10] Magnesium acts as a Ca^{++} channel blocker and is the generally accepted therapy for torsades de pointes in the acquired long QT syndromes.[67] These observations regarding therapeutic efficacy are compatible with the role of I_{CaL} or Ca^{++} loading and I_{NCX} in the generation of EADs in the long QT syndrome.

MAP recordings trace the time course of repolarization with reasonable fidelity, but they do not reflect accurately the true Em. Therefore, it is not possible to determine from such recordings the Em at which EADs are generated. However, from the time of appearance of the EADs, and from the relationship between the configuration of EAD and MAP, it is possible to infer that EADs are generating either during phase 2 or phase 3 of repolarization. In most of the recordings published, EADs appeared to be generated during phase 3 of repolarization; however, there are examples of EADs that appear to be occurring during or near phase 2 of repolarization.[58] Thus, there is evidence for EADs that could be generated by I_{CaL} and for EADs that must be generated by another current such as I_{NCX}.

In LTQ3, the variety of the long QT syndrome produced by a mutation in the Na^+ channel gene SCN5A that results in a defect in inactivation of I_{Na}, it has been proposed that adrenergic stimulation may not be a potent trigger of arrhythmias.[68] This observation, if validated, could suggest a lesser role for Ca^{++} channel support in this variety of the syndrome. It is possible that enhanced Na^+ current could be directly involved in EAD generation in this syndrome and that the influence of adrenergic stimulation may be reduced. Recent observations indicate that Na^+ channel blockade with mexiletine can shorten the QT interval in LQT3, but the effect on arrhythmias is not yet known.[69]

Echocardiographic determinations of the contraction pattern in patients with the congenital long QT syndrome indicate that there is more rapid initial shortening, a prolonged contraction phase, and sometimes indication of a secondary shortening before relaxation.[70] These findings have been interpreted to suggest an abnormality in Ca^{++} transport that involves prolonged elevation of cytosolic Ca^{++} and/or secondary increase in cytosolic Ca^{++}. The contractile abnormalities were reversed by verapamil.[71] These findings fit with either a reactivation of I_{CaL} during EADs or a spontaneous release of Ca^{++} from the SR during EADs. They also indicate contractility in these patients reflected in the more rapid initial contraction.

In summary, observations in patients with long QT syndromes implicate EAD as the trigger mechanism for ventricular tachyarrhythmias in the syndromes. The response to β-blockers and Ca^{++} channel blockers supports the hypotheses that I_{CaL}- or I_{NCX}-activated spontaneous Ca^{++} release from Ca^{++}-loaded myocytes are the current underlying EAD generation. Echocardiographic contractile abnormalities observed in the long QT syndromes also fit with the hypotheses of abnormal Ca^{++} transport in EAD generation.

References

1. Cranefield PF. Action potentials, afterpotentials, and arrhythmias. *Circ Res* 1977;41:415-423.
2. El-Sherif N, Craelius W, Boutjdir M. Early afterdepolarizations and arrhythmogenesis. *J Cardiovasc Electrophysiol* 1990;1:145-160.
3. Rajagopalan CV, Szabo B, Lazzara R. Use of phase plane plots for the evaluation of early afterdepolarizations in cardiac action potentials. *J Cardiovasc Electrophysiol* 1992;25(suppl):1571.
4. Szabo B, Rajagopalan CV, Lazzara R. The role of $Na^+:Ca^{2+}$ exchange in generation of early afterdepolarizations in cardiac action potentials. *FASEB J* 1992;6:A1164.
5. Szabo B, Sweidan R, Rajagopalan CV, Lazarra R. Role of $Na^+:Ca^{2+}$ exchange current in Cs^+-induced early afterdepolarizations in Purkinje fibers. *J Cardiovasc Electrophysiol* 1994;5:933-944.
6. Paes de Carvalho A, Nascimento JHM. Ionic current and conductance estimated from the time course of action potentials: Measurement, display, and interpretation of dV/dt. In Rosen M, Janse MJ, Wit AL (eds): *Cardiac Electrophysiology: A Textbook*. Mount Kisco, NY: Futura Publishing Co, Inc.; 1990:439-458.
7. Jenerick HP. Phase plane trajectories of the muscle spike potential. *Biophys J* 1963;3:363-377.
8. Boutjdir M, Restivo M, Wei Y. Early afterdepolarization formation in cardiac myocytes: Analysis of phase plane patterns, action potential, and membrane currents. *J Cardiovasc Electrophysiol* 1994;5:609-620.
9. Aliot E, Szabo B, Sweidan R, et al. Prevention of torsades de pointes with calcium channel blockade in an animal model. *J Am Coll Cardiol* 1985;5:492.

10. Jackman WM, Szabo B, Friday KJ, et al. Ventricular tachyarrhythmias related to early afterdepolarizations and triggered firing: Relationship to QT interval prolongation and potential therapeutic role for calcium channel blocking agents. *J Cardiovasc Electrophysiol* 1990;1:170-195.

11. Damiano BP, Rosen MR. Effects of pacing on triggered activity induced by early afterdepolarizations. *Circulation* 1984;69:1013-1025.

12. Roden DM, Lazzara R, Rosen M, et al. Multiple mechanisms in the long-QT syndrome. Current knowledge, gaps, and future directions. *Circulation* 1996;94:1996-2012.

13. Marban E, Robinson SW, Wier WG. Mechanisms of arrhythmogenic delayed and early afterdepolarizations in ferret ventricular muscle. *J Clin Invest* 1986;78:1185-1192.

14. January CT, Shorofsky SR. Early afterdepolarizations: Newer insights into cellular mechanisms. *J Cardiovasc Electrophysiol* 1990;1:161-169.

15. Hirano Y, Moscucci A, January CT. Direct measurement of L-type Ca^{2+} window current in heart cells. *Circ Res* 1992;70:445-455.

16. January CT, Riddle JM. Early afterdepolarizations: Mechanism of induction and block. A role for L-type Ca^{2+} current. *Circ Res* 1989;64:977-990.

17. January CT, Moscucci A. Cellular mechanisms of early afterdepolarizations. *Ann N Y Acad Sci* 1992;644:23-32.

18. Hodgkin AL, Huxley AF. A quantitative description of membrane current and its application to conduction and excitation in nerve. *J Physiol* 1952;117:500-544.

19. El-Sherif N, Fozzard HA, Hanck DA. Dose-dependent modulation of the cardiac sodium channel by sea anemone toxin ATXII. *Circ Res* 1992;70:285-301.

20. January CT, Riddle JM, Salata JJ. A model for early afterdepolarizations: Induction with the Ca^{2+} channel agonist Bay K 8644. *Circ Res* 1988;62:563-571.

21. Zeng J, Rudy Y. Early afterdepolarizations in cardiac myocytes: Mechanism and rate dependence. *Biophys J* 1995;68:949-964.

22. Luo CH, Rudy Y. A dynamic model of the cardiac ventricular action potential. II. Afterdepolarizations, triggered activity, and potentiation. *Circ Res* 1994;74:1097-1113.

23. Antzelevitch C, Sicouri S. Clinical relevance of cardiac arrhythmias generated by afterdepolarizations. Role of M cells in the generation of U waves, triggered activity and torsade de pointes. *J Am Coll Cardiol* 1994;23:259-277.

24. Sicouri S, Antzelevitch C. Electrophysiologic characteristics of M cells in the canine left ventricular free wall. *J Cardiovasc Electrophysiol* 1995;6:591-603.

25. Liu DW, Antzelevitch C. Characteristics of the delayed rectifier current (I_{Kr} and I_{Ks}) in canine ventricular epicardial, midmyocardial, and endocardial myocytes. A weaker I_{Ks} contributes to the longer action potential of the M cell. *Circ Res* 1995;76:351-365.

26. Jafri MS, Rice JJ, Winslow RL. Cardiac Ca^{2+} dynamics: The role of ryanodine receptor adaptation and sarcoplasmic reticulum load. *Biophys J* 1998;74:1149-1168.

27. Grantham CJ, Cannell MB. Ca^{2+} influx during the cardiac action potential in guinea pig ventricular myocytes. *Circ Res* 1996;79:194-200.

28. deLeon M, Wang Y, Jones L, et al. Essential Ca^{2+}-binding motif for Ca^{2+}-sensitive inactivation of L-type Ca^{2+} channels. *Science* 1995;270:1502-1506.

29. Imredy JP, Yue DT. Submicroscopic Ca^{2+} diffusion mediates inhibitory coupling between individual Ca^{2+} channels. *Neuron* 1992;9:197-207.

30. Gutnick MJ, Lux HD, Swandulla D, et al. Voltage-dependent and calcium-dependent inactivation of calcium channel current in identified snail neurones. *J Physiol* 1989;412:197-220.

31. Santana LF, Cheng H, Gomez AM, et al. Relationship between the sarcolemmal Ca^{2+} current and Ca^{2+} sparks and local control theories for cardiac excitation-contraction coupling. *Circ Res* 1996;78:166-171.

32. Imredy JP, Yue DT. Mechanism of Ca^{2+}-sensitive inactivation of L-type Ca^{2+} channels. *Neuron* 1994; 12:1301-1318.

33. Yue DT, Backx PH, Imredy JP. Calcium-sensitive inactivation in the gating of single calcium channels. *Science* 1990;250:1735-1738.

34. McDonald TF, Pelzer S, Trautwein W, et al. Regulation and modulation of calcium channels in cardiac, skeletal, and smooth muscle cells. *Physiol Rev* 1994;74:365-507.

35. Szabo B, Kovacs T, Banyasz T. Cesium increases intracellular uptake of $^{45}Ca^{2+}$ uptake and increases force development in cardiac ventricular muscle during the evolution of early afterdepolarization. *J Am Coll Cardiol* 1990;15:77A.

36. Szabo B, Kovacs T, Lazzara R. Role of calcium loading in early afterdepolarizations generated by Cs^+ in canine and guinea pig Purkinje fibers. *J Cardiovasc Electrophysiol* 1995;6:796-812.

37. Marchi S, Szabo B, Lazzara R. Membrane potential oscillations induced by small inward currents in isolated cardiac myocytes. *Am Fed Clin Res* 1989;37:277A.

38. Szabo B, Sweidan R, Fugate R, et al. Ca^{2+} transients during generation of early afterdepolarizations in Cs^+ treated canine ventricular myocytes. *Circulation* 1990;82(III):746.

39. Yamada KA, Corr PB. Effects of β-adrenergic receptor activation on intracellular calcium and membrane potential in adult cardiac myocytes. *J Cardiovasc Electrophysiol* 1992;3:209-224.

40. Priori SG, Corr PB. Mechanisms underlying early and delayed afterdepolarizations induced by catecholamines. *Am J Physiol* 1990;258:H1796-H1805.

41. Volders PG, Kulcsar A, Vos MA, et al. Similarities between early and delayed afterdepolarizations induced by isoproterenol in canine ventricular myocytes. *Cardiovasc Res* 1997;34:348-359.

42. Kass RS, Tsien RW. Fluctuations in membrane current driven by intracellular calcium in cardiac Purkinje fibers. *Biophys J* 1982;38:259-269.

43. Szabo B, Sweidan R, Scherlag BJ, et al. Cesium-induced late-coupled, triggered action potentials in Purkinje fibers. *J Am Coll Cardiol* 1986;7:52A.

44. Szabo B, Marchi S, Scherlag BJ, et al. Simultaneous demonstration of early- and delayed afterdepolarization in Ca^{2+} loaded cardiac cells. *J Am Coll Cardiol* 1989;13:185A.

45. Patterson E, Szabo B, Scherlag BJ, et al. Early and delayed afterdepolarizations associated with cesium chloride-induced arrhythmias in the dog. *J Cardiovasc Pharmacol* 1990;15:323-331.

46. Levine JH, Spear JF, Guarnieri T, et al. Cesium chloride-induced long QT syndrome: Demonstration of afterdepolarizations and triggered activity in vivo. *Circulation* 1985;72:1092-1103.

47. Dolphin AC. Regulation of calcium channel activity by GTP binding proteins and second messengers. *Biochem Biophys Acta* 1991;1091:68-80.

48. Egan TM, Noble D, Noble SJ, et al. An isoprenaline activated sodium-dependent inward current in ventricular myocytes. *Nature* 1987;328:634-637.

49. Han X, Ferrier GR. Contribution of Na$^+$-Ca^{2+} exchange to stimulation of transient inward current by isoproterenol in rabbit cardiac Purkinje fibers. *Circ Res* 1995;76:664-674.

50. Callewaert G, Cleemann L, Morad M. Epinephrine enhances Ca^{2+} current-regulated Ca^{2+} release and Ca^{2+} reuptake in rat ventricular myocytes. *Proc Natl Acad Sci U S A* 1988;85:2009-2013.

51. Janiak R, Lewartowski B. Early after-depolarisations induced by noradrenaline may be initiated by calcium released from sarcoplasmic reticulum. *Mol Cell Biochem* 1996;164:125-130.

52. Xu J, Pelleg A. A novel guinea pig heart model for studying AV nodal conduction and triggered activity in vivo. *Am J Physiol* 1996;270:H1850-H1857.

53. Xu J, Zaim S, Pelleg A. Effects of pinacidil, verapamil, and heart rate on afterdepolarization in guinea pig heart in vivo. *Heart Vessels* 1996;11:289-302.

54. Gavrilescu S, Luca C. Right ventricular monophasic action potentials in patients with long QT syndrome. *Br Heart J* 1978;40:1014-1018.

55. Bonatti V, Botti G. Recording of monophasic action potentials of the right ventricle in long QT syndromes, complicated by severe ventricular arrhythmias. *Eur Heart J* 1983;4:168-179.

56. Bonatti V, Botti G. Monophasic action potential studies in human subjects with prolonged ventricular repolarization and long QT syndromes. *Eur Heart J* 1985;D(suppl):131-143.

57. El-Sherif N, Bekheit SS, Henkin R. Quinidine-induced long QTU interval and torsade de pointes: Role of bradycardia-dependent early afterdepolarizations. *J Am Coll Cardiol* 1989;14:252-257.

58. Habbab MA, El-Sherif N. Drug-induced torsades de pointes: Role of early afterdepolarizations and dispersion of repolarization. *Am J Med* 1990;89:241-246.

59. Shimizu W, Ohe T, Kurita T, et al. Early afterdepolarizations induced by isoproterenol in patients with congenital long QT syndrome. *Circulation* 1991;84:1915-1923.

60. Shimizu W, Tanaka K, Suenaga K, et al. Bradycardia-dependent early afterdepolarizations in a patient with QTU prolongation and torsade de points in association with marked bradycardia and hypokalemia. *PACE* 1991;14:1105-1111.

61. Zhou JT, Shong LR, Liu Y. Early afterdepolarizations in the familiar long QTU syndrome. *J Cardiovasc Electrophysiol* 1992;3:431-436.

62. Kurita T, Ohe T, Shimizu W, et al. Early afterdepolarization in a patient with complete atrioventricular block and torsade de points. *PACE* 1998;13:33-38.

63. Shimizu W, Ohe T, Kurita T. Effects of verapamil and propranolol on early afterdepolarizations and ventricular arrhythmias induced by epinephrine in congenital long QT syndrome. *J Am Coll Cardiol* 1995;26:1299-1309.

64. Levine SA, Woodworth CR. Congenital deaf-mutism, prolonged QT interval, syncopal attacks and sudden death. *N Engl J Med* 1958;259:412-417.

65. Jervell A, Thingstad R, Endsjo T. The surdo-cardiac syndrome: Three new cases of congenital deafness with syncopal attacks and Q-T prolongation in the electrocardiogram. *Am Heart J* 1966;72:582-593.

66. Jackman WM, Clark M, Friday KJ, et al. The long QT syndromes: A critical review, new clinical observations and a unifying hypothesis. *Prog Cardiovasc Dis* 1988;31:115-172.

67. Fazekas T, Scherlag BJ, Vos MA, et al. Magnesium and the heart: Antiarrhythmic therapy with magnesium. *Clin Cardiol* 1993;16:768-774.

68. Schwartz PJ. *The Long QT Syndrome.* Armonk, NY: Futura Publishing Co, Inc.; 1997:56-57.

69. Schwartz PJ, Priori SG, Locati EH. Long QT syndrome patients with mutations on the SCN5A and HERG genes have differential responses to Na$^+$ channel blockade and to increases in heart rate. Implications for gene-specific therapy. *Circulation* 1995;92:3381-3386.

70. Nador F, Beria G, deFerrari GM. Unsuspected echocardiographic abnormality in the long QT syndrome: Diagnostic, prognostic, and pathogenetic implications. *Circulation* 1991;84:1530-1542.

71. deFerrari GM, Nador F, Beria G. Effect of calcium channel block on the wall motion abnormality of the idiopathic long QT syndrome. *Circulation* 1994;89:2126-2132.

32

Early Afterdepolarizations in the In Situ Canine Heart:

Mechanistic Insights into Acquired Torsades de Pointes Arrhythmias

Marc A. Vos, PhD, S. Cora Verduyn, PhD and Hein J. Wellens, MD, PhD

Introduction

In recent years, different genes have been shown to be responsible for the transcription of specific cardiac proteins that encode ionic channels that have been related to the congenital and possibly acquired long QT syndrome.[1-3] In patients treated with class III drugs, the incidence of torsades de pointes (TdP) is between 1% and 10%[4,5] and is partly dependent on synergistic circumstances such as bradycardia, cascade of ectopic beats, hypokalemia, and/or hypomagnesemia.[6] Study of the circumstances leading to TdP arrhythmias has been accomplished through use of drugs that increase the action potential duration (APD) in animal models, and multicellular preparations.[7-22] For example, the application of I_{kr} blockers such as dofetilide, almokalant, or d-sotalol might be linked in their electrocardiographic presentation to the congenital LQT2 syndrome.

The cause of TdP has been suggested to be early afterdepolarizations (EADs) and/or dispersion of repolarization.[23] Both parameters can possibly

This study was supported by grants from the Netherlands Heart Foundation (#91.104 and #94.010).

From Franz MR (ed): *Monophasic Action Potentials: Bridging Cell and Bedside.* ©Futura Publishing Company, Inc., Armonk, NY, 2000.

be visualized in the intact canine heart with the use of monophasic action potential (MAP) catheters. In our canine model of TdP, the occurrence of both pacing-induced and spontaneously occurring acquired TdP has been associated with 1) EADs; 2) ectopic beats; and 3) interventricular dispersion of repolarization (ΔAPD = LV APD$_{endo}$ - RV APD$_{endo}$).

This chapter will discuss the following: 1) the difficulties underlying the registration of EADs, including a possible alternative explanation for these humps; 2) the possible contribution of EADs to interventricular dispersion (ΔAPD); and 3) their role in the genesis of TdP.

In Situ Registration of EADs: Definition, Evidence, Assumptions, and Pitfalls

The MAP signal can be seen as a summation of the electrical changes of different myocardial cells and/or layers beneath the recording catheter.[24,25] In our experience, the MAP duration (left ventricular [LV] APD) correlates well with global repolarization (QT time) during baseline (r^2= 0.7).[17] To what extent different cell types and/or layers contribute to the endocardial APD is not yet known, but the different possibilities are discussed at the end of this chapter.

Among the first investigators to record MAP signals in the hearts of patients with congenital and acquired long QT syndrome were Gavrilescu and Luca.[26] A later report by Bonatti et al[27] yielded similar observations by positioning the endocardial MAP catheter at different sites in the right ventricle (RV): regional differences in APD at the separate RV sites, and "humps" in the morphology of the MAPs with the longer APDs (Fig. 1).[26,27] Nowadays, we refer to these humps as EADs, while the spatial difference in APD is referred to as dispersion— in this case, intraventricular dispersion.

EADs have been defined by Cranefield and Aronson[28] as "*depolarizing afterpotentials that begin prior to completion of repolarization and cause (or constitute) an interruption or retardation of normal repolarization.*" In vitro, with use of transmembrane action potentials, EADs have been described to occur particularly under circumstances that prolong repolarization, such as slow frequencies and certain APD-increasing drugs. Simultaneous measurements of action potentials by transmembrane action potential and MAP recordings in tissue have shown similar deflections (Fig. 2).[12,13] These deflections preceded the occurrence of ectopic beats (triggered EADs). The coupling interval between the EADs and the ectopic beats in the study by Levine et al[13] not only showed a close correlation, but was nearly identical. Following these experiments, more groups have used the MAP technique to record EADs. Two similar methods of quantifi-

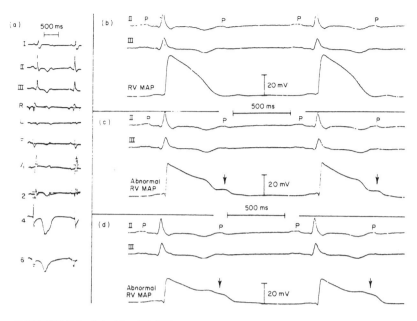

V. BONATTI ET AL, Eur. H. J. vol 4, pg 168, 1983

Figure 1. Recording of a MAP signal in a patient with bradycardia- (2:1 atrioventricular block) induced long QT. Electrocardiogram on the left side (**a**) and 3 expanded endocardial right ventricular MAP (RV MAP) recordings at the right side (**b**, **c**, and **d**) are shown. In b, a MAP is seen with an apparent normal morphology, while in c and d, recorded at different sites in the RV, prominent humps (arrows) can be seen, possibly reflecting early afterdepolarizations (EADs). Moreover, these EADs increase action potential duration nonuniformly, causing dispersion in repolarization. Reproduced from Reference 27, with the approval of the European Society of Cardiology.

cation have been proposed by the same group: relative amplitude, and relative area.[15] In both instances the amplitude or area beneath the EAD was related to total MAP amplitude (defined as the difference between phases 2 and 4) or total MAP area. These parameters can be used to quantify the response to different interventions and demonstrate a good correlation with the occurrence of polymorphic ventricular tachycardias.[14,15] Therefore, these measurements were in agreement with the concept that the EADs measured with the MAPs reflected true EADs and not motion artifacts (see also below).

To optimize the registration of EADs in the MAPs, we use the following criteria: 1) the MAP catheter should be placed by experienced investigators to ensure contact with the endocardium through properly applied pressure; 2) in the control state, the MAP contour should be smooth, with a minimum amplitude of 15 mV, and should possess a stable baseline (direct current coupling of the amplifier); 3) consecutive beats should have an identical

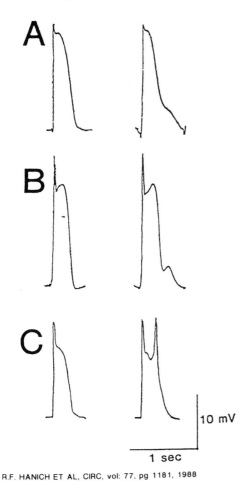

Figure 2. Occurrence of different early afterdepolarizations (EADs) on the MAP after cesium administration in dogs. At left baseline conditions are shown, illustrating a smooth MAP signal. Administration of cesium resulted in either high membrane deflections (EADs) as seen in **A** and **B**, or a low membrane EAD as observed in **C**. Reproduced from Reference 12, with permission of the American Heart Association.

R.F. HANICH ET AL, CIRC, vol: 77, pg 1181, 1988

MAP morphology and duration; and 4) visualization of EADs in the MAP after the administration of class III agents should disappear after interventions that lead to EAD suppression in vitro, such as medication and continuous pacing at higher frequency.

In regard to medication, magnesium, which is often used to treat patients with congenital and acquired TdP,[29-32] has been validated in several animal models to suppress EADs and TdP.[14,18,19,33,34] Also, the I_{KATP} openers pinacidil, levcromakalim, and nicorandil have been used in animal studies of TdP[35,36] or have been implemented in the treatment of TdP in patients with congenital long QT syndrome.[37] Furthermore, agents that interact with intracellular calcium handling such as ryanodine and flunarizine have been shown to suppress EADs and EAD-related TdP.[16]

Another accepted way to suppress the EAD and related arrhythmias is pacing at cycle lengths (CLs) shorter than the intrinsic heart rate.[38] In Figure

3 a representative example of the occurrence and disappearance of EADs is shown with the changing of the paced CL in a dog with chronic, complete atrioventricular (AV) block. Three paced frequencies were applied after administration of d-sotalol. At the slow steady state rhythm of 1500 milliseconds, an EAD is clearly visible in both the LV and in the RV MAP (Fig. 3, left part of panel 1, arrows). The amplitudes of the EADs decrease when a steady state with a CL of 1000 milliseconds has been reached (left part of panel 2). Finally, at a steady state of 500 milliseconds, the EADs have completely disappeared (left part of panel 3). After the pacing CL has returned to 1500 milliseconds, the EADs will return in time. After 90 seconds, the EAD reap-

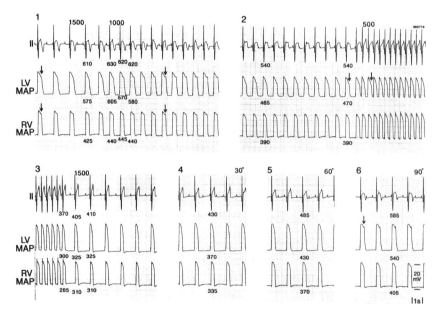

Figure 3. Frequency dependence of early afterdepolarizations (EADs) and interventricular dispersion. In this figure, different paced cycle lengths are present after d-sotalol (2 mg/kg) in the dog with chronic, complete atrioventricular block. Each panel consist of a lead II surface electrocardiogram and two endocardial MAP signals: one in the left and one in the right ventricle (LV and RV MAP) at a paper speed of 10 mm/s. Steady state is achieved after pacing for at least 3 minutes. In panel **1** the paced cycle length is changed from 1500 to 1000 milliseconds, while in panel **2** a shift from 1000 to 500 milliseconds is illustrated. In panels **3** through **6**, the temporal behavior (at 0, 30, 60, and 90 seconds) of the reversal from 500 to 1500 milliseconds is shown. Three important observations can be made: 1) Disappearance of EADs (arrows) on decreasing the paced cycle length (right side of panel 2) and the slow return after switching back to 1500 milliseconds in the left ventricle (panel 6). 2) This is associated with disappearance and reappearance of the U wave and a reduction in dispersion from 150 (panel 1) to 15 milliseconds (panel 3) followed by a slow recovery (panels 4 through 6). 3) Acceleration-induced EADs directly after the cycle length switch temporarily increase the amplitude of the EAD and interventricular dispersion from 150 to 165 milliseconds (panel 1).

pears first in the LV (panel 6). Because in this example criteria 1 through 4 have been fulfilled, we consider this deflection in the MAP an EAD.

Interventricular Dispersion

In Figure 3, another important observation can be made in regard to differences in repolarization between the LV and the RV in this dog with chronic AV block. We refer to ΔAPD as the difference between two randomly placed endocardial MAP signals, one in the LV and the other in the RV. Randomly placed signals allow a good estimation of the ΔAPD, because the response of the APD within the ventricles (intraventricular dispersion) to interventions is rather homogenous.[18] ΔAPD is influenced by bradycardia (Fig. 3), by class III drugs (see Figs. 3 through 8),[18,20,39] and possibly by pathophysiologic circumstances such as cardiac hypertrophy.[20] As illustrated in Figure 3, ΔAPD decreases with a decrease in CL from 150 milliseconds at a CL of 1500 milliseconds, to 75 to 80 milliseconds at a CL of 1000 milliseconds and 15 milliseconds at a CL of 500 milliseconds, which closely resembles the CL of the former sinus rhythm.

EADs, Ectopic Beats, and ΔAPD in the Genesis of TdP

In the anesthetized dog with chronic AV block, after intravenous administration of class III drugs, TdP can occur spontaneously or can reproducibly be induced by pacing. An example of both forms of TdP can be seen in Figures 4, 5 and 6. After almokalant (0.12 mg/kg per 5 minutes), most TdP occur spontaneously, preceded by a specific sequence of events (Fig. 4). First, the

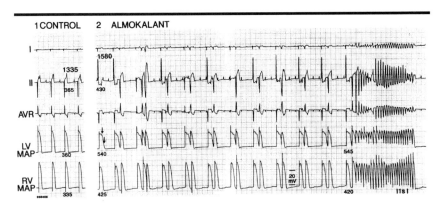

Figure 4. Development of early afterdepolarizations (EADs), ectopic beats, and spontaneous torsades de pointes (TdP) after almokalant. The control situation, consisting of 3 electrocardiogram leads and 2 endocardial MAP recordings (RV

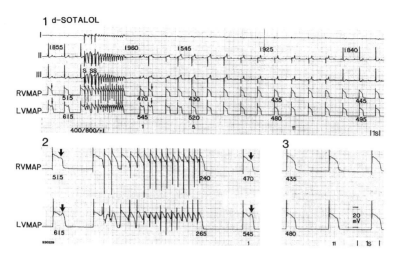

Figure 5. Initiation and spontaneous termination of pacing-induced torsades de pointes (TdP) after d-sotalol. Three electrocardiogram leads are shown simultaneously with 2 MAP registrations, one in the left and the other in the right ventricle (LV and RV MAP). Prior to TdP induction by pacing, the cycle length of the idioventricular rhythm amounts to 1855 milliseconds with a QT time of 550 milliseconds. The left ventricular action potential duration (LV APD) measures 615 milliseconds and the right ventricular APD (RV APD) 515 milliseconds, resulting in an interventricular dispersion (ΔAPD) of 100 milliseconds. In both the LV APD and the RV APD a clear early afterdepolarization (EAD) (arrow) is seen. In panel **2**, the MAP signals have been enlarged. A pacing mode (400/800/400 milliseconds, indicated by S) is interrupted by an ectopic beat and after the extrastimulus the TdP starts. The last beat of the TdP has a ΔAPD of 25 milliseconds and the EADs have disappeared. In the first beat after the TdP the EAD is back in both MAPs (panel 2). In subsequent beats the EAD gradually decreases. In the 5th beat the EAD from the RV has disappeared and the EAD in the LV has clearly diminished. In the 10th beat post termination the EAD on the LV has also disappeared (shown enlarged in panel **3**). In line with the disappearance of the EADs, the ΔAPD decreases (90 milliseconds in the 5th to 45 milliseconds in the 10th beat).

(Figure 4 *continued.*) and LV MAP), is shown at a paper speed of 10 mm/s. At baseline the cycle length-idioventricular rhythm amounts to 1335 milliseconds with a QT time of 365 milliseconds. Both MAP signals are smooth and the interventricular dispersion is 35 milliseconds (LV - RV action potential duration [APD]). After almokalant (0.12 mg/kg per 10 minutes), there is an increase in cycle length to 1580 milliseconds, an increase in QT time, and a nonuniform increase in the APDs leading to an increased dispersion of 115 milliseconds. Moreover, there is the development of EADs (arrows) in the left ventricle occurring at both the plateau level and phase 3 (arrows). The ectopic beats arise before the end of the left ventricular APD, while the second ectopic beat seems to arise from the phase 3 EAD. This cascade of events leads to a spontaneous episode of TdP which is self-terminating.

APD will increase. Often this will occur nonuniformly (more in the LV than in the RV) leading to a more pronounced ΔAPD. Thereafter, EADs appear, also contributing to dispersion. The EADs are followed by ectopic beats, further contributing to ΔAPD by causing different responses to the frequency change in the LV than in the RV. This sequence sets the stage for TdP, which normally appear for 15 to 25 minutes after the start of a single bolus of almokalant. Thereafter, TdP can still be induced by a specific pacing protocol (PES)[17-19] for another 20 minutes. Not all class III drugs will cause a high incidence of spontaneous TdP in this model. For instance, 2 mg/kg per 5 minutes d-sotalol will only result in TdP in 5% to 8% of dogs, while this occurrence can be increased to 50% after PES (Figs. 5 and 6). A major difference in the electrophysiologic effects of the two drugs is their effect on ΔAPD: almokalant increased ΔAPD to 110±60 milliseconds versus 80±45 milliseconds after d-sotalol in the same dog tested serially.[17] When comparing the different magnitude of ΔAPD at baseline, after class III agent administration that does not result in spontaneous TdP with spontaneous acquired TdP, it is clear that ΔAPD plays an important role in the generation of TdP (Fig. 7,

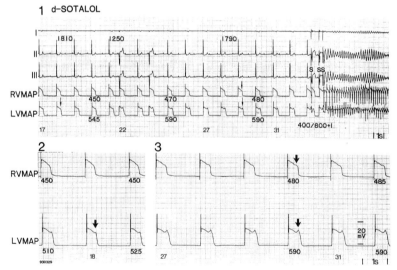

Figure 6. Return of early afterdepolarizations (EADs) and dispersion leading to reinduction of torsades de pointes (TdP). This registration was recorded after that in Figure 5 and has the same composition. It starts 17 beats after spontaneous termination of the TdP. A minor EAD is present in the left ventricular MAP (LV MAP) and becomes more pronounced in the following beats (see the enlargement in panel **2**). With the increase in height of the EAD in the LV MAP, the ΔAPD also gradually starts to increase from 60 (beat 17) to 110 milliseconds (beat 30, see enlargement in panel **3**), just before the resumption of the pacing mode (panel **1**). Panel 3 shows the return of the EAD in right ventricular MAP (RV MAP) returns around the 25th beat (panel 3). The same pacing mode performed as in Figure 5 after 32 beats again induces TdP.

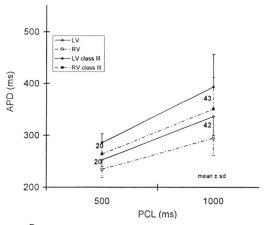

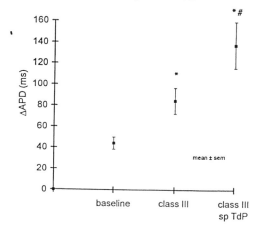

Figure 7. Interventricular dispersion. **A**. Response of the left and right ventricular action potential duration (APD) (LV and RV; y axis) to pacing at 500 and 1000 milliseconds (x axis) before (open symbols) and after class III agents (closed symbols) in the absence of early afterdepolarizations (EADs) on the MAPs. An increase in cycle length from 500 to 1000 milliseconds increases the APD but also interventricular dispersion (ΔAPD = LV APD – RV APD) from 20 to 40 milliseconds. Administration of a class III agent (either d-sotalol or almokalant) increases APD in both ventricles significantly. However, EADs are not observed and the ΔAPD remains similar at both cycle length. **B**. ΔAPD is shown during idioventricular rhythm at baseline, after administration of class III agents in experiments with and without the development of spontaneous torsades de pointes (TdP). ΔAPD shows an increase with class III drugs that is most pronounced for those animals that developed spontaneous TdP. (*$P<0.05$ versus baseline and #$P<0.05$ versus class III).

panel B). ΔAPD is bradycardia-dependent after d-sotalol, as can be seen in panel A of Figure 7. EADs and ectopic beats seem to contribute to a lesser extent because they also occur frequently in noninducible dogs.[19]

The TdP episodes (both spontaneous and PES-induced) terminated spontaneously within 10 seconds in about two thirds of the cases. The other one third of episodes that lasted longer than 10 seconds were externally cardioverted with approximately 50 to 70 J to prevent degeneration in ventricular fibrillation and/or deterioration of cardiac function. The mean duration of self-terminating episodes of *PES-induced* TdP after d-sotalol or almokalant (from consecutive experiments) was found to be 15±9 beats (range 5 to 35; n=20) with a mean CL of 240±20 milliseconds. The duration of *spontaneous episodes of TdP* was comparable (range 5 to 35, 10.5±7; n=36) with a mean CL of 275±32 milliseconds. In both instances the last beat of the TdP had a significantly shorter APD and almost no ΔAPD was present. In addition no EADs were observed (see Figs. 4 and 5).

Relation Between EADs and ΔAPD

Administration of class III agents increases the APD but surprisingly does not seem to alter the ΔAPD at the specific paced CLs when no EADs are visible (see Fig. 7, panel A). Therefore, an increase in ΔAPD after administration of class III drugs during spontaneous rhythm can be based on either slowing of the idioventricular rate, as is often seen with these drugs, and/or by the occurrence of EADs. This relation between EADs and ΔAPD is not completely clear, because both are bradycardia-dependent and appear in similar tissue under similar conditions. To unravel this contribution of EADs to ΔAPD, we examined two situations in which the presence or absence of the EADs in the MAP was well controlled.

First, we evaluated in 14 dogs the frequency (500 and 1000 milliseconds) dependency of ΔAPD under baseline circumstances and after administration of class III drugs (almokalant or d-sotalol) in the absence of EADs (Fig. 7, panel A).[18] When EADs do occur after class III drugs, there is an increase in ΔAPD at most CLs in which they appear, as is illustrated in panel B of Figure 8 for the group comparison as well as for an individual

---

Figure 8. Left ventricular (LV) pacing at 500 and 1000 milliseconds in the presence and absence of class III agents. In this figure we have plotted the differences between the left and right ventricular action potential duration (APD) (LV and RV) at different frequencies of 500 and 1000 milliseconds before (**A**) and after (**B**) administration of class III agents. In the left part, electrocardiogram lead II is visualized at a paced cycle length of 500 milliseconds (panel 1) and 1000 milliseconds (panel 2) together with the two MAP signals, which have been synchronized for the beginning of activation time in panel 3. The length of the APD is shown together with the difference (ΔAPD) of 20 milliseconds at a cycle length of

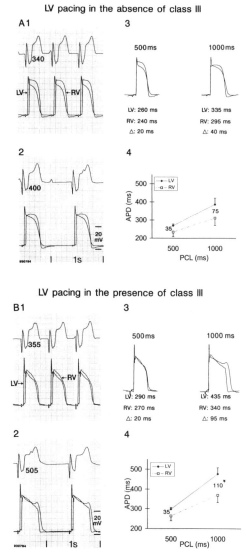

Figure 8 *(continued)*. 500 milliseconds which increases to 40 milliseconds at a cycle length of 1000 milliseconds. In panel 4, the mean frequency-dependent LV and RV APD is plotted for a group of 6 dogs showing a bradycardia dependent increase in ΔAPD from 35 to 75 milliseconds. In B, similar plots have been made after administration of a class III agent (in this particular animal d-sotalol). At 500 milliseconds (panels 1 and 3) the LV and RV APD is prolonged uniformly, resulting in a similar ΔAPD. At 1000 milliseconds (panels 2 and 3), a clear EAD is present in the LV, leading to a nonuniform APD increase that results in a ΔAPD of 95 milliseconds at a cycle length of 1000 milliseconds. The average increase in ΔAPD for the group of 6 dogs with the development of EADs was 75 milliseconds (from 35 to 110 milliseconds), which was significant.

dog. At 500 milliseconds there is an increase in APD due to class III drugs, but not in ΔAPD. At 1000 milliseconds, however, there is the clear presence of an EAD, which increases the difference between the two ventricles from 45 milliseconds at baseline to 95 milliseconds after class III drugs (in this case d-sotalol). Such an increase in ΔAPD at a certain CL was observed only when EADs were present.

A second way to analyze the relationship between EADs and ΔAPD was found in the behavior of these parameters after termination and reinduction of PES-induced episodes of TdP. Self-terminating episodes of PES-induced TdP were analyzed, with special attention paid to 1) the beat before PES resulting in TdP; 2) the last beat of the TdP; and 3) the beats following spontaneous termination. The advantage of PES-induced TdP is that the time of reinduction can be determined by the investigator, ie, that the onset of the TdP can be better controlled.

In each of these beats the LV and RV APD were measured and the absence or presence of EADs was registered. The results are summarized in Table 1. Before the TdP, the ΔAPD amounted to 80 ± 55 milliseconds, and EADs were present in half of the MAPs. TdP occurred either in or directly after the paced stimuli. The EADs had all disappeared in the last beat of the TdP (Figs. 4 and 5) in combination with a decrease in the LV and RV APD, reducing the ΔAPD to 10 ± 15 milliseconds. In the beats following termination, the APD and the presence of an EAD showed a biphasic pattern, ie, in the first beat an EAD was often observed with a relatively long APD. Thereafter the APD shortened and the EAD disappeared (Figs. 5 and 6). No major changes in the rate of the idioventricular rhythm took place. After this initial decrease, the APD gradually started to increase (Figs. 5 and 6) and the EAD reappeared. Such a biphasic pattern

Table 1

Electrophysiologic Parameters (mean + SD) Measured before Class III Drug Administration (Control), Just Before Pacing-Induced Acquired Torsades de Pointes (TdP), the Last Beat and Several Beats After a Spontaneously Terminating Episode of TdP

	Control	Before TdP	Last Beat of TdP	1st Beat After TdP	5th Beat After TdP
CL-IVR (ms)	1645 ± 295	1870 ± 255	250 ± 30	1920 ± 420	1935 ± 315
LV APD (ms)	365 ± 45	460 ± 80	$250 \pm 25^*$	$430 \pm 55^*$	$390 \pm 55^{**}$
RV APD (ms)	325 ± 30	380 ± 50	$235 \pm 15^*$	$370 \pm 50^*$	$345 \pm 40^{**}$
ΔAPD (ms)	40 ± 25	80 ± 55	$10 \pm 15^*$	$60 \pm 50^*$	45 ± 30
EAD	0	20/40	0/40^*	23/40	9/40^{**}

*$P<0.05$ versus before TdP**, $P<0.05$ versus 1st beat after TdP; CL-IVR = cycle length of the idioventricular rhythm; LV = left ventricle; RV = right ventricle; APD = action potential duration; ΔAPD = difference between LV and RV action potential duration; EAD = early afterdepolarization.

was a general finding in all dogs following spontaneous termination of PES-induced TdP. Reinduction of TdP follows PES when the APD, ΔAPD, and EAD have returned to their pre-TdP level (Fig. 6 and Table 2). If this is not the case, repetition of PES does not result in TdP (Table 2).

Table 2
Electrophysiologic Parameters in Relation to Either
Successful Reinduction or Failure to Reinduce TdP

	CL IVR (ms)	LV APD (ms)	RV APD (ms)	Δ APD (ms)	EAD
First episode n=8	1810±295	455±90	380±70	70±30	8/16
Reinducible	1790±290	455±75	385±60	70±35	7/16
First episode n=7	1965±220	445±85	370±40	75±65	5/14
Not reinducible	1995±150	420±70*	370±45	50±40*	2/14

*$P<0.05$ versus TdP first episode; Abbreviations same as in Table 1.

Controversy Surrounding the Visualization of EADs: Alternative Explanation

In recent years, different myocardial cell types have been described that respond differently to frequency changes and to APD-increasing drugs. In addition to the different response of Purkinje fibers,[34,38] the M cells located in the mid myocardium of the ventricular wall show a different sensitivity in comparison to endocardial and epicardial ventricular cells.[11,21,22] The nonuniform increase of the APD in the different cell types results in transmural differences in repolarization, as has been clearly demonstrated in isolated cells and in multicellular preparations from the dog, guinea pig, and human.[40,41] Similar differences in cell types between the ventricles can also explain our ΔAPD. This transmural dispersion has been implicated as a second or alternative explanation for the humps in the MAP registration. Because both phenomena, EADs and dispersion, occur in similar cell types (Purkinje or M cells) under similar conditions, it is difficult to distinguish between the two. Until now, conflicting results have been reported in relation to the existence of transmural differences in the APD in vivo. Specifically, the discussion about whether a bell-shaped curve can be observed transmurally, explaining the M cell contribution, is still a matter of discussion.

Using the activation recovery intervals (ARIs) of local electrograms with high doses of anthopleurin-A, El-Sherif et al[7] were able to describe a nonuniform gradient with the highest value within the myocardium, whereas Anyukhovsky et al[10,11] could not confirm this with quinidine, using ARI and/or ventricular effective refractory period measurements. An alternative would be to use a needle MAP electrode.[42] Also with this methodology, conflicting preliminary reports have been published. Our own experience with this technique points to a gradual decline in interventricular or transseptal dispersion going from the endocardial LV site with the longest APD to the endocardial RV site with the shortest APD.[43]

Are there arguments in favor of the EAD or the transmural dispersion hypothesis? Whereas Cranefield and Aronson[28] include both retardation and interruption of the normal repolarization in their definition of EAD, we are in favor of the exclusion of retardation and, by this, a possible contribution of transmural differences. We consider true interruption of repolarization accompanied by a depolarizing current to be the true definition of an EAD (see Fig. 2, panels B and C). In this way, it is also understandable that the ectopic beats that precede TdP are caused by triggered activity. When EADs are responsible, they should occur before the repolarization has completed. As observed in panel 2 of Figure 4 and concluded from an analysis of 20 experiments with spontaneous ectopic beats after administration of class III agents, we could demonstrate that in greater than 75% of the beats, the coupling interval was well within the duration of the LV endocardial MAP. An alternative explanation would be phase 2 reentry.

Second, we have demonstrated that EADs (and related ectopic beats) can be induced by pacing or, better, by an abrupt change in CL (acceleration-induced EADs). As can be seen in Figure 3, a sudden change in paced CL will increase the APD and increase ΔAPD before the parameters diminish as a result of the higher frequency. The prolongation is accompanied by the appearance of an EAD (see Figure 5 in Reference 19), which can be prevented by the administration of drugs such as flunarizine and ryanodine, suggesting a role of intracellular calcium handling. Similar observations with an EAD exclusively in the M cell region have been made in vitro by Sicouri et al.[22] In our opinion, this relation with intracellular calcium and possibly the $Na^+:Ca^{++}$ exchanger, points to focal activity and, less likely, to phase 2 reentry to explain the accompanying ectopic beats.

Conclusion

The role of EADs in the onset of TdP is still not clear, although triggered activity seems to be the most probable cause for the appearance of ectopic beats preceding TdP. Furthermore, we have tried to demonstrate that EADs can contribute to ΔAPD in a direct and indirect way by the formation of ectopic beats. The mechanism of TdP continuation is also unresolved, although reentry and/or focal activity with shifting pathways on the basis of dispersion are the most likely causes. ΔAPD can contribute to TdP in both theories: it can make a focal ventricular tachycardia behave as a polymorphic one on the basis of activation fronts which have to travel different routes because they encounter different regions of repolarization. Similarly, ΔAPD as part of a reentry circuit is also acceptable on the basis of transseptal differences in which the different APDs are in close proximity to create unidirectional block.

However, it is perhaps more important to discuss the contribution of the MAP technique to electrophysiology than to argue about its limitations. Dispersion, which can be measured by the MAP technique, represents a phenomenon that is directly linked to the occurrence of TdP. Therefore it can be used to study and predict proarrhythmic and antiarrhythmic behavior of drugs in the intact human heart. The original investigators should be credited for that!

Acknowledgments The authors would like to thank Mrs. Jet Leunissen for performing the experiments and the realization of the pictures, and Jurren van Opstal, MD for analysis of part of the data.

References

1. Duggal P, Vesely MR, Wattanasirichaigoon D, et al. Mutation of the gene for IsK associated with both Jervell and Lange-Nielsen and Romano-Ward forms of long-QT syndrome. *Circulation* 1998;97:142-146.
2. Moss AJ, Zareba W, Benhorin J, et al. ECG T-wave patterns in genetically distinct forms of the hereditary long QT syndrome. *Circulation* 1995;92:2929-2934.
3. Donger C, Denjoy I, Berthet M, et al. KVLQT1 C-terminal missense mutation causes a form fruste long-QT syndrome. *Circulation* 1997;96:2778-2781.
4. Hohnloser SH, Singh BN. Proarrhythmia with class III antiarrhythmic drugs: Definition, electrophysiologic mechanisms, incidence, predisposing factors, and clinical implications. *J Cardiovasc Electrophysiol* 1995;6:920-936.
5. Singh BN, Sarma JM, Zhang ZH, Takanaka C. Controlling cardiac arrhythmias by lengthening repolarization: Rationale from experimental findings and clinical considerations. *Ann N Y Acad Sci* 1992;644:187-209.
6. Stratmann HG, Kennedy HL. Torsades de pointes associated with drugs and toxins: Recognition and management. *Am Heart J* 1987;113:1470-1482.
7. El-Sherif N, Caref EB, Yin H, Restivo M. The electrophysiological mechanism of ventricular arrhythmias in the long QT syndrome. Tridimensional mapping of activation and recovery patterns. *Circ Res* 1996;79:474-492.
8. Shimizu W, Antzelevitch C. Sodium channel block with mexiletine is effective in reducing dispersion of repolarization and preventing torsade des pointes in LQT2 and LQT3 models of the long-QT syndrome. *Circulation* 1997;96:2038-2047.
9. Priori SG, Napolitano C, Cantu F, et al. Differential response to Na+ channel blockade, beta-adrenergic stimulation, and rapid pacing in a cellular model mimicking the SCN5A and HERG defects present in the long-QT syndrome. *Circ Res* 1996;78:1009-1015.

10. Anyukhovsky EP, Sosunov EA, Feinmark SJ, Rosen MR. Effects of quinidine on repolarization in canine epicardium, midmyocardium, and epicardium II. In vivo study. *Circulation* 1997;96:4019-4026.

11. Anyukhovsky EP, Sosunov EA, Rosen MR. Regional differences in electrophysiological properties of epicardium, midmyocardium, and endocardium: In vitro and in vivo correlations. *Circulation* 1996;96:1981-1988.

12. Hanich RF, Levine JH, Spear JF, Moore EN. Autonomic modulation of ventricular arrhythmia in cesium chloride-induced long QT syndrome. *Circulation* 1988;77:1149-1161.

13. Levine JH, Spear JF, Guarnieri T, et al. Cesium chloride-induced long QT syndrome: Demonstration of afterdepolarizations and triggered activity in vivo. *Circulation* 1985;72:1092-1103.

14. Bailie DS, Inoue H, Kaseda S, et al. Magnesium suppression of early afterdepolarizations and ventricular tachyarrhythmias induced by cesium in dogs. *Circulation* 1988;77:1395-1402.

15. Ben David J, Zipes DP. Differential response to right and left ansae subclaviae stimulation of early after depolarizations and ventricular tachycardia induced by cesium in dogs. *Circulation* 1988;78:1241-1250.

16. Verduyn SC, Vos MA, Gorgels AP, et al. The effect of flunarizine and ryanodine on acquired torsades de pointes arrhythmias in the intact canine heart. *J Cardiovasc Electrophysiol* 1995;6:189-200.

17. Verduyn SC, Vos MA, Wellens HJ, et al. Further observations to elucidate the role of interventricular dispersion of repolarization and early afterdepolarizations in the genesis of acquired torsade de pointes arrhythmias. A comparison between almokalant and d-sotalol using the dog as its own control. *J Am Coll Cardiol* 1997;30:1575-1584.

18. Verduyn SC, Vos MA, van der Zande J, et al. Role of interventricular dispersion of repolarization in acquired torsade-de-pointes arrhythmias: Reversal by magnesium. *Cardiovasc Res* 1997;34:453-463.

19. Vos MA, Verduyn SC, Gorgels AP, et al. Reproducible induction of early afterdepolarizations and torsade de pointes arrhythmias by d-sotalol and pacing in dogs with chronic atrioventricular block. *Circulation* 1995;91:864-872.

20. Vos MA, de Groot S, Verduyn SC, et al. Enhanced susceptibility for acquired torsade de pointes arrhythmias in the dog with chronic complete atrioventricular block is related to cardiac hypertrophy and electrical remodeling. *Circulation* 1998;98:1125-1135.

21. Sicouri S, Antzelevitch C. A subpopulation of cells with unique electrophysiological properties in the deep subepicardium of the canine ventricle. The M cell. *Circ Res* 1991;68:1729-1741.

22. Sicouri S, Moro S, Elizari MV. d-Sotalol induces marked action potential prolongation and early afterdepolarization in M but not in epicardial or endocardial cells of the canine ventricle. *J Cardiovasc Pharmacol Therapeut* 1997;2:27-38.

23. Surawicz B. Electrophysiologic substrate of torsade de pointes: Dispersion of repolarization or early afterdepolarizations? *J Am Coll Cardiol* 1989;14:172-184.

24. Franz MR. Method and theory of monophasic action potential recording. *Prog Cardiovasc Dis* 1991;33:347-368.

25. Ino T, Karagueuzian HS, Hong K, et al. Relation of monophasic action potential recorded with contact electrode to underlying transmembrane action potential properties in isolated cardiac tissues: A systematic microelectrode validational study. *Cardiovasc Res* 1988;22:255-264.

26. Gavrilescu S, Luca C. Right ventricular monophasic action potentials in patients with long QT syndrome. *Br Heart J* 1978;40:1014-1018.
27. Bonatti V, Rolli A, Botti G. Recording of monophasic action potentials of the right ventricle in long QT syndromes complicated by severe ventricular arrhythmias. *Eur Heart J* 1983;4:168-179.
28. Cranefield PF, Aronson RS. *Cardiac Arrhythmias: The Role of Triggered Activity and Other Mechanisms.* Mount Kisco, New York: Futura Publishing, Inc.; 1988.
29. Banai S, Tzivoni D. Drug therapy for torsade de pointes. *J Cardiovasc Electrophysiol* 1993;4:206-210.
30. Garcia-Rubira JC, Garcia-Aranda VL, Cruz FJM. Magnesium sulphate for torsade de pointes in a patient with congenital long QT syndrome. *Int J Cardiol* 1990;27:282-283.
31. Kurita T, Ohe T, Shimizu W, et al. Early afterdepolarization in a patient with complete atrioventricular block and torsades de pointes. *PACE* 1993;16:33-38.
32. Tzivoni D, Banai S, Schuger C, et al. Treatment of torsade de pointes with magnesium sulfate. *Circulation* 1987;77:392-397.
33. Carlsson L, Almgren O, Duker G. QTU-prolongation and torsades de pointes induced by putative class III antiarrhythmic agents in the rabbit: Etiology and interventions. *J Cardiovasc Pharmacol* 1990;16:276-285.
34. Kaseda S, Gilmour-RF J, Zipes DP. Depressant effect of magnesium on early afterdepolarizations and triggered activity induced by cesium, quinidine, and 4-aminopyridine in canine cardiac Purkinje fibers. *Am Heart J* 1989;118:458-466.
35. Carlsson L, Abrahamsson C, Drews L, Duker G. Antiarrhythmic effects of potassium channel openers in rhythm abnormalities related to delayed repolarization. *Circulation* 1992;85:1491-1500.
36. Vos MA, Gorgels AP, Lipcsei GC, et al. Mechanism-specific antiarrhythmic effects of the potassium channel activator levcromakalim against repolarization-dependent tachycardias. *J Cardiovasc Electrophysiol* 1994;5:731-742.
37. Sato T, Hata Y, Yamamoto M, et al. Early afterdepolarization abolished by potassium channel opener in a patient with idiopathic long QT syndrome. *J Cardiovasc Electrophysiol* 1995;6:279-282.
38. Davidenko JM, Cohen L, Goodrow R, Antzelevitch C. Quinidine-induced action potential prolongation, early afterdepolarizations, and triggered activity in canine Purkinje fibers. Effects of stimulation rate, potassium, and magnesium. *Circulation* 1989;79:674-686.
39. Vos MA, Gorgels AP, Leunissen JD, et al. Further observations to confirm the arrhythmia mechanism-specific effects of flunarizine. *J Cardiovasc Pharmacol* 1992;19:682-690.
40. Antzelevitch C, Sicouri S, Litovsky SH, et al. Heterogeneity within the ventricular wall. Electrophysiology and pharmacology of epicardial, endocardial, and M cells. *Circ Res* 1991;69:1427-1449.
41. Drouin E, Charpentier F, Gauthier C, et al. Electrophysiologic characteristics of cells spanning the left ventricular wall of human heart: Evidence for presence of M cells. *J Am Coll Cardiol* 1995;26:185-192.
42. Weissenburger J, Nesterenko VV, Antzelevitch C. M cells contribute to transmural dispersion of repolarization and to the development of torsade de pointes in the canine heart in vivo. *PACE* 1996;19:707. Abstract.
43. van der Hulst FF, Vos MA, Leunissen HDM, Wellens HJJ. Transseptal dispersion in the dog with chronic AV-block: Distribution and frequency dependence. *Eur Heart J* 1998;19:72 (P567). Abstract.

33

Delayed Afterdepolarizations in the In Situ Canine Heart:

The Role of the Diastolic Upslope

Marc A. Vos, PhD,
S. H. Marieke de Groot, MD, PhD and
Hein J. Wellens, MD, PhD

Introduction

Although the monophasic action potential (MAP) recording technique has been used clinically for more than 30 years,[1] relatively few articles have been published dealing with the registration of delayed afterdepolarizations (DADs) and related cardiac arrhythmias in vivo.[2-13] In recent reviews by Yuan et al[14] and Franz[15] about the (clinical) use of the MAP technique, no information about the recording of DADs in the in situ heart was presented. This scarcity of data could lead to doubts regarding the clinical importance of DAD-dependent triggered activity as one of the basic mechanisms of cardiac arrhythmias. Most articles present examples of early afterdepolarizations (EADs) and EAD-dependent triggered activity. This is surprising because, in contrast to EADs, the etiology, registration, and characteristics of DADs are no matter of discussion (see further). Moreover, since their discovery in the early 1970s, DADs have been implicated in many pathophysiologic conditions leading to ventricular arrhythmias, such as digitalis

This study was supported by grants from the Wynand N. Pon Foundation and the Netherlands Organisation for Scientific Research (NWO #902-16-214).

intoxication, stretch, cardiac hypertrophy, catecholamines, ischemia, and reperfusion. This chapter describes the current expertise in registering DADs by the MAP technique, the criteria available to distinguish between a true DAD and an artifact, and quantification of (the amplitude of) the DADs by their slope in order to predict the occurrence or suppression of DAD-dependent triggered arrhythmias.

Definition DAD and Identification of Triggered Arrhythmias

DADs are abnormal, low-amplitude, secondary afterdepolarizations that occur after repolarization has ended. The mechanism underlying the generation of DADs is complex but is related to intracellular calcium overload or to improper calcium handling.[16,17] The elegant work of Yamada and Corr[17] nicely illustrated that aftercontractions, visualized by calcium transients, were related to DADs. Most interventions aimed at improving cardiac function (digitalis, isoprenaline, hypertrophy, phosphodiesterase inhibitors, etc) can therefore lead to the occurrence of DADs. When a DAD is of sufficient amplitude, it will give rise to a triggered ectopic beat. This phenomenon can be repetitive, causing sustained atrial or ventricular tachycardias (VTs). Until direct proof became available with the use of MAP catheters, we and others had been using different criteria to identify DADs and, more specifically, DAD-dependent triggered arrhythmias[18-20]: 1) their response to programmed electrical stimulation (their frequency dependency and concordant relation to the coupling interval of stimulated beats), and 2) their reaction to mechanism-specific drugs such as flunarizine. Already in those days, controversy existed about the specificity of using overdrive stimulation to terminate DAD-dependent tachycardias.[3,18]

MAP Criteria and DAD Identification

Under normal circumstances, a typical ventricular MAP (Fig. 1, upper right panel) should have a stable diastolic baseline (direct-current–coupled differential amplifier), a sharp positive directed overshoot of at least 15 mV during early depolarization (phase 0), a short-lasting deflection followed by the plateau phase (phases 1 and 2), and a downward repolarization (phase 3) returning to the diastolic baseline (phase 4). To optimize the registration of DADs in the MAP, we use the following criteria: 1) the MAP catheter should be placed by experienced investigators to control contact with the endocardium and appropriate pressure of the catheter; 2) consecutive beats should have an identical MAP morphology and duration; 3) there

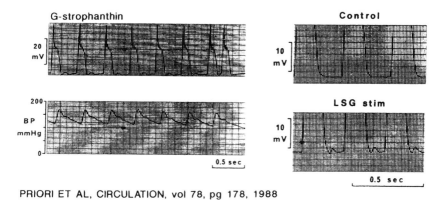

PRIORI ET AL, CIRCULATION, vol 78, pg 178, 1988

Figure 1. Tracings showing delayed afterdepolarizations (DADs) in the left ventricular endocardial MAP of a cat. Left panel: Simultaneous recording of MAP and blood pressure (BP) after administration of calcium and strophanthin. Note the presence of DADs and the occurrence of one ectopic, triggered beat. Right panel: MAP recording at high amplification in control (upper) and after stimulation of the left stellate ganglion (lower) when DADs are present. Reproduced with permission of the American Heart Association.

should be corresponding changes between the MAP and other recordings (eg, the electrocardiogram recording or a pressure signal[5]; 4) the observed arrhythmia should bear the characteristics of triggered arrhythmias; and 5) the occurrence of DADs in the MAP (and related arrhythmias) should disappear after interventions that lead to DAD and DAD-related arrhythmia suppression in vitro.

In Vivo Registration of DADs

One of the first groups to reproducibly register a DAD in an intact feline heart was that of Priori et al.[2] At the endocardium of the left ventricle, they recorded DADs and DAD-dependent ectopic activity after administration of G-strophanthin together with calcium gluconate (Fig. 1, left upper panel), and after left stellate ganglion stimulation (Fig. 1, right lower panel). In the following years, focal triggered activity was recorded at the left ventricular (LV) endocardium in dogs after intracoronary application of ouabain,[3] after intravenous and intracoronary cesium,[4] and at the LV and right ventricular (RV) endocardium after intravenous application of ouabain.[8,10] Also in rabbits, DADs were recorded at the endocardium of the RV after application of methoxamine and class III drugs.[6] Finally, the data from animal experiments include the recording of DADs and DAD-related triggered arrhythmias in the mid myocardium of the LV of guinea pigs after treatment with digoxin.[9,11] Similar observations, presented in abstract, were made in dogs by Levine et al[12] (acetylstrophanthidin) and Brachmann et al[13] (left stellate ganglion stimulation). In order to exclude mechanical effects as the cause of the DADs, some investigators repeated the experiments in similar positive inotropic conditions; Xu and coworkers[9,11] showed that isoprenaline had positive inotropic effects similar to those of digoxin but did not cause DADs.

In humans, we found two published reports: 1) in the hypertrophied left ventricle of patients with aortic stenosis, Paulus et al[5] recorded DADs and DAD-induced ectopic beats in half of the investigated patients, and 2) in adult patients with atrial tachycardia, Chen et al[7] recorded DADs in the right atrium (Fig. 2). It is important to mention that Paulus

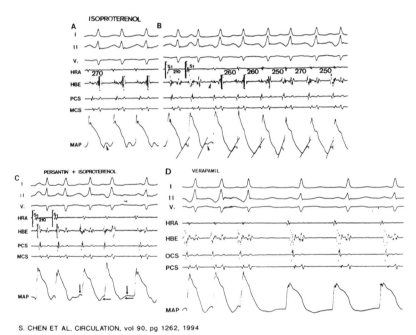

S. CHEN ET AL. CIRCULATION, vol 90, pg 1262, 1994

Figure 2. Tracings showing delayed afterdepolarization (DAD)-dependent atrial tachycardia (AT) in a patient. **A.** A sinus tachycardia (cycle length 270 milliseconds) can be seen with DADs in the MAP recordings after isoproterenol i.v. **B.** The induction of AT can be seen after atrial pacing (S1-S1: cycle length 210 milliseconds) in combination with isoproterenol. The slope is indicated with the lines in the MAP. **C.** The response after persantin and isoproterenol i.v. can be seen. Two atrial beats were induced by triggered DADs, while the third DAD shows a less steep slope (horizontal arrow) and a smaller amplitude (vertical arrow) than the first DAD. **D.** Termination of DAD-dependent AT can be seen after administration of verapamil followed by sinus rhythm and stable MAP recordings. HRA = high right atrium; HBE = His bundle area; PCS = proximal coronary sinus; MCS = middle coronary sinus; OCS = coronary sinus orifice. Reproduced with permission of the American Heart Association.

et al[5] recorded DADs that could be associated with changes in the diastolic pressure curve. Often the DADs and related arrhythmias were induced with the assistance of programmed electrical stimulation[3,4,5,8,10] and effectively suppressed by the administration of drugs such as verapamil (Fig. 2),[7,8,9,12] $MgSO_4$,[8] or lidocaine.[10] The fact that the MAP catheter can be provided with pacing capabilities enables the investigator to pace and record from proximal sites. In other experiments, Hariman and Gough[21] showed that unipolar recordings are also capable of detecting DADs and triggered arrhythmias in ouabain-intoxicated or infarcted canine hearts.

Quantification of DADs: Amplitude or Slope

One of the disadvantages of using the MAP technique in comparison to the transmembrane action potential is the absence of information concerning the absolute amplitude. Some investigators have calculated the amplitude of the DAD either absolute or in relation to the total amplitude. For instance, Priori et al[2] calculated the DAD to be 1.2 mV or about 6% of the MAP amplitude of around 20 mV. The amplitude became taller when the pacing rate was increased; Xu and coworkers[9] calculated an amplitude of 0.5 mV at 200 milliseconds to 2.7 mV at 130 milliseconds, going from 3% to 20% of the MAP amplitude.

In vitro, investigators have used the diastolic upslope to quantify the DAD.[22,23] A major advantage of this quantification method is that it can be measured during triggering of DADs, ie, during atrial or VT (Fig. 2). On the other hand, it still provides the opportunity to measure DADs that are subthreshold. The slope is calculated as the mean rate of rise (dV/dt) of the ascending limb of the DAD[22,23] or as the mean change in diastolic potential of 5 paced beats or 5 beats of a tachycardia.[10] In some cases, the DAD follows an initial phase of hyperpolarization. This hyperpolarization was excluded in the calculation of the slope. Application of this approach to our MAP data recorded in anesthetized dogs with chronic, complete atrioventricular block (CAVB) revealed the following: 1) temporary increase in the diastolic upslope during pacing was related to the induction of DADs and DAD-dependent arrhythmias; 2) concordant behavior of the slope angle with the interstimulus interval, 3) decrease in slope prior to spontaneous or drug induced termination of ouabain-induced ventricular arrhythmias; 4) depressed diastolic upslope after antiarrhythmic drugs, in accordance with the time course of elimination (half-life) of these drugs; and 5) increased slope under circumstances of improved cardiac function.

Value of the Slope to Predict Triggered Arrhythmias Post Pacing

In CAVB dogs, the diastolic upslope was calculated at the end of the pacing train to relate this value to the ability to induce triggered ectopic activity.[10] Under control circumstances, a "flat" diastolic upslope can be measured (2 mV/s). After treatment with ouabain in a dose that causes VTs in these dogs (45 µg/kg), the slope at the end of a pacing train increased to 26 mV/s, and DADs could be seen postpacing in 74% of the pacing trains while VT could be induced in 33% (Fig. 3).[10] To ensure the applicability of the slope during circumstances of normally conducted sinus rhythm, we have repeated the ouabain experiments in dogs with normal atrioventricular (AV) conduction and found similar results.

Concordant Behavior of the Slope with Interstimulus Interval

When comparing different interstimulus intervals, it became clear that shorter interstimulus intervals will result in steeper slopes and more arrhythmogenic activity; eg, pacing with a paced cycle length of 300 milliseconds caused a slope of 20 mV, an incidence of 80% DADs and related VTs, while a paced cycle length of 400 milliseconds resulted in a slope of 13 mV/s and an incidence of 36% DADs with 21% VTs.[10]

Decrease in Slope Prior to Spontaneous or Drug-Induced Termination of Triggered Arrhythmias

The behavior of the diastolic upslope during ouabain-induced VT was followed over time. As can be seen in Figure 3, at the start of the VT the slope had a value of 11 mV/s. This value either stabilized (perpetuation of the VT) or decreased in time. In case of the latter, spontaneous termination of the VT occurred, as can be seen in the bottom part of Figure 3. Similar observations have been made with drug- (lidocaine, ryanodine, and verapamil) induced termination of these VTs.

Preventive Action of Antiarrhythmic Drugs (Depressed Diastolic Upslope)

After lidocaine administration in the presence of ouabain, the pacing-induced increase in diastolic upslope was no longer seen (4 mV/s). This was associated with a decrease in the incidence of DADs and the inability

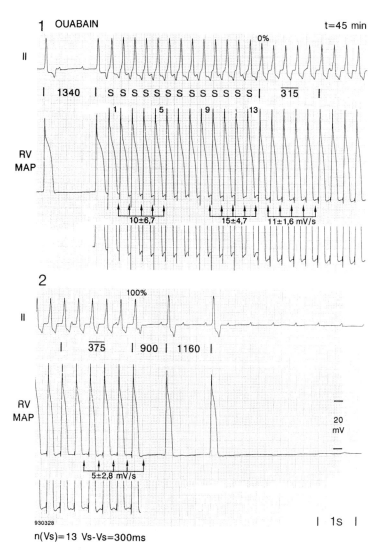

Figure 3. The induction and the spontaneous termination of a delayed afterdepolarization (DAD)-dependent ventricular tachycardia (VT) in a dog with chronic complete AV block. Electrocardiogram lead II is presented together with a MAP recording in the right ventricle (RV) at a paper speed of 25 mm/s. The lower part of the MAP is enlarged underneath the RV MAP. **1.** The combination of ouabain and pacing (S) with 13 stimuli and an interstimulus interval of 300 milliseconds results in the induction of a VT. Note the appearance of DADs in the MAP during pacing with an increase in slope from 10 to 15 mV/s. The VT starts with a slope of 11 mV/s which gradually decreases until 5 mV/s just prior to spontaneous termination of this VT. This is accompanied with an increase in cycle length of the VT from 315 to 375 milliseconds. After termination, two spontaneous beats occur before overdrive suppression can be seen.

to induce VT. After washout of lidocaine, all the ouabain-induced changes returned and VTs could again be induced.

Increased Slope Under Circumstances of Improved Cardiac Function

Currently, we are relating the occurrence of DADs to potentiation of cardiac function. Using pacing trains, we are calculating the effect of pacing on LV systolic function, in particular + LV dP/dt. In this way, we have demonstrated that the induction of DAD-dependent triggered arrhythmias is related to postpacing potentiation. The occurrence of DADs is frequently seen after CAVB (Fig. 4) but never at acute AV block (Fig. 5). Chronic AV block will, in time, lead to biventricular hypertrophy, electrical remodeling, and improved cardiac function.[24]

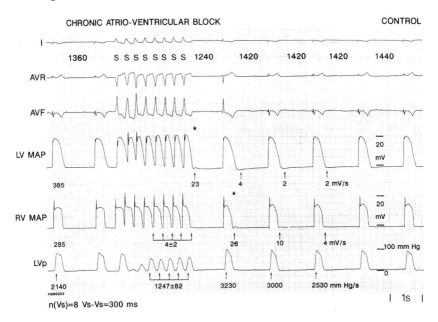

Figure 4. Delayed afterdepolarization (DAD) occurrence during a pacing protocol in a dog with chronic atrioventricular block. Three electrocardiogram leads with two MAP recordings and a left ventricular pressure (LVp) signal are shown. Pacing (S) is performed using 8 stimuli at an interstimulus interval of 300 milliseconds. Due to the absence of a clear diastolic interval, the slope cannot be measured during pacing in the left ventricular MAP (LV MAP). Before pacing, the maximum LV dP/dt was 2140 mm Hg/s. Directly after pacing, LV dP/dt had increased to 3230 mm Hg/s normalizing during the following beats. A DAD appeared directly after pacing in the LV MAP and 1 beat later in the right ventricular (RV) MAP. Also, the slope diminished in time from 26 mV/s for the RV MAP to 4 mV/s after postpacing beat 3.

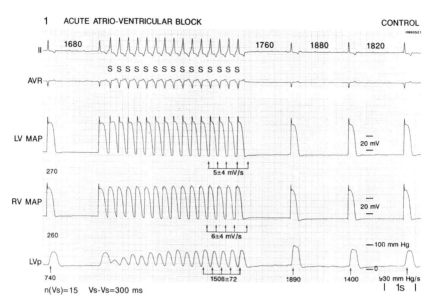

Figure 5. Performance of a pacing protocol during acute atrioventricular block. Two electrocardiogram leads, 2 MAPs, and 1 left ventricular pressure (LVp) signal can be seen. Pacing is performed using 15 stimuli with an interstimulus interval of 300 milliseconds (S). Pacing leads to an increase in the maximum LV dP/dt from 740 to 1890 mm Hg/s. However, no change is seen in the slope during or after pacing.

Of course, there are also limitations in the use of the diastolic slope. During very fast rhythms, there is no measurable LV diastolic interval (see Fig. 4). Moreover, there are huge interindividual differences in the steepness of the slope. Therefore, until normal values have been established, the slope can be used best to evaluate changes over time (after interventions).

Site of Localization of DADs and the "Reach" of the MAP Catheter

In the early studies of the 1970s, DADs were induced in Purkinje fibers.[23] It is known that Purkinje fibers have a higher sensitivity for drugs than do ventricular myocardium. More recently, Sicouri and Antzelevitch[25] also described increased sensitivity of M cells for the induction of DADs after drugs. In the intact canine heart, predilection sites for the induction of DADs have been described after global digitalis intoxication.[26] However, Furakawa et al[3] clearly demonstrated that local application of ouabain results in the local formation of DADs and DAD-dependent ventricular arrhythmias (Fig. 6). Similarly, Priori et al[2] demonstrated that left stellate ganglion stimulation did not always induce DADs at each recording site, whereas Xu and coworkers[9,11] demonstrated that a midmyocardial plunge electrode is also capable of registering DADs and related ectopic activity. Therefore, from these data it is unclear to what depth the MAP catheter can detect electrical signals and to what extent Purkinje cells or M cells contribute to the genesis of DADs. Drug delivery studies given at different sites in the myocardial wall must be performed to answer these questions.

Another limitation of the lack of information concerning the MAP viewing window is the difficulty differentiating afterdepolarizations. Are the recordings reflections of true DADs, or is there communication between the different cellular layers so that phase 3 EADs appear as an electronically modified DAD. This subject is further complicated by the fact that certain interventions (eg, cesium[4] and certain class III agents in combination with methoxamine[6]) seem to induce both EADs and DADs.

In conclusion, we have presented evidence that, with use of the MAP technique, DADs and DAD-related triggered arrhythmias can be detected in the intact beating heart. The use of the diastolic upslope provides the

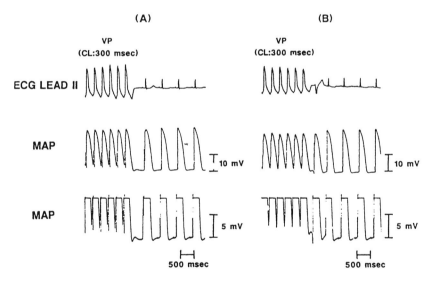

T. FURUKAWA ET AL, CIRCULATION, vol 82, pg 549, 1990

Figure 6. Site-specific registration of delayed afterdepolarizations (DADs) after local application of ouabain through the septal catheter. One electrocardiogram lead is presented with two endocardial MAP recordings: one from the septal site (lower MAP) and one from the posterior wall. Tracings of induced DADs (**A**) and ectopic beats (**B**) at the septal site can only be seen after a ventricular pacing (VP) protocol. Note that the triggered ectopic beat has the same coupling interval as the DAD. Reproduced with permission of the American Heart Association.

investigator with the possibility to quantify this arrhythmogenic parameter. This will allow us to obtain in the intact heart better insights in the role of DADs in the genesis of clinically occurring arrhythmias.

References

1. Korsgen M, Leskinen E, Sjostrand U, Varnauskas E. Intracardiac recording of monophasic action potentials in the human heart. *Scand J Clin Lab Invest* 1966;18:561-564.
2. Priori SG, Mantica M, Schwartz PJ. Delayed afterdepolarizations elicited in vivo by left stellate ganglion stimulation. *Circulation* 1988;78:178-185.
3. Furukawa T, Kimura S, Castellanos A, et al. In vivo induction of focal triggered ventricular arrhythmias and responses to overdrive pacing in the canine heart. *Circulation* 1990;82:549-559.
4. Patterson E, Szabo B, Scherlag BJ, Lazzara R. Early and delayed afterdepolarizations associated with cesium chloride induced arrhythmias in the dog. *J Cardiovasc Pharmacol* 1990;15:323-331.
5. Paulus WJ, Goethals MA, Sys SU. Failure of myocardial inactivation: A clinical assessment in the hypertrophied heart. *Basic Res Cardiol* 1992;87(2):145-161.
6. Buchanan LV, Kabell G, Brunden MN, Gibson JK. Comparative assessment of ibutilide, d-sotalol, clofilium, E-4031, and UK-68,798 in a rabbit model of pro-arrhythmia. *J Cardiovasc Pharmacol* 1993;220:540-549.
7. Chen SA, Chiang CE, Yang CJ, et al. Sustained atrial tachycardia in adult patients. Electrophysiological characteristics, pharmacological response, possible mechanisms, and effects of radiofrequency ablation. *Circulation* 1994;90:1262-1278.
8. Vos MA, Fazekas T, Gorgels APM, et al. The action of MgSO4 differs from moricizine and verapamil on ouabain-induced ventricular tachycardia in normomagnesemic conscious dogs. *J Cardiovasc Pharmacol* 1994;23:252-258.
9. Xu J, Hurt CM, Pelleg A. Digoxin induced ventricular arrhythmias in the guinea pig heart in vivo: Evidence for a role of endogenous catecholamines in the genesis of delayed afterdepolarizations and triggered activity. *Heart Vessels* 1995;10:119-127.
10. de Groot SHM, Vos MA, Gorgels APM, et al. Combining monophasic action potential recordings with pacing to demonstrate delayed afterdepolarizations and triggered arrhythmias in the intact heart. The value of the diastolic slope. *Circulation* 1995;92:2697-2704.
11. Xu J, Pelleg A. A novel guinea pig heart model for studying AV-nodal conduction and triggered activity in vivo. *Am J Physiol* 1996;270:H1850-H1857.
12. Levine JH, Weisfeldt ML, Burkhoff D, et al. Delayed afterdepolarizations in MAPs in vivo. *Circulation* 1984;70:II-88. Abstract.
13. Brachmann J, Beyer T, Seller W, et al. Non-pharmacologic induction of delayed afterdepolarizations generated by adrenergic stimulation in chronically ischaemic canine heart *Eur Heart J* 1990;11:477. Abstract.
14. Yuan S, Blomstrom-Lundquist C, Olsson SB. Monophasic action potentials: Concepts to practical applications. *J Cardiovasc Electrophysiol* 1994;5:287-308.
15. Franz MR. Bridging the gap between basic and clinical electrophysiology: What can be learned from monophasic action potential recordings? *J Cardiovasc Electrophysiol* 1994;5:699-710.

16. Berlin JR, Canell MB, Lederer WJ. Cellular origins of the transient inward current in cardiac myocytes. Role of fluctuations and waves of elevated intracellular calcium. *Circ Res* 1989;65:115-126.
17. Yamada KA, Corr PB. Effects of β-adrenergic receptor activation on intracellular calcium and membrane potential in adult cardiac myocytes. *J Cardiovasc Electrophysiol* 1992;3:209-224.
18. Rosen MR. Is the response to programmed electrical stimulation diagnostic of mechanisms for arrhythmias? *Circulation* 1986;73(II):18-27.
19. Gorgels APM, Vos MA, Leunissen HDM, et al. Flunarizine as a specific drug to identify triggered activity based on delayed afterdepolarizations. In Josephson ME, Wellens HJJ (eds): *Tachycardias: Mechanisms and Management.* Mount Kisco, NY: Futura Publishing Co., Inc.; 1993:87-97.
20. Cranefield PF, Aronson R. *Cardiac Arrhythmias: The Role of Triggered Activity and Other Mechanisms.* Mount Kisco, NY: Futura Publishing Co., Inc.; 1988.
21. Hariman RJ, Gough WB. Delayed afterdepolarization induced triggered activity as a mechanism of ventricular arrhythmias in vivo. In Rosen MR, Janse MJ, Wit AL (eds): *Cardiac Electrophysiology: A Textbook.* Mount Kisco, NY: Futura Publishing Co., Inc.; 1990:323-332.
22. Felzen B, Lotan R, Binah O. Interspecies variations in myocardial responsiveness to cardiac glycosides: Possible relations to the thyroid status. *J Mol Cell Cardiol* 1989;21:165-174.
23. Rosen MR, Danilo P. Effects of tetrodotoxin, lidocaine, verapamil and AHR-2666 on ouabain induced delayed afterdepolarizations in canine Purkinje fibers. *Circ Res* 1980;46:117-124.
24. Vos MA, de Groot SHM, Verduyn SC, et al. Enhanced susceptibility for acquired torsade de pointes arrhythmias in the dog with chronic, complete AV block is related to cardiac hypertrophy and electrical remodeling. *Circulation* 1998;98:1125-1135.
25. Sicouri S, Antzelevitch C. Afterdepolarizations and triggered activity develop in a select population of cells (M-cells) in canine ventricular myocardium: The effects of acetylstrophanthidin and Bay K 8644. *PACE* 1991;14(Pt. II):1714-1720.
26. Gorgels APM, de Wit B, Beekman HDM, et al. Effects of different modes of stimulation on the morphology of the first QRS-complex following pacing during digitalis induced ventricular tachycardia: Observations in the conscious dog with chronic, complete AV-block. *PACE* 1986;9:842-859.

34

Electrophysiologic Characteristics of M Cells and Their Role in Arrhythmias

Charles Antzelevitch, PhD, Gan-Xin Yan, MD, PhD, Wataru Shimizu, MD, PhD, Serge Sicouri, MD, Geoffrey Eddlestone, PhD and Andrew C. Zygmunt, PhD

The existence of regional differences in the electrical properties of ventricular myocardium is now well recognized.[1-5] Electrical and pharmacologic distinctions between endocardium and epicardium of the canine, feline, rabbit, rat, and human heart have been described.[6-15] Differences in the electrophysiologic characteristics and pharmacologic responsiveness of M cells located in the deep structures of the canine, guinea pig, and human ventricles are also well documented.[2,12,16-30]

Epicardial cells, endocardial cells, and M cells differ principally with respect to the early and late repolarization of the action potential (Fig. 1). Ventricular epicardium and M cells usually display action potentials with a prominent notch, due to a conspicuous phase 1 that is largely mediated by a 4-aminopyridine- (4-AP) sensitive transient outward current (I_{to}). The absence of a prominent notch in the endocardial action potential is due to a much smaller I_{to} in that tissue. Regional differences in I_{to}, first suggested

Supported by grants from the National Institutes of Health (HL 47678), the American Heart Association, New York State Affiliate, and the Masons of New York State and Florida.
From Franz MR (ed): *Monophasic Action Potentials: Bridging Cell and Bedside.* ©Futura Publishing Company, Inc., Armonk, NY, 2000.

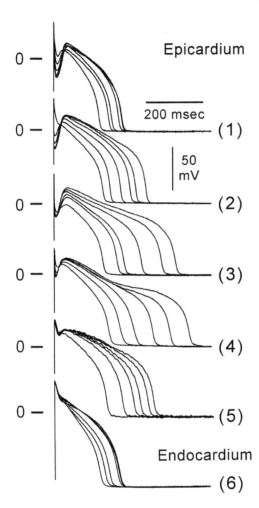

Figure 1. Transmembrane action potentials recorded from myocytes disaggregated from epicardial, midmyocardial, and endocardial regions of the canine left ventricle. Basic cycle lengths are varied over a range of 300 to 8000 milliseconds. Epicardial cells (1) and endocardial cells (6) were isolated from their respective tissues. M cells (longer action potentials) and transitional cells (2 through 5) were isolated from the midmyocardial region. From Reference 12, with permission.

on the basis of action potential data,[7] have now been demonstrated using whole-cell patch clamp techniques in canine,[12] feline,[31] rabbit,[9] rat,[32] and human[33,34] ventricular myocytes. In addition to transmural differences, major differences have been demonstrated in the magnitude of I_{to} and action potential notch in right versus left ventricular epicardium.[35] This chapter focuses on recent experimental data that have advanced our knowledge of the electrical heterogeneity that exists in ventricular myocardium, with an emphasis on the role of the M cell.

Characteristics of the M Cell

The hallmark of the M cell is the ability of its action potential to prolong disproportionately in response to a slowing of rate and/or in response to

APD-prolonging agents (Fig. 1, Table 1).[1,16,26] The ionic basis for these features of the M cell includes the presence of a smaller slowly activating delayed rectifier current (I_{Ks}) (Fig. 2),[21] but a larger late sodium current (late I_{Na}) (Fig. 3).[36] The rapidly activating delayed rectifier current (I_{Kr}) and the inward rectifier current (I_{K1}) are similar in the 3 transmural cell types, near the base of the canine heart. It is noteworthy that apicobasal differences in the density of I_{Kr} channels in the ferret heart have been described.[37] Histologically, M cells are similar to epicardial and endocardial cells. Electrophysiologically and pharmacologically, they are more akin to Purkinje cells, although a number of important distinctions exist between Purkinje cells and M cells (Table 2).[38,39]

The precise location of M cells within the ventricular wall has been investigated in detail only in the left ventricle of the canine heart. Transitional cells are found throughout the wall in the canine left ventricle; M cells displaying the longest action potentials (at basic cycle lengths [BCLs] ≥2000 milliseconds) are commonly localized in the deep subepicardium to mid myocardium in the lateral wall, in the deep subendocardium to mid myocardium in the anterior wall, and throughout the wall in the region of the outflow tracts. The extent to which transmural dispersion of repolarization (TDR) can be observed across the ventricular wall depends on the methodology used to record this parameter. In the absence of drugs but at slow rates, tissue slices isolated from the M region display action potential durations (APDs) more than 100 milliseconds longer than those recorded from endocardium or epicardium (Table 3).[16] Myocytes enzymatically dissociated from the respective regions of the wall show a much larger dispersion.[12,13,21] When recorded from the intact left ventricular wall of arterially perfused wedge preparations, in which the 3 cell types are electrotonically

Table 1

Early Afterdepolarization-Induced Triggered Activity and/or
Prominent Action Potential Prolongation

	Epicardium	Endocardium	M cells
Quinidine (3.3 μM)	−	−	+++
4-Aminopyridine (2.5–5 mM)	−	−	+++
Amiloride (1–10 μM)	−	−	++
Clofilium (1 μM)	−	−	+++
Bay K 8644 (1 μM)	−	−	++
Cesium (5–10 mM)	−	−	++
Sotalol (100 μM)	−	−	+++
Erythromycin (10–100 μg/mL)	−	−	+++
ATX-II (10–20 nM)	+	++	++++
E-4031 (1–5 μM)	−	−	+++
Azimilide (5–20 μM)	+	++	+++
Chromanol 293B (10–100 μM)	+++	+++	+++

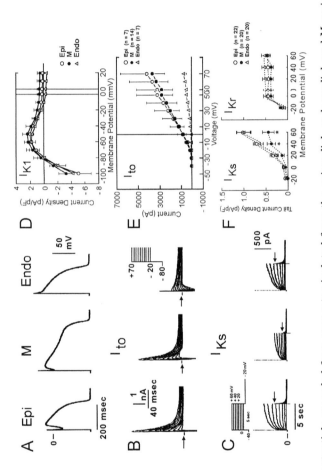

Figure 2. **A.** Action potentials recorded from myocytes isolated from the epicardial, endocardial, and M regions of the canine left ventricle. **B.** Transient outward current (I_{to}) recorded from the 3 cell types (current traces recorded during depolarizing steps from a holding potential of -80 mV to test potentials ranging between -20 and +70 mV). **C.** Voltage-dependent activation of the slowly activating component of the delayed rectifier K+ current (I_{Ks}) (currents were elicited by the voltage pulse protocol shown in the inset; Na+, K+- and Ca++-free solution). **D.** Current-voltage (I-V) relations for I_{K1} in epicardial, endocardial, and M region myocytes. Values are mean ± SD. **E.** The average peak I-V relationship for I_{to} for each of the 3 cell types. Values are mean ± SD. **F.** Voltage dependence of I_{Ks} (current remaining after exposure to E-4031) and I_{Kr} (E-4031-sensitive current). Values are mean ± SE. *$P<0.05$ compared with Epi or Endo. From References 12 and 21, with permission.

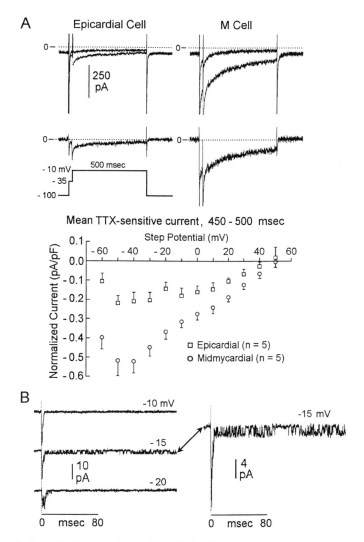

Figure 3. Late I_{Na} is larger in the M cell. **A.** Shown are whole-cell voltage clamp traces of sodium current. The upper panels show epicardial (left) and M cell (right) currents recorded in response to steps from –100 to –10 mV before and after the addition of 5 μM TTX. The TTX-sensitive currents are shown in the middle panels. Data from 5 cells of each type indicate consistently larger late sodium current in the M cell. Current-voltage (I-V) plots of the average current density during the last 50 milliseconds of each 500-millisecond voltage step are shown in the lower panels. **B.** Traces represent the activity of sodium channels in a cell-attached patch experiment conducted in an M cell. The bursting behavior observed with a step to –15 mV (from a holding potential of –100 mV; trace is amplified in the right panel) is similar to that reported for the ΔKPQ deletion of SCN5A (LQT3 syndrome). This bursting behavior, more commonly observed in M cells, is thought to contribute to the larger late I_{Na} of the M cells.

Table 2
Electrophysiologic Distinctions Among Epicardial Cells, Endocardial Cells, M Cells, and Purkinje Fibers

	Purkinje	M	Epi	Endo
Long APD, steep APD-rate	yes	yes	no	no
Develop EADs in response to agents with class III action	yes	yes	no	no
Develop DADs in reponse to digitalis, high Ca^{2+}, catechols	yes	yes	no	no
α_1-Agonist-induced change in APD	↑	↓	↔	↔
V_{max}	high	intermediate	low in surface tissues	
Phase 4 depolarization	yes	no	no	no
Depolarize in low $[K+]_o$	yes	no	no	no
Develop DADs with Bay K8644	no	yes	no	no
Found in bundles	yes	no	no	no

APD = action potential duration; DAD = delayed afterdepolarization; EAD = early afterdepolarization.

Table 3
Transmural Dispersion of Action Potential Duration Among Isolated Myocytes, Tissue Slices, and Arterially Perfused Canine Left Ventricular Wedge Preparations

	Control	I_{Kr} Block (D-Sotalol, 100 μM)	ATX-II (10–30 nM)
Myocytes	170±51 80–300 ms	–	–
Tissues	105±45 90–220 ms	286±129 140–450 ms	481±155 130–715 ms
Perfused Wedge	67±15 44–83 ms	87±16 72–112 ms	178±44 127–237 ms

Values are mean ± standard deviation (in ms). APD_{90} = action potential duration measured at 90% repolarization using floating microelectrodes. Range of values is indicated below each mean.

well coupled, the dispersion of APD is reduced to 64±25 milliseconds and dispersion of repolarization is reduced to 45±25 milliseconds (at a BCL of 2000 milliseconds; Table 4). In the wedge, electrotonic forces act to abbreviate the M cell action potential below its intrinsic duration and to prolong the APD of epicardial and endocardial cells beyond their intrinsic values.[28,40,41] A similar dispersion of repolarization (30 to 40 milliseconds at a BCL of 1400 to 1500 milliseconds; anesthetized young dog) is recorded in the canine heart in vivo with transmural monophasic action potential

Table 4

Action Potential Durations Measured in Different Regions of the
Arterially Perfused Canine Left Ventricular Wedge

	APD_{90} (ms)		Transmural Dispersion of APD_{90} (ms)		Transmural Dispersion of Repolarization Time (ms)	
BCL (msec)	1000	2000	1000	2000	1000	2000
Epicardium	207±20 (n=15)	217±24 (n=15)				
M cell	260±21 (n=15)	281±25 (n=15)	51±19 (n=15)	64±25 (n=15)	34±18 (n=15)	45±25 (n=15)
Endocardium	249±18 (n=15)	266±21 (n=15)				
Subendocardial Purkinje fiber	299±17 (n=14)	326±19 (n=14)				

Values are Mean ± standard deviation (in ms). APD_{90} = action potential duration measured at 90% repolarization using floating microelectrodes. BCL = Basic cycle length. From Reference 40 with permission.

(MAP) recordings[23,42] or when unipolar electrodes recordings are used to estimate the activation-recovery interval (ARI).[29]

Unipolar ARI and MAP measurements generally provide a reasonable approximation of APD at a local site. The TDR observed under control conditions in the canine heart in vivo and in the wedge preparations increases dramatically in the presence of agents with class III actions, such as d-sotalol, erythromycin, ATX-II, and anthopleurin-A, due to the preferential action of these agents to prolong the APD of the M cell.[28,29,40-42] Transmural repolarization gradients as large as 150 milliseconds can be observed under these conditions (Fig. 4). Unipolar electrograms provide an ARI that can be interpreted on the basis of biophysical theory,[43-46] and correlate well with APD under a variety of conditions. Bipolar electrograms, on the other hand, provide a repolarization complex that is not as readily interpretable because it represents the difference in the activity of two sites. Consequently, it is difficult to make a distinction between repolarization times at the two sites, and when differences exist, they are usually obscured. Irrespective of their placement within the wall, ARI values of bipolar electrograms, measured as the interval between the negative peak of the QRS and the *latest* peak of the T wave of the differentiated electrogram,[26] can greatly underestimate TDR.

The extent to which TDR is observed in vivo can vary dramatically as a function of the anesthetic used. Recent studies have shown dispersion of repolarization measured across the anterior canine left ventricular wall (transmural MAP recordings) to be considerably less when sodium pento-

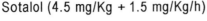

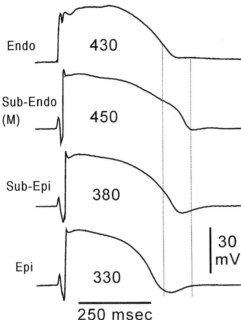

Sotalol (4.5 mg/Kg + 1.5 mg/Kg/h)

Endo   430

Sub-Endo (M)   450

Sub-Epi   380

Epi   330

30 mV

250 msec

Figure 4. MAPs recorded from 4 intramural sites in the anterior region of the left ventricular wall 48 minutes after the start of sotalol infusion (basic cycle length of 1000 milliseconds). Data were obtained from an open-chest dog under halothane anesthesia, with use of a recently developed method for MAP recording.[113] Numbers denote MAP duration measured from the middle of upstroke to 90% repolarization. In the anterior left wall M cells were found to reside preferentially in subendocardial layer. MAP recorded from this site had the longest duration. Overall transmural dispersion of repolarization totaled 120 milliseconds in this experiment. From Reference 114, with permission.

barbital is used for general anesthesia than when halothane is used. This difference in control is still more exaggerated when an I_{Kr} blocker like d-sotalol is infused (Fig. 4).[23,42] d-Sotalol produces a dramatic increase in TDR with halothane, but not with sodium pentobarbital anesthesia.[42] Abbreviation of the M cell APD but prolongation of the APD of epicardium and endocardium (secondary to block of I_{Ks} and late I_{Na}) contributes to these effects of sodium pentobarbital to reduce transmural dispersion.[47] The effects of other anesthetics remain to be studied.

Such differences in methodology are likely to account for the failure of some studies to discern significant repolarization gradients across the canine left ventricular wall in vivo[26,48,49] and the ability of others to demonstrate them consistently.[29,42,50] A relatively small TDR has been reported (at slow rates) in in vivo studies that have used pentobarbital for anesthesia[26,42,48,51] versus studies that have used other agents including isoflurane[29,50] or halothane.[42] Concordant with these findings, the development of in vivo models of torsades de pointes (TdP) has met with failure when sodium pentobarbital or α-chloralose, were used for anesthesia,[42,52] whereas TdP could be readily induced when halothane or isoflurane was used[29,42,50,53] or when no anesthesia was used.[54,55] Although TDR is much smaller with sodium pentobarbital than with halothane anesthesia, and TdP occurs only under halothane anesthesia, it is not as yet clear whether halothane and isoflurane also reduce TDR and thus lead to an underestimation of the transmural gradients present in the awake state.

These observations may help to explain the inability of earlier studies to detect the M cell. These issues are gradually coming into better focus and appear to involve the use by earlier studies of either 1) relatively fast stimulation rates; 2) bipolar recording techniques to estimate ARI; or 3) sodium pentobarbital anesthesia, or a combination of these. One of the few early studies to infer delayed repolarization in the deep layers of the canine left ventricle was that by Burgess et al,[56] in which repolarization was estimated by local measurement of refractoriness.

What purpose do the M cells serve and why did they evolve? One possibility is that they evolved for the purpose of improved pump efficiency, especially at slow rates where long depolarizations permit more efficient contractions. Epicardium and endocardium may have developed to electrically stabilize the M region, preventing excessive prolongation of the M cell action potential and/or the development of afterdepolarizations. There seems little doubt that epicardium and endocardium serve to electrically stabilize and abbreviate the APD of the M cells.[26,28,40,57,58] Removal or infarction of either would be expected to lead to a prolongation of the APD of the M cell.[15] In support of this hypothesis, the QT interval and QT dispersion (QTd) are reported to increase in some patients (2nd and 3rd day following an infarct) presenting with non–Q-wave infarction in which a thin margin of the endocardium is infarcted.[59] The effect of infarction to transiently augment transmural repolarization gradients may be still more exaggerated in patients receiving agents with class III antiarrhythmic actions or in patients manifesting congenital or acquired long QT. A highly arrhythmogenic substrate capable of maintaining both monomorphic and polymorphic arrhythmias would be expected to develop.

Role of the M Cell in Inscription of the Electrocardiographic T Wave

Transmural voltage gradients that develop as a result of the imposition of an M cell layer in the midmyocardial region of the ventricular wall play an important role in the inscription of the electrocardiographic T wave. Data from the perfused wedge have provided valuable new insights into the cellular basis of the T wave as well as the "pathophysiologic" U wave. These data point to transmural voltage gradients at the level of the action potential plateau as well as during phase 3, as the predominant forces governing the inscription of the T wave (Figs. 5 and 6). The results provide direct evidence in support of the hypothesis that voltage gradients between epicardium and the M region and between endocardium and the M region contribute prominently to the inscription of the electrocardiographic T

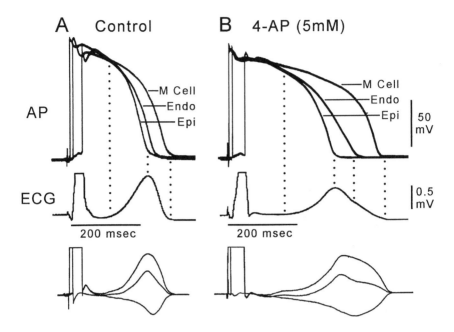

Figure 5. Voltage gradients at the level of the action potential plateau contribute prominently to inscription of the electrocardiographic T wave. **Top:** Action potentials simultaneously recorded from endocardial, epicardial, and M region sites of an arterially perfused canine left ventricular wedge preparation. **Middle:** Electrocardiogram (ECG) recorded across the wedge. **Bottom:** Computed voltage differences between the epicardium and M region action potentials ($\Delta V_{M\text{-}Epi}$) and between the M region and endocardium responses ($\Delta V_{Endo\text{-}M}$). If these traces are representative of the opposing voltage gradients on either side of the M region, responsible for inscription of the T wave, then the weighted sum of the two traces should yield a trace (middle trace in bottom grouping) resembling the ECG, which it does. **A.** Under control conditions the T wave begins when the plateau of epicardial action potential separates from that of the M cell. As epicardium repolarizes, the voltage gradient between epicardium and the M region continues to grow, giving rise to the ascending limb of the T wave. The voltage gradient between the M region and epicardium ($\Delta V_{M\text{-}Epi}$) reaches a peak when the epicardium is fully repolarized—this marks the peak of the T wave. On the other side of the ventricular wall, the endocardial plateau deviates from that of the M cell, generating an opposing voltage gradient ($\Delta V_{Endo\text{-}M}$) that limits the amplitude of the T wave and contributes to the initial part of the descending limb of the T wave. The voltage gradient between the endocardium and the M region reaches a peak when the endocardium is fully repolarized. The gradient continues to decline as the M cells repolarize. All gradients are extinguished when the longest M cells are fully repolarized. **B.** 4-Aminopyridine (4-AP) prolongs the action potential of the M cell more than those of the epicardial and endocardial cells, giving rise to a widening of the T wave and a prolongation of the QT interval. The greater separation of epicardial and endocardial repolarization times also gives rise to a notch in the descending limb of the T wave. Once again, the T wave begins when the plateau of epicardial action potential diverges from that of the M cell. The same relationships as described for A are observed

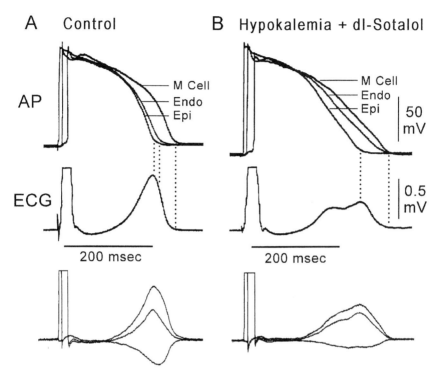

Figure 6. Shift of voltage gradients on either side of the M region results in T wave bifurcation. The format of the traces are the same as in Figure 5. For definition of traces, please see Figure 5. **A.** Control. **B.** In the presence of hypokalemia ($[K^+]_o$ = 1.5 mM), the I_{Kr} blocker dl-sotalol (100 μM) prolongs the QT interval and produces a bifurcation of the T wave, a morphology some authors refer to as T-U complex. The rate of repolarization of phase 3 of the action potential is slowed, giving rise to smaller opposing voltage gradients that cross over, producing a lower amplitude bifid T wave. Initially, the voltage gradient between the epicardium and M regions (M-Epi) is greater than that between endocardium and M region (Endo-M). When endocardium pulls away from the M cell, the opposing gradient (Endo-M) increases, interrupting the ascending limb of the T wave. Predominance of the M-Epi gradient is restored as the epicardial response continues to repolarize and the Epi-M gradients increases, thus resuming the ascending limb of the T wave. Full repolarization of epicardium marks the peak of the T wave. Repolarization of both endocardium and the M region contribute importantly to the descending limb. Basic cycle length = 1000 milliseconds. From Reference 114, with permission.

Figure 5 *(continued).* during the remainder of the T wave. The 4-AP–induced increase in dispersion of repolarization across the wall is accompanied by a corresponding increase in the T_{peak}-T_{end} interval in the pseudo-ECG. From Reference 114, with permission.

wave under normal conditions, and to the widened or bifurcated T wave and long QT interval observed under long QT conditions.

A number of theories have been advanced to explain the U wave. The most popular of these ascribes it to the delayed repolarization of the His-Purkinje system.[60] The small mass of the specialized conduction system is often difficult to reconcile with the sometimes very large U wave deflections reported in the literature, especially in cases of acquired and congenital long QT syndrome (LQTS). Consequently, we suggested that the M cells, more abundant in mass and possessing repolarization characteristics similar to those of Purkinje cells, may be responsible for the inscription of the pathophysiologic U wave.[22] Our recent findings derived from the wedge clearly indicate that what many clinicians refer to as an accentuated or inverted U wave is not a U wave but rather a component of the T wave whose descending or ascending limb (especially during hypokalemia) is interrupted (Fig. 6).[28,61,62] Variation in current flow across the wall due to shifting voltage gradients between epicardium and the M region and between endocardium and the M region appear to underlie these phenomena. The data suggest that the "pathophysiologic" U which develops under conditions of acquired or congenital LQTS is actually part of the T wave and that the various hump morphologies represent different levels of interruption of the ascending limb of the T wave, arguing for use of the term T2 in place of U to describe these events, as previously suggested by Lehmann et al.[63]

What then is responsible for the normal U wave, the very small distinct deflection following the T wave? The repolarization of the His-Purkinje system, as previously suggested by Watanabe,[60] seems the most plausible hypothesis.

Role of the M Cell in the LQTS

LQTS is characterized by the appearance of long QT intervals in the electrocardiogram (ECG) and atypical polymorphic ventricular arrhythmias displaying features of TdP that can lead to sudden cardiac death.[64-66] Genetic linkage analysis has identified 4 forms of congenital LQTS caused by mutations in ion channel genes located on chromosomes 3, 7, 11, and 21,[67-70] responsible for defects in the sodium channel (*SCN5A*, LQT3),[67] I_{Kr} (*HERG*, LQT2),[71] and I_{Ks} (*KvLQT1*, LQT1 or *KCNE1*, LQT5), respectively.[70,72,73] A brief discussion of the role of the M cell in LQTS follows.

As previously noted, electrical heterogeneity secondary to the presence of M cells within the ventricular wall contributes to the manifestation of the both normal and abnormal T waves in the ECG.[2-4,22,28,57,62,74,75] Preferential prolongation of cells in the M region is thought to underlie LQTS, contributing to the development of long QT intervals, the phenotypic appearance of abnormal T waves, and the development of TdP.

Direct lines of evidence in support of these hypotheses have been advanced, by use of the arterially perfused wedge preparation.[28,40,57,61,62,76] The wedge is capable of developing and sustaining a variety of arrhythmias, including TdP. We have used this experimental model to assess the contribution of electrical heterogeneity across the ventricular wall to the manifestation of the T wave under conditions of "acquired" LQTS mimicking the 4 genetic defects that have been linked to the congenital syndrome.

To mimic LQT1, we used chromanol 293B, an I_{Ks} blocker, and the β-adrenergic agonist isoproterenol. I_{Ks} block alone produced a homogeneous prolongation of repolarization and refractoriness across the ventricular wall and never induced arrhythmias. The addition of isoproterenol caused abbreviation of epicardial and endocardial APD with little or no change in the APD of the M cell, resulting in a marked augmentation of TDR and the development of spontaneous and stimulation-induced TdP.[76] These cellular changes give rise to a broad-based T wave and a long QT interval, characteristic of LQT1. The development of TdP in the model is exquisitely sensitive to β-adrenergic stimulation, consistent with the sensitivity of congenital LQTS, LQT1 in particular, to sympathetic stimulation.[64-66,77-81]

The I_{Kr} blocker d-sotalol was used to mimic LQT2 and acquired (drug-induced) forms of LQTS. A greater prolongation of the M cell action potential and slowing of phase 3 of the action potential of all 3 cell types results in a low-amplitude T wave, long QT interval, large TDR, and the development of spontaneous and stimulation-induced TdP. The addition of hypokalemia gives rise to low-amplitude T waves with a deeply notched or bifurcated appearance, similar to those commonly seen in patients with the LQT2 syndrome.[28,62]

ATX-II, an agent that augments late I_{Na} by slowing the inactivation of the sodium channel, was used to mimic the LQT3 syndrome.[28] ATX-II markedly prolongs the QT interval, delays the onset of the T wave, in some cases also widening it, and causes a sharp rise in TDR as a result of a greater prolongation of the APD of the M cell. The differential effect of ATX-II to prolong the M cell is likely due to the presence of a larger late sodium current in the M cell.[36] ATX-II produces a marked delay in onset of the T wave due to relatively large effects of the drug on epicardial and endocardial APD, consistent with the late-appearing T wave pattern observed in patients with the LQT3 syndrome. Also concordant with the clinical syndrome, the LQT3 model exhibits a steep rate dependence of the QT interval and develops TdP at slow rates. TdP, an atypical polymorphic ventricular tachycardia, is associated with prolongation of the QT interval in congenital and acquired LQTS. TdP has often been reported in patients receiving quinidine who develop hypokalemia and present with slow heart rates or long pauses. Such a combination of predisposing factors is common in the clinic. These conditions are similar to those under which quinidine and other agents induce EADs and triggered activity in isolated Purkinje fibers and M cells, suggesting a role for EAD-induced triggered activity in the genesis of TdP. While EADs may underlie the premature beat that initiates TdP, recent studies have provided considerable evidence in support of circus-movement reentry as the mechanism responsible for the maintenance of the arrhythmia.[2,29,50,82-84]

In the clinic, the onset of TdP has long been known to follow a short-long cycle length sequence.[85,86] Recent clinical reports indicate that a sudden moderate acceleration from an initially slow heart rate when followed by an intrinsic or extrinsic extrasystole holds the highest risk for induction of TdP in LQTS patients[87] as well as in animal models with acquired LQTS.[53,88-90] Similar characteristics are observed in isolated M cell preparations as well as in wedge preparations pretreated with APD-prolonging agents.[91] These observations suggest that the short of the short-long sequence may be as important or more important than the long.

Role of the M Cell in QTd

Interlead variation of the QT interval is thought to provide an index of the degree of heterogeneity of repolarization within the ventricles of the heart. This parameter, known as QTd, is generally defined as the difference between the longest and the shortest QT interval among the leads of a 12-lead standard ECG, and, in some instances, as the difference among the 6 precordial leads.[92,93] QTd has been proposed as a marker of heterogeneous repolarization and electrical instability because experimental studies have shown that increased dispersion of ventricular repolarization reduces the ventricular fibrillation threshold and facilitates the induction of reentrant ventricular arrhythmias.[94,95]

QTd in normal subjects usually ranges between 40 and 50 milliseconds; a 65-millisecond value is regarded by some as an upper normal limit.[93] QTd has been quantitated in a variety of clinical conditions, including congenital[96-99] and acquired[100] LQTS (>75 milliseconds), acute myocardial infarction,[101-106] congestive heart failure,[107,108] and hypertrophic cardiomyopathy.[109] Patients with congenital LQTS who fail to respond to β-adrenergic blockers (possibly LQT3 patients) have been reported to exhibit markedly increased (>130 milliseconds) QTd values.[98]

The cellular basis for the dispersion of the QT interval recorded at the body surface is not completely understood. Contributing to QTd are heterogeneities of repolarization time in the 3-dimensional structure of the ventricular myocardium; these are secondary to regional differences in APD and activation time. While differences in APD occur along the apicobasal and antero-postero axes in both epicardium and endocardium of many species, transitions are usually gradual.[110,111] Studies of the type documented above have also demonstrated important APD gradients along the transmural axis. Because transmural heterogeneities in repolarization time are more abrupt than those recorded along the surfaces of the heart, they are likely to represent a more onerous substrate for the development of arrhythmias, and their quantitation may provide a valuable tool for evaluation of arrhythmia risk. Data from the arterially perfused canine left ventricular wedge preparation have shown that the start of the T wave is caused by a more rapid decline of the plateau or phase 2 of the epicardial action potential, creating a voltage gradient across the wall. The gradient increases as the epicardial action potential continues to repolarize, reaching a maximum with full repolarization of epicardium; this juncture marks the peak of the T wave. The next region to repolarize is endocardium, giving rise to the initial descending limb of the upright T wave. The last region to repolarize is the M region, contributing to the final segment of the T wave. Full repolarization of the M region marks the end of the T wave (Figs. 5 and 6). The time interval between the peak and the end of the T wave represents the TDR. Conditions known to augment corrected QT (QTc) dispersion, including acquired LQTS (class Ia or III antiarrhythmics), lead to an augmentation of TDR in the wedge due to a preferential effect of the drugs to prolong the M cell action potential. Agents known to diminish QTc dispersion, such as amiodarone, also diminish TDR in the wedge by causing a preferential prolongation of APD in epicardium and endocardium. These data point to intraventricular differences in the repolarization of cells in the M region as the basis for QTd under normal and long QT conditions. When augmentation of QTd is due to amplified TDR, it is likely to correlate well with arrhythmic risk. When secondary to differences in repolarization at widely spaced sites, it is unlikely to be prognostic of risk. The available experimental data suggest that the interval delimited by the peak to the end of the T wave, because it represents an accurate measure of regional dispersion of repolarization across the ventricular wall, may also prove to be a valuable index for assessment of arrhythmia risk.[112]

References

1. Antzelevitch C, Sicouri S, Litovsky SH, et al. Heterogeneity within the ventricular wall: Electrophysiology and pharmacology of epicardial, endocardial and M cells. *Circ Res* 1991;69:1427-1449.
2. Antzelevitch C, Sicouri S. Clinical relevance of cardiac arrhythmias generated by afterdepolarizations: The role of M cells in the generation of U waves, triggered activity and torsade de pointes. *J Am Coll Cardiol* 1994;23:259-277.
3. Antzelevitch C, Sicouri S, Lukas A, et al. Clinical implications of electrical heterogeneity in the heart: The electrophysiology and pharmacology of epicardial, M and endocardial cells. In Podrid PJ, Kowey PR (eds): *Cardiac Arrhyth-*

mia: Mechanism, Diagnosis and Management. Baltimore: Williams & Wilkins; 1995:88-107.

4. Antzelevitch C, Sicouri S, Lukas A, et al. Regional differences in the electrophysiology of ventricular cells: Physiological and clinical implications. In Zipes DP, Jalife J (eds): *Cardiac Electrophysiology: From Cell to Bedside*. Philadelphia: W. B. Saunders Co.; 1995:228-245.

5. Antzelevitch C. The M cell. Invited Editorial Comment. *J Cardiovasc Pharmacol Ther* 1997;2:73-76.

6. Gilmour RF, Zipes DP. Different electrophysiological responses of canine endocardium and epicardium to combined hyperkalemia, hypoxia, and acidosis. *Circ Res* 1980;46:814-825.

7. Litovsky SH, Antzelevitch C. Transient outward current prominent in canine ventricular epicardium but not endocardium. *Circ Res* 1988;62:116-126.

8. Krishnan SC, Antzelevitch C. Sodium channel blockade produces opposite electrophysiologic effects in canine ventricular epicardium and endocardium. *Circ Res* 1991;69:277-291.

9. Fedida D, Giles WR. Regional variations in action potentials and transient outward current in myocytes isolated from rabbit left ventricle. *J Physiol (Lond)* 1991;442:191-209.

10. Krishnan SC, Antzelevitch C. Flecainide-induced arrhythmia in canine ventricular epicardium: Phase 2 reentry? *Circulation* 1993;87:562-572.

11. Di Diego JM, Antzelevitch C. Pinacidil-induced electrical heterogeneity and extrasystolic activity in canine ventricular tissues: Does activation of ATP-regulated potassium current promote phase 2 reentry? *Circulation* 1993; 88:1177-1189.

12. Liu DW, Gintant GA, Antzelevitch C. Ionic bases for electrophysiological distinctions among epicardial, midmyocardial, and endocardial myocytes from the free wall of the canine left ventricle. *Circ Res* 1993;72:671-687.

13. Lukas A, Antzelevitch C. Differences in the electrophysiological response of canine ventricular epicardium and endocardium to ischemia: Role of the transient outward current. *Circulation* 1993;88:2903-2915.

14. Di Diego JM, Antzelevitch C. High [Ca^{2+}]-induced electrical heterogeneity and extrasystolic activity in isolated canine ventricular epicardium: Phase 2 reentry. *Circulation* 1994;89:1839-1850.

15. Yan GX, Antzelevitch C. Cellular basis for the electrocardiographic J wave. *Circulation* 1996;93:372-379.

16. Sicouri S, Antzelevitch C. A subpopulation of cells with unique electrophysiological properties in the deep subepicardium of the canine ventricle: The M cell. *Circ Res* 1991;68:1729-1741.

17. Sicouri S, Antzelevitch C. Drug-induced afterdepolarizations and triggered activity occur in a discrete subpopulation of ventricular muscle cell (M cells) in the canine heart: Quinidine and digitalis. *J Cardiovasc Electrophysiol* 1993;4:48-58.

18. Sicouri S, Fish J, Antzelevitch C. Distribution of M cells in the canine ventricle. *J Cardiovasc Electrophysiol* 1994;5:824-837.

19. Sicouri S, Antzelevitch C. Electrophysiologic characteristics of M cells in the canine left ventricular free wall. *J Cardiovasc Electrophysiol* 1995;6:591-603.

20. Drouin E, Charpentier F, Gauthier C, et al. Electrophysiological characteristics of cells spanning the left ventricular wall of human heart: Evidence for the presence of M cells. *J Am Coll Cardiol* 1995;26:185-192.

21. Liu DW, Antzelevitch C. Characteristics of the delayed rectifier current (I_{Kr} and I_{Ks}) in canine ventricular epicardial, midmyocardial and endocardial myocytes:

A weaker I_{Ks} contributes to the longer action potential of the M cell. *Circ Res* 1995;76:351-365.

22. Antzelevitch C, Nesterenko VV, Yan GX. The role of M cells in acquired long QT syndrome, U waves and torsade de pointes. *J Electrocardiol* 1996;28(suppl):131-138.

23. Weissenburger J, Nesterenko VV, Antzelevitch C. Intramural monophasic action potentials (MAP) display steeper APD-rate relations and higher sensitivity to class III agents than epicardial and endocardial MAPs: Characteristics of the M cell in vivo. *Circulation* 1995;92:I300. Abstract.

24. Sicouri S, Quist M, Antzelevitch C. Evidence for the presence of M cells in the guinea pig ventricle. *J Cardiovasc Electrophysiol* 1996;7:503-511.

25. Li GR, Feng J, Carrier M, Nattel S. Transmural electrophysiologic heterogeneity in the human ventricle. *Circulation* 1995;92:I158. Abstract.

26. Anyukhovsky EP, Sosunov EA, Rosen MR. Regional differences in electrophysiologic properties of epicardium, midmyocardium and endocardium: In vitro and in vivo correlations. *Circulation* 1996;94:1981-1988.

27. Rodriguez-Sinovas A, Cinca J, Tapias A, et al. Lack of evidence of M-cells in porcine left ventricular myocardium. *Cardiovasc Res* 1997;33:307-313.

28. Shimizu W, Antzelevitch C. Sodium channel block with mexiletine is effective in reducing dispersion of repolarization and preventing torsade de pointes in LQT2 and LQT3 models of the long-QT syndrome. *Circulation* 1997;96:2038-2047.

29. El-Sherif N, Caref EB, Yin H, Restivo M. The electrophysiological mechanism of ventricular arrhythmias in the long QT syndrome: Tridimensional mapping of activation and recovery patterns. *Circ Res* 1996;79:474-492.

30. Weirich J, Bernhardt R, Loewen N, et al. Regional- and species-dependent effects of K^+-channel blocking agents on subendocardium and mid-wall slices of human, rabbit, and guinea pig myocardium. *Pflügers Arch* 1996;431:R 130. Abstract.

31. Furukawa T, Myerburg RJ, Furukawa N, et al. Differences in transient outward currents of feline endocardial and epicardial myocytes. *Circ Res* 1990;67:1287-1291.

32. Clark RB, Bouchard RA, Salinas-Stefanon E, et al. Heterogeneity of action potential waveforms and potassium currents in rat ventricle. *Cardiovasc Res* 1993;27:1795-1799.

33. Wettwer E, Amos GJ, Posival H, Ravens U. Transient outward current in human ventricular myocytes of subepicardial and subendocardial origin. *Circ Res* 1994;75:473-482.

34. Nabauer M, Beuckelmann DJ, Uberfuhr P, Steinbeck G. Regional differences in current density and rate-dependent properties of the transient outward current in subepicardial and subendocardial myocytes of human left ventricle. *Circulation* 1996;93:168-177.

35. Di Diego JM, Sun ZQ, Antzelevitch C. I_{to} and action potential notch are smaller in left vs. right canine ventricular epicardium. *Am J Physiol* 1996;271:H548-H561.

36. Eddlestone GT, Zygmunt AC, Antzelevitch C. Larger late sodium current contributes to the longer action potential of the M cell in canine ventricular myocardium. *PACE* 1996;19:II569. Abstract.

37. Brahmajothi MV, Morales MJ, Reimer KA, Strauss HC. Regional localization of ERG, the channel protein responsible for the rapid component of the delayed rectifier, K^+ current in the ferret heart. *Circ Res* 1997;81:128-135.

38. Burashnikov A, Antzelevitch C. α-Agonists produce opposite effect on action potential duration in Purkinje and M cells isolated from the canine left ventricle. *PACE* 1995;18:II935. Abstract.

39. Burashnikov A, Antzelevitch C. Mechanisms underlying early afterdepolarization activity are different in canine Purkinje and M cell preparations. Role of intracellular calcium. *Circulation* 1996;94:I527. Abstract.

40. Antzelevitch C, Sun ZQ, Zhang ZQ, Yan GX. Cellular and ionic mechanisms underlying erythromycin-induced long QT and torsade de pointes. *J Am Coll Cardiol* 1996;28:1836-1848.

41. Yan GX, Antzelevitch C. Delayed repolarization of M cells underlies the manifestation of U waves, notched T waves and long QT intervals in the electrocardiogram (ECG). *Circulation* 1995;92:I480. Abstract.

42. Weissenburger J, Nesterenko VV, Antzelevitch C. M cells contribute to transmural dispersion of repolarization and to the development of torsade de pointes in the canine heart in vivo. *PACE* 1996;19:II-707. Abstract.

43. Plonsey R. Action potential sources and their volume conductor fields. *Proc IEEE* 1977;65:601-611.

44. Spach MS, Barr RC, Serwer GA, et al. Extracellular potentials related to intracellular action potentials in the dog Purkinje system. *Circ Res* 1972;30:505-519.

45. Haws CW, Lux RL. Correlation between in vivo transmembrane action potential durations and action-recovery intervals from electrograms. Effects of interventions that alter repolarization time. *Circulation* 1990;81:281-288.

46. Steinhaus BM. Estimating cardiac transmembrane activation and recovery times from unipolar and bipolar extracellular electrograms: A simulation study. *Circ Res* 1989;64:449-462.

47. Sun ZQ, Eddlestone GT, Antzelevitch C. Ionic mechanisms underlying the effects of sodium pentobarbital to diminish transmural dispersion of repolarization. *PACE* 1997;20:1116. Abstract.

48. Friegang KD, Becker R, Bauer A, et al. Electrophysiological properties of individual muscle layers in the in vivo canine heart. *J Am Coll Cardiol* 1996;27(suppl A):124A. Abstract.

49. Anyukhovsky EP, Sosunov EA, Feinmark SJ, Rosen MR. Effects of quinidine on repolarization in canine epicardium, midmyocardium, and endocardium. II. In vivo study. *Circulation* 1997;96:4019-4026.

50. El-Sherif N, Chinushi M, Caref EB, Restivo M. Electrophysiological mechanism of the characteristic electrocardiographic morphology of torsade de pointes tachyarrhythmias in the long-QT syndrome. Detailed analysis of ventricular tridimensional activation patterns. *Circulation* 1997;96:4392-4399.

51. Sosunov EA, Anyukhovsky EP, Rosen MR. Comparison of repolarization of cells from different layers of myocardium in vitro and in vivo. *Biophys J* 1996;70(Pt. 2):A276. Abstract.

52. Duker GD, Linhardt GS, Rahmberg M. An animal model for studying class III-induced proarrhythmias in the halothane-anesthetized dog. *J Am Coll Cardiol* 1994;23:326A. Abstract.

53. Vos MA, Verduyn SC, Gorgels APM, et al. Reproducible induction of early afterdepolarizations and torsade de pointes arrhythmias by d-sotalol and pacing in dogs with chronic atrioventricular block. *Circulation* 1995;91:864-872.

54. Weissenburger J, Davy JM, Chezalviel F, et al. Arrhythmogenic activities of antiarrhythmic drugs in conscious hypokalemic dogs with atrioventricular block: Comparison between quinidine, lidocaine, flecainide, propranolol and sotalol. *J Pharmacol Exp Ther* 1991;259:871-883.

55. Weissenburger J, Davy JM, Chezalviel F. Experimental models of torsade de pointes. *Fundam Clin Pharmacol* 1993;7:29-38.

56. Burgess MJ, Green LS, Millar K, et al. The sequence of normal ventricular recovery. *Am Heart J* 1972;84:660-669.

57. Yan GX, Shimizu W, Antzelevitch C. Characteristics and distribution of M cells in arterially perfused canine left ventricular wedge preparations. *Circulation* 1998;98:1921-1927.

58. Van Capelle FJL. Propagation and reentry in two dimensions. In Zipes DP, Jalife J (eds): *Cardiac Electrophysiology: From Cell to Bedside*. Philadelphia: W. B. Saunders Co.; 1990:175-182.

59. Chauhan VS, Skanes AC, Tang ASL. Dynamics and dispersion of QT intervals: Q-wave versus non Q-wave myocardial infarction. *Circulation* 1996;94:I433. Abstract.

60. Watanabe Y. Purkinje repolarization as a possible cause of the U wave in the electrocardiogram. *Circulation* 1975;51:1030-1037.

61. Shimizu W, Antzelevitch C. Characteristics of spontaneous as well as stimulation-induced torsade de pointes in LQT2 and LQT3 models of the long QT syndrome. *Circulation* 1997;96:I554. Abstract.

62. Yan GX, Antzelevitch C. Cellular basis for the normal T wave and the electrocardiographic manifestations of the long QT syndrome. *Circulation* 1998; 98:1928-1936.

63. Lehmann MH, Suzuki F, Fromm BS, et al. T-wave "humps" as a potential electrocardiographic marker of the long QT syndrome. *J Am Coll Cardiol* 1994;24:746-754.

64. Schwartz PJ. The idiopathic long QT syndrome: Progress and questions. *Am Heart J* 1985;109:399-411.

65. Moss AJ, Schwartz PJ, Crampton RS, et al. The long QT syndrome: Prospective longitudinal study of 328 families. *Circulation* 1991;84:1136-1144.

66. Zipes DP. The long QT interval syndrome: A Rosetta stone for sympathetic related ventricular tachyarrhythmias. *Circulation* 1991;84:1414-1419.

67. Wang Q, Shen J, Splawski I, et al. *SCN5A* mutations associated with an inherited cardiac arrhythmia, long QT syndrome. *Cell* 1995;80:805-811.

68. Curran ME, Splawski I, Timothy KW, et al. A molecular basis for cardiac arrhythmia: *HERG* mutations cause long QT syndrome. *Cell* 1995;80:795-803.

69. Wang Q, Curran ME, Splawski I, et al. Positional cloning of a novel potassium channel gene: *KVLQT1* mutations cause cardiac arrhythmias. *Nat Genet* 1996;12:17-23.

70. Splawski I, Tristani-Firouzi M, Lehmann MH, et al. Mutations in the hminK gene cause long QT syndrome and suppress I_{Ks} function. *Nat Genet* 1997;17:338-340.

71. Sanguinetti MC, Jiang C, Curran ME, Keating MT. A mechanistic link between an inherited and an acquired cardiac arrhythmia: *HERG* encodes the I_{Kr} potassium channel. *Cell* 1995;81:299-307.

72. Sanguinetti MC, Curran ME, Zou A, et al. Coassembly of KvLQT1 and minK (IsK) proteins to form cardiac I_{Ks} potassium channel. *Nature* 1996;384:80-83.

73. Barhanin J, Lesage F, Guillemare E, et al. KvLQT1 and IsK (minK) proteins associate to form the I_{Ks} cardiac potassium current. *Nature* 1996;384:78-80.

74. Lukas A, Antzelevitch C. The contribution of K+ currents to electrical heterogeneity across the canine ventricular wall under normal and ischemic conditions. In Dhalla NS, Pierce GN, Panagia V (eds): *Pathophysiology of Heart Failure*. Boston: Academic Publishers; 1996:440-456.

75. Antzelevitch C. Repolarizing currents in canine ventricular myocardium. Regional differences and similarities. In Vereecke J, Verdonck F, van Boagaert P-P (eds): *Potassium Channels in Normal and Pathological Conditions. In honor of Professor Edward Carmeliet.* Leuven: Leuven University Press; 1996:256-259.
76. Shimizu W, Antzelevitch C. Cellular basis for the ECG features of the LQT1 form of the long QT syndrome: Effects of beta-adrenergic agonists, antagonists and sodium channel blockers on transmural dispersion of repolarization and torsade de pointes. *Circulation* 1998;98:2314-2322.
77. Crampton RS. Another link between the left stellate ganglion and the long Q-T syndrome. *Am Heart J* 1978;96:130-132.
78. Crampton RS. Preeminence of the left stellate ganglion in the long Q-T syndrome. *Circulation* 1979;59:769-778.
79. Timothy KW, Zhang L, Meyer KJ, Vincent GM. Differences in precipitators of cardiac arrest and sudden death in chromosome 11 versus 7 genotype long QT syndrome patients. *Circulation* 1996;94:I204. Abstract.
80. Ali RH, Zareba W, Rosero SZ, et al. Adrenergic triggers and non-adrenergic factors associated with cardiac events in long QT syndrome patients. *PACE* 1997;20:1072. Abstract.
81. Schwartz PJ, Malteo PS, Moss AJ, et al. Gene-specific influence on the triggers for cardiac arrest in the long QT syndrome. *Circulation* 1997;96:I-212. Abstract.
82. Shimizu W, Ohe T, Kurita T, et al. Early afterdepolarizations induced by isoproterenol in patients with congenital long QT syndrome. *Circulation* 1991;84:1915-1923.
83. Shimizu W, Ohe T, Kurita T, et al. Effects of verapamil and propranolol on early afterdepolarizations and ventricular arrhythmias induced by epinephrine in congenital long QT syndrome. *J Am Coll Cardiol* 1995;26:1299-1309.
84. Akar FG, Yan GX, Antzelevitch C, Rosenbaum DS. Optical maps reveal reentrant mechanism of torsade de pointes based on topography and electrophysiology of mid-myocardial cells. *Circulation* 1997;96(8):I355. Abstract.
85. Coumel P. Early afterdepolarizations and triggered activity in clinical arrhythmias. In Rosen MR, Janse MJ, Wit AL (eds): *Cardiac Electrophysiology: A Text Book.* Mount Kisco, NY: Futura Publishing Co., Inc.; 1990:387-411.
86. Moss AJ. Long QT syndrome. In Podrid PJ, Kowey PR (eds): *Cardiac Arrhythmia: Mechanisms, Diagnosis and Management.* Baltimore: Williams & Wilkins; 1995:1110-1120.
87. Locati EH, Maison-Blanche P, Dejode P, et al. Spontaneous sequences of onset of torsade de pointes in patients with acquired prolonged repolarization: Quantitative analysis of Holter recordings. *J Am Coll Cardiol* 1995;25:1564-1575.
88. Cobbe SM, Hoffman E, Ritzenhoff A, et al. Action of sotalol on potential reentrant pathways and ventricular tachyarrhythmias in conscious dogs in the late postmyocardial infarction phase. *Circulation* 1983;68:865-871.
89. Habbab MA, El-Sherif N. TU alternans, long QTU, and torsade de pointes: Clinical and experimental observations. *PACE* 1992;15:916-931.
90. Sasyniuk BI, Brunet S. Torsade de pointes induced by quinidine, d-sotalol, and E-4031 in the isolated rabbit heart: Importance of interval dependent dispersion of repolarization. *PACE* 1995;18:II-904. Abstract.
91. Burashnikov A, Antzelevitch C. Mechanism of acceleration-induced early afterdepolarization activity and action potential prolongation in tissues isolated from the M region of the canine ventricule. *PACE* 1996;19:II645. Abstract.

92. Statters DJ, Malik M, Ward DE, Camm AJ. QT dispersion: Problems of methodology and clinical significance. *J Cardiovasc Electrophysiol* 1994;5:672-685.

93. Surawicz B. Will QT dispersion play a role in clinical decision-making? *J Cardiovasc Electrophysiol* 1996;7:777-784.

94. Han J, Moe GK. Nonuniform recovery of excitability in ventricular muscle. *Circ Res* 1964;14:44-60.

95. Kuo CS, Munakata K, Reddy CP, Surawicz B. Characteristics and possible mechanism of ventricular arrhythmia dependent on the dispersion of action potential durations. *Circulation* 1983;67:1356-1367.

96. Day CP, McComb JM, Campbell RWF. QT dispersion: An indication of arrhythmia risk in patients with long QT intervals. *Br Heart J* 1990;63:342-344.

97. Linker NJ, Colonna P, Kekwick CA, et al. Assessment of QT dispersion in symptomatic patients with congenital long QT syndromes. *Am J Cardiol* 1992;69:634-638.

98. Priori SG, Napolitano C, Diehl L, Schwartz PJ. Dispersion of the QT interval: A marker of therapeutic efficacy in the idiopathic long QT syndrome. *Circulation* 1994;89:1681-1689.

99. Shimizu W, Kamakura S, Ohe T, et al. Diagnostic value of recovery time measured by body surface mapping in patients with congenital long QT syndrome. *Am J Cardiol* 1994;74:780-785.

100. Hii JTY, Wyse DG, Gillis AM, et al. Precordial QT interval dispersion as a marker of torsade de pointes. Disparate effects of class Ia antiarrhythmic drugs and amiodarone. *Circulation* 1992;86:1376-1382.

101. Loo AVD, Arendts W, Hohnloser SH. Variability of QT dispersion measurements in the surface electrocardiogram in patients with acute myocardial infarction and in normal subjects. *Am J Cardiol* 1994;74:1113-1118.

102. Zareba W, Moss AJ, Cessie SL. Dispersion of ventricular repolarization and arrhythmic cardiac death in coronary artery disease. *Am J Cardiol* 1994;74:550-553.

103. Perkiomaki JS, Koistinen MJ, Mayry S, Huikuri HV. Dispersion of QT interval in patients with and without susceptibility to ventricular tachyarrhythmias after previous myocardial infarction. *J Am Coll Cardiol* 1995;26:174-179.

104. Moreno FL, Villanueva MT, Karagounis LA, Anderson JL, the TEAM-2 Study Investigators. Reduction in QT interval dispersion by successful thrombolytic therapy in acute myocardial infarction. *Circulation* 1994;90:94-100.

105. Glancy JM, Garratt CJ, Woods KL, Bono DPD. QT dispersion and mortality after myocardial infarction. *Lancet* 1995;345:945-948.

106. Leitch J, Basta M, Dobson A. QT dispersion does not predict early ventricular fibrillation after acute myocardial infarction. *PACE* 1995;18:45-48.

107. Barr CS, Naas A, Freeman M, et al. QT dispersion and sudden unexpected death in chronic heart failure. *Lancet* 1994;343:327-329.

108. Davey PP, Bateman J, Mulligan IP, et al. QT interval dispersion in chronic heart failure and left ventricular hypertrophy: Relation to autonomic nervous system and Holter tape abnormalities. *Br Heart J* 1994;71:268-273.

109. Buja G, Miorelli M, Turrini P, et al. Comparison of QT dispersion in hypertrophic cardiomyopathy between patients with and without ventricular arrhythmias and sudden death. *Am J Cardiol* 1993;72:973-976.

110. Zabel M, Portnoy S, Franz MR. Electrocardiographic indexes of dispersion of ventricular repolarization: An isolated heart validation study. *J Am Coll Cardiol* 1995;25:746-752.

111. Franz MR, Bargheer K, Costard-Jaeckle A, et al. Human ventricular repolarization and T wave genesis. *Prog Cardiovasc Dis* 1991;33:369-384.
112. Antzelevitch C, Shimizu W, Yan GX, Sicouri S: Cellular basis for QT dispersion. *J Electrocardiol* 1998;30(suppl):168-175.
113. Nesterenko VV, Weissenburger J. Experimental evidence for re-interpretation of basis for the monophasic action potential: A new technique with large amplitude and stable transmural signals. *Circulation* 1995;92:I299. Abstract.
114. Antzelevitch C, Nesterenko VV, Shimizu W, Di Diego JM. Electrophysiological characteristics of the M cell. In Franz MR, Schmitt C, Zrenner B (eds): *Monophasic Action Potentials*. Berlin: Springer; 1997:212-226.

35

Monophasic Action Potentials and Torsades de Pointes:

Bridging the Gap Between Experimental Studies and Clinical Data

Lars Eckardt, MD, Robert Johna, MD, Martin Borggrefe, MD, FESC, Günter Breithardt, MD, FESC, FACC and Wilhelm Haverkamp, MD

Introduction

Literally translated from French as *"twisting of the points,"* torsades de pointes (TdP), as initially described by Dessertenne,[1] is a distinct form of life-threatening polymorphic ventricular tachycardia (VT). The tachyarrhythmia is characterized by the electrocardiographic configuration of a progressively changing ventricular axis and spontaneous termination, with the exception of rare degeneration into ventricular fibrillation in the presence of abnormal QT prolongation and/or abnormal TU complexes (Fig. 1). It may be associated with a wide variety of clinical entities including the congenital long QT syndrome (LQTS),[2] and acquired abnormal QT prolongation (Table 1). The majority of cases of acquired TdP occur due to treatment with class Ia and class III antiarrhythmic agents, which prolong the QT interval by delaying repolarization.[3-5] TdP related to these antiarrhythmic drugs has been estimated to occur in 1% to 8% of patients treated.

From Franz MR (ed): *Monophasic Action Potentials: Bridging Cell and Bedside.*
©Futura Publishing Company, Inc., Armonk, NY, 2000.

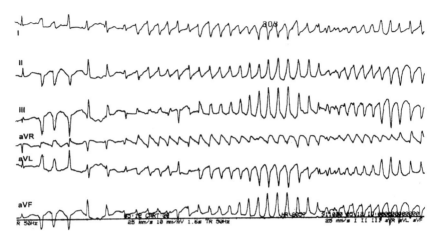

Figure 1. Typical example of torsades de pointes induced by quinidine (3rd day of treatment). Paper speed: 25mm/s.

QT prolongation seems to be an essential but not sufficient factor to provoke TdP. In many cases, concomitant triggers such as hypokalemia and bradycardia are of major importance,[3,4,6,7] as they increase the propensity toward the development of TdP.

Whereas the QT interval in the surface electrocardiogram (ECG) measures the duration of repolarization of the whole ventricular myocardium, monophasic action potential (MAP) recordings have been demonstrated to provide more precise information on local repolarization and activation because MAPs derive from a limited area not more than 5 mm in diameter.[8] MAPs can be used to measure accurately the time course of repolarization[8-10] because they are similar to transmembrane action potentials with respect to duration and shape. Thus, they may be of particular importance in repolarization-related arrhythmias such as TdP.

Mechanism of TdP

The mechanisms that cause QT prolongation, T(U) abnormalities, and TdP are far from being completely understood. Dessertenne[1] suggested that the unusual configuration of the tachycardia was due to ventricular activation by at least two autonomic foci firing at slightly different rates. This hypothesis could be replicated in an early experimental animal model.[11] During recent years, there has been growing evidence that early afterdepolarizations (EADs) are one, or even the most important, mechanism underlying triggered activity as the electrophysiologic substrate of TdP.[12,13] EADs are cellular depolarizations that occur during phases 2 and 3 of the transmembrane potential before repolarization is completed. These

Table 1
Clinical Conditions Associated with
Repolarization Abnormalities and Torsades de Pointes

Congenital forms
  Jervell and Lange-Nielsen syndrome
  Romano-Ward syndrome

Drugs and chemicals
  antiarrhythmics

class Ia agents	quinidine
	procainamide
	disopyramide
class III agents	amiodarone
	d, l sotalol
	N-acetylprocainamide
	sematilide
	new "pure" class" III agents (eg, dofetilide, ibutilide d-sotalol)
class IV agents	bepridil
	lidoflazine, prenylamine
psychotropic agents	phenothiazines (eg, thioridazine, chlorpromazine)
	haloperidol
	droperidol
	chloral hydrate
	tri- and tetracylic antidepressants (eg, amitryptiline, imipramine, doxepin, maprotiline)
	pimozide
antimicrobial agents	erythromycin
	spiramycin
	trimethoprim-sulfamethoxazole
antimalarial drugs	halofantrine
antihistamines	terfenadine
	astemizole
	amantadine
hypolipidemic agents	probucol
serotonin antagonists	ketanserin, zimeldine
miscellaneous	terodiline
	cisapride
	trimetaphan
	pentamidine

Bradyarrhythmias
  sinus bradycardia
  AV block

Metabolic disturbances
  hypokalemia
  hypocalcemia
  hypomagnesemia
  hypothyroidism

Nutritional deficits
  anorexia nervosa
  liquid protein diets

Cerebrovascular disorders
  subarachnoidal hemorrhage
  intracranial trauma

AV = atrioventricular. Reproduced from Reference 18, with permission.

depolarizations may give rise to premature action potentials or even to trains of potentials that have been referred to as *triggered activity*.[14] Apart from or next to EAD-related ectopic beats, the nonuniform prolongation of action potentials that is a substrate for reentry has been proposed as the underlying mechanism of TdP ("dispersion hypothesis").[15] In a 3-dimensional analysis of activation patterns, El-Sherif et al[16] recently showed that the initial beat of TdP arose as focal activity from a subendocardial site whereas subsequent beats were due to successive subendocardial focal activity, reentrant excitation, or a combination of both mechanisms. In addition, Gray et al[17] favored the concept of several coexisting spiral waves drifting rapidly through the ventricles and giving rise to the complex pattern of TdP. Thus, more than one mechanism may be implicated in the genesis of TdP and it appears possible that TdP has multiple causes serving as a final common pathway for the electrocardiographic pattern viewed as characteristic of TdP. Furthermore, the mechanism that initiates TdP might differ from that which maintains it.

MAPs and TdP

The insights into the basic mechanisms of TdP are, to a great extent, based on experimental and clinical studies. MAPs have been demonstrated to be of particular value, as they may be useful to investigate both EADs and dispersion of repolarization.

Experimental Studies of TdP Using MAPs

Numerous experimental models have been developed to study TdP and its mechanisms.[18] The following paragraphs concentrate one those studies in which MAP recording has provided valuable information.

MAPs, EADs, and TdP

EADs have been recorded in transmembrane potentials in isolated cardiac tissue under various conditions, such as during administration of cesium chloride,[19-21] anthopleurin-A,[22] and quinidine.[23] When a bolus of intravenous cesium chloride is administered to dogs, bradycardia-dependent QTU prolongation and polymorphic ventricular tachyarrhythmias resembling TdP occur.[19] Levine et al[21] as well as Sato et al[24] recorded MAPs in this model of drug-related TdP. They described interruptions of the smooth contour of phase 2 or 3 of the action potential that corresponded to a prolonged QT interval and gave rise to ectopic ventricular beats. A typical example is given in Figure 2. The MAP deflections were interpreted to represent EADs. Both the MAP deflections and the ventricular arrhythmias resolved simultaneously during overdrive pacing. Numerous other investigators have observed changes in the MAP contour which were often described as "humps." Although the recordings in many cases showed only slight changes in the MAP contour rather than marked deflections, they were almost always interpreted to represent EADs. This assumption could not be proved by intracellular recordings. Bailie et al[25] demonstrated that magnesium diminishes or even suppresses cesium-related arrhythmias and EAD-like changes in right ventricular endocardial MAP recordings in a canine cesium model. This provided experimental support and a possible explanation for the clinical use of magnesium in patients with TdP. In addition, it nicely correlated to transmembrane potential recordings that demonstrated suppression of EADs by magnesium (Fig. 3).

The sea anemone toxin anthopleurin-A belongs to a different class of drugs which has also been demonstrated to induce action potential prolongation and EADs in vitro and bradycardia-dependent QT prolongation, as well as TdP in dogs in vivo.[22] It markedly delays sodium inactivation and, thus, may represent a pharmacologic model for the genetic variant of LQTS with a mutation for the gene that encodes the voltage-gated sodium channel α subunit ($SCN5A$).[26] MAP recordings strongly suggested that the prominent U wave in the surface ECG

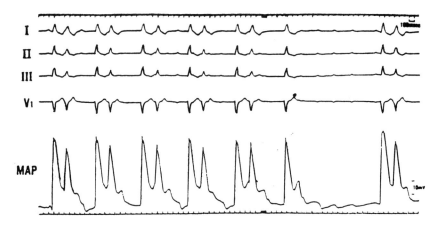

Figure 2. Ventricular ectopy after administration of cesium chloride in a dog and an example of possible early afterdepolarizations (EADs) in the MAPs. MAPs were recorded with use of the Franz electrode catheter. When the amplitude of the EAD reached a threshold potential, ventricular ectopic beats appeared. As the deflection of the 6th ventricular beat did not result in a ventricular ectopic, Sato et al[24] assumed that the amplitude of the EAD was below the threshold potential, and so the EAD did not fire. Reproduced from Reference 24, with permission.

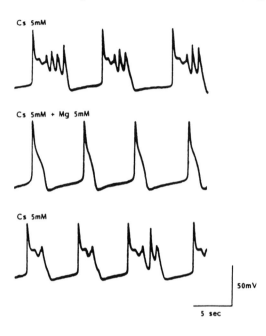

Figure 3. Effect of magnesium chloride on early afterdepolarizations (EADs) in transmembrane potential recordings. EADs were induced by cesium in canine cardiac Purkinje fibers (upper panel). Five minutes after superfusion with 5 mM MgCl₂ added to the cesium-low potassium solution, EADs were abolished (middle panel). Bottom panel: After washout of magnesium and resumption of superfusion with cesium-low potassium Tyrode's solution, EADs recurred. Reproduced from Reference 25, with permission.

induced by anthopleurin-A is due to EADs generated in Purkinje fibers and that at least the initiating beats of TdP are due to triggered activity arising from EADs. The deflections on MAP recordings were very similar to EADs on transmembrane action potentials with regard to shape and timing. As noted by El-Sherif et al,[13] the relation between the EAD and the U wave was further strengthened by the observation that when U wave alternans was seen in surface leads, it was associated with 2:1 alteration of the deflections in MAP recordings. Carlsson et al[27] described similar results in an in vivo rabbit model in which a pause-dependent polymorphic VT resembling TdP developed after administration of the class III agent clofilium in the presence of the α-agonist methoxamine. Preceding the onset of the VT, a marked prolongation of MAP duration as well as EAD-like deflections were observed during phase 3 of epicardial MAP recordings. These correlated to simultaneous typical alterations in the morphology of the QT(U) segment. Prominent U waves occurred which were synchronous with the changes in MAP shape.

Our group[28,29] has recently developed an experimental model to study TdP in isolated Langendorff-perfused rabbit hearts. Conditions and circumstances that are clinically known to be associated with an increased propensity toward the development of TdP, such as bradycardia and hypokalemia, were simulated. The class III agent clofilium (1 μM) and d,l-sotalol (10 μM) as well as the antibiotic erythromycin (30 to 150 μM), which is also known to have proarrhythmic potential, were infused in the presence of either normal or low potassium concentration. Under these conditions, TdP spontaneously emerged in the clofilium-, d,l-sotalol-, and erythromycin-treated hearts. The episodes showed typical features of TdP found in humans (Fig. 4). They developed within 4 to 12 minutes after the onset of infusion, were normally nonsustained, and only rarely degenerated into ventricular fibrillation. Electrical stimulation at cycle lengths shorter than 600 milliseconds and perfusion with $MgSO_4$ suppressed arrhythmic activity. In the d,l-sotalol- and erythromycin-treated hearts, TdP only occurred in the presence of hypokalemia and bradycardia whereas in the presence of clofilium, bradycardia alone caused TdP. Johna et al[28] recently demonstrated that high concentrations of clofilium (10 μM) do even induce marked action potential prolongation in MAP recordings and TdP in isolated sinus-driven rabbit hearts in the presence of low potassium. Typical bursts of erythromycin-related TdP in the presence of hypokalemia are shown in Figure 5. Although we registered MAPs epicardially and endocardially during episodes of TdP, EADs were mainly endocardially but only occasionally epicardially recorded. Approximately 30% of the endocardial MAP recordings demonstrated EADs that corresponded to a marked T(U) prolongation or even to the initiation of TdP. This may be explained by the fact that we recorded MAPs from sites and/or cell groups different from those of TdP origin. Of note is that clofilium has been shown to produce EAD-induced triggered activity in canine subepicardial (M cells)

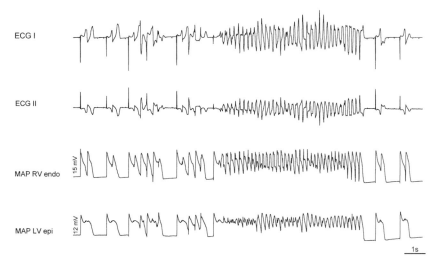

ECG I

ECG II

MAP RV endo

MAP LV epi

Figure 4. d,l-Sotalol- (10 μM) related torsades de pointes in the isolated atrioventricular-blocked rabbit heart in the presence of low potassium perfusion (1.5 mM). Two volume-conducted electrocardiographs and 2 MAPs are shown. MAPs were recorded in the apex of the right ventricle (RV endo) and the left lateral free wall (LV epi). Both recordings demonstrate early afterdepolarizations. Reproduced from Reference 29, with permission.

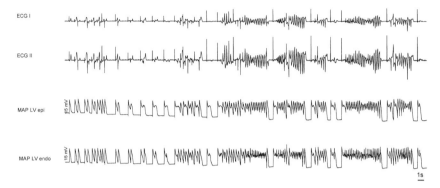

Figure 5. Example of erythromycin- (150 μM) induced torsades de pointes in the isolated atrioventricular-blocked rabbit heart in the presence of low potassium perfusion (1.5 mM). MAPs were recorded in the apex of the left ventricle (LV endo) and the left lateral free wall (LV epi). Both recordings demonstrate early afterdepolarizations. Reproduced from Reference 29, with permission.

cells of the left ventricular free wall, but not in endocardial or epicardial cells.[30] This may favor the hypothesis of an endocardial origin of TdP. With erythromycin, however, EADs could be reproducibly demonstrated both endocardially and epicardially (Fig. 5). Our results of the d,l-sotalol–treated hearts are in accordance with a very recent publication by Zabel et al,[31] who used a similar protocol and demonstrated reproducible induction of TdP and EADs in MAP recordings in rabbit hearts treated with 10 μM d-sotalol, which causes maximal I_{Kr} block.

MAP, Dispersion of Repolarization, and TdP in Experimental Studies

As MAPs represent the local repolarization at the recording site, the spatial time difference of MAP duration, activation time, and repolarization time (equal to activation time + MAP duration) measured at multiple sites, as well as their changes after electrical or pharmacologic interventions, are unique for evaluating dispersion of repolarization.

Using MAP recordings of the left and right ventricles, Verduyn et al[32] demonstrated bradycardia dependence of intraventricular dispersion of MAP duration, with the interventricular dispersion of MAP duration being larger in dogs with d,l-sotalol-related TdP compared to control dogs without arrhythmias. They observed EAD-like changes in MAP recordings more predominately in the left ventricle than in the right ventricle. Moreover, suppression or prevention of TdP by $MgSO_4$ was related to diminution of interventricular dispersion of MAP duration and disappearance of the MAP deflections. A similar increase in dispersion of repolarization measured as the maximal difference of 10 simultaneous MAPs was reported by Zabel et al[31] in their isolated rabbit heart model of TdP.

Clinical Studies of TdP Using MAPs

Although endocardial mapping has become a valuable and essential study to localize the area of interest during catheter ablation and preoperatively, few electrophysiologic studies have been done in patients presenting with TdP in congenital or acquired LQTS. This is because the majority of episodes of TdP are transient, and a role for programmed electrophysiologic stimulation in patients with LQTS or TdP could not be demonstrated.[33] As many patients acutely presenting with TdP are in an unstable situation, only few instances of MAP recordings in the acute phase of presentation of TdP have been described. In addition, the origin of the tachycardia is difficult to determine because of its polymorphic and self-terminating nature. Thus, studies including diagnosis and management of patients presenting with TdP have been mainly dependent on the patients' history, ECG recording, and, more recently, on a detailed genetic analysis.

MAPs in the Acute Phase of TdP

Figure 6 shows MAP recordings in a patient with acquired LQTS and recurrent episodes of TdP secondary to marked serum and total body hypomagnesemia. The first ectopic beat (#1) and a second ventricular couplet (#2) arose from a deflection that may represent a high-amplitude EAD or a "triggered upstroke" at the end of the action potential plateau. The presence of the triggered upstroke and the EAD coincided with a prominent and markedly widened negative T(U) wave in lead II of the surface ECG. Their peaks were synchronous with the peak of the T(U) waves. In the absence of a triggered upstroke or EAD, a positive T wave was recorded. Similar action potential and ECG changes were reported by Miwa and Inoue,[34] who evaluated the shape and duration of MAPs using a standard bipolar catheter in 4 patients in the acute phase of TdP. Their patients were all shown to have prolonged action potential duration, greater dispersion of action potential duration and of repolarization, and deflections during phase 3 of MAP. Of note is that these findings were suppressed or normalized by rapid right ventricular pacing. Unfortunately, the bipolar catheter recordings were not compared with standard suction or contact MAP catheters or with transmembrane action potentials. Habbab and El-Sherif[12] reported a case of procainamide-related TdP with two simul-

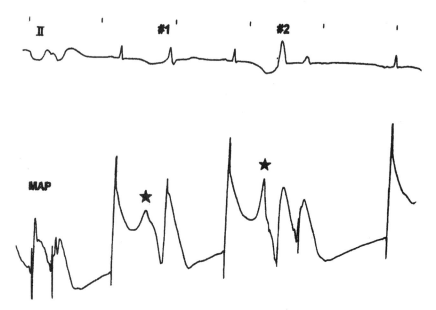

Figure 6. Spontaneous arrhythmias and corresponding MAP changes resembling early afterdepolarizations in a patient with hypomagnesemia. Reproduced with permission, from Haverkamp et al. Role of drugs in torsade de pointes and triggered activity. In Breithardt G, Borggrefe M, Camm J, Shenasa M (eds): *Antiarrhythmic Drugs.* Berlin: Springer; 1995:263.

taneous MAP recordings from right and left ventricular endocardial sites. They found a markedly prolonged MAP duration and EAD-like deflections on the repolarization phase. They also found a marked dispersion of repolarization, ranging from 180 to 280 milliseconds, and a marked dispersion of local activation time between right and left ventricular recording sites during TdP. The persistent dispersion of repolarization in subsequent short cycles and a marked dispersion of repolarization between right and left ventricular MAP recording sites may create the electrophysiologic prerequisites for TdP. El-Sherif et al[13] recorded MAPs from the right ventricle of a patient with quinidine-related LQTS and TdP. Figure 7 illustrates the effect of rapid ventricular pacing at a cycle length of 600 milliseconds on the amplitude of the first postpacing T(U) wave and the EAD-like MAP deflections. The last beat of the pacing train in the lower panel was spontaneous. The amplitude of both the T(U) wave and the EAD is larger after longer postpacing cycles (compare the lower and upper panels). The amplitude of both is also larger in the first postpacing beat than in other beats at approximately similar cycle lengths. Suppression of quinidine-related TdP by rapid ventricular pacing was associated with disappearance of the deflections in MAP recordings, the U wave on surface ECG, and ventricular ectopic beats.

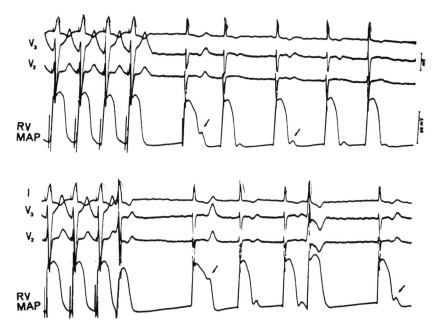

Figure 7. Simultaneous recording of electrocardiogram leads I, V_2, and V_3 and MAPs from the endocardial surface of the right ventricle (RV-MAP) showing the effect of a 20-second train of rapid pacing. The last beat of the pacing train in the lower panel was spontaneous and probably mechanically induced by the pacing electrode. For details see text. Reproduced from Reference 13, with permission.

EADs in Clinical Studies with MAPs

Several studies recorded MAPs in patients with a history of LQTS outside the acute phase of TdP presentation. The presence of deflections in MAP recordings and their possible relations with TdP have repeatedly been reported.[13,35-39] Figure 8 shows an example of such a deflection in a right ventricular MAP in a patient with LQTS recorded with suction electrodes outside the acute phase of TdP.[39] Arrows point at MAP deflections of varying amplitude and duration in the falling phase of the MAP preceding completion of repolarization which are interpreted by Bonatti et al[39] as abnormalities in repolarization rather than as motion artifacts. In a similar series of 3 patients with TdP, 1 caused by quinidine and 2 with congenital LQTS, Gavrilescu and Luca[36] also reported deformities in the terminal phase of repolarization. Right ventricular MAPs recorded with suction electrodes were excessively prolonged and were of varying shapes. Similar to the above-mentioned experimental data, the observed deflections in MAP recordings coincided with a distinct U wave on the surface ECG. Sakurada et al[38] confirmed the findings of regional differences in MAP durations in recordings from

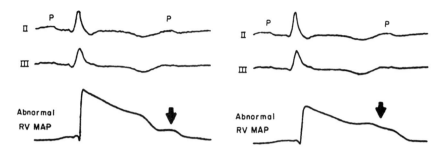

Figure 8. Example of possible afterdepolarizations in the MAP recorded with suction electrodes. Surface electrocardiogram and MAP from two different regions of the right ventricle (RV) in an 82-year-old woman with the long QT syndrome and 2:1 atrioventricular block. Arrows point at MAP deflections of varying amplitude and duration that were attributed by Bonatti et al[39] to abnormalities of repolarization. Reproduced from Reference 39, with permission.

the right ventricular outflow tract in a patient with LQTS. They demonstrated that the appearance of MAP deflections was associated with ST-T alternans in the surface ECG. Increasing the pacing rate suppressed the EAD-like deflections on right ventricular outflow tract MAP recordings. They reappeared after the stimulation was stopped, and correlated with ST-T alternans in the surface ECG. In a more comprehensive study, Ohe et al[33] studied 26 patients with a history of documented TdP who presented with a long QT interval at the time of TdP. Five patients suffered from LQTS, in 15 patients TdP was caused by antiarrhythmic drugs, and in 6 patients TdP was interpreted to be due to bradycardia. MAPs were recorded from the endocardium of the right (apex, upper septum) and left ventricle (apex). In 3 patients with congenital LQTS and TdP and in 2 patients with antiarrhythmic drug-related TdP, isoproterenol could induce a hump in phase 3 of repolarization on the MAP that corresponded to T(U) abnormalities in the surface ECG. Of note is that the QT prolongation associated with class Ia drug administration was significantly larger in patients with class Ia antiarrhythmic-related TdP than in those without TdP, and disopyramide injection also induced a deflection in MAP phase 3 only in patients with class Ia drug-related TdP. Shimizu et al[40] and Chinushi et al[41] reported two similar patients with LQTS and premature ventricular beats induced by epinephrine in whom administration of verapamil alone or in combination with propanolol[42] and nicorandil[41] reduced or even resulted in complete disappearance of the EAD-like deflections in right ventricular MAP recordings. Of note is that several clinical reports have demonstrated the suppression of premature ventricular beats and TdP by verapamil in patients with LQTS.[43]

MAP, Dispersion of Repolarization, and TdP in Clinical Studies

Numerous studies have shown that in healthy humans there is a normal degree of dispersion of repolarization, and dispersion is particularly increased in patients with LQTS. Gavrilescu and Luca[36] assessed dispersion of repolarization in one patient with quinidine-induced TdP and in two patients with LQTS, by recording MAPs from various right ventricular endocardial sites. Differences in MAP duration were between 120 and 175 milliseconds in patients with LQTS, while no difference was observed in the patient with acquired TdP. In the above-mentioned studies, Bonatti et al[37,39] also found important variations in the extent of dispersion of ventricular repolarization. A marked difference in the duration of MAP was observed between different areas of the right ventricle which, however, never exceeded 40 milliseconds in normal subjects whereas it ranged from 100 to 270 milliseconds in patients with QT prolongation and a history of TdP. In comparison, Linker et al[44] performed right ventricular endocardial mapping from 4 and 6 sites in 2 patients with congenital LQTS and demonstrated significant dispersion of repolarization, which was excessive compared to the reference values.[45] Similar results were recently reported by Shimizu et al,[40] who recorded MAPs from the left and right ventricular endocardium in 6 patients with LQTS and in 8 control patients. The MAP duration was significantly prolonged in LQTS patients but was shortened in control patients. Furthermore, dispersion of MAP duration was increased by isoproterenol infusion in LQTS patients whereas no change was found in the control group. These results further confirmed the existence of primary repolarization abnormalities in patients with congenital LQTS, and suggested an important role of sympathetic activity in the exaggeration of these repolarization abnormalities.

Limitations of MAP-Related Data in Studies Investigating TdP

The experimental and clinical studies that have indicated the presence of repolarization abnormalities in MAP have raised interest in the potential value of this technique. There has been extensive discussion regarding whether deflections ('humps') on MAP recordings represent true EADs or rather motion artifacts. As mere local differences in repolarization between Purkinje and adjacent muscle, or even motion artifacts of the MAP catheter, may result in similar or even identical MAP changes,[46] the above-described deflections in MAP recordings may mimic EADs or may result in EAD-like changes due to the summation of the electrical activity of cells with different action potential duration in different structures of the heart.[30] It is impossible to prove that all EAD-like MAP deflections represent true EADs. However, as changes in amplitude of the MAP deflections and oscillations were often closely correlated with changes in the late component of the T(U) waves, these humps are likely to represent an important cellular phenomenon. This may be local EAD activity or it may represent local differences in repolarization that result in increased dispersion of repolarization, which may favor reentrant mechanisms. In conclusion, due to the lack of large studies and often the lack of control groups, artifacts are unlikely but can still not be excluded with certainty.

As MAP recording is limited to a small endocardial and subendocardial area, it may underestimate the role of M cells, which are located in the deep subepicardium and have been demonstrated to be the primary targets of repolarization-prolonging agents in various animal models.[47,48] Thus, the M cell region may be of particular importance for the initiation of TdP.

Conclusions and Clinical Relevance

The in vivo applicability of MAPs has been demonstrated in several studies to assist in bridging the gap between data from experimental TdP models and those from patients with LQTS and TdP. As EADs, which are easily inducible by agents that result in TdP in experimental models as well as humans, are relatively slow waveforms, they cannot be detected by conventional intracardiac or surface ECG recordings. MAP recordings have therefore proven to be particularly valuable means for examining basic electrophysiologic mechanisms. Thanks to MAP recordings, there has been a growing body of evidence that local abnormalities of repolarization play an important role in the development of TdP in patients with congenital and acquired LQTS. The close similarity of EADs in in vitro animal experiments and deflections in MAP recordings of LQTS patients supports the theory that EADs are the primary mechanism, or at least one possible mechanism, for the repolarization abnormalities in LQTS. Recording of MAPs during electrophysiologic studies might be useful not only for study of the basic mechanisms of TdP but also for evaluation of possible therapeutic strategies that may result in suppression of TdP due to a loss of EAD and/or decreased regional dispersion of repolarization. As there is growing interest in the development of novel selective class III antiarrhythmics, the knowledge that such agents may induce or exacerbate cardiac arrhythmias such as TdP underlines the important role of MAP recordings in experimental as well as in clinical studies.

References

1. Dessertenne F. La tachycardie ventriculaire à deux foyers opposés variables. *Arch Mal Coeur* 1966;59:263-272.
2. Schwartz PJ, Periti M, Malliani A. The long Q-T syndrome. *Am Heart J* 1975;89:378-390.
3. Jackman WM, Friday KJ, Anderson JL, et al. The long QT syndromes: A critical review, new clinical observations and a unifying hypothesis. *Prog Cardiovasc Dis* 1988;31:115-172.
4. Haverkamp W, Shenasa M, Borggrefe M, Breithardt G. Torsade de pointes. In Zipes DP, Jalife J (eds): *Cardiac Electrophysiology: From Cell to Bedside.* Philadelphia; W. B. Saunders Company; 1995:885-899.
5. Ben David J, Zipes DP. Torsades de pointes and proarrhythmia. *Lancet* 1993;341:1578-1582.
6. Roden DM, Thompson KA, Hoffman BF, Woosley RL. Clinical features and basic mechanisms of quinidine-induced arrhythmias. *J Am Coll Cardiol* 1986;8:73A-78A.
7. Haverkamp W, Martinez Rubio A, Hief C, et al. Efficacy and safety of d,l-sotalol in patients with ventricular tachycardia or survivors of cardiac arrest. *J Am Coll Cardiol* 1997;30:487-495.
8. Franz MR, Burkhoff D, Spurgeon H, et al. In vitro validation of a new cardiac catheter technique for recording monophasic action potentials. *Eur Heart J* 1986;7:34-41.
9. Franz MR. Long-term recording of monophasic action potentials from human endocardium. *Am J Cardiol* 1983;51:1629-1634.
10. Franz MR, Bargheer K, Rafflenbeul W, et al. Monophasic action potential mapping in human subjects with normal electrocardiograms: Direct evidence for the genesis of the T wave. *Circulation* 1987;75:379-386.
11. Naumann D, Alnoncourt C, Zierhut W, Lüderitz B. "Torsade de pointes" tachycardia: Reentry or focal activity? *Br Heart J* 1982;48:213-216.
12. Habbab MA, El-Sherif N. Drug-induced torsades de pointes: Role of early afterdepolarizations and dispersion of repolarization. *Am J Med* 1990;89:241-246.
13. El-Sherif N, Bekheit SS, Henkin R. Quinidine-induced long QTU interval and torsade de pointes: Role of bradycardia-dependent early afterdepolarizations. *J Am Coll Cardiol* 1989;14:252-257.
14. Cranefield PF. Action potentials, afterpotentials, and arrhythmias. *Circ Res* 1977;41:415-423.
15. Surawicz B. Electrophysiologic substrate of torsade de pointes: Dispersion of repolarization or early afterdepolarizations? *J Am Coll Cardiol* 1989;14:172-184.
16. El-Sherif N, Caref EB, Yin H, Restivo M. The electrophysiological mechanism of ventricular arrhythmias in the long QT syndrome: Tridimensional mapping of activation and recovery patterns. *Circ Res* 1996;79:474-492.
17. Gray RA, Jalife J, Panfilov A, et al. Nonstationary vortexlike reentrant activity as a mechanism of polymorphic ventricular tachycardia in the isolated rabbit heart. *Circulation* 1995;91:2454-2469.
18. Eckardt L, Haverkamp W, Borggrefe M, Breithardt G. Experimental models of torsade de pointes. *Cardiovasc Res* 1998;39:178-193.
19. Brachmann J, Scherlag BJ, Rosenshtraukh LV, Lazzara R. Bradycardia-dependent triggered activity: Relevance to drug-induced multiform ventricular tachycardia. *Circulation* 1983;68:846-856.

20. Damiano BP, Rosen MR. Effects of pacing on triggered activity induced by early afterdepolarizations. *Circulation* 1984;69:1013-1025.
21. Levine JH, Spear JF, Guarnieri T, et al. Cesium chloride-induced long QT syndrome: Demonstration of afterdepolarizations and triggered activity in vivo. *Circulation* 1985;72:1092-1103.
22. El-Sherif N, Zeiler RH, Craelius W, et al. QTU prolongation and polymorphic ventricular tachyarrhythmias due to bradycardia-dependent early afterdepolarizations. Afterdepolarizations and ventricular arrhythmias. *Circ Res* 1988;63:286-305.
23. Davidenko JM, Cohen L, Goodrow R, Antzelevitch C. Quinidine-induced action potential prolongation, early afterdepolarizations, and triggered activity in canine Purkinje fibers. Effects of stimulation rate, potassium, and magnesium. *Circulation* 1989;79:674-686.
24. Sato T, Hirao K, Hiejima K. The relationship between early afterdepolarization and the occurrence of torsades de pointes: An in vivo canine model study. *Jpn Circ J* 1993;57:543-552.
25. Bailie DS, Inoue H, Kaseda S, et al. Magnesium suppression of early afterdepolarizations and ventricular tachyarrhythmias induced by cesium in dogs. *Circulation* 1988;77:1395-1402.
26. Wang Q, Shen J, Splawski I, et al. SCN5A mutations associated with an inherited cardiac arrhythmia, long QT syndrome. *Cell* 1995;80:805-811.
27. Carlsson L, Almgren O, Duker G. QTU-prolongation and torsades de pointes induced by putative class III antiarrhythmic agents in the rabbit: Etiology and interventions. *J Cardiovasc Pharmacol* 1990;16:276-285.
28. Johna R, Mertens H, Haverkamp W, et al. Clofilium in the isolated perfused rabbit heart: A new model to study proarrhythmia by class III antiarrhythmic drugs. *Basic Res Cardiol* 1998;93:127-135.
29. Eckardt L, Haverkamp W, Mertens H, et al. Drug-related torsade de pointes in the isolated rabbit heart: Comparison of clofilium, d,l-sotalol and erythromycin. *J Cardiovasc Pharmacol* 1998;32:425-434.
30. Antzelevitch C, Sicouri S, Lukas A, et al. Regional differences in the electrophysiology of ventricular cells: Physiological and clinical implications. In Zipes, Jalife J (eds): *Cardiac Electrophysiology: From Cell to Bedside*. Philadelphia; W. B. Saunders; 1994:228-245.
31. Zabel M, Hohnloser SH, Behrens S, et al. Electrophysiologic features of torsades de pointes: Insights from a new isolated rabbit heart model. *J Cardiovasc Electrophysiol* 1997;8:1148-1158.
32. Verduyn SC, Vos MA, van der Zande J, et al. Role of interventricular dispersion of repolarization in acquired torsade-de-pointes arrhythmias: Reversal by magnesium. *Cardiovasc Res* 1997;34:453-463.
33. Ohe T, Kurita T, Aihara N, et al. Electrocardiographic and electrophysiologic studies in patients with torsades de pointes. Role of monophasic action potentials. *Jpn Circ J* 1990;54:1323-1330.
34. Miwa S, Inoue T. Monophasic action potential in patients with torsades de pointes. *Circulation* 1989;80:II660.
35. Shimizu W, Tanaka K, Suenaga K, Wakamoto A. Bradycardia-dependent early afterdepolarizations in a patient with QTU prolongation and torsade de pointes in association with marked bradycardia and hypokalemia. *PACE* 1991;14:1105-1111.
36. Gavrilescu S, Luca C. Right ventricular monophasic action potentials in patients with long QT syndrome. *Br Heart J* 1978;40:1014-1018.

37. Bonatti V, Rolli A, Botti G. Monophasic action potential studies in human subjects with prolonged ventricular repolarization and long QT syndromes. *Eur Heart J* 1985;6:131-143.
38. Sakurada H, Tejima T, Hiyoshi Y, et al. Association of humps on monophasic action potentials and ST-T alternans in a patient with Romano-Ward syndrome. *PACE* 1991;14:1485-1491.
39. Bonatti V, Rolli A, Botti G. Recording of monophasic action potentials of the right ventricle in long QT syndromes complicated by severe ventricular arrhythmias. *Eur Heart J* 1983;4:168-179.
40. Shimizu W, Ohe T, Kurita T, et al. Epinephrine-induced ventricular premature complexes due to early afterdepolarizations and effects of verapamil and propranolol in a patient with congenital long QT syndrome. *J Cardiovasc Electrophysiol* 1994;5:438-444.
41. Chinushi M, Aizawa Y, Furushima H, et al. Nicorandil suppresses a hump on the monophasic action potential and torsade de pointes in a patient with idiopathic long QT syndrome. *Jpn Heart J* 1995;36:477-481.
42. Shimizu W, Ohe T, Kurita T, et al. Epinephrine-induced ventricular premature complexes due to early afterdepolarizations and effects of verapamil and propranolol in a patient with congenital long QT syndrome. *J Cardiovasc Electrophysiol* 1943;5:438-444.
43. Jackman WM, Szabo B, Friday KJ, et al. Ventricular tachyarrhythmias related to early afterdepolarizations and triggered firing: Relationship to QT interval prolongation and potential therapeutic role for calcium channel blocking agents. *J Cardiovasc Electrophysiol* 1990;1:170-195.
44. Linker NJ, Camm AJ, Ward DE. Dynamics of ventricular repolarisation in the congenital long QT syndromes. *Br Heart J* 1991;66:230-237.
45. Morgan JM, Cunningham D, Rowland E. Dispersion of monophasic action potential duration: Demonstrable in humans after premature ventricular extrastimulation but not in steady state. *J Am Coll Cardiol* 1992;19:1244-1253.
46. Habbab MA, El-Sherif N. TU alternans, long QTU, and torsade de pointes: Clinical and experimental observations. *PACE* 1997;15:916-931.
47. Antzelevitch C, Nesterenko VV, Yan G, et al. Role of M cells in acquired long QT syndrome, U waves, and torsade de pointes. *J Electrocardiol* 1995;28:131-137.
48. Sicouri S, Antzelevitch C. Electrophysiologic characteristics of M cells in the canine left ventricular free wall. *J Cardiovasc Electrophysiol* 1995;6:591-603.

36

Disorders of Cardiac Repolarization and Arrhythmogenesis

Nabil El-Sherif, MD and Edward B. Caref, PhD

Introduction

Disorders of ventricular repolarization have long been recognized as an important electrophysiologic substrate for reentrant ventricular tachyarrhythmias.[1] These disorders can be due to differences in active or passive membrane properties of myocardial fibers and/or of intercellular resistance.[2] Spatial dispersion of refractoriness is a prerequisite for reentrant excitation. When an activation wave front encounters regions of dispersion of repolarization, the result can be slowed conduction and functional unidirectional conduction block, which set the stage for circus-movement reentry. However, no practical technique has been available to measure the tridimensional distribution of repolarization in vivo with sufficient spatial and temporal resolution. The most common approach to mapping repolarization is indirect, through measurements of refractory periods.[3] A disadvantage of this technique is that the measurements must be obtained at individual sites in a sequential manner, thereby making it unsuitable for evaluation of dynamic changes in refractoriness. Furthermore, the definition of refractory period depends on the amplitude, duration, and polarity of the stimulating current.[4] Intracellular microelectrode recordings and

Supported in part by Department of Veterans Affairs Medical Research funds to NES and EBC.
From Franz MR (ed): *Monophasic Action Potentials: Bridging Cell and Bedside.* ©Futura Publishing Company, Inc., Armonk, NY, 2000.

the surrogate in vivo technique of monophasic action potential (MAP) recording can provide accurate measurements of action potential duration (APD).[5] However, measurements can only be obtained from a number of limited sites and mostly from endocardial or epicardial surfaces. In the last few years it became evident that a better insight into the role of dispersion of repolarization and arrhythmogenesis can only be realized if we are able to measure the ventricular tridimensional pattern of repolarization and to correlate this pattern with the tridimensional activation pattern. This chapter briefly reviews the advantages and limitations of the various techniques that have been proposed to measure ventricular repolarization as well as the role of dispersion of ventricular repolarization in arrhythmogenesis.

The Nature of the MAP

Unlike intracellular microelectrode recordings, the MAP is measured with an extracellular catheter tip electrode that has a diameter of approximately 1 to 2 mm. Although arguments continue to exist regarding the nature of the MAP, the following is the most plausible hypothesis[6]: mechanical pressure (or suction) exerted against the myocardium depolarizes and inactivates the group of cells subjacent to the electrode while leaving the adjacent cells largely unaffected. Because these adjacent normal cells retain their ability to depolarize and repolarize actively, there is an electrical gradient between the depolarized and inexcitable cells subjacent to the electrode and the adjacent normal cells. During electrical diastole, this gradient results in a source current emerging from the normal cells and a sink current descending into the depolarized cells subjacent to the MAP electrode. Under the volume conductor conditions provided by the surrounding tissue and pool, the sink current near the MAP electrode results in a negative electrical field that is proportional to the strength of current flow, which again is proportional to the potential gradient between the subjacent depolarized cells and the adjacent nondepolarized cells. During electrical systole, the normal cells adjacent to the MAP electrode undergo complete depolarization which overshoots the zero potential by some 30 mV, whereas the already depolarized, and therefore refractory, cells subjacent to the MAP electrode cannot further depolarize and maintain their potential at the former reference level. As a result, the former current sink reverses to a current source, producing an electrical field of opposite polarity. The strength and polarity of the boundary current and the resulting electrical field reflect the potential gradient between the (depolarized and refractory) reference potential in the cells subjacent to the electrode and voltage changes in the normal adjacent cells undergoing periodic depolarization and repolarization. According to this hypothesis, the MAP recording reflects the voltage time course of the normal cells that bound the surface of the volume of cells depolarized by the contact pressure. Thus, both depolarized (injured) and active (uninjured) cells contribute equally to the genesis of the boundary current that produces the MAP field potential. It would be of theoretical interest to test the above given hypothesis on the genesis of the contact MAP by directly measuring the membrane potential of cells beneath the depolarizing electrode. This might further clarify the source of the electromotive force which gives rise to the MAP. This concept becomes important when we later discuss a proposed alternative technique to record the MAP.

There is a general consensus that the MAP recording reflects local electrical activity at the recording site,[7] although the actual spatial resolution of the MAP is still not well defined. There is extensive literature that suggests that the recording can faithfully reproduce the duration and configuration of the local transmembrane action potential (TAP).[6] The MAP reasonably approximates the duration of local repolarization under a variety of pathophysiologic situations. However, the recording may correlate with APD but not with the refractory period in situations where postrepolarization refractoriness exists (eg, in the setting of ischemia). Theoretically, this is also possible when there are significant electronic interactions that distort the smooth repolarization phase of the action potential (AP), a situation that is more likely to occur in the long QT syndrome (LQTS).[8] These limitations equally apply, however, to other techniques of recording local repolarization including optical AP mapping and activation-recovery intervals (ARIs) calculated from unipolar electrograms.

A more controversial interpretation of the endocardial MAP recording in experimental models of LQTS and in patients with either the congenital or acquired LQTS is the assumption that certain deflections or "humps" that distort the repolarization phase of the recording may actually represent genuine early afterdepolarizations (EADs). We and other investigators have made these assumptions in the past. For example, Figure 1 illustrates an endocardial MAP recording from a dog following anthopleurin-A (AP-A) administration, a surrogate experimental model of LQT3. The recordings show prominent deflections on phase 3 of the MAP that were interpreted to represent EADs. Alternation of the QT segment of the surface electrocardiogram (ECG) that was associated with 2:1 recording of those deflections was interpreted to be due to 2:1 conduction block of a local EAD.[9] These same recordings are now more correctly interpreted to be due to electrotonic interactions between contiguous myocardial tissue with disparate APDs reflected in the MAP recording. Similar deflections in the endocardial MAP were also frequently recorded in patients with the LQTS either on phase 3 of the MAP

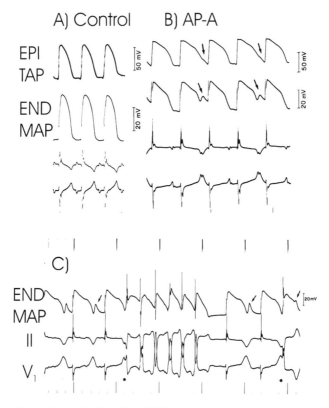

Figure 1. Recordings of epicardial (EPI) transmembrane action potential (TAP), endocardial (END) MAP, and surface electrocardiogram showing QTU alternans in the canine anthopleurin-A model of the long QT syndrome. **A.** Control recordings. **B.** Recordings obtained 14 minutes after the administration of AP-A (4 μg/kg) showing QTU alternans due to 2:1 alternation of an early afterdepolarization ([EAD] marked by arrows) that was more prominent in the endocardial MAP. Cardiac cycle during the alternans was 450 milliseconds. Both epicardial and endocardial recordings were repositioned in panels B and C. **C.** Cardiac cycle length was increased to 700 to 750 milliseconds by vagal stimulation. Epicardial TAP could not be maintained. There was further prolongation of the endocardial MAP and QTU segment with disappearance of the QTU alternans. Every action potential was followed by an EAD. Amplitude of the EAD significantly increased, and the deflection occurred during late phase 3 to simulate a delayed afterdepolarization. A short run of monomorphic ventricular tachycardia occurred and was initiated by an ectopic beat with different QRS configuration. First ectopic action potential arose from the peak of the EAD and was followed by 5 action potentials with relatively monomorphic configuration. The arrhythmia terminated by full repolarization of the last action potential, which did not show an EAD. QTU interval was markedly prolonged, and the QTU segment showed a terminal prominent deflection synchronous with the EAD in the endocardial MAP. Reproduced from Reference 9, with permission. N.B. The deflections interpreted as EAD are, at present, considered to represent electrotonic interaction between contiguous cardiac tissues with disparate action potential durations.

recording (Fig. 2)[10] or at the end of phase 2 (Fig. 3),[11] and were interpreted to represent EADs. Examples of T wave alternans associated with alternation of configuration and location of those "humps" have also been reported (Fig. 4).[12]

Even though it is almost certain that most of the humps in endocardial MAPs represent electrotonic interactions, the nature of the cardiac tissue contributing to the recording is not clear. One interpretation is that the endocardial MAP recording represents a summation of the local activity of Purkinje and subendocardial myocardial tissue. Investigators from our laboratory[13] and from other laboratories[14] studied this hypothesis by measuring the relative contribution of Purkinje fiber and ventricular muscle fiber activity to the MAP recorded in vivo from canine endocardium. Be-

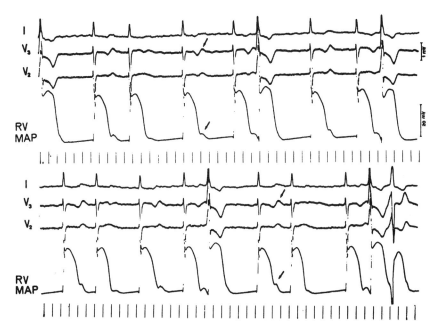

Figure 2. Simultaneous recording of surface electrocardiogram (ECG) leads I, V_2, and V_3 and a MAP from the endocardial surface of the posterior paraseptal region of the right ventricle (RV-MAP) in a patient with quinidine-induced long QTU and torsades de pointes. The MAP shows a distinct hump on phase 3 repolarization (arrow) characteristic of EAD. The peak of the EAD is synchronous with the peak of the U wave, and the amplitude of both waves (arrows) varies significantly with the length of the preceding RR interval. Ventricular ectopic beats occur only after RR intervals of greater than 1000 milliseconds, and seem to arise close to the peak of the U wave and the EAD. ECG leads are recorded at twice the standard amplitude. Reproduced from Reference 10, with permission. N.B. As in Figure 1, the deflections interpreted as EADs are at present considered to represent electrotonic interactions between contiguous cardiac tissues with disparate action potential durations.

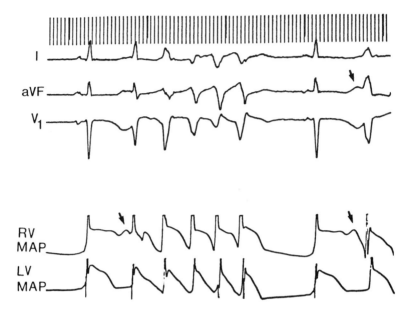

Figure 3. Simultaneous recording of MAP from apical sites in the right ventricle (RV) and left ventricle (LV) in a patient with acquired long QTU and torsades de pointes who was receiving procainamide. The MAP from the RV site was markedly prolonged (640 milliseconds) and showed a deflection at the end of the plateau consistent with early afterdepolarization (EAD), which corresponded to a prominent late deflection in the long QTU segment (both marked by arrows). On the other hand, the MAP recording from the LV site had a much shorter duration (380 milliseconds) and failed to show an EAD. The dispersion of repolarization between RV and LV sites was 260 milliseconds. The torsades de pointes tachycardia was initiated by a premature depolarization that seemed to arise from the peak or on the descending limb of the EAD in the RV MAP. The premature action potential occurred 200 milliseconds after the end of repolarization of the LV MAP. Reproduced from Reference 11, with permission. N.B. As in Figures 1 and 2, the deflections interpreted as EAD are at present considered to represent electrotonic interactions between contiguous cardiac tissues with disparate action potential durations.

cause the Purkinje fibers have longer APDs compared to myocardial fibers, their contribution to the local endocardial MAP appeared as a slow deflection on phase 3 of the MAP that may simulate what has been described as phase 3 EAD (Fig. 5). Some investigators, however, have questioned whether, in vivo, Purkinje fibers can contribute significantly to the MAP recording in comparison to the much larger mass of subendocardial myocardium.[6] In other words, the issue is whether the electrotonic interactions are between contiguous Purkinje and myocardial tissue with disparate APDs or are mainly between contiguous myocardial tissue with disparate APDs.

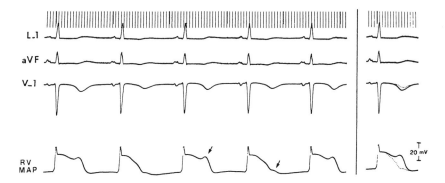

Figure 4. Endocardial MAP recording from the right ventricle (RV) showing alternation of the configuration and duration of MAP associated with subtle but definite alternation of the TU wave at a constant cycle length of 1140 milliseconds. The right panel illustrates a superimposed recording of two consecutive beats. The arrows point to deflections consistent with early afterdepolarization. Reproduced from Reference 12, with permission. N.B. As in Figures 1 through 3, the deflections interpreted as early afterdepolarization are at present considered to represent electrotonic interactions between contiguous cardiac tissues with disparate action potential durations.

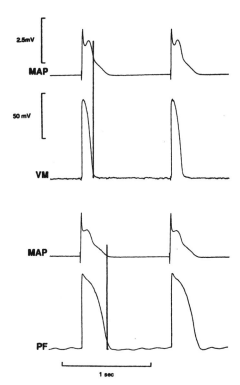

Figure 5. Simultaneous recordings from a superfused in vitro canine endocardial preparation of a MAP, and transmembrane action potential from a myocardial fiber with minimally overlying Purkinje fibers (VM, top panel) and a MAP and transmembrane action potential from a subendocardial Purkinje fiber strand (PF, bottom panel). Note the difference in action potential duration (APD) between VM and PF. The inflection on phase 3 of the MAP occurs after complete repolarization of the shorter APD of VM and reflects the contribution of the longer repolarization of PF.

Are There Alternative Techniques to Record MAPs?

In a preliminary report, Nesterenko and Weissenburger[15] described a new technique to record MAPs. The method consisted of a thin (300 Å [30 nm]) silver wire, isolated except for the tip (0.5 mm), that has been placed in contact with the myocardium or inserted intramurally and referenced to a KCl electrode placed at a separate location and used to depolarize a discrete region of the myocardium. The assumption was that the membrane potentials of cells at the KCl electrode were depolarized close to 0 mV and that the recording obtained from the exploring electrode would more accurately reflect the local TAP at this site. These assumptions are largely unproven. As shown in Figure 6, the recording at the KCl electrode is in fact an injury potential and the recording of the exploring electrodes represents the subtraction of this injury potential from the local unipolar electrogram; however, the recording can simulate a TAP and can be stable for a long period of time. Figure 7 illustrates recordings from a canine AP-A experiment in which recordings from 8 unipolar electrodes (separated by 1 mm), which were mounted on a plunge needle inserted across the left ventricular wall, were referenced to the same KCl electrode. The recording illustrates simultaneous MAP recordings along the epicardial-endocardial axis of the left ventricle and shows an increase in APD from epicardial to midmyocardial/endocardial zones. A more abrupt increase in APD appears to occur between electrode sites 5 and 4. Panel A of Figure 7 shows two spontaneous premature beats, the first of which had a longer coupling interval to the basic beat and conducted to all 8 electrode sites. On the other hand, the second premature beat, with a shorter coupling interval, appears to block between electrode sites 5 and 4 in conjunction with the greater dispersion of repolarization between these two sites. Similarly, panel B shows two premature beats, of which the second beat, with shorter coupling, also blocked between sites 5 and 4 and initiated a torsades de pointes tachyarrhythmia. Although use of a single KCl electrode for reference would allow simultaneous tridimensional recording of MAP as shown in Figure 7, the MAP is really a hybrid recording, and is susceptible to distortion of the AP-like configuration. This is clearly seen in the recordings shown in panel C of Figure 6 and in Figure 7.

Tridimensional Recording of Ventricular Repolarization

Two major techniques have been proposed for the simultaneous measurment of cardiac repolarization at multiple sites. One is an imaging tech-

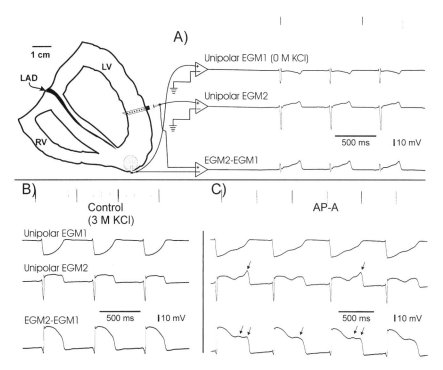

Figure 6. The technique for recording MAPs with use of a KCl reference electrode. Shown are the electrogram at the reference electrode (Unipolar EGM1), at the exploring electrode (the most epicardial electrode of a multielectrode plunge needle across the left ventricular wall; Unipolar EGM2), and the recording obtained by subtracting EGM1 from EGM2. **A.** Control recording before application of 3 M KCl to the reference electrode site. Both EGM1 and EGM2 show typical unipolar electrogram configuration, while the composite recording resembles a bipolar electrogram. **B.** Following application of 3 M KCl to the reference electrode site, the EGM1 recording reveals the development of an injury potential, while the EGM2 recording remains unchanged from control. The composite recording (EGM2-EGM1) now records a MAP. **C.** Following administration of anthopleurin-A, there was a marked prolongation of both the injury current recording at EGM1 and the local unipolar electrogram, EGM2, which shows alternation of the configuration of the terminal component of the local T wave (marked by arrows). The composite MAP shows the development alternatively, of 1 or 2 inflections on phase 2 that simulate early afterdepolarizations.

nique that uses a potentiometric fluorescent dye to image AP patterns optically with a photodiode array,[16] and the second is signal processing of extracellular electrograms.[17] With use of optical mapping techniques, the time of the peak second derivative of the AP has been shown to coincide with the end of the effective refractory period (ERP).[18] However, it is important to recognize that this technique measures the summed responses of hundreds of cells contributing to a photodiode signal, and its validity

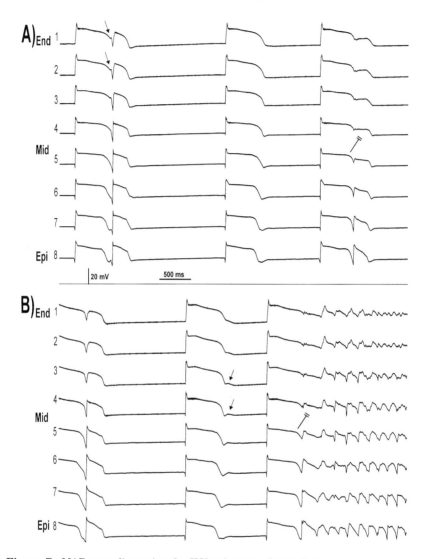

Figure 7. MAP recording using the KCl reference electrode from a canine experiment following the administration of anthopleurin-A. Shown are simultaneous recordings of 8 MAPs recorded from a multielectrode plunge needle inserted across the left ventricular free wall as shown in Figure 6. Note the shorter action potential duration (APD) at epicardial (Epi) compared to midmyocardial (Mid) and endocardial (End) sites. **A.** The long coupled premature beat conducted to all sites, while the second short-coupled premature beat resulted in conduction block between electrode sites 5 and 4 due to the presence of a greater degree of dispersion of APD between these two sites. **B.** The second short-coupled premature beat resulted in intramural conduction block and initiated a torsades de pointes tachyarrhythmia. The arrows refer to inflections on the MAP that simulate phase 2 EAD (A) or late phase 3 EAD (B). These most probably represent electrotonic interactions.

in the presence of steep dispersion of refractoriness has not been tested. Presently, the primary limitation of optical AP mapping is that recordings can only be obtained from a bidimensional surface, most commonly the epicardium.

The ARI in unipolar electrograms, defined as the time interval between the minimum temporal derivative (dV/dt_{min}) of the QRS and the maximum temporal derivative (dV/dt_{max}) of the local T wave, has been proposed as a useful measure of the duration of repolarization.[17] The validity of the measurement has also been demonstrated with respect to refractory periods. Millar et al[17] showed that ARIs from unipolar electrograms correlated closely with ventricular refractory periods under conditions of varying cycle length (CL) and adrenergic stimulation. Blanchard et al[19] concluded that the ARI measures local events since the measurement was not significantly altered by changing the timing of distant electrical events. Wyatt[20] examined the relation between ARIs and APDs during changes in CL and coronary occlusion. Haws and Lux[21] provided an analytic derivation of the theoretical basis for the correlation between times of dV/dt_{min} of the QRS and dV/dt_{max} of the AP upstroke and times of dV/dt_{max} of the T wave and dV/dt_{min} of the AP downstroke, as well as evidence for the correlation between ARI and in vivo TAP duration under a variety of conditions. On the other hand, simulation studies by Steinhaus,[22] while upholding the value of ARI measurements from unipolar electrograms, also showed that potential errors in estimation of activation and recovery times from electrograms can occur. Factors responsible for those errors included nonuniform coupling resistance, nonuniform membrane properties, and alterations in recording site relative to activation sequence. The technique of ARI has been widely applied to measure the dispersion of refractoriness on the epicardial surface in the human heart,[23] from the body surface in patients with congenital LQTS,[24] and from the epicardial surface in various in vivo animal models.[25,26]

We used the ARI technique to perform high-resolution tridimensional mapping of the repolarization pattern in the canine AP-A model of LQTS and to correlate this pattern with the tridimensional activation pattern, in an attempt to study the in vivo electrophysiologic substrate of arrhythmogenesis in the LQTS.[27] Although previous experimental studies have shown that ARIs derived from unipolar electrograms reasonably approximate the local ERP, there was compelling evidence that, in the presence of AP-A, large differences in repolarization occur over short distances. Since none of the previous studies analyzed ARIs in the presence of large spatial differences in repolarization, we performed an analysis of the relationship of ARI to refractoriness during control and in the presence of AP-A, in order to validate the technique of ARI determination in this model. Figure 8 illustrates one such experiment and shows that ARI and ERP at each of multiple sites correlated within ±15 milliseconds.

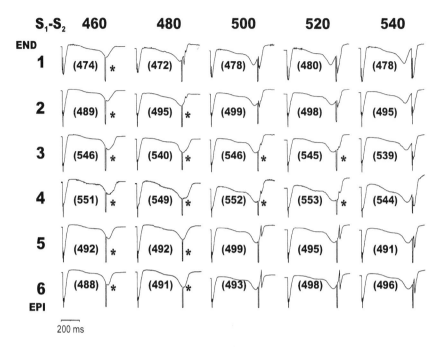

Figure 8. Relation between activation-recovery interval (ARI) and effective refractory period (ERP) across the epicardial (EPI)-endocardial (END) axis of the left ventricular wall after anthopleurin-A infusion in the dog as determined by field stimulation from a central stimulating electrode. The first unipolar complex in each of the 5 panels represents the last S1 beat in a train of 50 cycles at a cycle length of 1000 milliseconds; the second complex is the premature stimulus (S2). The numbers on top are the S1-S2 coupling intervals, and the numbers in brackets are the calculated ARIs at each site. The asterisks denote blocked local responses to the S2 stimulus. The ARI and ERP at each site correlated within ±15 milliseconds. Note the significantly longer ARIs and ERPs at midmyocardial sites 3 and 4 compared with EPI sites 5 and 6 and END sites 1 and 2. Reproduced from Reference 27, with permission.

Microelectrode studies in transmural preparations have shown that subepicardial, midmyocardial, and subendocardial cells respond differently to changes in CL.[2,28,29] Midmyocardial M cells had the steepest APD-CL relationship, followed by transitional cells. The least steep APD-CL relationship was observed in subepicardial cells. We studied the relationship between ARI and CL at steady state across the left ventricular free wall during control conditions and during AP-A infusion. The difference in the ARI-CL relation along the epicardial-endocardial axis was markedly exaggerated during AP-A infusion. This is illustrated in Figure 9, which shows 8 transmural unipolar electrograms recorded across the basolateral wall of the left ventricle.

Tridimensional mapping of ventricular repolarization from ARIs allowed the first in vivo demonstration of the existence of spatial dispersion

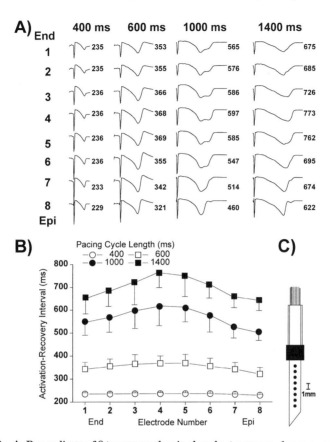

Figure 9. A. Recordings of 8 transmural unipolar electrograms, 1 mm apart, across the basolateral wall of the left ventricle at cycle lengths (CLs) of 400, 600, 1000, and 1400 milliseconds, from a canine heart following anthopleurin-A (AP-A) infusion. The calculated activation-recovery interval (ARI) is shown next to each electrogram (in milliseconds). The figure illustrates the steep ARI-CL relation of midmyocardial sites compared with subepicardial (Epi) and subendocardial (End) sites, resulting in steep gradients of ARI at the transition zones at the longer CL. **B**. Composite data of ARI distribution collected from 12 unipolar plunge needle recordings in the basolateral wall of the left ventricle in a 4×10 mm section from the same experiment. After AP-A, ARIs increased 2 to 3 times compared with control at similar CLs. The steepest increase occurred at midmyocardial zones. At 600 milliseconds, ARIs were slightly longer in midmyocardial zones, but the differences were not statistically significant. At 1000 and 1400 milliseconds, a significant increase in ARIs was apparent in midmyocardial electrodes 3 to 6 compared with both subendocardial electrodes 1 and 2 and subepicardial electrodes 7 and 8. There was, however, marked variation in ARI dispersion at the two transitional zones between midmyocardial sites and both Epi and End sites. Differences in ARIs of up to 80 milliseconds (at a CL of 1400 to 1500 milliseconds) between contiguous sites, 1 mm apart, at the transition zones were not uncommon. **C**. Diagrammatic illustration of the plunge needle electrode used to collect ARI data. Modified from Reference 27, with permission.

of repolarization in the ventricular wall and differences in regional recovery in response to CL changes that were markedly exaggerated after AP-A administration. Simultaneous analysis of tridimensional repolarization and activation patterns showed that the initial beat of torsades de pointes ventricular tachycardia consistently arose as focal activity from a subendocardial site, whereas subsequent beats were due to reentrant excitation. The latter was due to infringement of a focal activity on the spatial dispersion of repolarization, resulting in functional conduction block and circulating wave fronts (Fig. 10).[27]

Further evidence of the role of dispersion of repolarization and arrhythmogenesis was recently reported in a study of the electrophysiologic basis of arrhythmogenicity of QT/T alternans in the LQTS.[30] The study investigated the phenomenon of QT/T alternans, which occurs during abrupt shortening of the CL in the canine AP-A model of LQTS, and showed that QT/T alternans was associated with a greater degree of dispersion of repolarization (estimated as differences in ARIs) compared with longer CLs with "longer QT interval" but no alternans (Fig. 11). The dispersion of ARI was most marked between midmyocardial and epicardial zones in the left ventricular free wall. In the presence of a critical degree of dispersion of ARI, propagation of the activation wave front during the basic impulse could be blocked between these zones to initiate reentrant excitation and polymorphic ventricular tachycardia. Two factors contribute to the modulation of ARI during QT/T alternans, resulting in a greater magnitude of dispersion of ARI between midmyocardial and epicardial zones at critical short CLs compared with basic rhythm. These are: 1) differences in restitution kinetics at midmyocardial sites, characterized by larger ΔARI and a slower time constant (τ) compared with epicardial sites; and 2) differences in the diastolic interval that would result in different input to the restitution curve at the same constant CL. The longer ARI of midmyocardial sites results in shorter diastolic intervals during the first short cycle and thus a greater degree of ARI shortening. Marked QT/T alternans could be present in local electrograms without manifest alternations of the QT/T segment in the surface ECG. This observation provides the electrophysiologic basis for the recent interest in the tachycardia-dependent subtle degrees of T wave alternans, detected by digital signal processing techniques, as a marker for the risk of malignant ventricular tachyarrhythmias.[31,32]

In summary, the ability to study the tridimensional pattern of ventricular repolarization using the ARI technique has already provided valuable insight into the role of dispersion of repolarization in arrhythmogenesis. Future investigations of the role of tridimensional dispersion of repolarization in other pathophysiologic states, such as ischemic heart disease, cardiomyopathy, and hypertrophy, are urgently needed.

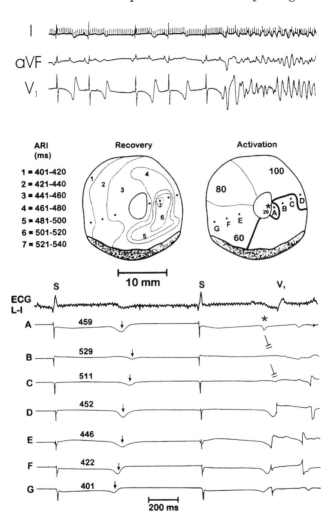

Figure 10. Recordings from a canine experiment after anthopleurin-A administration that resulted in the development of the long QT syndrome (LQTS) and torsades de pointes ventricular tachycardia (top tracing). Shown are the isochronal activation and recovery maps of the apical section of the dog's heart of the penultimate sinus beat that preceded the V_1 beat that initiated the tachyarrhythmia shown on top. The recovery isochrones are drawn as closed contours at 20-millisecond intervals. The electrograms at the bottom of the maps illustrate the calculated activation-recovery interval ([ARI] in milliseconds) at selected sites. The arrows mark the maximum temporal derivative (dV/dt_{max}) of the local T wave used to calculate the ARI. The asterisk marks the subendocardial site of origin of the V_1 beat. Note the longer ARI at midmyocardial sites compared to epicardial sites. Also note that the lines of functional conduction block in the activation map correspond largely to sites with steep gradient of ARIs. The development of functional conduction block sets the stage for the initiation of reentrant excitation. Modified from Reference 27, with permission.

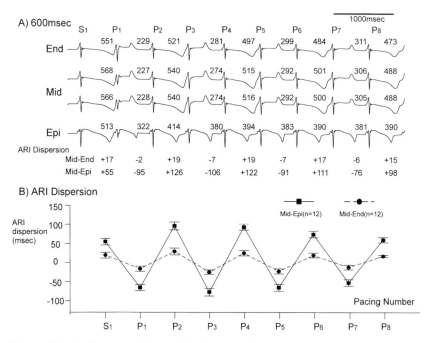

Figure 11. A. Transmural recording from a plunge needle electrode in the left ventricular free wall of a dog during infusion of anthopleurin-A (AP-A). The recording illustrates unipolar electrograms from endocardial (End), midmyocardial (Mid), and epicardial (Epi) sites. QT alternans was induced by abrupt decrease of the cardiac cycle length (CL) from 1000 milliseconds (S1) to 600 milliseconds (P1, P2, P3, etc.). The numbers represent the activation-recovery interval (ARI) in milliseconds. Note that even though the overall QT interval is shorter at 600 milliseconds compared to 1000 milliseconds, the degree of ARI dispersion between Epi and Mid sites was greater at 600 milliseconds. Also note the reversal of the gradient of ARI between Epi and Mid sites, with a consequent reversal of polarity of the intramyocardial QT wave in alternate cycles. **B**. Graphic illustration of mean ± SEM of ARI dispersion between Mid and Epi sites and between Mid and End sites during successive short CLs of 600 milliseconds from 12 different sites from the left ventricular free wall in the same experiment. Reproduced from Reference 30, with permission.

References

1. Han J, Moe GK. Nonuniform recovery of excitability in ventricular muscle. *Circ Res* 1964;14:44-60.
2. Restivo M, Gough WE, El-Sherif N. Ventricular arrhythmias in the subacute myocardial infarction period: High-resolution activation and refractory patterns of reentrant rhythms. *Circ Res* 1990;66:1310-1327.
3. Hoffman BF, Kao CY, Suckling EE. Refractoriness in cardiac muscle. *Am J Physiol* 1957;190:473-482.
4. Michelson EL, Spear JF, Moore EN. Electrophysiological and anatomical correlates of sustained ventricular tachyarrhythmias in a model of chronic myocardial infarction. *Am J Cardiol* 1980;45:583-590.

5. Franz MR. Long-term recording of monophasic action potentials from human endocardium. *Am J Cardiol* 1983;51:1629-1634.

6. Franz MR. Method and theory of monophasic action potential recording. *Prog Cardiovasc Dis* 1991;6:347-368.

7. Franz MR, Burkhoff D, Spurgeon H, et al. In vitro validation of a new cardiac catheter technique for recording monophasic action potentials. *Eur Heart J* 1986;7:34-41.

8. Antzelevitch C, Sicouri S. Clinical relevance of cardiac arrhythmias generated by afterdepolarizations. The role of M cells in the generation of U waves, triggered activity and torsade de pointes. *J Am Coll Cardiol* 1994;23:259-277.

9. El-Sherif N, Zeiler RH, Craelius W, et al. QTU prolongation and polymorphic ventricular tachyarrhythmias due to bradycardia-dependent early afterdepolarizations. *Circ Res* 1988;63:286-305.

10. El-Sherif N, Bekheit SS, Henkin R. Quinidine-induced long QTU interval and torsades de pointes: Role of bradycardia-dependent early afterdepolarizations. *J Am Coll Cardiol* 1989;14:252-257.

11. Habbab MA, El-Sherif N. Drug induced torsades de pointes. Role of early afterdepolarizations and dispersion of repolarization. *Am J Med* 1990;89:241-246.

12. Habbab MA, El-Sherif N. TU alternans, long QTU, and torsades de pointes: Clinical and experimental observations. *PACE* 1992;15:916-931.

13. Gough WB, Henkin R. The early afterdepolarization as recorded by the monophasic action potential technique: Fact or artifact? *Circulation* 1989;80:II130. Abstract.

14. Ino T, Karaguezian HS, Hong K, et al. Relation of monophasic action potential recorded with contact electrode to underlying transmembrane action potential properties in isolated cardiac tissues: A systematic microelectrode validation study. *Cardiovasc Res* 1988;22:255-264.

15. Nesterenko VV, Weissenburger J. Experimental evidence for re-interpretation of basis for the monophasic action potential: A new technique with large amplitude and stable transmural signals. *Circulation* 1995;92:I299. Abstract.

16. Salama G, Morad M. Merocyanine-540, as an optical probe of transmembrane electrical activity in the heart. *Science* 1976;101:485-487.

17. Millar CK, Kralios FA, Lux RL. Correlation between refractory periods and ARIs from electrograms: Effects of rate and adrenergic interventions. *Circulation* 1985;72:1372.

18. Salama G, Kanai A, Efimov IR. Subthreshold stimulation of Purkinje fibers interrupts ventricular tachycardia in intact hearts: Experimental study with voltage-sensitive dyes and imaging techniques. *Circ Res* 1994;74:604-619.

19. Blanchard SM, Smith WM, Damiano RJ, et al. The effects of distant events on ARIs. *Circulation* 1986;74:II258. Abstract.

20. Wyatt RF. *Comparison of Estimates of Activation and Recovery Times from Bipolar and Unipolar Electrograms to In Vivo Transmembrane APDs.* Washington DC: Proc IEEE Eng Med Biol Soc, 2nd annual conference; Sept 1980:22-25.

21. Haws CW, Lux RL. Correlation between in vivo transmembrane action potential durations and activation recovery intervals from electrograms. Effects of interventions that alter repolarization time. *Circulation* 1991;81:281-288.

22. Steinhaus BM. Estimating cardiac transmembrane activation and recovery times from unipolar and bipolar extracellular electrograms: A simulation study. *Circ Res* 1989;64:449.

23. D'Alche P, Morel M, Gauthier V, et al. Mapping of activation, recovery and activation-recovery intervals in the human heart. *Physiol Res* 1993;42:77-79.

24. Shimizu W, Kamakura S, Ohe T, et al. Diagnostic value of recovery time measured by body surface mapping in patients with congenital long QT syndrome. *Am J Cardiol* 1994;74:780-785.

25. Dhein S, Gerwin R, Ziskoven V, et al. Propranolol unmasks class III-like electrophysiological properties of norepinephrine. *Arch Pharmacol* 1993;348:643-649.

26. Dhein S, Muller A, Gerwin R, Klauss W. Comparative study on the proarrhythmic effects of some antiarrhythmic agents. *Circulation* 1993;87:617-630.

27. El-Sherif N, Caref EB, Yin H, Restivo M. The electrophysiological mechanism of ventricular tachyarrhythmias in the long QT syndrome: Tridimensional mapping of activation and recovery patterns. *Circ Res* 1996;79:474-492.

28. Antzelevitch C, Sicouri S, Litovsky SH, et al. Heterogeneity within the ventricular wall: Electrophysiology and pharmacology of epicardial, endocardial, and M cells. *Circ Res* 1991;69:1427-1449.

29. Sicouri S, Antzelevitch C. Electrophysiologic characteristics of M cells in the canine left ventricular free wall. *J Cardiovasc Electrophysiol* 1995;6:591-603.

30. Chinushi M, Restivo M, Caref EB, El-Sherif N. The electrophysiological basis of arrhythmogenicity of QT/T alternans in the long QT syndrome. Tridimensional analysis of the kinetics of cardiac repolarization. *Circ Res* 1998;83:614-628.

31. Rosenbaum DS, Jackson LE, Smith JM, et al. Electrical alternans and vulnerability to ventricular arrhythmias. *N Engl J Med* 1994;330:235-241.

32. Estes NAM III, Michaud G, Zipes DP, et al. Electrical alternans during rest and exercise as predictors of vulnerability to ventricular arrhythmias. *Am J Cardiol* 1997;80:1314-1318.

37

Early Afterdepolarizations and Polymorphic Ventricular Arrhythmias in Acquired and Congenital Long QT Syndrome:

Observations from Clinical and Experimental Studies

Wataru Shimizu, MD, PhD, Tohru Ohe, MD and Charles Antzelevitch, PhD

The Long QT Syndrome

The long QT syndrome (LQTS) is characterized by the appearance of long QT intervals in the electrocardiogram (ECG) and an atypical life-threatening polymorphic ventricular arrhythmia known as torsades de pointes (TdP).[1-4] The LQTS can be subdivided into two major categories: congenital (hereditary) and acquired. Genetic linkage analysis has identified 4 forms of congenital LQTS caused by mutations in ion channel genes located on chromosomes 3, 7, 11, and 21.[5-8] Chromosome 3-linked LQT3

Supported by grants from the National Institutes of Health (HL 47678), the Medtronic Japan, the American Heart Association, New York State Affiliate, and the Masons of New York State and Florida.

From Franz MR (ed): *Monophasic Action Potentials: Bridging Cell and Bedside.* ©Futura Publishing Company, Inc., Armonk, NY, 2000.

is linked to mutations in *SCN5A*, a gene that encodes for the α subunit of the sodium channel in heart,[5] whereas chromosome 7-linked LQT2 is associated with mutations in *HERG*, a gene that encodes for the channels that carry the rapidly activating delayed rectifier potassium currents (I_{Kr}).[9] Chromosome 11-linked LQT1 is caused by a mutation in *KvLQT1* which encodes for the slowly activating delayed rectifier potassium currents (I_{Ks}),[10,11] and chromosome 21-linked LQT5 is the result of a mutation in *KCNE1* (*minK*), whose product coassembles with that of *KvLQT1* to form the I_{Ks} channel.[8,10,11] It has long been appreciated that some forms of congenital LQTS are very sensitive to adrenergic stimulation. On the other hand, the acquired form of LQTS is often associated with a variety of pharmacologic agents and electrolyte imbalances, usually coupled with bradycardia or long pauses. Most but not all agents that are capable of prolonging the QT interval are capable of causing TdP. They include widely prescribed antibiotics, antihistaminics, antifungal agents, and antiarrhythmic drugs (class Ia and class III antiarrhythmics).[12,13] Among these, antiarrhythmic agents appear to be the most common causes of acquired LQTS.[14]

The chief aim of this chapter is to review clinical and experimental data that have advanced our knowledge of the cellular basis for the long QT interval and abnormal T waves, of the mechanism of TdP, and of possible therapeutic approaches to the treatment of congenital and acquired LQTS. Monophasic action potential (MAP) recordings discussed in this chapter are from clinical studies of patients with LQTS.[15-22] Experimental data are from studies involving our recently developed arterially perfused preparations that consist of wedges of canine left ventricle.[23-28]

Phenotypic Appearance of Abnormal T Waves in LQTS

It was recently suggested that differences in the phenotypic appearance of T wave patterns in the ECG vary as a function of the genotype.[29] LQT3 patients show distinctive late-appearing T waves, whereas LQT1 or LQT2 patients display broad-based prolonged T waves or low-amplitude T waves with a notched or bifurcated appearance, respectively. Several clinical studies report the appearance of notched or bifurcated T waves and long QT interval just preceding an episode of TdP in patients with antiarrhythmic drug-induced acquired LQTS.[21]

The discovery of the M cell[30] unveiled a subpopulation of cells in the deep structures of the canine ventricle that display electrical characteristics and responses to drugs consistent with the electrocardiographic manifestations that attend the development of long QT and TdP. Electrical heterogeneity introduced by the presence of M cells within the ventricle contributes to the manifestation of both the normal and abnormal T waves in the ECG.[12,28,31-33] Preferential prolongation of cells in the M region is believed to underlie LQTS, contributing to the development of long QT intervals, the phenotypic appearance of abnormal T waves, and the development of TdP.

Evidence that supports this hypothesis has been advanced through use of the arterially perfused canine left ventricular (LV) wedge preparations, in which transmembrane action potentials are simultaneously recorded from epicardial, M, and endocardial or subendocardial Purkinje sites along the transmural surface of the ventricular wall by use of floating glass microelectrodes.[23-28] A pseudo-ECG recorded concurrently along the same vector permits correlation of transmembrane and electrocardiographic activity. The wedge is capable of developing a variety of arrhythmias, including TdP. We have used this experimental model to assess the contribution of electrical heterogeneity across the ventricular wall to the manifestation of the T wave in the ECG under normal conditions as well as under conditions of "acquired" LQTS mimicking 4 genetic defects that have been linked to the congenital syndrome (Fig. 1).[5,6,8-11] It is noteworthy that the peak of the T wave is coincident with the repolarization of the epicardial action potential and that the end of the T wave coincides with repolarization of the M cell action potential. Repolarization of endocardial action potentials is intermediate. The transmural dispersion of repolarization across the ventricular wall is therefore defined by the difference in repolarization time (activation time + action potential duration [APD]) between the M cell and epicardial cell. In the ECG, the time interval between the peak and the end of the T wave represents the transmural dispersion of repolarization, and can be a valuable electrocardiographic index (Fig. 1). Increased sympathetic activity due to physical or emotional stress has long been known to produce a QT prolongation, which is often accompanied by an increase in QT dispersion, cardiac arrhythmias, and sudden cardiac death in patients with congenital LQTS.[1-3,34] This relation appears to be more common in the LQT1 syndrome than in either the LQT2 or the LQT3.[35] In the presence of chromanol 293B, a relatively specific I_{Ks} blocker[36] which can be used to mimic the LQT1 (and LQT5) syndrome,[25] β-adrenergic stimulation with isoproterenol increases transmural dispersion of repolarization as a result of an abbreviation of the APD of epicardial and endocardial cells but not of M cells. This results in a long QT interval with a broad-based T wave (Fig. 1, panel B), consistent with the phenotypic appearance of the ECG of patients afflicted with the LQT1 syndrome. It is noteworthy that chromanol 293B alone produces a homogeneous prolongation of APD across the canine ventricular wall and that transmural dispersion of repolarization is not augmented until a β-adrenergic agonist is introduced. The differential response of the 3 cell types to isoproterenol may be due to their intrinsic differences in I_{Ks}. A larger augmentation of remaining I_{Ks} by isoproterenol in epicardial and endocardial cells than that in M cells, where

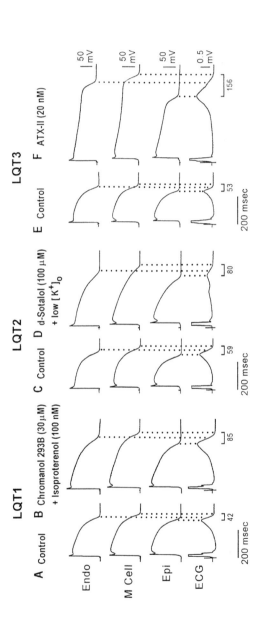

Figure 1. Transmembrane action potentials and transmural electrocardiogram (ECG) in the LQT1 (**A** and **B**), LQT2 (**C** and **D**), and LQT3 (**E** and **F**) models in arterially perfused canine left ventricular wedge preparations. Isoproterenol + chromanol 293B - an I_{Ks} blocker, d-sotalol + low $[K^+]_o$, and ATX-II, an agent that slows inactivation of late I_{Na}, were used to mimic the LQT1, LQT2, and LQT3 syndrome, respectively. Panels **A** through **F** depict action potentials simultaneously recorded from endocardial (Endo), M, and epicardial (Epi) sites together with a transmural ECG. Basic cycle length = 2000 milliseconds. **B**. Isoproterenol (100 nmol/L) in the presence of chromanol 293B (30 μmol/L) produced a preferential prolongation of action potential of the M cell greater than that of epicardial and endocardial cells, resulting in an accentuated transmural dispersion of repolarization and broad-based T waves as commonly seen in LQT1 patients. **D**. d-Sotalol (100 μmol/L) in the presence of low potassium (2 mmol/L) gave rise to low-amplitude T waves with a notched or bifurcated appearance due to a very significant slowing of repolarization as commonly seen in LQT2 patients. **F**. ATX-II (20 nmol/L) markedly prolonged the QT interval, widened the T wave, and caused a sharp rise in the transmural dispersion of repolarization. ATX-II also produced a marked delay in onset of the T wave due to relatively large effects of the drug on the epicardial and endocardial action potentials, consistent with the late-appearing T wave pattern observed in LQT3 patients. Modified from References 24 and 25, with permission.

I_{Ks} is intrinsically weak, would be expected to abbreviate the epicardial and endocardial responses but not that of the M cell, giving rise to a broad-based T wave and a large transmural dispersion of repolarization.

I_{Kr} blockers such as d-sotalol can be used to mimic LQT2 as well as acquired (drug-induced) forms of LQTS. In such a model, a greater prolongation of the M cell APD and the slowing of phase 3 repolarization of the 3 cell types results in a long QT intervals, increased transmural dispersion of repolarization, and low-amplitude T waves. Because M cells have a weaker I_{Ks} than endocardial and epicardial cells,[37] making I_{Kr} the main repolarizing current, block of I_{Kr} in the M cell exerts a greater prolongation in this cell type. The addition of hypokalemia to I_{Kr} block leads to a very significant slowing of repolarization due to a more potent drug-induced inhibition of I_{Kr} and a smaller I_{K1} at the lower $[K^+]_o$ (Fig. 1, panel D).[38] In this case, long QT intervals are accompanied by low-amplitude T waves with a deeply notched or bifurcated appearance, as commonly seen in patients with the LQT2 syndrome (Fig. 1, panel D).

ATX-II, an agent that augments late sodium current (I_{Na}) by slowing the inactivation of the sodium channel, is used to mimic the LQT3 syndrome.[24] ATX-II markedly prolongs the QT interval, delays the onset of the T wave, in some cases also widening it, and causes a sharp rise in transmural dispersion of repolarization as a result of a greater prolongation of the APD of the M cell (Fig. 1, panel F). The differential effect of ATX-II to prolong the M cell is most likely due to the presence of a larger late I_{Na} in the M cell.[39] ATX-II produces a marked delay in onset of the T wave due to relatively large effects of the drug on epicardial and endocardial APD, consistent with the late-appearing T wave pattern observed in patients with the LQT3 syndrome (Fig. 1, panel F).

These results highlight the important contribution of transmural electrical heterogeneity to the distinctive phenotypic appearance of the T wave in both congenital and acquired (drug-induced) forms of the LQTSs. The concordance of the results in the wedge preparations with the phenotypic electrocardiographic and pharmacologic manifestation of congenital forms of the LQTS observed in patients suggests that these drugs are a reasonable surrogate for the congenital and acquired forms of LQTS.

Mechanism of TdP

TdP is an atypical polymorphic ventricular tachycardia associated with prolongation of the QT interval in the ECG. Historically, the most noteworthy examples of TdP occurred in patients on quinidine who developed hypokalemia and presented with slow heart rates or long pauses. Such a combination of predisposing factors is commonly encountered in the clinic. These conditions are similar to those under which APD-prolonging drugs such as quinidine induce early afterdepolarizations (EADs) and triggered activity in isolated Purkinje fibers and M cells.[40,41] Recent clinical studies using MAP recordings techniques have demonstrated EAD-like activity in both congenital and acquired LQTS.[15-22,42,43] These experimental and clinical observations suggested a role for EAD-induced triggered activity in the genesis of TdP, although the role of EADs and triggered activity in the genesis and maintenance of TdP is not well defined. It has been suggested that TdP at times may be initiated and maintained by triggered activity simultaneously originating at two independent foci. Others have suggested that TdP may be initiated by a triggered beat but maintained by a circus-movement reentry mechanism.[16,19,20,22,31,44,45]

In clinical studies of patients with congenital LQTS, MAP recordings indicated that the initiating beats (ventricular premature complexes [VPCs]) of TdP are closely related to triggered activity arising from EADs.[19,20,22] Panel A of Figure 2 shows a 12-lead ECG recording from a 23-year-old female patient with congenital LQTS that displays marked QT prolongation (QT = 0.68 s) and low-amplitude T waves with a notched or bifurcated appearance (leads V_3 through V_6). Several episodes of spontaneous TdP were documented (CM5 lead) after the patient was awakened by a noise of an alarm clock or excited by a ringing telephone (Fig. 2, panel B). The morphology of the initiating beats is always one of right bundle branch block (RBBB) (Fig. 2, panel B; see *). Because syncope and TdP were always preceded by exercise or emotional stress, the response to epinephrine infusion was examined. Epinephrine infusion (5 μg/min) reproducibly induces VPCs with RBBB morphology and left axis deviation (LAD), suggesting that the VPCs originate near the LV inferior wall (Fig. 2, panel C). Figure 3 includes MAP traces simultaneously recorded from the right ventricular (RV) anterior wall (RV ant MAP), the RV septum (RV sep MAP), and the LV mid-base inferior wall (LV mid-base inferior MAP) together with 6-lead ECG during epinephrine infusion (5 μg/min) in the same patient. EADs are recorded in the LV mid-base inferior MAP and are associated with an increased amplitude of the second component of T waves in lead V_3 (Fig. 3, see arrows). Epinephrine also induces VPCs with RBBB and LAD morphology that arise from the peak of the EAD (Fig. 3, see *). The upstroke of the MAP (phase 0) in the LV mid-base inferior wall precedes QRS onset of the VPC by approximately 30 milliseconds (Fig. 3, see *), indicating that the MAP catheter is positioned very close to the origin of the VPC and that the VPC is closely related to the EADs. In recent MAP studies, Kurita and coworkers[21] have also demonstrated a significant role of EADs in the generation of the long QT interval and in the development of TdP in class Ia drug-induced LQTS.

In experimental studies, Verduyn et al[46] and Volders et al[47] have documented the appearance of EADs as well as the development of a marked interventricular dispersion of repolarization in response to agents with

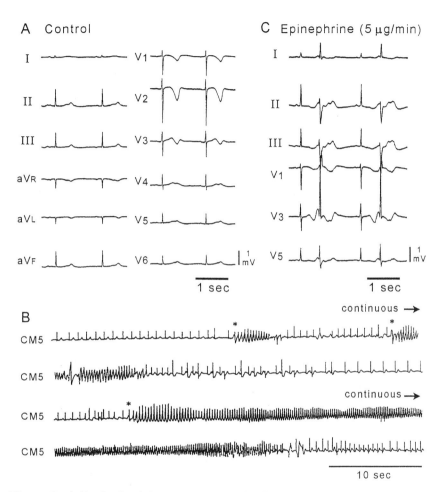

Figure 2. A. Twelve-lead electrocardiogram (ECG) of a 23-year-old female patient with congenital form of the long QT syndrome, showing marked QT prolongation (QT = 0.68 seconds) and low-amplitude T waves with a notched or bifurcated appearance (leads V_3 through V_6). **B.** Typical features of torsades de pointes (TdP) on monitor ECG (CM5 leads) after the patient was awakened by the noise of an alarm clock (upper two tracings) and excited by a ringing telephone (lower two tracings). Note that the morphology of initiating beats of TdP always showed a right bundle branch block (RBBB) pattern (*). **C.** Epinephrine-induced ventricular premature complexes (VPCs) on the 6-leads ECG. Epinephrine infusion (5 µg/min) induced VPCs with RBBB morphology and left axis deviation, indicating that the origin of the VPCs was near the left ventricular inferior wall. Modified from Reference 19, with permission.

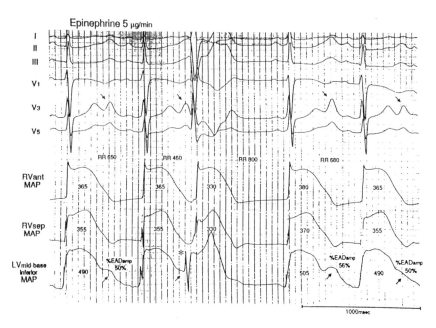

Figure 3. Epinephrine-induced early afterdepolarizations (EADs) and ventricular premature complex (VPC) during MAP recording in the same patient with congenital form of long QT syndrome as shown in Figure 2. Shown are electrocardiogram leads I, II, III, V_1, V_3, and V_5, and MAP recorded simultaneously from the right ventricular (RV) anterior wall (RVant), the RV septum (RVsep), and the left ventricular (LV) mid-base inferior wall (LV mid-base inferior). Epinephrine infusion (5 μg/min) induced VPC with right bundle branch block morphology and left axis deviation that arose from the peak of the EADs (*) recorded in the LV mid-base inferior MAP. Note that the upstroke of the MAP (phase 0) in the LV mid-base inferior wall preceded the QRS onset of the VPC by approximately 30 milliseconds, indicating that the VPC was closely related to the EADs. From reference 19 with permission.

class III action in the canine heart in vivo. While there is general agreement that the initiating event in TdP is an EAD-induced triggered response,[44,45] still in question is the origin of the triggered beats, as both Purkinje fibers[48] and M cells[49] are capable of generating EADs under similar conditions.

Consensus is also building that the maintenance of TdP is due to reentry; in addition, the substrate responsible for the development of the arrhythmia is not fully understood.[31,50,51] El-Sherif and coworkers,[44,45] using high-resolution tridimensional isochronal maps of activation and repolarization patterns, concluded that the initial beat of the TdP arises from a focal subendocardial site, whereas subsequent beats are due to reentrant excitation.

Studies involving the arterially perfused canine LV wedge preparations have provided further evidence to support this hypothesis. TdP develops spontaneously in some wedge preparations (Fig. 4, panel A), and can, by use of programmed electrical stimulation (Fig. 4, panel B), be induced in

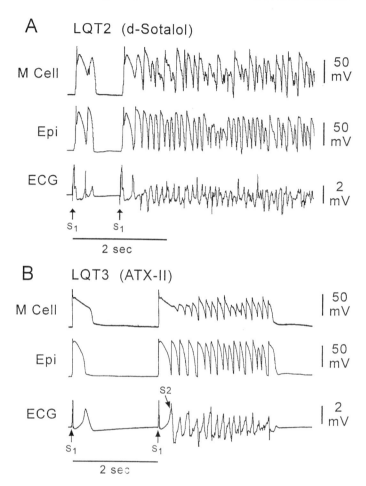

Figure 4. Polymorphic ventricular tachycardia displaying features of torsade de pointes (TdP) in the LQT2 (**A**) and LQT3 (**B**) models of arterially perfused canine left ventricular wedge preparations. d-Sotalol was used to mimic LQT2, and ATX-II was used to mimic LQT3, respectively. Each trace shows action potentials simultaneously recorded from M and epicardial (Epi) cells together with a transmural electrocardiogram (ECG). The preparation was paced from the endocardial surface at a basic cycle length of 1000 or 2000 milliseconds (S1). **A.** Spontaneous torsades de pointes (TdP) induced in the LQT2 model. First grouping shows spontaneous ventricular premature beat that failed to induce TdP, and second grouping shows spontaneous premature beat that succeeded. Premature response appears to originate from deep subendocardium (M or Purkinje). **B.** Programmed electrical stimulation-induced TdP in the LQT3 model. ATX-II produced very significant transmural dispersion of repolarization (first grouping). A single extrastimulus (S2) applied to the epicardial surface at an S1-S2 interval of 320 milliseconds initiated TdP (second grouping). Modified from Reference 24, with permission.

a majority of the preparations studied in models of the LQT1, LQT2, and LQT3 syndromes[24-26,28] as well as acquired forms of LQTS.[23] The fact that episodes of spontaneous TdP were induced in the wedge preparations suggests that the first extrasystole to initiate TdP originates in the deep subendocardium either in the Purkinje or M cells in all 3 models of the LQTS (Fig. 4, panel A).[24-26] Both cell types are capable of developing EAD-induced triggered activity. The following lines of evidence point to reentry as a likely mechanism for TdP developing in the wedge[23-26]: 1) the prerequisite of a marked dispersion of repolarization and refractoriness; 2) the ability to most easily induce the arrhythmia using a single extrastimulus introduced at the site of earliest repolarization (epicardium); 3) the occurrence of maintained arrhythmic activity only in larger preparations; and 4) the ability of several pharmacologic agents to suppress TdP by reducing the vulnerable window during which a single extrastimulus can induce TdP (as described below). These are all well established hallmarks of circus-movement reentry. Direct evidence for intramural reentry as the basis for TdP in the wedge was recently provided by Akar and coworkers,[52] who used optical recording techniques.

Possible Pharmacologic Therapy for the LQTS

A direct link of gene mutations to ion channel dysfunction suggests the possibility of gene-specific therapy for congenital LQTS. Schwartz and coworkers[53] have shown that sodium channel block with mexiletine is much more effective in abbreviating QT interval in LQT3 patients—those manifesting the sodium channel defect—than in LQT2 patients.[53] Exogenously administered potassium has been reported to correct repolarization abnormalities in congenital (LQT2) and acquired LQTS patients.[54,55]

In recent clinical studies, we used MAP recording techniques to assess the effects of several antiarrhythmic agents on MAP duration at 90% repolarization ($MAPD_{90}$), interventricular dispersion of $MAPD_{90}$, as well as the QT interval in patients with congenital forms of LQTS.[19,20,22] Most of our congenital LQTS patients were recently found to have chromosome 11-linked LQT1 syndrome[22] (and unpublished data). Our MAP data showed that verapamil, a Ca^{++} channel blocker, and nicorandil, a K^+ channel opener, suppress EADs and prolongation of $MAPD_{90}$ induced by epinephrine, indicating that these drugs may be of therapeutic value for congenital LQTS patients (Figs. 5 and 6). Our data also suggest that propranolol, a β-blocker, dramatically suppresses the effects of epinephrine, which include inducing EADs, prolonging the $MAPD_{90}$, and increasing the interventricular dispersion of $MAPD_{90}$ (Fig. 6).

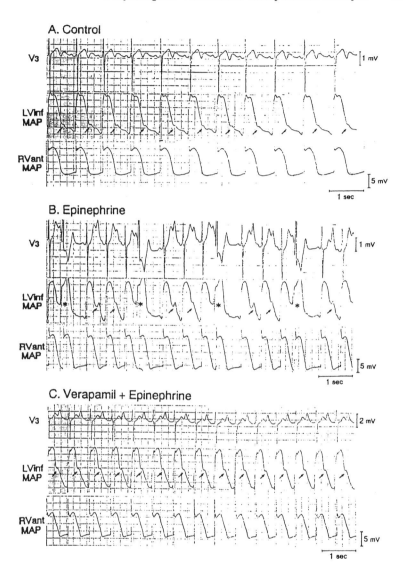

Figure 5. Effects of verapamil on epinephrine-induced early afterdepolarization (EAD) and ventricular premature complexes (VPCs) in a patient with congenital form of long QT syndrome. Each panel shows electrocardiographic lead V_3 and MAP recorded simultaneously from the left ventricular inferior wall (LVinf) and the right ventricular anterior wall (RVant). **A.** There was no ventricular arrhythmia, although EADs were recorded in the LVinf MAP (arrows). **B.** Epinephrine infusion (0.5 μg/min) increased the amplitude of EADs (arrows), and induced VPCs that arose from the peak (*) of the EADs, suggesting that the VPCs were closely related to the EADs. **C.** Verapamil injection (5 mg) during epinephrine infusion totally abolished the VPCs, although EADs were still present (arrows). From Reference 20, with permission.

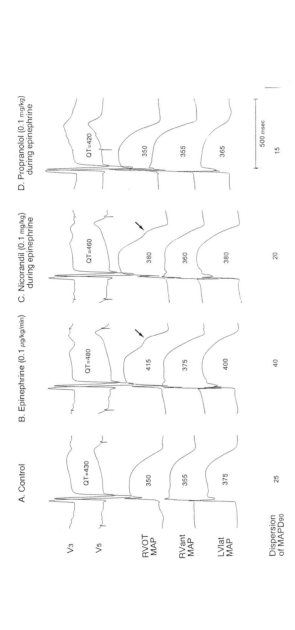

Figure 6. Effects of nicorandil and propranolol on epinephrine-induced prolongation of 90% monophasic action potential duration (MAPD$_{90}$) and early afterdepolarization (EAD) during MAP recording in a patient with congenital form of LQT1 syndrome with *KvLQT1* defect. Shown are electrocardiographic leads V3 and V5, and MAP recorded simultaneously from the right ventricular outflow tract (RVOT), the RV anterior wall (RVant), and the left ventricular lateral wall (LVlat) at a constant atrial pacing (cycle length 600 milliseconds). **B.** Epinephrine infusion (0.1 μg/kg/min) induced EAD in the RVOT MAP (arrow), prolonged the QT interval and the MAPD$_{90}$ in all sites, and increased the interventricular dispersion of MAPD$_{90}$ defined as the difference between the longest and the shortest MAPD$_{90}$. **C.** Nicorandil injection (0.1 mg/kg) abbreviated the QT interval and the MAPD$_{90}$ in all sites and decreased the interventricular dispersion of MAPD$_{90}$. **D.** Addition of propranolol injection (0.1 mg/kg) abolished the EAD and completely reversed the effects of epinephrine to the control level. The numbers in each MAP recording show the MAPD$_{90}$, and those at the bottom of the MAP recordings show the interventricular dispersion of MAPD$_{90}$. From Reference 22, with permission.

Although these clinical studies evaluate the effects of the antiarrhythmic agents on the QT interval and APD, they do not assess their actions on *transmural* dispersion of repolarization or on the relative risk for development of life-threatening arrhythmias, such as TdP. Experimental models involving the wedge preparation are able to evaluate these parameters quantitatively. The available data are presented in Table 1.

β-Blockers are widely reported to reduce the incidence of syncope and sudden cardiac death in patients with congenital LQTS.[2] Among the 3 forms of congenital LQTS, LQT1 is especially responsive to β-blockers.[35] Consistent with these observations, therapeutic concentrations of the β-blocker propranolol completely inhibit the ability of isoproterenol to increase transmural dispersion of repolarization and to produce spontaneous as well as stimulation-induced TdP in the LQT1 model in the wedge preparations.[25] Our data also point to a diminution of transmural dispersion of repolarization during normal sympathetic tone or prevention of an augmentation in transmural dispersion in response to strong sympathetic stimulation as the basis for the antiarrhythmic effectiveness of β-blockers. Although the relative effectiveness of β-blockers in the LQT2 and LQT3 models remain to be studied in the wedge, recent data from isolated tissues suggest that LQT2 but not LQT3 may be prominently influenced by the β-adrenergic system.

The class Ib antiarrhythmic mexiletine is an agent which, like lidocaine, shows rapid dissociation kinetics from the sodium channel. At relatively slow rates, it significantly blocks the late I_{Na} at the level of the action potential plateau, although its effects on fast I_{Na} and on normal conduction are negligible at the lower concentrations. Studies employing the arterially perfused wedge show that, while mexiletine is more effective in abbreviat-

Table 1
Effects of Pacing and Antiarrhythmic Agents

	LQT1 (and LQT5)	LQT2	LQT3
Rate dependence of QT interval	++	++	+++++
Sensitivity to catecholamines	+++++	+++	–
Effect of β-blockers	+++++	+++	–
Effect of Ca^{2+} channel blockers	+++	+++	?
Effect of Na^+ channel blockers	+++	++++	+++++
Effect of K^+ channel openers	++	++	–

ing the QT interval in the LQT3 (ATX-II) model than in either the LQT1 (chromanol 293B) or the LQT2 (d-sotalol) model, the sodium channel blocker reduces transmural dispersion of repolarization and prevents the development of spontaneous as well as stimulation-induced TdP equally in the 3 models.[24,25] The similar ability of mexiletine to decrease the transmural dispersion of repolarization and to suppress TdP in the LQT1 and LQT2 models as well as in the LQT3 model may be due to the relatively significant tendency of the drug to abbreviate the APD of the M cell, in which the late I_{Na} is relatively large, and the very insignificant tendency to abbreviate the APD of the epicardial and endocardial cells, in which the late I_{Na} is smaller. These results suggest that sodium channel block may be of value in the treatment of the LQT1 and LQT2 as well as the LQT3 syndrome.

Preliminary data suggest that nicorandil, a K^+ channel opener, is capable of abbreviating long QT, reducing transmural dispersion of repolarization, and preventing spontaneous and stimulation-induced TdP when LQTS is secondary to reduced I_{Ks} (LQT1) or I_{Kr} (LQT2) but not when it is due to augmented late I_{Na} (LQT3); however, relatively high concentrations of nicorandil are required.

The preventive effects of these antiarrhythmic agents on TdP may be due to 1) suppression of the triggered activity responsible for initiation of TdP, and/or 2) elimination of the substrate for reentry via a reduction of transmural and other dispersions of repolarization.

Pacing Therapy for the Long QT Syndrome

The value of pacemaker therapy for patients with congenital LQTS that is resistant to antiadrenergic therapy (eg, β-blockers, left cervicothoracic sympathetic ganglionectomy) has long been appreciated.[56] Schwartz et al[53] indicated that increases in heart rate recorded during exercise testing or on Holter recording are effective in significantly abbreviating the QT interval in LQT3 but not LQT2 patients. In contrast, we demonstrate using MAP recordings that both the $MAPD_{90}$ and the interventricular dispersion of $MAPD_{90}$ are attenuated more in patients with congenital LQTS than in control patients when heart rate is increased by atrial pacing.[57] Most of our LQTS patients are linked to LQT1.[22] In the wedge preparations, APD-rate, QT-rate, and transmural dispersion of repolarization-rate relations are generally much steeper in the LQT3 (ATX-II) model than in either the LQT1 (chromanol 293B) or the LQT2 (d-sotalol) model, probably because of the very slow kinetics of reactivation of sodium current. The rate relations, however, are all steeper than under control conditions.[24,25] These results suggest that although pacemaker therapy is likely to be very effective for the treatment of LQT3, its usefulness in LQT1 and LQT2 should not be discounted (Table 1).

References

1. Schwartz PJ. The idiopathic long QT syndrome: Progress and questions. *Am Heart J* 1985;109:399-411.
2. Moss AJ, Schwartz PJ, Crampton RS, et al. The long QT syndrome: Prospective longitudinal study of 328 families. *Circulation* 1991;84:1136-1144.
3. Zipes DP. The long QT interval syndrome: A Rosetta stone for sympathetic related ventricular tachyarrhythmias. *Circulation* 1991;84:1414-1419.
4. Roden DM, Lazzara R, Rosen MR, et al, and The SADS Foundation Task Force on LQTS. Multiple mechanisms in the long-QT syndrome: Current knowledge, gaps, and future directions. *Circulation* 1996;94:1996-2012.
5. Wang Q, Shen J, Splawski I, et al. *SCN5A* mutations associated with an inherited cardiac arrhythmia, long QT syndrome. *Cell* 1995;80:805-811.
6. Curran ME, Splawski I, Timothy KW, et al. A molecular basis for cardiac arrhythmia: *HERG* mutations cause long QT syndrome. *Cell* 1995;80:795-803.
7. Wang Q, Curran ME, Splawski I, et al. Positional cloning of a novel potassium channel gene: *KVLQT1* mutations cause cardiac arrhythmias. *Nat Genet* 1996;12:17-23.
8. Splawski I, Tristani-Firouzi M, Lehmann MH, et al. Mutations in the *hminK* gene cause long QT syndrome and suppress I_{Ks} function. *Nat Genet* 1997;17:338-340.
9. Sanguinetti MC, Jiang C, Curran ME, Keating MT. A mechanistic link between an inherited and an acquired cardiac arrhythmia: *HERG* encodes the I_{Kr} potassium channel. *Cell* 1995;81:299-307.
10. Sanguinetti MC, Curran ME, Zou A, et al. Coassembly of KvLQT1 and minK (IsK) proteins to form cardiac I_{Ks} potassium channel. *Nature* 1996;384:80-83.
11. Barhanin J, Lesage F, Guillemare E, et al. KvLQT1 and IsK (minK) proteins associate to form the I_{Ks} cardiac potassium current. *Nature* 1996;384:78-80.
12. Antzelevitch C, Sicouri S, Lukas A, et al. Clinical implications of electrical heterogeneity in the heart: The electrophysiology and pharmacology of epicardial, M and endocardial cells. In Podrid PJ, Kowey PR (eds): *Cardiac Arrhythmia: Mechanism, Diagnosis and Management.* Baltimore, MD: Williams & Wilkins; 1995:88-107.
13. Roden DM, George AL, Bennett PB. Recent advances in understanding the molecular mechanisms of the long QT syndrome. *J Cardiovasc Electrophysiol* 1995;6:1023-1031.
14. Kay GN, Plumb VJ, Arciniegas JG, et al. Torsade de pointes: The long-short initiating sequence and other clinical features: Observations in 32 patients. *J Am Coll Cardiol* 1983;2:806-817.
15. Ohe T, Kurita T, Aihara N, et al. Electrocardiographic and electrophysiologic studies in patients with torsades de pointes: Role of monophasic action potentials. *Jpn Circ J* 1990;54:1323-1330.
16. Shimizu W, Ohe T, Kurita T, et al. Early afterdepolarizations induced by isoproterenol in patients with congenital long QT syndrome. *Circulation* 1991;84:1915-1923.
17. Shimizu W, Tanaka K, Suenaga K, Wakamoto A. Bradycardia-dependent early afterdepolarizations in a patient with QTU prolongation and torsade de pointes

in association with marked bradycardia and hypokalemia. *PACE* 1991;14:1105-1111.

18. Kurita T, Ohe T, Shimizu W, et al. Early afterdepolarization in a patient with complete atrioventricular block and torsades de pointes. *PACE* 1993;16:33-38.

19. Shimizu W, Ohe T, Kurita T, et al. Epinephrine-induced ventricular premature complexes due to early afterdepolarizations and effects of verapamil and propranolol in a patient with congenital long QT syndrome. *J Cardiovasc Electrophysiol* 1994;5:438-444.

20. Shimizu W, Ohe T, Kurita T, et al. Effects of verapamil and propranolol on early afterdepolarizations and ventricular arrhythmias induced by epinephrine in congenital long QT syndrome. *J Am Coll Cardiol* 1995;26:1299-1309.

21. Kurita T, Ohe T, Shimizu W, et al. Early afterdepolarization like activity in patients with class IA induced long QT syndrome and torsade de pointes. *PACE* 1997;20:695-705.

22. Shimizu W, Kurita T, Matsuo K, et al. Improvement of repolarization abnormalities by a K^+ channel opener in the LQT1 form of congenital long QT syndrome. *Circulation* 1998;97:1581-1588.

23. Antzelevitch C, Sun ZQ, Zhang ZQ, Yan GX. Cellular and ionic mechanisms underlying erythromycin-induced long QT and torsade de pointes. *J Am Coll Cardiol* 1996;28:1836-1848.

24. Shimizu W, Antzelevitch C. Sodium channel block with mexiletine is effective in reducing dispersion of repolarization and preventing torsade de pointes in LQT2 and LQT3 models of the long-QT syndrome. *Circulation* 1997;96:2038-2047.

25. Shimizu W, Antzelevitch C. Cellular basis for the ECG features of the LQT1 form of the long-QT syndrome: Effects of beta-adrenergic agonists and antagonists and sodium channel blockers on transmural dispersion of repolarization and torsade de pointes. *Circulation* 1998;98:2314-2322.

26. Shimizu W, Antzelevitch C. Characteristics of spontaneous as well as stimulation-induced torsade de pointes in LQT2 and LQT3 models of the long QT syndrome. *Circulation* 1997;96:I554. Abstract.

27. Yan GX, Shimizu W, Antzelevitch C. The characteristics and distribution of M cells in arterially perfused canine left ventricular wedge preparations. *Circulation* 1998;98:1921-1927.

28. Yan GX, Antzelevitch C. Cellular basis for the normal T wave and the electrocardiographic manifestations of the long-QT syndrome. *Circulation* 1998;98:1928-1936.

29. Moss AJ, Zareba W, Benhorin J, et al. ECG T-wave patterns in genetically distinct forms of the hereditary long QT syndrome. *Circulation* 1995;92:2929-2934.

30. Sicouri S, Antzelevitch C. A subpopulation of cells with unique electrophysiological properties in the deep subepicardium of the canine ventricle: The M cell. *Circ Res* 1991;68:1729-1741.

31. Antzelevitch C, Sicouri S. Clinical relevance of cardiac arrhythmias generated by afterdepolarizations: The role of M cells in the generation of U waves, triggered activity and torsade de pointes. *J Am Coll Cardiol* 1994;23:259-277.

32. Antzelevitch C, Sicouri S, Lukas A, et al. Regional differences in the electrophysiology of ventricular cells: Physiological and clinical implications. In Zipes DP, Jalife J (eds): *Cardiac Electrophysiology: From Cell to Bedside*. Philadelphia: W. B. Saunders Co.; 1995:228-245.

33. Antzelevitch C, Nesterenko VV, Yan GX. The role of M cells in acquired long QT syndrome, U waves and torsade de pointes. *J Electrocardiol* 1996;28(suppl):131-138.
34. Crampton RS. Preeminence of the left stellate ganglion in the long Q-T syndrome. *Circulation* 1979;59:769-778.
35. Schwartz PJ, Malteo PS, Moss AJ, et al. Gene-specific influence on the triggers for cardiac arrest in the long QT syndrome. *Circulation* 1997;96:I212. Abstract.
36. Busch AE, Suessbrich H, Waldegger S, et al. Inhibition of I_{Ks} in guinea pig cardiac myocytes and guinea pig I_{sK} channels by the chromanol 293B. *Pflügers Arch* 1996;432:1094-1096.
37. Liu DW, Antzelevitch C. Characteristics of the delayed rectifier current (I_{Kr} and I_{Ks}) in canine ventricular epicardial, midmyocardial and endocardial myocytes: A weaker I_{Ks} contributes to the longer action potential of the M cell. *Circ Res* 1995;76:351-365.
38. Yang T, Roden DM. Extracellular potassium modulation of drug block of I_{Kr}. Implications for torsade de pointes and reverse use-dependence. *Circulation* 1996;93:407-411.
39. Eddlestone GT, Zygmunt AC, Antzelevitch C. Larger late sodium current contributes to the longer action potential of the M cell in canine ventricular myocardium. *PACE* 1996;19:II569. Abstract.
40. Roden DM, Hoffman BF. Action potential prolongation and induction of abnormal automaticity by low quinidine concentrations in canine Purkinje fibers: Relationship to potassium and cycle length. *Circ Res* 1986;56:857-867.
41. Davidenko JM, Cohen L, Goodrow RJ, Antzelevitch C. Quinidine-induced action potential prolongation, early afterdepolarizations, and triggered activity in canine Purkinje fibers. Effects of stimulation rate, potassium, and magnesium. *Circulation* 1989;79:674-686.
42. Bonatti V, Rolli A, Botti G. Recording of monophasic action potentials of the right ventricle in the long QT syndromes complicated by severe ventricular arrhythmias. *Eur Heart J* 1983;4:168-179.
43. Jackman WM, Szabo B, Friday KJ, et al. Ventricular tachyarrhythmias related to early afterdepolarizations and triggered firing: Relationship to QT interval prolongation and potential therapeutic role for calcium channel blocking agents. *J Cardiovasc Electrophysiol* 1990;2:170-195.
44. El-Sherif N, Caref EB, Yin H, Restivo M. The electrophysiological mechanism of ventricular arrhythmias in the long QT syndrome: Tridimensional mapping of activation and recovery patterns. *Circ Res* 1996;79:474-492.
45. El-Sherif N, Chinushi M, Caref EB, Restivo M. Electrophysiological mechanism of the characteristic electrocardiographic morphology of torsade de pointes tachyarrhythmias in the long-QT syndrome. Detailed analysis of ventricular tridimensional activation patterns. *Circulation* 1997;96:4392-4399.
46. Verduyn SC, Vos MA, van der Zande J, et al. Role of interventricular dispersion of repolarization in acquired torsade-de-pointes arrhythmias: Reversal by magnesium. *Cardiovasc Res* 1997;34:453-463.
47. Volders PGA, Kulcsar A, Vos MA, et al. Early afterdepolarizations and aftercontractions induced by isoproterenol in canine ventricular myocytes are fast-pacing dependent! *J Am Coll Cardiol* 1997;29:329A. Abstract.
48. January CT, Riddle JM, Salata JJ. A model for early afterdepolarizations: Induction with the Ca^{2+} channel agonist BAY K 8644. *Circ Res* 1988;62:563-571.
49. Sicouri S, Antzelevitch C. Electrophysiologic characteristics of M cells in the canine left ventricular free wall. *J Cardiovasc Electrophysiol* 1995;6:591-603.

50. Antzelevitch C, Sicouri S, Litovsky SH, et al. Heterogeneity within the ventricular wall: Electrophysiology and pharmacology of epicardial, endocardial and M cells. *Circ Res* 1991;69:1427-1449.
51. Surawicz B. Electrophysiologic substrate of torsade de pointes: Dispersion of repolarization or early afterdepolarizations? *J Am Coll Cardiol* 1989;14:172-184.
52. Akar FG, Yan GX, Antzelevitch C, Rosenbaum DS. Optical maps reveal reentrant mechanism of torsade de pointes based on topography and electrophysiology of mid-myocardial cells. *Circulation* 1997;96(8):I355. Abstract.
53. Schwartz PJ, Priori SG, Locati EH, et al. Long QT syndrome patients with mutations of the *SCN5A* and *HERG* genes have differential responses to Na$^+$ channel blockade and to increases in heart rate: Implications for gene-specific therapy. *Circulation* 1995;92:3381-3386.
54. Compton SJ, Lux RL, Ramsey MR, et al. Genetically defined therapy of inherited long-QT syndrome. Correction of abnormal repolarization by potassium. *Circulation* 1996;94:1018-1022.
55. Choy AM, Lang CC, Chomsky DM, et al. Normalization of acquired QT prolongation in humans by intravenous potassium. *Circulation* 1997;96:2149-2154.
56. Moss AJ, Liu JE, Gottlieb S, et al. Efficacy of permanent pacing in the management of high-risk patients with long QT syndrome. *Circulation* 1991;84:1524-1529.
57. Hirao H, Shimizu W, Kurita T, et al. Frequency-dependent electrophysiologic properties of ventricular repolarization in patients with congenital long QT syndrome. *J Am Coll Cardiol* 1996;28:1269-1277.

38

Gender as a Risk Factor for Acquired Torsades de Pointes

Steven N. Ebert, PhD, Xiao-Ke Liu, MD and Raymond L. Woosley, MD, PhD

Introduction

Torsades de pointes (TdP) is a clinical arrhythmia that was first described in 1966 by the French cardiologist Dessertenne.[1] The name *torsades de pointes* derives from the characteristic electrocardiographic pattern, ie, "twisting of the points" of the QRS, or constantly changing morphology as the QRS axis rotates around the isoelectric line. The first reported cases were predominantly in patients who had been treated with the antiarrhythmic drug, quinidine. However, clinical cases of TdP have been subsequently shown to occur with many other categories of drugs and in individuals with congenital prolongation of the QT interval on their electrocardiogram (ECG) (see below). The diagnostic feature of *drug-induced* or acquired TdP is marked prolongation of the QT interval in the beats preceding the initiation of the arrhythmia. Arrhythmias that resemble TdP can be induced in animal models by drugs that block one or more potassium channels and by drugs or toxins that open or slow inactivation of sodium and/or calcium currents.[2-4] It is generally recognized that the drugs that are known to induce TdP in humans have in common the ability to block the rapid component of the delayed rectifier potassium current (I_K), termed I_{Kr}.

Non–drug-induced TdP is seen in patients who have the congenital long QT syndrome (LQTS) and in a rare group of individuals who have a

From Franz MR (ed): *Monophasic Action Potentials: Bridging Cell and Bedside.*
©Futura Publishing Company, Inc., Armonk, NY, 2000.

normal QT interval and a characteristically short-coupled variant of the arrhythmia.[5] Recently, studies of the molecular mechanisms responsible for the congenital LQTS have provided pathophysiologic insights into the potential mechanisms responsible for drug-induced arrhythmias. There are at least 6 chromosomal loci that have been linked to the LQTS (chromosomes 3, 4, 7, 11, 21, and undetermined).[6-9] Like the targets for the drugs and toxins that are known to cause TdP, the known mutations associated with the congenital LQTS also affect either potassium or sodium channels to lengthen action potential duration (APD) and QT interval. Although the autosomal inheritance of the known LQTS mutations would suggest otherwise, an increased incidence has been described in females.[10] Additionally, a preliminary analysis has found female bias mainly in patients with *LQT2* or *HERG* mutations that alter I_{Kr}.[11] These observations may be relevant to the reports of an increased incidence of TdP in females treated with antiarrhythmic drugs, especially those drugs that block I_{Kr}. As discussed below, ventricular cardiomyocytes isolated from female rabbits have a lower I_{Kr} density than those isolated from male rabbits.[12] We therefore hypothesize that I_{Kr} is a primary candidate current for gender-based differences in cardiac repolarization.

TdP and Gender

TdP is an often overlooked cause of syncope and sudden death.[13] The small number of cases presenting to any one physician makes it difficult to determine patterns or etiologic factors. However, as early as 1983 Abinader and Shahar[14] recognized that women might be at an increased risk of TdP when treated with the drug prenylamine. Ten years elapsed before it was generally accepted that female gender is a predisposing factor for drug-induced TdP. In 1993, Makkar et al[15] published an analysis of the gender distribution of 332 cases of TdP induced by antiarrhythmic drugs. From their analysis, it was clear that women were at an increased risk of developing TdP with every antiarrhythmic drug that they surveyed except procainamide. While the predicted incidence was 41%, women comprised ~70% of the 332 cases of TdP evaluated. Another publication from this group reported that 15 of the 16 cases of TdP with probucol in the Food and Drug Administration (FDA) Medwatch database were women.[16] In 1995, Kawasaki et al[17] reported an increased propensity in women for TdP during complete heart block not associated with congenital LQTS or drugs that prolong QT. Additionally, the SWORD trial, a large international trial with the d-isomer of sotalol, found female gender to be the major risk factor associated with increased risk of arrhythmic death in a post–myocardial-infarction population.[18]

The mechanisms responsible for the predisposition of women to TdP are unknown but may be related to the fact that the baseline electrocardiographic QT interval is naturally longer in women than in men.[19] Only recently has it become clear that this is because the QT interval in males begins to shorten at puberty and returns to equal that of women at about age 50.[20] This period of QT shortening occurs at the time when androgens are highest in males and, suggests that one or more of the male hormones may be responsible for the QT shortening and the relatively lower risk of drug-induced TdP in men. Interestingly, Lehmann et al[21] showed a similar effect for individuals who are "genotype positive" at the 7q (*HERG*) and 11p (*KVLQT1*) loci for LQTS, both potassium channel mutations; thus, despite having significantly longer baseline QT values than genotype-negative individuals, mean corrected QT (QTc) values in males were significantly shorter than those in females only after the onset of puberty (age > 16 years). Lehmann et al[21] also showed that the QTc is shorter in genotype-negative males after puberty. These results suggest that the gender difference in QTc is the result of changes that occur during and/or after male puberty (eg, increases in circulating androgens).

An understanding of the role that gender plays in modulating cardiac repolarization and influencing arrhythmia frequency could lead to potential approaches for reducing the risk of, or possibly preventing, drug-induced TdP. In addition to the obvious medical benefit, this would also have a tremendous impact on the ability of the pharmaceutical industry to develop new drugs. The risk of drug-induced arrhythmias has effectively halted the development of almost all new antiarrhythmic drugs,[18,22] and is complicating the development of new antihistamines, neuroleptics, calcium channel blockers, and miscellaneous drugs such as terodiline and cisapride. Furthermore, because TdP may be a model for other causes of sudden arrhythmic death, an understanding of the role of gender in TdP may lead to the identification of potential mechanisms for prevention of sudden death in high-risk populations such as those with congestive heart failure or ischemic heart disease.

Mechanisms of Drug-Induced TdP

It is important to make the obvious point that not all patients who are taking drugs that prolong the QT interval develop TdP. In fact, many of these drugs were developed as antiarrhythmic agents. Additional factors must be contributory, and some of these factors have been suggested by the clinical setting in which patients develop TdP. There are drug-specific characteristics of the clinical presentation, and, in addition to gender, there are risk factors that are common to all of the inciting drugs. The relationship of TdP to plasma concentration is an example of a drug-specific factor.

The incidence of TdP is dependent on plasma concentration in the case of the antiarrhythmic drug sotalol.[23] On the other hand, quinidine-induced TdP is usually associated with low- or subtherapeutic plasma concentrations.[24,25] TdP with the nonsedating antihistamines terfenadine or astemizole is highly dependent on the dose or the occurrence of drug interactions that lead to higher than usual plasma concentrations.[26,27] Drug-induced TdP is generally associated with the degree of QT prolongation and one or more of the following factors: low serum potassium, low serum magnesium, female gender, and a sudden increase or decrease in heart rate.[13,28,29] The risk of TdP seems greater when more than one of these factors is present. These factors, with the exception of gender, have been examined in experimental models and clinical studies, suggesting a general understanding of the pathogenesis of TdP.[2-4]

Although QT prolongation by drugs alone is not adequate to cause TdP, it is considered to be the first of several steps in the development of drug-induced TdP.[13] QT prolongation is usually caused by drugs that reduce outward potassium currents (Fig. 1), but it can also be caused by toxins or drugs that increase inward currents such as the sodium current.[2,3] Since APD is normally inversely related to the heart rate, a slow heart rate can contribute to the degree of baseline QT prolongation. An initial difference

Elements of TdP

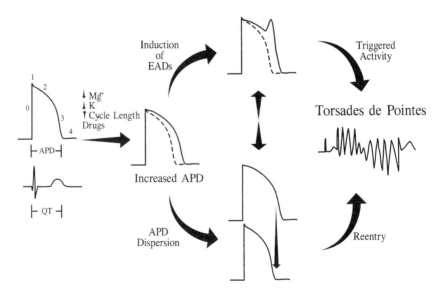

Figure 1. Potential mechanisms leading to the development of torsades de pointes ventricular arrhythmias.

in QT between individuals of opposite sexes is due to the naturally longer, rate-corrected QT interval seen in women.[19,20] Reduction in serum potassium or magnesium, often due to diuretic therapy, can also increase APD and QT. When the QT interval is excessively prolonged by one or more of these factors, cardiac tissue can develop early afterdepolarizations (EADs) during repolarization.[30] Clinically, these appear as markedly lengthened, distorted, alternating, notched, and/or bipolar T waves.[31] If occurring during phase 2, EADs are thought to be caused by increased inward current through L-type calcium channels[32] or through the sodium-calcium exchanger.[33] Depolarizing currents occurring late in phase 3 are thought to be due to inward currents through T-type calcium channels or sodium channels.[34] If these EADs reach threshold and propagate to the entire heart, they can elicit premature action potentials. When repetitive and sustained, such activity precipitates the TdP form of ventricular tachycardia. The sequence of these events is displayed in Figure 1. Alternatively, dispersion of electrical activity can lead to regional current sinks and sources of sufficient magnitude that triggered action potentials develop, and these may induce a reentrant tachyarrhythmia that migrates throughout the ventricle. Consequently, there are multiple sites in the cascade that can influence the potential for developing TdP.

Clinical Studies

Drug-induced arrhythmias have been a recognized problem with antiarrhythmic drugs for more than 40 years. In 1986, we summarized the clinical characteristics of TdP induced by quinidine.[24] Of the 24 patients with quinidine-induced LQTS and TdP that we studied, 16 were women: ie, 66% females compared to the predicted incidence of 45% based on actual prescriptions.[15] We have since collaborated with epidemiologists at the FDA and analyzed the reports of TdP and cardiovascular adverse reactions to drugs known to cause TdP in the FDA's Spontaneous Reporting System (SRS).[26] In our initial published analysis of 25 cases of TdP reported with the nonsedating antihistamine terfenadine, we found that 15 of the 25 patients in the SRS reports were female.[26] In a similar analysis of the FDA database, we found that a greater number of women than men have been reported to develop TdP with the antimalarial halofantrine. We found 20 reports of serious cardiac events in adult women and only 12 in males. Of the 12 males reported, 6 were less than 17 years of age (mean = 9 years). We have also analyzed 346 cases of serious cardiac reactions in FDA reports of patients treated with erythromycin, a commonly used antibiotic that also blocks potassium channels and has been associated with TdP arrhythmias. Although roughly equal numbers of males and females were treated with erythromycin, 65% of the FDA reports involved females.[35] These results, obtained through use of drugs from many therapeutic classes, suggest that women are more likely than men to develop TdP arrhythmias following exposure to these drugs that have in common the ability to block potassium channels.

To determine whether prospective administration of potassium channel blocking drugs might preferentially prolong the QT in women, we recently completed a study of 12 men and 12 women who were given infusions of quinidine gluconate or placebo in randomized order.[36] ECGs and plasma samples were obtained for blinded analysis of QT interval and free and total quinidine concentration 12 times during the 24 hours after each dose. As seen in Figure 2, women had a greater average slope for their response to quinidine than did men. The men had a significantly lower average slope (0.026 versus 0.033 ms/μg/mL; $P<0.001$) for the relationship, indicating a lower sensitivity to the potassium channel blocking actions of quinidine. There were no significant differences between quinidine pharmacokinetics or plasma protein binding in men and women. These data show that women appear to be more sensitive to quinidine-induced QT prolongation than do men. Since QT lengthening is a known risk factor for the induction of TdP cardiac arrhythmias, these studies suggest that women would be more likely to develop such arrhythmias following exposure to drugs that increase QT. However, the fact that none of these women developed TdP suggests that additional contributory factors are involved.

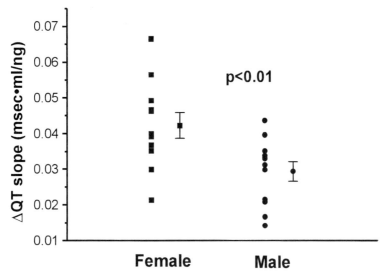

Figure 2. Comparison of slopes for quinidine concentration effect in 12 men and 12 women.

The Isolated, Perfused (Langendorff) Rabbit Heart Model

To identify the factors involved in TdP induction, we examined the ability of various drugs to prolong the QT interval in isolated, perfused rabbit hearts (Langendorff technique). Initially, we chose drugs known to be associated clinically with TdP. As seen in Figure 3, both quinidine and d-sotalol preferentially lengthened QT intervals in female hearts more so than in male hearts. These data suggest that the Langendorff rabbit heart can mimic some of the clinical findings seen with these drugs, and it can therefore serve as a model system for examining some of the electrophysiologic and biochemical foundations of gender-biased drug responses in the heart.

We have used this model system to test the hypothesis that females have longer QT intervals and greater sensitivity to QT-prolonging drugs than males, because of intrinsic differences in cardiac ion current densities. As shown in Figure 4, age- and weight-matched female rabbit hearts had longer baseline QT values than their male counterparts. In fact, the degree of gender difference is similar in normal human subjects and isolated rabbit hearts (Fig. 4, panels A and B, respectively). This gender difference in QT in rabbit hearts is most pronounced during pacing at slow rates.[12] This is similar to the rate dependence that we and others have seen in the gender difference in QT intervals.[20,37] The normal difference in resting QTc between men and women is lost when the heart rate is increased by exercise or isoproterenol infusion.[37] However, adult male hearts, both human and rabbit, have shorter QT intervals than female hearts. Consequently, females may be at greater risk of developing TdP arrhythmias, because drugs that induce QT lengthening might be more likely to extend their already longer QT intervals beyond a hypothetical "threshold" value critical for the induction of TdP, especially at slow heart rates.

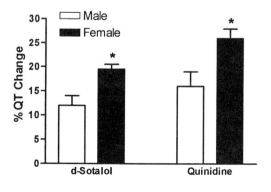

Figure 3. Effects of potassium channel blocking drugs on the degree of QT prolongation in isolated male and female rabbit hearts. The hearts were paced at fixed cycle lengths of either 1200 or 400 milliseconds and perfused with either d-sotalol (10 μM) or quinidine (3.3 μM), respectively.

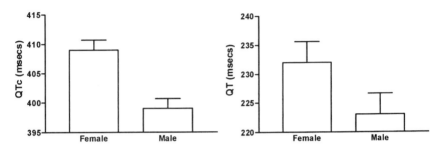

A. Normal Human Subjects   B. Isolated Rabbit Hearts

Figure 4. Baseline QTc and QT values in (**A**) men (n=6) and women (n=5), and (**B**) male and female rabbit hearts. The pacing cycle length for the isolated rabbit heart experiments was 2.3 seconds.[12]

The isolated, perfused rabbit heart model has also provided evidence that suggests that one of the mechanisms responsible for the observed gender difference in susceptibility to drug-induced TdP occurs subsequent to QT prolongation (see Fig. 1 for flow diagram of TdP development). For example, TdP can be reliably and preferentially induced in female rabbit hearts when they are challenged with 4-aminopyridine (4-AP) and abrupt changes in pacing cycle length while being perfused with Tyrode's buffer containing low concentrations of K^+ and Mg^{++}.[38] Male rabbit hearts subjected to the same treatment paradigm are relatively resistant to the development of TdP despite the fact that they display a similar degree of QT prolongation in response to 4-AP.[38] It is not clear why 4-AP does not induce gender differences in QT responsiveness, but part of the reason may be that 4-AP primarily blocks the transient outward potassium current, I_{to}. In contrast, quinidine and d-sotalol primarily block I_K. Nevertheless, drug-induced TdP occurs more than twice as frequently in female hearts than it does in male rabbit hearts in this model system.

As mentioned previously, one of the events that is thought to be involved in the triggering of TdP is the generation of EADs. Indeed, by continuously recording monophasic action potentials (MAPs) from isolated, perfused female rabbit hearts subjected to TdP induction by 4-AP, low K^+/Mg^{++}, and abrupt pacing cycle length changes as described above, we have observed EADs immediately preceding an episode of TdP (Fig. 5). In fact, it appears that EADs are generated during TdP as well as during the period immediately preceding it. Another example of drug-induced (4-AP, 1 mM) EAD production is shown in Figure 6. Prominent EADs are visible from the MAP recording. It appears that the first EAD immediately precedes extrasystoles. In contrast, the EAD that appears in the rightmost

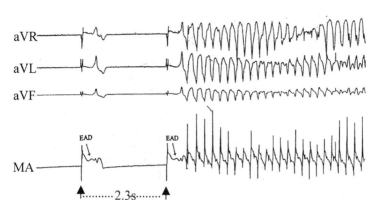

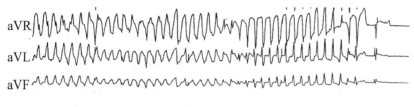

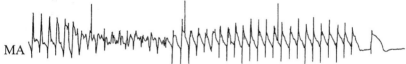

Figure 5. Electrocardiogram (ECG) and MAP recordings of a long episode of torsades de pointes (TdP) induced in an isolated female rabbit heart perfused with Tyrode's buffer containing low K⁺/Mg⁺⁺ concentrations and 1 mM 4-aminopyridine (4-AP).[38] TdP was triggered by switching the pacing cycle length from 0.3 to 2.3 seconds. ECG and MAP recordings are from the left ventricular endocardium. Note the typical twisting of the axis of the QRS complexes and the undulating patterns. Prominent early afterdepolarizations ([EADs] arrows) were recorded in the MAP of the initiating beat.

MAP signal, though prominent, is not associated with any extrasystoles. Thus, while EADs are often associated with extrasystoles and TdP, they can appear in the absence of such events. This caveat notwithstanding, the appearance of EADs, particularly in combination with drug-induced QT prolongation and increased MAP duration, indicates that conditions are conducive for the development of TdP. Since acquired TdP occurs more frequently in females than in males, the electrophysiologic mechanisms responsible for the production of EADs could prove to be a fertile area of investigation into the biological nature of the female preponderance for developing acquired TdP.

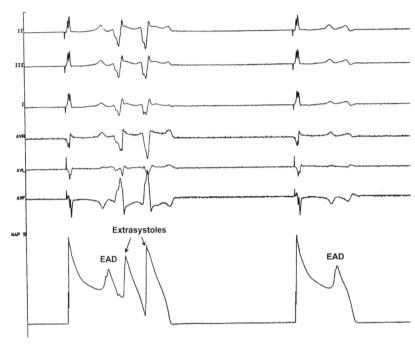

Figure 6. Early afterdepolarizations (EADs) induced by 4-aminopyridine (4-AP) (1 mM) in the MAP signal from an isolated perfused female rabbit heart. The top 6 traces represent electrocardiogram recordings and the bottom tracing is a MAP recording from the left ventricular endocardium.

Repolarizing Potassium Currents in Isolated Cardiomyocytes

As indicated above, several of the drugs known to lengthen QT intervals and elicit TdP arrhythmias are also known to block cardiac potassium currents. Thus, since females have longer baseline QT intervals and display greater QT lengthening when exposed to potassium channel blocking agents, we have hypothesized that female ventricular cardiomyocytes may have less cardiac potassium currents than do male cells. To test this hypothesis, we have measured the current densities of several specific potassium channels in rabbit ventricular cardiomyocytes isolated from male and female hearts. Multiple cells from at least 3 different hearts were analyzed for each sex, and the Student t test was used to compare current densities at a given voltage. All values are presented as mean ± SEM.

I_{Kr} is one of the major repolarizing currents in rabbit ventricular cardiomyocytes, and it has been implicated as a target in TdP.[21,26,39,40] To determine whether a gender difference in I_{Kr} may contribute to the observed gender difference in QT, I_{Kr} was compared in isolated male and female rabbit ventricular cardiomyocytes. Female cells had significantly less ($P<0.05$) I_{Kr} density compared with male cells (Fig. 7), yet no significant differences were observed in either the voltage dependence or the activation and deactivation kinetics of I_{Kr}.[12] These data demonstrate that despite similarities in voltage dependence and activation/deactivation kinetics, a significantly higher I_{Kr} density exists, on average, in ventricular cardiomyocytes isolated from male versus female rabbit hearts. These differences were most apparent at more positive test potentials, and represent a maximum difference in current density of approximately 20%.

To determine whether other outward potassium currents also display a gender difference, we next examined the I_{K1} density in female and male ventricular myocytes. Although there was no significant difference in the inward portion of I_{K1} between male and female cells, the outward component of I_{K1} (that responsible for regulating repolarization) was significantly less in female than in male cells ($P<0.05$). Peak outward I_{K1} at -50 mV was 1.46 ± 0.06 pA/pF in female cells versus 1.67 ± 0.08 pA/pF in male cells ($P<0.05$). This difference represents I_{K1} density of approximately 14% greater in male cells compared with female cells at its peak.

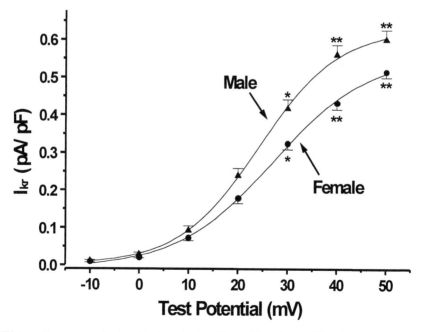

Figure 7. Average I_{Kr} density in male (n=37) and female (n=45) rabbit ventricular myocytes.[12] I_{Kr} tail currents are shown at various test potentials. Female cells had significantly less I_{Kr} at the indicated test potentials: *$P<0.05$; **$P<0.01$. Reprinted from Reference 12, with permission.

We have therefore concluded that small but significant differences in I_{Kr} and I_{K1} exist in randomly isolated cells from rabbit ventricular muscle. In both examples, current densities were significantly less in females compared to males. These small changes, when magnified throughout the ventricular muscle, could conceivably lead to significant alterations in APD. To estimate how these changes might influence APD, we performed a computer simulation, using the HEART (version 3.3) software program.[41] We used our patch clamp results showing maximum differences in current densities for I_{Kr} and I_{K1} of 20% and 14%, respectively, in female ventricular myocytes compared to those found in male myocytes (Figs. 7 and 8) to determine the effect that the magnitude of these differences would have on ventricular APD. The results of this simulation are shown in Figure 9. Bearing in mind the inherent limitations of this simulation (eg, the assumption that all other currents are unchanged), it nevertheless predicts that the observed differences in I_{Kr} and I_{K1} densities would result in a 9% increase

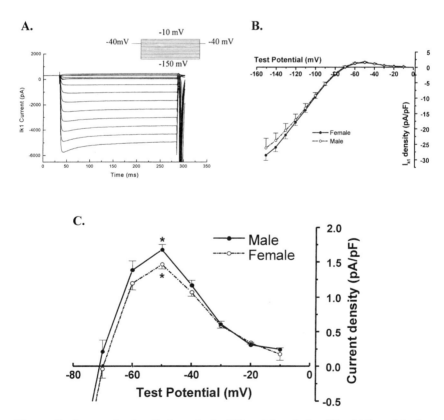

Figure 8. Average I_{K1} density in male (n=27) and female (n=46) rabbit ventricular myocytes at various test potentials.[12] A significant gender difference in the peak I_{K1} density was seen at -50 mV. *$P<0.05$. Reprinted from Reference 12, with permission.

Computer simulation of APD following 20% reduction of I_{Kr} and 14% reduction of I_{K1}

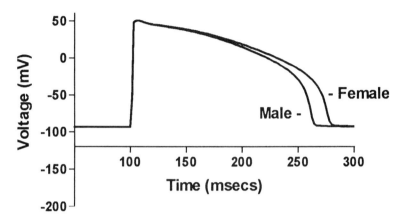

Figure 9. Computer simulated effect of decreased I_{Kr} and I_{K1} densities on the ventricular action potential using the HEART (version 3.3) software program.[41]

of APD in female cells compared to male cells. Approximately two thirds of this projected increase is predicted to come solely from the difference in I_{Kr} density. This model serves as an indicator of how changes in specific currents could potentially alter APD and, consequently, QT.

A Role for Sex Steroid Hormones?

The underlying causes of these observed gender differences are not known, but one hypothesis is that sex steroid hormones influence the activities of specific cardiac ion channels (reflected by current densities as noted above). We have begun to examine this hypothesis by manipulating these hormone levels in sexually mature rabbits and measuring expression of the mRNAs encoding for specific cardiac ion channel genes.[42] We observed a strong downregulation of mRNA concentrations encoding for the I_{sK} and *HK2* (Kv1.5), but not *HERG*, potassium channel genes in the presence of either 17-β-estradiol (E2) or dihydrotestosterone (DHT).[42] Although it is not clear at this time why E2 and DHT acted similarly in this model, these results provide strong evidence to suggest that sex steroid hormones can modulate expression of specific cardiac ion channel genes. Other cardiac ion channels and their currents will need to be examined to determine if differential regulation occurs and whether the current activities (in addition to gene and/or protein expression) of the channels are affected.

Compelling evidence that channel activities can be influenced by sex steroid hormones comes from our examination of the QT response to quinidine in the isolated, perfused rabbit heart model.[42] Female rabbits were ovariectomized and then implanted with pellets that provided sustained release of either E2 or DHT. The hearts from control and E2-treated rabbits responded similarly to quinidine, but the hearts from animals treated with DHT displayed an attenuated response (Fig. 10).

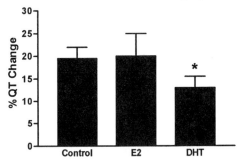

Figure 10. Quinidine response of isolated rabbit hearts for control, E2-treated, and dihydrotestosterone- (DHT)-treated ovariectomized rabbits. The DHT group showed a significantly smaller increase in response to quinidine than either the control or the E2 groups ($P<0.02$). Reprinted from Reference 42, with permission.

DHT significantly ($P<0.02$) reduced the degree of QT prolongation induced by quinidine in these experiments. This result is consistent with the clinical data discussed earlier[21] that suggest that postpubescent males have shorter QT intervals and are more resistant to the effects of I_K blocking drugs.

Summary and Future Directions

The clinical data indicate that women have a longer baseline QTc than men, and when exposed to drugs such as quinidine or sotalol, greater prolongation of the QTc occurs in women than in men. Since lengthening of QTc is a well established prerequisite for the development of TdP cardiac arrhythmias, women are at higher risk for the development of these life-threatening arrhythmias than are men. Indeed, it has been shown that many more women than men develop these arrhythmias following exposure to a diverse array of drugs. In most of these cases, the drugs have been shown to block one or more of the repolarizing potassium currents in the heart.

To uncover the biological basis for these observed gender differences, we have used the Langendorff rabbit heart model. Some of the advantages offered by this model system are the exquisite control of heart rate and drug concentration, and that it allows for the evaluation of direct cardiac effects without the potentially confounding influences of nervous system activity, circulating hormones, and other secondary factors. With use of this system, we have shown that clinical data for both the baseline and drug-induced gender differences in QT can be mimicked in the Langendorff-perfused rabbit heart. Moreover, the study of specific ion current densities in ventricular myocytes isolated from these hearts has led to the recent finding that females have, on average, lower I_{Kr} and I_{K1} densities than males. Since these currents contribute to the repolarization phase of the QT interval, their relatively lower abundance in female cells could help to explain why females have longer baseline QT intervals than males. I_{Kr}, in particular, is an attractive candidate because many of the drugs that produce TdP arrhythmias clinically have been shown to block this current.

To date, however, few cardiac ion currents have been examined for possible gender differences. Another important consideration is the potential contributory role of regional differences in specific cardiac current densities. Regional variation could play an important role in the dispersion of repolarization which, in turn, could also lead to the genesis of TdP arrhythmias (see Fig. 1). In addition, once the specific currents and regions of the heart that are responsible for the observed gender differences in cardiac repolarization have been identified, it will be necessary to determine the underlying reason for these differences. The best evidence currently available suggests that male hormones may play a role in regulating the QT interval, but the way that this is achieved is still unknown. Are the responsible currents controlled by differences in gene expression? Post-transcriptional or post-translational modifications? Interaction with different coupling factors? If so, how do these potential molecular differences (eg, different number of channel proteins versus differential gating properties of a similar number of channels) lead to the observed gender differences in current densities, lengthening of APD and QT, and, ultimately, to the increased risk of developing TdP cardiac arrhythmias? These are just a few of the many outstanding questions that need to be addressed. Clearly, however, progress is being made, and with the further development of clinically relevant experimental model systems, the answers to these questions will be within reach. Elucidation of the biochemical and electrophysiologic mechanisms responsible for the female preponderance of TdP cardiac arrhythmias should help in the prescription and design of better and safer drugs for women and men.

References

1. Dessertenne F. La tachycardie ventriculaire a deux foyes oposes variables. *Arch Mal Coeur* 1966;59:263-272.

2. Asano Y, Davidenko JM, Baxter WT, et al. Optical mapping of drug-induced polymorphic arrhythmias and torsade de pointes in the isolated rabbit heart. *J Am Coll Cardiol* 1997;29:831-842.

3. El-Sherif N, Caref EB, Yin H, Restivo M. The electrophysiological mechanism of ventricular arrhythmias in the long QT syndrome. Tridimensional mapping of activation and recovery patterns. *Circ Res* 1996;79:474-492.

4. Carlsson L, Almgren O, Duker G. QTU-prolongation and torsade de pointes induced by putative class III antiarrhythmic agents in the rabbit: Etiology and interventions. *J Cardiovasc Pharmacol* 1990;16:276-285.

5. Leenhardt A, Glaser E, Burguera M, et al. Short-coupled variant of torsade de pointes. *Circulation* 1994;89:206-215.

6. Curran ME, Splawski I, Timothy KW, et al. A molecular basis for cardiac arrhythmia: *HERG* mutations cause long QT syndrome. *Cell* 1995;80:795-803.

7. Sanguinetti MC, Jiang C, Curran ME, Keating MT. A mechanistic link between an inherited and an acquired cardiac arrhythmia: HERG encodes the I_{Kr} potassium channel. *Cell* 1995;81:299-307.

8. Wang Q, Curran ME, Splawski I, et al. Positional cloning of a novel potassium channel gene: KVLQT1 mutations cause cardiac arrhythmias. *Nat Genet* 1996;12:17-23.

9. Duggal P, Vesely MR, Wattanasirichaigoon D, et al. Mutation of the gene for IsK associated with both Jervell and Lange-Nielsen and Romano-Ward forms of long-QT syndrome. *Circulation* 1998;97:142-146.

10. Moss AJ, Schwartz PJ, Crampton RS, et al. The long QT syndrome. Prospective longitudinal study of 328 families. *Circulation* 1991;84:1136-1144.

11. Zareba W, Moss AJ, Le Cessie S, et al. Risk of cardiac events in family members of patients with long QT syndrome. *J Am Coll Cardiol* 1995;26:1685-1691.

12. Liu XK, Katchman A, Drici MD, et al. Gender difference in the cycle length-dependent QT and potassium currents in rabbits. *J Pharmacol Exp Ther* 1998;285:672-679.

13. Lazzara R. Mechanisms and management of congenital and acquired long QT syndromes. *Arch Mal Coeur Vaiss* 1996;89:51-55.

14. Abinader A, Shahar B. Possible female preponderance in prenylamine-induced "torsades de pointes" tachycardia. *Cardiology* 1983;70:37-40.

15. Makkar RR, Fromm BS, Steinman RT, et al. Female gender as a risk factor for torsades de pointes associated with cardiovascular drugs. *JAMA* 1993; 270:2590-2597.

16. Reinoehl J, Frankovich D, Machado C, et al. Probucol-associated tachyarrhythmic events and QT prolongation: Importance of gender. *Am Heart J* 1996;131:1184-1191.

17. Kawasaki R, Machado C, Reinoehl J, et al. Increased propensity of women to develop torsades de pointes during complete heart block. *J Cardiovasc Electrophysiol* 1995;6:1-7.

18. Waldo AL, Camm AJ, deRuyter H, et al. Effect of d-sotalol on mortality in patients with left ventricular dysfunction after recent and remote myocardial infarction. The SWORD Investigators. Survival With Oral d-Sotalol. *Lancet* 1996;348:7-12.

19. Bazett HC. An analysis of the time relationship of electrocardiograms. *Heart* 1920;7:353-370.

20. Rautaharju PM, Zhou SH, Wong S, et al. Sex differences in the evolution of the electrocardiographic QT interval with age. *Can J Cardiol* 1992;8:690-695.

21. Lehmann MH, Timothy KW, Frankovich D, et al. Age-gender influence on the rate-corrected QT interval and the QT-heart rate relation in families with genotypically characterized long QT syndrome. *J Am Coll Cardiol* 1997; 29:93-99.

22. Woosley RL. CAST: Implications for drug development. *Clin Pharmacol Ther* 1990;47:553-556.

23. MacNeil DJ. The side effect profile of class III antiarrhythmic drugs: Focus on d,l- sotalol. *Am J Cardiol* 1997;80:90G-98G.

24. Roden D, Woosley R, Primm R. Incidence and clinical features of the quinidine-associated long-QT syndrome: Implications for patient care. *Am Heart J* 1986;111:1088-1093.

25. Thompson KA, Murray JJ, Blair IA, et al. Plasma concentrations of quinidine, major metabolites, and dihydroquinidine in patients with torsades de pointes. *Clin Pharmacol Ther* 1988;43:636-642.

26. Woosley RL, Chen Y, Freiman JP, Gillis RA. Mechanism of the cardiotoxic actions of terfenadine. *JAMA* 1993;269:1532-1536.

27. Woosley RL. Do H1 blockers astemizole (Hismanal) and terfenadine (Seldane) cause torsades de pointes? *Eur J Cardiac Pacing Electrophysiol* 1994;4:15.

28. Selzer A, Wray HW. Quinidine syncope: Paroxysmal ventricular fibrillation occurring during treatment of chronic atrial arrhythmias. *Circulation* 1964;30:17-26.

29. Locati EH, Maison-Blanche P, Dejode P, et al. Spontaneous sequences of onset of torsades de pointes in patients with acquired prolonged repolarization: Quantitative analysis of Holter recordings. *J Am Coll Cardiol* 1995;25:1564-1575.

30. Roden DM. Early after-depolarizations and torsade de pointes: Implications for the control of cardiac arrhythmias by prolonging repolarization. *Eur Heart J* 1993;14(suppl H):56-61.

31. El-Sherif N, Bekheit SS, Henkin R. Quinidine-induced long QTU interval and torsade de pointes: Role of bradycardia-dependent early afterdepolarizations. *J Am Coll Cardiol* 1989;14:252-257.

32. January CT, Riddle JM. Early afterdepolarizations: Mechanism of induction and block: A role for L-type Ca^{++} current. *Circ Res* 1989;64:977-990.

33. Szabo B, Sweidan R, Rajagopalan CV, Lazzara R. Role of Na+:Ca2+ exchange current in Cs+-induced early afterdepolarizations in Purkinje fibers. *J Cardiovasc Electrophysiol* 1995;5:933-944.

34. Roden DM, Lazzara R, Rosen M, et al. Multiple mechanisms in the long QT syndrome. Current knowledge, gaps, and future directions. *Circulation* 1996;94:1996-2012.

35. Drici MD, Knollmann B, Wang W-X, Woosley RL. Cardiac actions of erythromycin: Influence of female sex. *JAMA* 1998;280:1774-1776.

36. Benton RE, Sale M, Flockhart DA, Woosley R. Greater quinidine induced QTc interval prolongation in women. 1996. Submitted to *N Engl J Med*.

37. Drici MD, Sale M, Burnett A, Woosley RL. RR-QT relationships differ during exercise- and isoproterenol-induced tachycardia. *Clin Pharmacol Ther* 1996;59:189. Abstract.

38. Liu X, Wang W-X, Ebert SN, et al. Female gender is a risk factor for torsades de pointes in an in vitro animal model. *Circulation* 1997;96:1555. Abstract.

39. Carlsson L, Almgren O, Duker G. QTU-prolongation and torsades de pointes induced by putative class III antiarrhythmic agents in the rabbit: Etiology and interventions. *J Cardiovasc Pharmacol* 1990;16:276-285.

40. Roden DM, Bennett PB, Snyders DJ, et al. Quinidine delays IK activation in guinea pig ventricular myocytes. *Circ Res* 1988;62:1055-1058.
41. Noble D, Noble SJ, Bett GC, et al. The role of sodium-calcium exchange during the cardiac action potential. *Ann N Y Acad Sci* 1991;639:334-353.
42. Drici MD, Burklow TR, Haridasse V, et al. Sex hormones prolong the QT interval and down-regulate potassium channel expression in the rabbit heart. *Circulation* 1996;94:1471-1474.

Section VI

Mechanoelectrical Feedback: Introduction

The electrical impulse of the heart (the action potential) has historically been viewed as the trigger for the mechanical heart beat and as a means to provide modulation of its strength by transmembrane and sarcoplasmic ion exchange mechanisms. This area of research is known as *excitation-contraction coupling* or *force-interval relation*. There is growing evidence that mechanical forces produced by the heart's contraction-relaxation cycle (or its hemodynamic consequences) feed back onto the electrophysiologic process that triggered them, either immediately or over the course of several ensuing beats. This phenomenon, known as *contraction-excitation coupling* or *mechanoelectrical feedback*, may be clinically relevant concerning the electrophysiologic mechanisms by which congestive heart failure or dilated cardiomyopathy may cause arrhythmias or sudden cardiac death.

Mechanoelectrical feedback is a relatively new area of research. With the use of the classic microelectrode technique it was nearly impossible to study this phenomenon in an intact heart, because mechanical forces sufficiently strong to produce mechanoelectrical feedback would dislodge the electrode from its intracellular position. Although not entirely free from the risk of movement artifacts, the monophasic action potential (MAP) technique has taken center stage in this important field of research. MAP recordings are able to track relative changes in transmembrane voltage and changes in action potential configuration even under excessive changes in ventricular pressure or volume loading and, as such, have helped this field of research to mature and gain credibility for explaining mechanically induced arrhythmias in patients with hemodynamic overload, ischemia, or myocardial failure.

39

Effect of Ventricular Dilatation on Conduction, Repolarization, and Defibrillation Thresholds in Isolated Rabbit Hearts

Michael J. Reiter, MD, PhD

Introduction

Electrophysiologic changes that occur as a result of acute alterations in muscle loading conditions have been referred to as *mechanoelectrical feedback* or *contraction-excitation coupling*. Recent studies have sparked an increased interest in these phenomena and have suggested their potential clinical importance.[1,2] Mechanoelectrical feedback probably comprises several different electrophysiologic phenomena. Acute dilatation can produce membrane potential depolarization, which, if of sufficient magnitude and rapidity, can precipitate spontaneous arrhythmias. Acute dilatation can also influence action potential duration (APD) and myocardial refractoriness. Changes in myocardial refractoriness can increase the tendency for reentry and ventricular fibrillation (VF), and may also influence the efficacy (and risk) of antiarrhythmic drugs and the energy required to terminate VF.

From Franz MR (ed): *Monophasic Action Potentials: Bridging Cell and Bedside.*
©Futura Publishing Company, Inc., Armonk, NY, 2000.

Effects of Mechanical Stretch on Conduction

Early observations suggested that stretch of myocardial tissue decreases conduction velocity. Penefsky and Hoffman[3] measured the conduction time between two carbon particles positioned on cat papillary muscle preparations from which they calculated conduction velocity before and after stretch. When the muscle was stretched to approximately 125% of its initial length, conduction velocity decreased; however, this degree of stretch is probably nonphysiologic, and when subjected to mild stretch, muscle conduction velocity was not changed.

Zabel et al[4] observed that when the left ventricular cavities of isolated rabbit hearts were dilated by 1 mL, the time between pacing stimulus and the upstroke of a recorded monophasic action potential (MAP) increased by approximately 12%, suggesting a decrease in conduction velocity. However, in earlier studies in which a similar preparation was used,[5,6] the conduction time between two epicardial electrodes was not influenced by the addition of similar volumes to the left ventricle. Conduction velocity in the intact heart is difficult to measure when the exact path followed by the impulse cannot be accurately determined. In order to obviate this difficulty, experiments were performed using a preparation consisting of only several cell layers of a Langendorff-perfused rabbit epicardium. When a ring of this rabbit epicardium was dilated, no change in conduction velocity was observed as evidenced by the constancy of the cycle length of tachycardia due to continuous reentrant propagation around the ring.[7] To directly measure conduction velocity, experiments in a 2-dimensional preparation of rabbit ventricular epicardium[8] demonstrated that dilatation, within a physiologic range, did not influence transverse or longitudinal velocity.

Effects of Mechanical Stretch on Refractoriness

Acute stretch or dilatation within a physiologic range decreases myocardial refractoriness by shortening APD. In isolated, Langendorff-perfused rabbit hearts, inflation of a balloon anchored within the left ventricle, which raised left ventricular end-diastolic pressure from 0 to 30 mm Hg, decreased left ventricular epicardial effective refractory period (ERP) by 23%, from 118 ± 4 to 91 ± 6 milliseconds ($P<0.01$).[5] The decrease in epicardial ERP was progressive, rapid, and reversible, and persisted for at least the duration of the experiments (several hours). In subsequent experiments,[8] the effects of dilatation appeared to be cycle length-dependent--dilatation having a greater effect in shortening refractoriness at rapid rates, with little effect at slow rates (Fig. 1).

Acute dilatation of isolated hearts decreases APD.[4,6,9-12] In experiments[6] in which the effects of acute dilatation on refractoriness were studied, the decrease in ERP (measured by the extrastimulus technique) is completely accounted for by the decrease in APD. In isolated rabbit hearts, when ERP decreased 13 ± 2 milliseconds (from 111 ± 4 to 98 ± 5 milliseconds at a potassium concentration of 4.9 mM), the monophasic APD at 90% repolarization ($MAPD_{90}$) decreased 15 ± 2 milliseconds (P=NS). At a lower potassium concentration, when ERP decreased 16 ± 2 milliseconds, monophasic action potential duration (MAPD) decreased 13 ± 4 milliseconds (P= NS). Franz et al[13] have demonstrated that the recording of a MAP accurately reflects the time course of membrane repolarization, and Michelson et al[14] have shown that ERP determined at twice diastolic threshold approximates the relative refractory period of the strength-interval curve.

A similar decrease in ventricular refractoriness has been in observed in a variety of animal models[9-12] and in humans.[15-18] A shortening of refractoriness has been observed in tissue preparations and in isolated hearts,[4,8,12] and in the in situ cross-circulated heart in both pigs[11] and canines.[9,10] In humans, Levine et al[16] found that the inflation of a balloon in the pulmonary outflow tract shortened the MAPD of the right ventricle, and that MAPD lengthened after successful valvuloplasty in patients with pulmonary stenosis. A qualitatively similar phenomenon has been observed in the human heart in vivo during withdrawal from cardiopulmonary bypass,[15] during transient aortic occlusion,[17] and with pharmacologic afterload reduction.[18]

In a study of isolated rabbit hearts,[5] when the left ventricle was dilated, the right ventricle, which was not dilated, did not show a significant decrease in ERP. Left and right epicardial refractoriness, while similar in the undilated state, were significantly different after left ventricular dilatation. When the left ventricle was dilated by a uniform increase in end-diastolic pressure, refractoriness and APD did not shorten in a homogeneous fashion over the whole left ventricle. For example, with balloon inflation, left apical epicardial refractoriness decreased by 17% while the ERP measured at a basilar site decreased by a statistically different 9%. In several experiments in which the temporal difference in ERP between two left ventricular sites was compared (either mid anterior versus apical left ventricle or mid anterior versus a lateral-basilar site), dilatation increased the mean of the absolute difference between the two sites from 168% to 240%. When MAPD from 5 to 6 epicardial sites was measured with Ag-AgCl contact MAP electrodes, balloon inflation within the left ventricle of isolated, Langendorff-perfused rabbit hearts shortened the $MAPD_{90}$ at some sites while lengthening it at other sites (Fig. 2), thus increasing the dispersion of APD measured during steady state pacing from 27 ± 5 milliseconds to 38 ± 6 milliseconds.[4] While this increase in dispersion of refractoriness is quantita-

A.

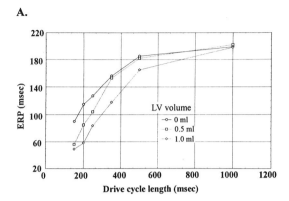

B.

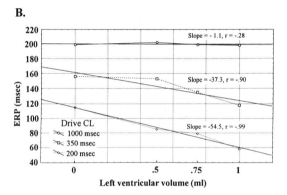

Figure 1. Influence of drive cycle length on left ventricular effective refractory period (ERP) for a typical experiment. ERP versus drive cycle length is plotted in panel **A**. For clarity, results are only shown for 3 different degrees of dilatation. **B**. Plot of ERP versus left ventricular volume during pacing at drive cycle lengths of 1000, 350, and 200 milliseconds. In the undilated preparation, as drive cycle length shortened (A), ERP decreased. This simply reflects the rate adaptation of refractoriness. After the addition of 0.5 mL into the left ventricular balloon, the ERP at cycle lengths ≥350 milliseconds was not different than the undilated ERP at the same cycle length. However, at shorter drive cycle lengths, the ERP was clearly decreased when the preparation was dilated. This effect was exaggerated with additional left ventricular dilatation (ie, 1.0 mL), since the ERP was shortened compared to the undilated state now at drive cycle lengths ≤500 milliseconds. Panel B illustrates data from the same preparation in a different format. Dilatation had no effect on refractoriness determined at a drive cycle length of 1000 milliseconds but caused a progressively greater decrease in ERP at shorter drive cycle lengths. The mean slopes of the ERP versus volume relationship as a function of basic drive cycle length demonstrate a progressively greater effect of increasing left ventricular volume on ERP as the cycle length decreases: at a cycle length of 1000 milliseconds the slope of this relationship was -2.8±1.6; at 500 milliseconds it was -10.1±4.1; at 350 milliseconds it was -14.5±8.0; at 250 milliseconds it was -25.4±8.1; and at 200 milliseconds it was -27.9±9.0. Reprinted from Reference 9, with permission.

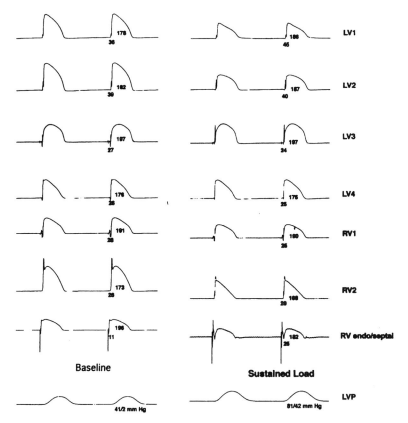

Figure 2. Example of MAP recordings during constant pacing (cycle length 600 milliseconds) comparing baseline (nondilated) and after the addition of 1 mL to a left ventricular balloon. Reprinted from Reference 5, with permission.

tively small, it may be enough to influence the arrhythmogenic substrate. In an open-chested dog model,[19] while the maximal difference between the longest and shortest recorded epicardial MAP associated with inducible arrhythmias was longer than those recorded in the isolated rabbit heart with dilatation, a change of only 17 milliseconds was associated with a change from a nonarrhythmogenic state to an arrhythmogenic state.

The explanation for the regionally heterogeneous change in refractoriness is unknown, but this change is likely related to the fact that wall compliance and thickness differ within the ventricle. Halperin et al[20] demonstrated that the primary determinant of the decrease in refractoriness is increased diastolic wall stress and, unlike interventricular pressure, which is equal throughout the left ventricle, wall stress is influenced by regional differences in circumference, wall thickness, and compliance.

The significance of these changes in refractoriness is related to the importance of reentry as a mechanism for ventricular arrhythmias. A decrease in refractoriness leads to a decrease in myocardial wavelength, which is an approximation of the length or duration of refractory tissue and mathematically is proportional to the product of the conduction velocity and refractoriness.[21] Because, as pointed out by Mines,[22] "*a closed circuit of muscle of considerably greater length than the excitation wave must be available...*[for reentry]," a shortening of myocardial wavelength increases the vulnerability of the tissue to a sustained reentrant arrhythmia and (because VF consists of multiple, continuous, chaotic wandering wavelets) increases the tendency for VF. Thus, reentry is favored by conditions that tend to slow conduction, shorten refractoriness, or increase regional differences in myocardial refractoriness.[19,23] Consistent with this hypothesis, increased inducibility of VF was observed when isolated rabbit hearts were dilated. The incidence of induced ventricular arrhythmias was 35% in preparations in which the ventricle was dilated (≥ 1.0 mL) compared to an inducibility of 3% when ventricular volume was ≤ 0.5 mL. The incidence of VF was correlated with the increase in the dispersion of refractoriness and the decrease in myocardial wavelength.

This arrhythmogenic effect of dilatation could act synergistically with other factors that might affect refractoriness or conduction velocity. In experiments which may have a clinical correlate, the interaction of ventricular dilatation and modification of the extracellular potassium concentration was studied.[6] Arrhythmias were not observed in undilated hearts at a normal extracellular potassium concentration (4.9 mM). In dilated hearts at similar potassium concentrations, the incidence of inducible VF was 38% while the wavelength shortened by 12% due to a decrease in refractoriness. In undilated hearts, under conditions of mild hypokalemia (3.5 mM), fibrillation was induced in 42% of experiments because hypokalemia decreased conduction velocity also decreasing myocardial wavelength by approximately 12% (in the absence of a change in refractoriness). In hearts subjected to both dilatation and hypokalemia, nearly all (92%) had inducible VF when the wavelength decreased by 28% because of a slowing of conduction and a decrease in ERP. These data are very comparable to experiments described by Rensma et al,[24] in which acetylcholine (which shortened atrial refractoriness) and class I antiarrhythmic agents (which slowed atrial conduction velocity) were used to influence wavelength of the atrial impulse in 19 dogs. Premature atrial stimuli provoked repetitive responses when the wavelength was shortened to less than 12.3 cm, but when further shortening was achieved, atrial extrastimuli induced either atrial flutter (when the wavelength was <9.7) or atrial fibrillation (when the wavelength was <7.8 cm).

The ventricular fibrillation threshold (VFT) is considered a measure of tendency of the myocardium for fibrillation, and is determined by scanning the vulnerable period with a train of impulses of increasing amplitude until VF is induced. VFT parallels susceptibility to spontaneous VF under a variety of conditions (eg, ischemia).[25,26] In the isolated heart, dilatation (to an end-diastolic pressure of approximately 30 mm Hg) decreased VFT by 30%.[27] Again, changes in VFT were correlated with the decrease in local refractoriness and excitation wavelength.

Effects of Mechanical Stretch on Defibrillation Threshold

The observation that acute dilatation decreases myocardial wavelength, increases inducibility of VF, and decreases the VFT suggested the possibility that dilatation may also influence the energy required to terminate VF (the "defibrillation threshold" [DFT]). An effect of acute dilatation on DFT could be clinically important. Implanted defibrillators deliver a fixed, limited, and sometimes marginal energy. If acute dilatation (eg, due to acute decompensation of congestive failure) raises DFT, a previously effective defibrillation energy may become ineffective, with important clinical consequences.

Lucy et al[28] showed that the development of congestive heart failure by chronic rapid pacing significantly increased DFT in a canine model. The DFT was fourfold higher in the animals with cardiomyopathy (13.3 ± 2.0 J compared to 3.3 ± 0.7 J). The development of failure was associated with myocardial hypertrophy and DFT was correlated with heart weight, but DFT remained significantly higher in the animals with congestive failure even when expressed as energy per gram of ventricle (0.086 ± 0.014 versus 0.032 ± 0.006 J/g), suggesting that the presence of failure had an effect independent of hypertrophy.

Although the factors that influence DFT in humans are significantly more complex, some data exist to suggest that intraoperative DFT increases with increasing left ventricular volume,[29] and that ejection fraction may be a better predictor of DFT than left ventricular mass.[30] In a prospective evaluation of factors that might predict a high (≥20 J) biphasic DFT in 114 consecutive patients,[29] multivariate analysis revealed only 2 independent predictors: echocardiographic measurement of left ventricular dilatation (odds ratio = 0.16, 95% confidence interval 0.05 to 0.53; $P=0.003$), and body size (odds ratio = 0.36, 95% confidence interval 0.17 to 0.73; $P=0.005$).

In order to examine the effect of dilatation in the absence of hypertrophy (or other histologic change), Ott and Reiter[31] dilated the left ventricle with a fluid-filled latex balloon in 19 isolated rabbit hearts. Dilatation (to an approximate end-diastolic pressure of 35 mm Hg) increased DFT an average of 30% (from 96 ± 4 to 125 ± 7 V; $P<0.001$) while decreasing left ventricular ERP by approximately 15% (from 116 ± 3 to 99 ± 3 milliseconds;

$P<0.001$). In one third of the preparations, the observed increase in DFT exceeded 150%.

In a subsequent series of experiments,[32] the effect of ventricular dilatation achieved by adding saline to a balloon secured within the left ventricle was compared to the effect of dilatation achieved by cannulating the left atrium and raising the left atrial pressure (and thereby left ventricular end-diastolic pressure) in working hearts. In all experiments, left ventricular end-diastolic pressures of 0 to 5 mm Hg (nondilated) and 20 to 25 mm Hg (dilated) were compared. In the working heart model, VF cycle length was recorded from sensing electrodes sutured onto the anterior lateral left and right ventricles. In these experiments two different defibrillating systems were also compared: epicardial and endocardial systems. After 10 seconds of VF, a monophasic shock of 12-millisecond pulse width was delivered between either a posterior patch electrode ($1.76\ cm^2$) in the epicardial system or an endocardial coil secured in the right ventricular apex (11 mm in length, 0.8 mm in diameter). The patch or coil electrodes served as the cathode, and a metallic aortic cannula as the anode.

Figure 3 illustrates the findings from this study. There was no significant difference in the nondilated DFT regardless of the method of dilatation or the defibrillation lead system used. Ventricular dilatation significantly increased the DFT in all 3 models. In the working heart with an epicardial lead, ventricular dilatation increased DFT by 57% (148 ± 8 V versus 233 ± 12 V; $P<0.001$; mean difference = 85 V). The

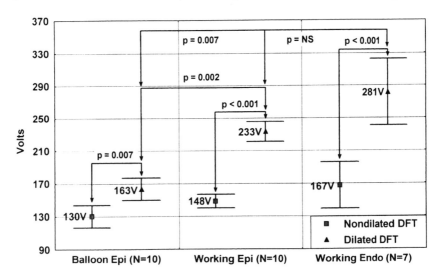

Figure 3. Effects of dilatation on defibrillation thresholds (DFTs) in balloon-dilated hearts with an epicardial defibrillating lead system, working hearts with an epicardial lead system, and working hearts with an endocardial coil as the cathode of the defibrillation electrode configuration.

increase in the DFT with dilatation in the working hearts with an endocardial lead was similar to that observed in the working hearts with an epicardial lead: increasing DFT by 68% (167 ± 28 V versus 281 ± 41 V; $P<0.001$; mean difference = 114 V). In the balloon-dilated model, ventricular dilatation increased DFT by 25% (130 ± 14 V versus 163 ± 14 V; $P=0.007$; mean difference = 33 V). The increase in the DFT in the working hearts regardless of the lead system was significantly greater than the increase in the DFT seen in the balloon-dilated hearts. In all experiments there was a significant reduction in left ventricular ERP with dilatation that was similar in balloon-dilated and working hearts. Mean left ventricular VF cycle length also decreased by 10% with dilatation (from 84.0 ± 3.4 milliseconds to 75.2 ± 1.5 milliseconds; $P=0.038$). There was no significant change in the right ventricular VF cycle length.

There was no significant difference in impedance between balloon-dilated and nondilated hearts (nondilated = $240\pm11.3 \geq$ versus dilated $241\pm13.8 \geq$; $P=NS$), but in both working heart models there was a statistically significant decrease in impedance between nondilated and dilated preparations (epicardial lead nondilated = $212\pm9.3 \geq$ versus $202\pm8.6 \geq$; $P=0.025$; endocardial lead nondilated = $195\pm15.8 \geq$ versus $184\pm11.8 \geq$; $P=0.045$). By multiple regression analysis, the dilatation-induced increase in DFT was significantly ($P=0.006$) correlated with the combination of VF cycle length and ERP determined at the shortest cycle length (250 milliseconds). A correlation between change in DFT and VF cycle length and impedance approached significance ($P=0.06$) in the working hearts.

The mechanisms by which congestive heart failure can influence DFT are no doubt complex, multiple, and largely unknown. These data suggest that in the balloon-dilated and working preparations, a change in the underlying arrhythmia (as manifested by a shorter average VF cycle length) and a decreased myocardial refractoriness (perhaps by increasing reinitiation of VF by surviving wavelets post shock) can influence DFT. In addition, in the working hearts, ventricular dilatation may also be associated with a "shunting" of energy through the intraventricular electrolyte solution, resulting in a lower myocardial energy gradient for defibrillation, thereby accounting for a greater increase in DFT than observed in balloon-dilated hearts (where the fluid is 'shielded" by the nonconductive latex balloon). This is supported by data reported by Strobel et al,[33] who evaluated the effect of volume on defibrillation efficacy in 8 pigs implanted with an endocardial lead system. These investigators compared a normal volume with a reduced volume achieved by inferior vena caval balloon occlusion. Reduction in ventricular volume significantly lowered defibrillation energy compared with normal volume (10.8 J versus 12.8 J; $P<0.05$) and was associated with significant increase in the impedance ($49.1 \geq$ versus $52.1 \geq$; $P<0.005$).

Conclusions

While its clinical significance is not known, mechanoelectrical feed-back may have important implications in those situations in which relatively rapid changes in ventricular volume occur clinically (eg, acute decompensation of congestive failure, acute mitral regurgitation). Hemodynamic decompensation, for example, appears to be associated with an increased risk of serious ventricular arrhythmias,[34] and dilatation can lead to degeneration of an initially stable tachyarrhythmia.[35] Pratt et al[35] published data from 15 patients who experienced VF during ambulatory ECG recordings. VF was initiated by ventricular tachycardia (VT) in all 15 cases (mean VT length before VF averaged 560 beats or approximately 2 minutes). These observations suggest that dramatic changes in rhythm may occur over a short period of time. Because even relatively slow VT may be associated with an increase in ventricular volume, mechanoelectrical feedback may offer a potential explanation for these observations. Development of tachycardia would normally lead to a shortening of refractoriness because of the rate adaptation of refractoriness. If, in addition, VT occurred in a dilated heart or led to dilatation, the increase in wall stress could cause an additional decrease in refractoriness. Because of the cycle-length–dependent nature of mechanoelectrical feedback, described above, the shortening of ERP associated with increased volume is likely to be greater during tachycardia than during sinus rhythm. These changes in refractoriness might explain why initially stable arrhythmias degenerate to VF.

It is well documented that patients with poor left ventricular function are less likely to respond to antiarrhythmic therapy. An agent may be "antiarrhythmic" by virtue of its effects in prolonging refractoriness, which could obliterate the excitable gap required for sustained reentrant arrhythmias and thus terminate (or prevent) the tachycardia. Dilatation by shortening refractoriness can widen the initial excitable gap, making any given refractoriness-prolonging effect of an antiarrhythmic agent less effective in eliminating the excitable gap. Figure 4 illustrates the effect of dilatation on average excitable gap and VT cycle length in preparations of a thin anisotropic ring of perfused rabbit epicardium.[7] In undilated preparations, VT cycle length averaged 190 ± 14 milliseconds, with an excitable gap of 91 ± 9 milliseconds. The class III antiarrhythmic agent d-sotalol, at 10 mg/L concentration, prolonged refractoriness from 99 ± 5 to 122 ± 6 milliseconds in the undilated hearts, decreasing the excitable gap 16 milliseconds. Dilatation of the untreated preparation shortened refractoriness and increased the excitable gap. But when the dilated preparation is treated with d-sotalol, the excitable gap is larger (92 ± 9 milliseconds) than in the undilated sotalol treated preparations (75 ± 7 milliseconds) and is essen-

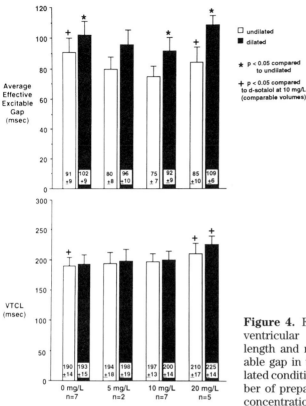

Figure 4. Effect of d-sotalol on ventricular tachycardia cycle length and mean effective excitable gap in the undilated and dilated conditions (n indicates number of preparations at each drug concentration). Reprinted from Reference 8, with permission.

tially identical to that in the untreated, undilated preparation (91 ± 9 milliseconds). Thus, the effect of dilatation in widening the excitable gap overwhelms the effect of sotalol in narrowing the excitable gap. This effect was not simply a function of drug level, nor could it be overcome by raising the final concentration of the drug (Fig. 4).

It is important to emphasize that the electrophysiologic effects of chronic dilatation may be different than those of acute dilatation. However, changes in refractoriness observed during acute dilatation, and their arrhythmogenic effects as described above, may have some relevance for the chronically dilated ventricle. It is interesting to note that in some studies,[36] end-diastolic volume is predictive of complex ventricular arrhythmias and it might be that a decrease in volume (and a decreasing mechanoelectrical feedback effect) can explain, in part, the mortality benefit of afterload-reducing agents in patients with congestive heart failure.[37,38] Additional studies, no doubt, will further clarify the nature and clinical significance of mechanoelectrical feedback.

References

1. Taggart P, Sutton P, Lab M. Interaction between ventricular loading and repolarisation: Relevance to arrhythmogenesis. *Br Heart J* 1992;67:213-215.

2. Reiter MJ. Effects of mechano-electrical feedback: Potential arrhythmogenic influence in patients with congestive heart failure. *Cardiovasc Res* 1996; 32:44-51.

3. Penefsky ZJ, Hoffman BF. Effects of stretch on mechanical and electrical properties of cardiac muscle. *Am J Physiol* 1963;204:433-438.

4. Zabel M, Portnoy S, Franz MR. Effect of sustained load on dispersion of ventricular repolarization and conduction time in the isolated rabbit heart. *J Cardiovasc Electrophysiol* 1996;7:9-16.

5. Reiter MJ, Synhorst DP, Mann DE. Electrophysiologic effects of acute ventricular dilatation in the isolated rabbit heart. *Circ Res* 1988;62:554-562.

6. Reiter MJ, Mann DE, Williams GR. Interaction of hypokalemia and ventricular dilatation in the isolated rabbit heart. *Am J Physiol* 1993;265(5 Pt. 2):H1544-H1550.

7. Reiter MJ, Zetelaki Z, Kirchhof CJH, et al. Acute ventricular dilatation decreases the class III effects of d-sotalol during sustained reentrant ventricular tachycardia around a fixed obstacle. *Circulation* 1994;89:423-431.

8. Reiter MJ, Zetelaki Z, Kirchhof CJH, Allessie MA. Electrophysiologic effects of acute dilatation in the isolated rabbit heart: Cycle length dependent effects on epicardial refractoriness and conduction velocity. *Circulation* 1997; 96:4050-4056.

9. Hansen DE. Mechanoelectrical feedback effects of altering preload, afterload, and ventricular shortening. *Am J Physiol* 1993;264(2 Pt. 2):H423-H432.

10. Lerman BB, Burkhoff D, Yue DT, Sagawa K. Mechanoelectrical feedback: Independent role of preload and contractility in modulation of canine ventricular excitability. *J Clin Invest* 1985;76:1843-1850.

11. Dean JW, Lab MJ. Effect of changes in load on monophasic action potential and segment length of pig heart in situ. *Cardiovasc Res* 1989;23:887-896.

12. Coulshed DS, Cowan JC. Contraction-excitation feedback in an ejecting whole heart model-dependence of action potential duration on left ventricular diastolic and systolic pressures. *Cardiovasc Res* 1991;25:343-352.

13. Franz MR, Burkhoff D, Spurgeon H, et al. In vitro validation of a new cardiac catheter technique for recording monophasic action potentials. *Eur Heart J* 1986;7:34-41.

14. Michelson EL, Spear JF, Moore EN. Strength-interval relations in a chronic canine model of myocardial infarction. Implications for the interpretation of electrophysiologic studies. *Circulation* 1981;63:1158-1165.

15. Taggart P, Sutton PMI, Treasure T, et al. Monophasic action potentials at discontinuation of cardiopulmonary bypass: Evidence for contraction excitation feedback in man. *Circulation* 1988;77:1266-1275.

16. Levine JH, Guarnieri T, Kadish AH, et al. Changes in myocardial repolarization in patients undergoing balloon valvuloplasty for congenital pulmonary stenosis: Evidence for contraction-excitation feedback in humans. *Circulation* 1988;77:70-77.

17. Taggart P, Sutton P, Lab M, et al. Effect of abrupt changes in ventricular loading on repolarization induced by transient aortic occlusion in humans. *Am J Physiol* 1992;263(3 Pt. 2):H816-H823.

18. Bashir Y, Sneddon JF, O'Nunain S, et al. Comparative electrophysiological effects of captopril or hydralazine combined with nitrate in patients with left ventricular dysfunction and inducible ventricular tachycardia. *Br Heart J* 1992;67:355-360.
19. Kuo CS, Munakata K, Reddy CP, Surawicz B. Characteristics and possible mechanism of ventricular arrhythmia dependent on the dispersion of action potential durations. *Circulation* 1983;67:1356-1367.
20. Halperin BD, Adler SW, Mann DE, Reiter MJ. Mechanical correlates of contraction- excitation feedback during acute ventricular dilatation. *Cardiovasc Res* 1993;27:1084-1087.
21. Wiener N, Rosenblueth A. The mathematical formulation of the problem of conduction of impulses in a network of connected excitable elements, specifically in cardiac muscle. *Arch Inst Cardiol Mex* 1946;16:205-265.
22. Mines GR. On dynamic equilibrium in the heart. *J Physiol* 1913;46:349-383.
23. Merx W, Yoon MS, Han J. The role of local disparity in conduction and recovery time on ventricular vulnerability to fibrillation. *Am Heart J* 1977;94:603-610.
24. Rensma PL, Allessie MA, Lammers WJEP, et al. Length of excitation wave and susceptibility to reentrant atrial arrhythmias in normal conscious dogs. *Circ Res* 1988;62:395-410.
25. Han J. Ventricular vulnerability during acute coronary occlusion. *Am J Cardiol* 1969;24:857-864.
26. Moore EN, Spear JF. Ventricular fibrillation threshold: Its physiological and pharmacological importance. *Arch Intern Med* 1975;135:446-453.
27. Jalal S, Williams GR, Mann DE, Reiter MJ. Effect of acute ventricular dilatation on fibrillation thresholds in the isolated rabbit heart. *Am J Physiol* 1992; 263:1306-1310.
28. Lucy SD, Jones DL, Klein GJ. Pronounced increase in defibrillation threshold associated with pacing induced cardiomyopathy in the dog. *Am Heart J* 1994;127:366-376.
29. Gold MR, Khalighi K, Kavesh NG, et al. Clinical predictors of transvenous biphasic defibrillation thresholds. *Am J Cardiol* 1997;79:1623-1627.
30. Chapman PD, Sagar KB, Wetherbee JN, Troup PJ. Relationship of left ventricular mass to defibrillation threshold for the implantable defibrillator. A combined clinical and animal study. *Am Heart J* 1987;114:274-278.
31. Ott P, Reiter MJ. Effect of ventricular dilatation on defibrillation threshold in the isolated perfused rabbit heart. *J Cardiovasc Electrophysiol* 1997;8:1013-1019.
32. Landers M, Reiter MJ. Ventricular dilatation in the isolated rabbit heart: Effect on the defibrillation threshold. *PACE* 1997;20:1174. Abstract.
33. Strobel JS, Kay GN, Walcott GP, et al. The effect of ventricular volume on ventricular defibrillation efficacy in pigs. *J Am Coll Cardiol* 1996;27:327A. Abstract.
34. Zado ES, Gottlieb CD, Marchlinski FE, et al. Exacerbation of heart failure precedes sudden death in patients with and without implantable defibrillators. *J Am Coll Cardiol* 1994;(suppl):393A. Abstract.
35. Pratt CM, Francis MJ, Luck JC, et al. Analysis of ambulatory electrocardiograms in 15 patients during spontaneous ventricular fibrillation with special reference to preceding arrhythmic events. *J Am Coll Cardiol* 1983;2:789-797.
36. Popovic AD, Neskovic AN, Pavlovski K, et al. Association of ventricular arrhythmias with left ventricular remodeling after myocardial infarction. *Heart* 1997;77:423-427.

37. Cohn JN, Archibald DG, Ziesche S, et al. Effect of vasodilator therapy on mortality in chronic congestive heart failure. Results of a Veterans Administration Cooperative study. *N Engl J Med* 1986;314:1547-1552.

38. The Consensus Trial Study Group. Effects of enalapril on mortality in severe congestive heart failure. Results of the Cooperative North Scandinavian Enalapril Survival Study (CONSENSUS). *N Engl J Med* 1987;316:1429-1435.

40

Mechanism of Load-Induced Changes in Ventricular Repolarization and Refractoriness

Bruce B. Lerman, MD and
Erica D. Engelstein, MD

Introduction

Patients with impaired left ventricular function, congestive symptoms, and increased ambient ventricular ectopy are at increased risk for sudden cardiac death.[1,2] The precise mechanism by which left ventricular dysfunction predisposes the myocardium to ventricular arrhythmias is unknown, but several factors are thought to play a role. These include acute ischemia, postinfarction remodeling, as well as metabolic and electrolytic disturbances and neurohumoral perturbations. Recent evidence suggests that alterations in gene expression for various voltage-dependent K$^+$ channels may be responsible for lethal arrhythmias in patients with congestive heart failure. For example, the densities of the transient outward current (I_{to}) and the inward rectifier (I_{K1}) are significantly reduced in these patients, resulting in action potential prolongation and early afterdepolarizations.[3]

This work was supported in part by a grant from the National Institutes of Health (RO1 HL56139).

The role of altered loading conditions in precipitating ventricular arrhythmias in heart failure patients is often underappreciated. The potential importance of this factor can perhaps be more fully understood by the recognition that mechanoelectrical feedback (or contraction-excitation coupling), defined as changes in myocardial mechanical state that precede and alter transmembrane potential, is the inverse process of excitation-contraction coupling, which is central to the biochemical processes governing cardiac function. The predominant effect of mechanical perturbations (increased load) on electrical properties relates to its effects on repolarization and refractoriness. The intent of this chapter is to review the experimental data that support this concept and to examine the mechanisms that mediate this process.

Background

The electrophysiologic effects of volume overload have been studied experimentally under two contrasting conditions: that related to transient diastolic stretch, and that due to steady state increases in stretch or volume. Initial studies in isolated myocardial tissue showed that transient stretch shortened action potential duration (APD) and elicited premature depolarizations.[4,5] These effects were subsequently confirmed in isolated mammalian hearts.[6,7] Several factors can potentiate the effects of transient stretch: an increase in steady state ventricular volume, an increment in both the amplitude and rate of stretch, and the diastolic timing of stretch.

The cellular mechanism(s) that mediate the electrical phenomena associated with transient diastolic stretch are thought to be related to stretch-activated channels. Among the better characterized cardiac stretch-activated channels are those isolated from rat ventricular myocytes, which are nonselective cation channels. These channels demonstrate an ohmic voltage-current relationship and a reversal potential of +30 mV.[8,9] Thus, at membrane potentials negative to the reversal potential, such as during diastole, activation of these channels can result in an inward or depolarizing current. Gadolinium (Gd^{3+}), a trivalent lanthanide and a blocker of stretch-activated ion channels in Xenopus oocytes,[10] also produces dose-dependent blockade of stretch-activated ventricular premature depolarizations in dog hearts.[11] Calcium channel blockers such as verapamil and nifedipine have no effect on stretch-activated premature depolarizations.

The second form of mechanoelectrical feedback is observed under conditions of steady state changes in preload and is the subject of the remainder of this chapter. In this model, increments in load occur gradually and are maintained over time, and primarily affect electrical repolarization and refractoriness.

Effect of Load on Repolarization and Refractoriness

Studies that commenced 15 years ago demonstrated that myocardial load alters the electrophysiologic responses in the intact mammalian ventricle.[12] To obviate potentially confounding variables such as neurohumoral influences, as well as the effects of ischemia and coronary artery perfusion pressure, many of these studies were performed in an isolated cross-circulated canine left ventricle, where ventricular pressure, volume, and coronary artery perfusion could be precisely controlled.

In such studies, measurement of load-induced refractoriness is performed using the techniques of extrastimulus testing. A more comprehensive measurement of myocardial excitability is assessed by the strength-interval relationship. Quantification of myocardial repolarization is, however, a more challenging task. Technical considerations preclude reliable long-term recordings with impaled floating microelectrodes and suction monophasic action potential (MAP) recordings. These limitations can be circumvented by recording MAPs deploying a contact electrode catheter consisting of two electrodes mounted on the distal end of the catheter.[13] One electrode is located at the tip of the catheter, whereas the other is 5 mm proximal to the tip. This catheter design and differential amplification allow for stable recordings of MAP duration from the ventricular epicardial surface throughout the course of an experiment. Importantly, recordings from this catheter reflect the time course of transmembrane depolarization and repolarization.[14]

With the use of this preparation several fundamental observations have been made. Increments in preload shorten ventricular refractoriness and increase electrical excitability.[12] This shifts the strength-interval curve to the left. A representative example is shown in Figure 1. This relationship holds whether the ventricle is beating isovolumically or is ejecting (Fig. 1, panel B). An increase in ventricular load also shortens MAP duration (Fig. 2). Since an approximate linear relationship exists between repolarization and refractoriness, load-induced changes in myocardial repolarization likely precede and account for shortening of refractoriness, as well as the leftward shift of the strength-interval curve. This concept is illustrated in Figure 3.

The mechanism mediating these phenomena are unknown; however, load-mediated activation of a K^+ repolarization current is consistent with experimental data. Further support for this hypothesis is derived from experiments examining the effects of the K^+ channel activator pinacidil. Pinacidil increases K^+ membrane conductance through augmentation of the ATP-regulated K^+ current $I_{K(ATP)}$.[15] Pinacidil, 0.5 to 1.0 mM, introduced into the isolated circuit of 6 isolated canine heart preparations depressed left ventricular contractility (Emax) by slightly more than 30%. Control measurements demon-

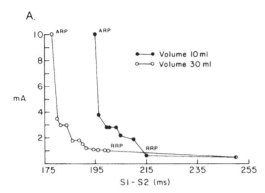

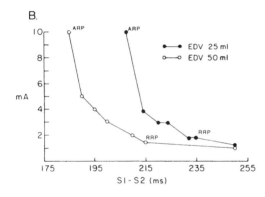

Figure 1. A. Representative effect of volume on the strength-interval relationship in an isovolumically beating left ventricle. Coupling intervals of the extrastimulus (S1-S2) are plotted versus the maximum milliamperage (mA) failing to capture the ventricle at that interval. Threshold excitability was unchanged by the increase in volume while the relative refractory period ([RRP] the longest coupling interval that required >0.1 mA increase in current for a 2-millisecond decrement in coupling interval to elicit a depolarization) and the absolute refractory period ([ARP] the longest coupling interval that failed to capture the ventricle at 10 mA) were decreased. **B.** Effect of volume on the strength-interval relationship in an ejecting left ventricle. Effects on threshold excitability, the RRP, and ARP were similar to those observed in isovolumically beating hearts. EDV = end-diastolic volume. Reproduced from Reference 12, with permission from *Journal of Clinical Investigation.* Copyright Rockefeller University Press.

strated that an increase in preload (two- to fourfold) was associated with a 6% shortening of MAP duration and a 3% decrease in the absolute refractory period. Pinacidil completely abolished the load-mediated decrease in MAP duration and the increase in ventricular excitability. These data are summarized in Figure 4. A representative strength-interval relationship for increased preload during control and in the presence of pinacidil is shown in Figure 5.

Experiments were also performed to evaluate the potential role of nonselective cation stretch channels in mediating these responses, since activation of these channels during phase 2 of the action potential would result in an outward current that would abbreviate APD (due to the reversal potential of these channels, +30 mV). Therefore, to determine the potential role of stretch-activated channels on load-induced changes in refractoriness and repolarization, the effects of Gd^{3+} were compared with control measurements (before Gd^{3+}) at low and high end-diastolic filling volumes in the isolated heart. Gd^{3+} was administered at a dose of 3 to 5 mg/kg

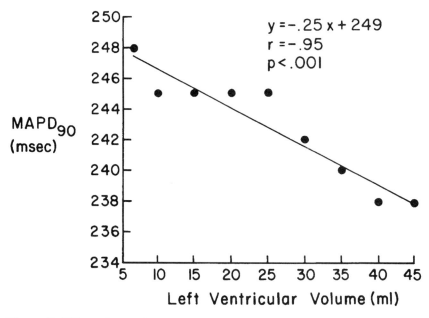

Figure 2. Effect of stepwise increases in left ventricular volume on ventricular MAP duration ($MAPD_{90}$) in an isovolumically beating canine left ventricle. Volume was sequentially changed by increments of 5 mL (5 to 45 mL). There was an inverse relationship between volume and $MAPD_{90}$. Reproduced from Reference 2, with permission.

(support dog body weight), which was based on the estimated volume of distribution of the support dog (13% of body weight) and circulatory circuit (1000 mL), and was calculated to achieve a minimum of a 10 mM concentration in the isolated heart perfusate.

Gd^{3+} increased contractility by slightly more than 40% and had minimal effects on left ventricular end-systolic or end-diastolic pressure. During control measurements, a fourfold increase in preload shortened MAP duration by 8% and decreased the absolute ventricular refractory period by 3%. Gd^{3+} increased MAP duration and the absolute refractory period at both low and high loads in all hearts (n=4). Despite the overall increase in APD and refractoriness, load-induced changes in these parameters were preserved in the presence of Gd^{3+}. For example, following pretreatment with Gd^{3+}, an increment in preload decreased the MAP duration by 7% and the absolute refractory period by 3%. Therefore, Gd^{3+}-sensitive stretch-activated channels do not appear to be responsible for steady state load-induced changes in repolarization and refractoriness. These data are summarized in Table 1.

It is likely that both forms of mechanoelectrical coupling (steady state increases in ventricular load and rapid diastolic stretch) act to synergisti-

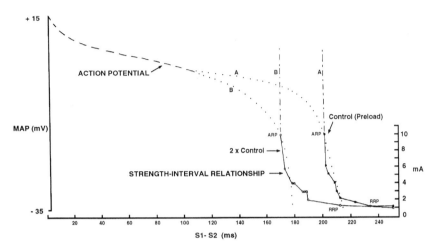

Figure 3. Superimposed on the strength-interval relationship at two different levels of preload are diagrammatic representations of the respective MAPs at the two levels of preload. Increased preload shortens the action potential duration (**B**) and allows membrane potential to recover earlier than the action potential associated with the lower preload (**A**). Therefore, because increased preload accelerates repolarization, premature extrastimuli are able to excite the ventricle at a coupling interval that would otherwise find the ventricle refractory at the lower preload. Reproduced and modified from Reference 12, with permission from *Journal of Clinical Investigation.* Copyright Rockefeller University Press.

cally enhance arrhythmogenesis. For example, stretch-induced arrhythmias are more likely to occur at higher rather than lower ventricular holding volumes.[6] It is also probable that each mechanical perturbation is independently arrhythmogenic, since steady state increases in ventricular load also enhance spontaneous ectopy,[12] increase the dispersion of repolarization,[16-19] increase inducibility of ventricular tachycardia with programmed stimulation,[16] and generate anodal current during accelerated repolarization, which can stimulate contiguous cells during their vulnerable period.[20]

The mechanoelectrical effects due to steady state increases in preload may in part be attributed to length-dependent activation of intracellular Ca^{++} ($[Ca^{++}]_i$).[12,21] The increase in $[Ca^{++}]_i$ due to mechanical stretch (load) and increment in sarcomere length is initially (30 seconds to 2 minutes) dependent on increased influx of Ca^{++}, whereas the subsequent increase in $[Ca^{++}]_i$ is related to enhanced Ca^{++} release from the sarcoplasmic reticulum.[22] Elevation of $[Ca^{++}]_i$ can activate several currents, some of which may prolong APD, and others which may abbreviate it. Increased transsarcolemmal Ca^{++} will prolong phase 2 of the action potential and increase the APD. Similarly, activation of the Na/Ca countertransport system exchanges 1 Ca^{++} for 3 Na^+ ions and therefore prolongs APD.[23] Intracellular

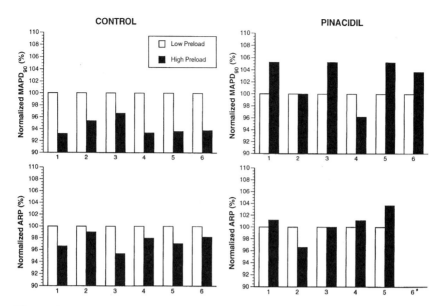

Figure 4. Effects of preload on MAP duration and the absolute refractory period (ARP) during control and in the presence of a potassium channel opener (pinacidil). Normalized MAP duration at 90% repolarization (MAPD$_{90}$) and the ARP are shown for each dog at low and high preload. During control, as previously shown, increases in preload decrease MAPD$_{90}$ and the ARP. Pinacidil abolished the effect of increased load on MAPD$_{90}$ and the ARP. *Dog No. 6 died following administration of pinacidil.

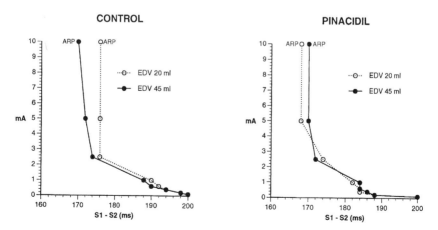

Figure 5. Representative effect of increased preload on the strength-interval relationship in an ejecting left ventricle during control and in the presence of pinacidil. Coupling intervals of the extrastimulus (S1-S2) are plotted versus the maximum milliamperage (mA) failing to capture the ventricle at that interval. Under control conditions, threshold excitability was unchanged by the increase in load while the ARP decreased. In the presence of pinacidil, the effects of increased load on ARP were abolished. EDV = end-diastolic volume. Abbreviations as previous described.

Table 1

Effects of Gadolinium on Mechanoelectrical Coupling

		Control	Gadolinium	
LVEDP (mm Hg)				
low preload	⌈	6.6±1.6	7.7±1.2	⌉
	$P<0.05$			$P<0.05$
high preload	⌊	27.4±2.8	31.5±5.4	⌋
LVESP (mm Hg)				
low preload	⌈	32±9.6	27±10	⌉
	$P<0.05$			$P<0.05$
high preload	⌊	97±23	105±25	⌋
ARP (ms)				
low preload	⌈	197±20	201±17	⌉
	$P<0.05$			$P<0.05$
high preload	⌊	190±20	195±17	⌋
MAPD$_{90}$ (ms)				
low preload	⌈	224±4	233±9	⌉
	$P<0.05$			$P<0.05$
high preload	⌊	206±8	217±10	⌋

ARP = absolute refractory period; LVEDP = left ventricular end-diastolic pressure; LVESP = left ventricular end-systolic pressure; MAPD$_{90}$ = monophasic action potential duration at 90% repolarization.

calcium overload can also activate a nonselective cationic channel, resulting in a transient inward current at the completion of repolarization.[24] In contrast, intracellular calcium can also activate outward currents that shorten APD. An example includes $I_{K(Ca)}$, a channel inhibited by charybdotoxin (CTX).

$I_{K(Ca)}$ has been identified in cardiac Purkinje fibers[25] and, more recently, in cardiac tissue from rabbits and humans.[26,27] This current is activated in myocytes by hypo-osmotic–induced membrane stretch and is abolished by chelation of intracellular Ca^{++}.[27] Activation of $I_{K(Ca)}$ results in diffusion of K^+ down its electrochemical gradient and the transfer of positive charge extracellularly, thereby abbreviating repolarization and APD.

Two predominant groups of $I_{K(Ca)}$ channels have been described: large K^+ conductance (BK) channels, with a very large single-channel conductance of 140 to 300 pS and high selectivity for K^+, and small conductance K^+ (SK) channels with a conductivity of ≤80 pS.[26-28] BK channels are also voltage-dependent, ie, at a given $[Ca^{++}]_i$, the probability of opening increases with the degree of depolarization.[29] BK channels are reversibly blocked with CTX ($K_d \sim 10$ nM), a protein component of the venom of the Israeli scorpion, *Leiurus quinquestriatus*.[30] CTX is thought to block the $I_{K(Ca)}$ channel by direct binding.[31]

Using the experimental preparation described earlier,[12] CTX (30 nM) abolished the changes in MAP duration and refractoriness observed with an increase in load. These results were confounded, however, by the unanticipated finding that CTX also resulted in load-independent shortening of the MAP duration in comparison with control. As a result, it is not possible to exclude the possibility that CTX may also activate an unidentified K^+ current. Therefore, the available evidence does not support a relationship between $I_{K(Ca)}$ and load-induced changes in repolarization and refractoriness.

Another possible mechanism by which load can mediate changes in repolarization and refractoriness involves the β-adrenergic receptor-effector coupling system. Activation of this system increases the slow-inward calcium current and also activates potassium (I_{Ks} and I_{to}) and chloride (I_{Cl}) currents, which accelerate repolarization.[32] To test the hypothesis that activation of the β-adrenergic system mediates this form of mechanoelectrical coupling, propranolol was infused into the perfusion system after control measurements were made. Of interest, propranolol completely abolished load-induced changes in repolarization and refractoriness.[33] To further corroborate these findings and to firmly establish the role of catecholamines in this process, hearts from dogs pretreated with reserpine over several days to produce catecholamine depletion failed to show load-induced changes in repolarization and refractoriness. These results suggest that myocardial stretch (or increased load) releases endogenous catecholamine stores that can activate β-adrenergic receptors. This in turn can activate repolarization currents that shorten repolarization and thereby decrease refractoriness.

Summary

Studies in the isolated left ventricle and the in vivo heart have clearly defined an inverse relationship between preload and ventricular refractoriness. This phenomenon is related to shortening of APD. This shortening is related to an abbreviation of phase 2 of the action potential and is likely due to an increase in a K^+ repolarizing current. These effects appear to be mediated by local release of norepinephrine and β-adrenergic stimulation, since load-induced changes in ventricular excitability and APD are abolished by propranolol or reserpine. Therefore, the cellular effects of mechanoelectrical coupling are in part due to load activation of the β-adrenergic-cAMP cascade. These effects appear to be mediated by an increase in activation of a cAMP-mediated repolarizing K^+ current (most likely the delayed rectifier I_{Ks}).

It is also likely that the process of mechanoelectrical feedback is a considerably more complex process than is generally appreciated and will involve not only interactions between K^+ and stretch-activated currents but also other currents not yet implicated. Just as important an issue will be whether mechanoelectrical effects actually potentiate clinical arrhythmias and, if so, by what mechanism? It has been noted that relatively large changes in load produce relatively small changes in refractoriness and repolarization, and that this finding alone would not likely have an arrhythmogenic effect. Therefore, it is of interest that increased load not only shortens APD but also perturbs it in a nonuniform manner,[16-19] thereby facilitating the induction of sustained ventricular tachycardia.[16,17] It is also noteworthy that increased load can also delay local activation time. Therefore, the wavelength of activation (conduction velocity × refractoriness) decreases, also potentiating the likelihood of a reentrant arrhythmia. These and other such findings should help delineate the ultimate significance of mechanoelectrical coupling in the initiation and perpetuation of clinical arrhythmias.

References

1. Gorgels AP, Vos MA, Smeets JL, et al. Ventricular arrhythmias in heart failure. *Am J Cardiol* 1992;70:37C-43C.
2. Lerman BB. Efficacy and risk of antiarrhythmic therapy in patients with asymptomatic ventricular arrhythmias and congestive heart failure. *J Cardiovasc Electrophysiol* 1991;2:S248-S254.
3. Tomaselli GF, Beuckelman DJ, Calkins HG, et al. Sudden cardiac death in heart failure: The role of abnormal repolarization. *Circulation* 1994;90:2534-2539.
4. Kaufmann R, Lab MJ, Hennekes, R, et al. Feedback interaction of mechanical and electrical events in the isolated ventricular myocardium (cat papillary muscle). *Pflügers Arch* 1971;332:96-116.
5. Lab MJ. Transient depolarisation and action potential alterations following mechanical changes in isolated myocardium. *Cardiovasc Res* 1980;14:624-637.
6. Hansen DE, Craig SC, Hondeghem LM. Stretch-induced arrhythmias in the isolated canine ventricle: Evidence for the importance of mechanoelectrical feedback. *Circulation* 1990;81:1094-1105.
7. Franz MR, Cima R, Wang D, et al. Electrophysiological effects of myocardial stretch and mechanical determinants of stretch activated arrhythmias. *Circulation* 1992;86:968-978.
8. Craelius W, Chen V, El-Sherif N. Stretch activated ion channels in ventricular myocytes. *Biosci Rep* 1988;407:407-414.
9. Craelius W. Stretch activation of rat cardiac myocytes. *Exp Physiol* 1993; 78:411-423.
10. Yang XC, Sachs F. Block of stretch activated ion channels in xenopus oocytes by gadolinium and calcium ions. *Science* 1989;243:1068-1071.
11. Hansen DE, Borganelli M, Stacey GP, et al. Dose-dependent inhibition of stretch-induced arrhythmias by gadolinium in isolated canine ventricles: Evidence for a unique mode of antiarrhythmic action. *Circ Res* 1991;69:820-831.
12. Lerman BB, Burkhoff D, Yue DT, et al. Mechanoelectrical feedback: Independent role of preload and contractility in modulation of canine ventricular excitability. *J Clin Invest* 1985;76:1843-1850.

13. Franz MR. Long-term recording of monophasic action potentials from human endocardium. *Am J Cardiol* 1983;51:1629-1634.
14. Franz MR, Burkhoff D, Spurgeon H, et al. In vitro validation of a new catheter technique for recording monophasic action potentials. *Eur Heart J* 1986;7:34-41.
15. Tseng GN, Hoffman BF. Actions of pinacidil on membrane currents in canine ventricular myocytes and their modulation by intracellular ATP and cAMP. *Pflügers Arch* 1990;415:414-424.
16. Reiter MJ, Synhorst DP, Mann DE, et al. Electrophysiological effects of acute ventricular dilatation in the isolated rabbit heart. *Circ Res* 1988;62:554-562.
17. Calkins H, Maughan WL, Weisman HF, et al. Effect of acute volume load on refractoriness and arrhythmia development in isolated chronically infarcted canine hearts. *Circulation* 1989;79:687-697.
18. Dean JW, Lab MJ. Regional changes in ventricular excitability during load manipulation of the in situ pig heart. *J Physiol (Lond)* 1990;429:387-400.
19. Zabel M, Portnoy S, Franz MR. Effect of sustained load on dispersion of ventricular repolarization and conduction time in the isolated intact rabbit heart. *J Cardiovasc Electrophysiol* 1996;7:9-16.
20. Brooks CM, Gilbert JL, Greenspan ME, et al. Excitability and electrical response of ischemic muscle. *Am J Physiol* 1960;198:1143-1147.
21. Lab MJ, Allen DG, Orchard CH. The effects of shortening on myoplasmic calcium concentration and on the action potential duration in mammalian ventricular muscle. *Circ Res* 1984;55:825-829.
22. Tatsukawa Y, Arite M, Kiyosue T, et al. Effects of mechanical stretch on intracellular calcium concentration in cultured rat ventricular cells. *Circulation* 1992;86:I822. Abstract.
23. Mullins LJ. The generation of electric currents in cardiac fibers by Na/Ca exchange. *Am J Physiol* 1979;236:C103-C110.
24. Colquhoun D, Neher E, Reuter H, et al. Inward current channels activated by intracellular Ca in cultured cardiac cells. *Nature* 1981;294:752-754.
25. Isenberg G. Cardiac Purkinje fibers. $[Ca^{2+}]_i$ controls steady state potassium conductance. *Pflügers Arch* 1977;371:71-76.
26. Krause PC, Rardon DP, Miles WM, et al. Characteristics of Ca^{2+}-activated K^+ channels isolated from the left ventricle of a patient with idiopathic long QT syndrome. *Am Heart J* 1993;126:1134-1141.
27. Hagiwara N, Matsude N, Shoda M, et al. Stretch induced calcium activated potassium current in single rabbit cardiac myocytes. *Circulation* 1992;86:I696. Abstract.
28. Latorre R, Oberhauser A, Labarca P, et al. Varieties of calcium-activated potassium channels. *Annu Rev Physiol* 1989;51:385-399.
29. Blatz AL, Magleby KL. Calcium-activated potassium channels. *Trends Neurosci* 1987;10:463-467.
30. Miller CH, Moczydlowski E, Latorre R, et al. Charybdotoxin, a protein inhibitor of single Ca^{2+}-activated K^+ channels from mammalian skeletal muscle. *Nature* 1985;313:316-318.
31. MacKinnon R, Miller C. Mechanism of charybdotoxin block of the high-conductance Ca^{2+}-activated K^+ channel. *J Gen Physiol* 1988;91:335-349.
32. Katz AM. Cardiac ion channels. *N Engl J Med* 1993;327:1244-1251.
33. Lerman BB, Todaka K, Engelstein E, et al. Beta-adrenergic mediation of mechanoelectrical feedback. *J Am Coll Cardiol* 1997;29:328A.

41

Time and Voltage Dependence of Electrophysiologic Stretch Effects in the Intact Heart

Markus Zabel, MD, Fred Sachs, PhD and Michael R. Franz, MD, PhD

Introduction

Ventricular arrhythmias and sudden cardiac death are frequently seen in patients with congestive heart failure.[1-4] Among other arrhythmogenic factors, it has been recognized that mechanical stretch can elicit ventricular arrhythmias in isolated tissues[5-7] as well as in intact heart models,[8-25] and may play an additional role in congestive heart failure. This association has been termed *mechanoelectrical* or *contraction-excitation* feedback.[9,26] The concept has recently been supported by the discovery of stretch-activated ion channels,[27-38] which help explain direct electrophysiologic effects of myocardial stretch. In patients or whole-heart animal models, the body surface electrocardiogram has been found to be too insensitive to detect the subtle changes induced by mechanical stretch. Therefore most data on electrophysiologic stretch effects have been acquired by use of monophasic action potential (MAP) recordings, usually with the contact electrode method.[39-41] This technique has been validated to yield signals identical in time course and shape with transmembrane electrode action

Supported in part by a Merck International Fellowship in Clinical Pharmacology and a Veterans Administration Merit Review Grant.
From Franz MR (ed): *Monophasic Action Potentials: Bridging Cell and Bedside.* ©Futura Publishing Company, Inc., Armonk, NY, 2000.

potentials[39,42] and has the advantage of being less prone to motion artifacts than intracellular recordings. This chapter reviews the various mechanisms of arrhythmia induction and facilitation by mechanical stretch that have been suggested in the literature,[8-25] and describes, with special emphasis, the opposing effects of very short, pulsatile stretch and prolonged, static mechanical stretch.

Electrophysiologic Effects of Acute Stretch

In early intracellular studies, mechanical stretch was found to shorten the action potential duration (APD).[5,7] In MAP recordings from the left ventricular epicardium of the isolated canine heart,[9,13,14] an acutely increased mechanical load was found to decrease both APD and refractory periods. Similar results were found in the isolated rabbit heart.[11] Other investigators, however, have reported lengthening of APD as a response to acute myocardial stretch.[8,12] Stretch-induced electrophysiologic changes also differed depending on whether acute mechanical stretch was applied in the form of an increased preload or increased afterload.[9,12,19,20] In addition, the repolarization level at which the APD is measured and the type of ventricular contraction seem to be factors that can help to explain the conflicting results. Franz et al[12] studied stretch-induced changes in the isovolumically beating canine ventricle, and demonstrated that an increase in ventricular volume load with a simultaneous increase in ventricular pressure shortened the APD at early repolarization levels, while lengthening APD at almost complete repolarization. Similar findings in isolated canine hearts were reported by Hansen.[19] Both investigators noted that the increase in the overall APD under increased isovolumic loads occurred in the shape of early afterdepolarizations (EADs).[12,19] Only recently, these results, which are opposing at first glance, could be explained by the time- and voltage-dependent stretch effects described below.[24] Franz et al[12,21] also reported a decrease in the resting potential as well as a decrease in the action potential amplitude under various conditions of isovolumic load in both dog[12] and rabbit[21] studies. The above-mentioned studies by Franz et al[12] and Hansen[19] also addressed the question of whether diastolic volume increase (preload) or rather systolic outflow impedance (afterload) is more important in the induction of stretch-induced electrophysiologic changes. Both investigators showed convincingly that only a preload increase leads to the acute stretch-induced electrophysiologic changes described above. For instance, changing the ventricular contraction mode from isovolumic to ejecting abolished EADs immediately.[12]

Electrophysiologic Effects of Short Transient Stretch

Franz et al[21] applied a series of rapid volume pulses of successively increasing amplitude to an isolated rabbit heart with atrioventricular block and rare escape beats. The volume pulses induced transient diastolic depolarizations that increased in amplitude with the parallel increase in pulse volume. Above a certain amplitude, each transient depolarization was associated with a premature ventricular response; ie, the preparation was 'paced" by the volume pulses. Similar stretch-induced premature ventricular contractions (PVCs) were reported in isolated frog,[8] pig,[15] and canine[17,18] hearts. Zabel et al[24] recently further investigated the effects of very short, differently timed pulsatile stretch in comparison to long, static stretch of the same amplitude in the intact, isolated rabbit heart. Stretch pulses of only 50 milliseconds" duration and flexible timing were applied by use of a servo-controlled piston pump connected to an intraventricular latex balloon (Fig. 1). In this study, both repolarizing and depolarizing responses were observed with a remarkable dependence on the timing of the stretch pulse with respect to the action potential phase. A short transient stretch pulse elicited either transient depolarizations when applied during late systole or diastole, or transient repolarizations when applied during the plateau of the MAP. A stretch pulse placed toward the end of the MAP caused depolarizations that mimicked EADs or, if placed after the MAP, delayed afterdepolarizations. When the depolarizations reached sufficient amplitude, PVCs resulted. The emergence of a stretch-induced PVC from a "take-off" potential that has reached threshold was first reported by Franz et al,[21] who investigated the effects of stretch velocity and amplitude in the isolated rabbit heart. Stacy et al[18] confirmed these results, but postulated that an accelerated phase 4 depolarization of Purkinje fibers is the mechanism of PVC induction. In contrast to "classic" early or delayed afterdepolarizations, the stretch-induced depolarizations did not depend on the trigger of a preceding action potential. The studies by Zabel et al[24] and Stacy et al[18] were able to demonstrate that the amplitude of a stretch-induced diastolic depolarization is linearly correlated with the amplitude of the underlying stretch pulse. In addition, Zabel et al[24] found that the amplitude of a stretch-related repolarization during the plateau phase of the MAP exhibits a linear relationship similar to the stretch pulse amplitude. Importantly, halfway between these opposing responses, a neutral response to stretch was found. A gradual crossover was seen between the two oppositely polarized stretch effects, as described above (Fig. 2). When the stretch pulse was applied during early phase 3 of the MAP, the repolarizing deflection was less than during the plateau of the action potential. Similarly, stretch-activated depolarizations became smaller when the pulse

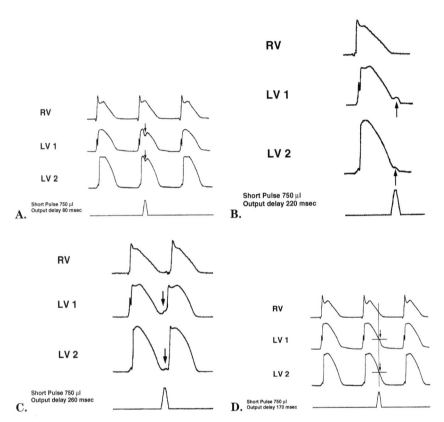

Figure 1. A. Example of a stretch-induced repolarization during early systole. Note that the timing of the repolarization is exactly coincident with the stretch pulse. No change is seen in the right ventricular MAP recording. **B**. Example of a stretch-induced depolarization during late systole/early diastole. **C**. Example of a stretch-induced premature ventricular contraction. Note that the highest amplitude is seen in the tracing where activation of the premature beat occurs earlier (LV2). **D**. Example of an absent response to myocardial stretch during phase 3 of depolarization. Note also that due to the slightly different shape of the two stretched action potentials (LV1 and LV2), there is a minimal depolarization left in LV1 whereas in LV2 there is already a minimal repolarization. When studying these individual leads these responses could be further minimized by changing output delays in steps of 1 millisecond. From Reference 24, with permission.

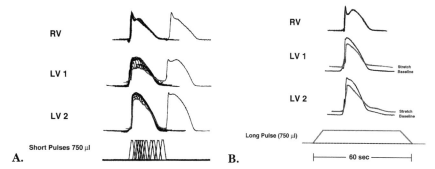

Figure 2. Plot of baseline MAP recordings with overlay of several MAPs during short transient stretch pulses (**A**) and the steady state MAP during a long static stretch pulse (60-second duration; **B**) of the same amplitude. Note that the enveloping line of the transient stretch pulses corresponds exactly to the real MAP during a long stretch pulse. From Reference 24, with permission.

was moved from full repolarization toward a less complete repolarization level. The study by Zabel et al[24] extended previous data by Lab[8] in isolated strips and whole frog ventricles, also demonstrating opposite electrophysiologic stretch effects that are dependent on the action potential phase.

Possibility of Motion Artifacts in MAP Recordings

In the earlier study by Lab,[8] action potentials were recorded with different techniques: either the insulated sucrose-gap technique, which cannot be used in the intact heart, or by the suction electrode method, which is more prone to artifact as compared to the contact electrode method. All of the referenced studies on stretch-induced electrophysiologic changes have raised the important question of whether some of the stretch-induced voltage changes represent motion artifacts. Unfortunately, no "gold standard" technique is available to prove that MAP recordings are artifact-free. However, for the following reasons it can be strongly argued that the electrical changes recorded are not artifacts. First, simultaneous MAP recordings from the right ventricle, which is not submitted to stretch, never showed any significant changes in response to short or sustained stretch pulses,[24] despite the fact that the right ventricular electrode, riding on the left ventricular septum, was subjected to a similar movement to that of the left ventricular electrodes. Second, the similarity between effects of short and long stretch pulses (Fig. 2) is of particular importance. There are no sudden mechanical perturbations of the heart during static stretch applied to the heart, yet the net effect on the MAP is almost identical to that of short stretch pulses. Third, there is no useful explanation as to why a motion artifact should change its polarity with different timings of the short stretch pulse. Fourth, PVCs emerging from a "take-off" potential—a finding confirmed in various models and species[8,15,17,18,21,24]—strongly support that these potentials are real.

Interpretation of Intact Heart Studies in View of Reported Characteristics of Stretch- Activated Ion Channels

Stretch-activated ion channels have been demonstrated in various noncardiac tissues[28,29,34,35,37] and subsequently in myocardial tissue.[27,30-32] The myocardium contains stretch-activated ion channels that allow both inward and outward currents.[27,30-32] The only available whole-cell recordings of mechanosensitive currents in the heart indicate a reversal potential in the range of –15 to –18 mV at room temperature.[38] These characteristics of stretch-activated ion channels from patch clamp studies were added to a computer heart model in order to simulate the effects of short pulsatile stretch on the MAP.[24] A remarkable similarity was found between the simulation and the actual results of the intact rabbit heart studies (Fig. 2).[24] The computer model predicted that activation of stretch-activated ion channels during the diastolic resting potential should result in an inward current (depolarization) and, conversely, that activation during the MAP plateau should result in an outward current (repolarization). The above-mentioned reversal potential also agrees well with the experimental MAP results shown here. Deviations between the experimental data and the computer simulation occur mainly in late repolarization when the time course is most sensitive to current changes. Because the MAP is identical in shape and relative voltage changes to the transcellularly recorded action potential,[39,42] one can assume a good correlation between voltage changes in the MAP and ion flow on a cellular level, given that all other factors remain constant. A striking similarity is then found between the voltage change to voltage relationship exhibited in the experimental study (Fig. 3) and the linear current-voltage relationship reported for many stretch-activated ion channels.[30-32]

Electrophysiologic Effects of Sustained Stretch

In accordance with the above characteristics of stretch-activated ion channels, the application of a sustained long stretch pulse in the study by

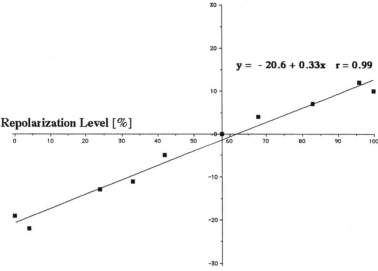

A.

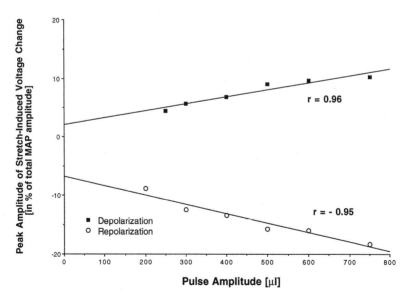

B.

Figure 3. **A.** Plot of stretch-induced voltage changes (in percent of MAP amplitude) against level of repolarization. A stretch pulse amplitude of 750 μL was applied. **B.** Relationship between the amplitude of short transient stretch pulses and the amplitude of stretch-induced depolarizations and repolarizations. The x intercept is the level of repolarization at which stretch induces no change in potential. From Reference 23, with permission.

Zabel et al[24] led to a similar effect on the MAP as the summation of an infinite number of very short pulses with different timing (Fig. 2, panel B). Although a direct measurement of voltage and MAP amplitude is not possible, this finding confirms earlier measurements by Franz et al,[12,21] who reported a decreased resting potential as well as a decreased action potential amplitude under stretch. It seems obvious that a slowly applied long stretch pulse is unable to trigger ventricular arrhythmias directly by one of the above-described mechanisms.[21,24] In an additional study by Zabel et al,[23] the electrophysiologic effects of sustained stretch were therefore further explored. This study showed that sustained, static load of the isolated rabbit ventricle influences several electrophysiologic parameters simultaneously and in a way that has been shown to facilitate the induction of sustained ventricular arrhythmias. As expected, average APD at 90% repolarization (APD_{90}) was shortened, particularly in the left ventricle. This translated into a shortening of refractoriness, which is generally believed to increase arrhythmogeneity.[43] While the average effect of mechanical loading was a shortening of APD and refractoriness, a lengthening of the action potential was also observed. The disparity of stretch effects between various locations of the ventricle, particularly between the stretched left ventricle and the unstretched right ventricle, led to an increased dispersion of ventricular repolarization. An increased dispersion of repolarization or refractoriness has been shown to be arrhythmogenic in many experimental models.[44-47] At the same time, activation time, measured as the longest interval between the pacing artifact and the fastest MAP upstroke in one of the MAP locations, was prolonged, particularly during premature extrastimulation. A prolongation of conduction time by stretch was also found by Calkins et al,[13] who used electrograms to determine activation time in the canine. Accordingly, a second arrhythmogenic condition is added to increased dispersion of repolarization. Unfortunately, the facilitation of inducible ventricular arrhythmias cannot be demonstrated in the isolated rabbit heart for the tendency of self-termination of such arrhythmias in the rabbit heart.[48] Such arrhythmogeneity of sustained stretch could be demonstrated in dog models.[13,14,17] In summarizing the experimental studies on sustained stretch, evidence is provided that this form of mechanical load alters electrophysiology and facilitates induction of sustained ventricular arrhythmias.

Summary

The electrophysiologic effects of very short, pulsatile stretch, acute stretch generated by increased preload and afterload, and sustained mechanical stretch can be explained by the existence of stretch-activated ion channels in the myocardium. As expected from the presumed characteristics of these channels, stretch generates a repolarizing response during electrical systole of the heart, a neutral response during phase 3 of repolarization (reversal potential), and a depolarizing response during diastole. The latter response can mimic EADs and, if reaching a threshold amplitude, can induce PVCs. Furthermore, sustained stretch can increase dispersion of ventricular repolarization and conduction times, and thereby facilitate reentry arrhythmias.

References

1. Bigger JT Jr. Why patients with congestive heart failure die: Arrhythmias and sudden cardiac death. *Circulation* 1987;75:IV28-IV35.
2. Parmley WW, Chatterjee K. Congestive heart failure and arrhythmias: An overview. *Am J Cardiol* 1986;57:34B-37B.
3. Pye MP, Cobbe SM. Mechanisms of ventricular arrhythmias in cardiac failure and hypertrophy. *Cardiovasc Res* 1992;26:740-750.
4. Singh SN. Congestive Heart Failure and arrhythmias: Therapeutic modalities. *J Cardiovasc Electrophysiol* 1997;8:89-97.
5. Dudel J, Trautwein W. Das Aktionspotential und Mechanogramm des Herzmuskels unter dem Einfluss der Dehnung. *Cardiologie* 1954;25:344.
6. Penefsky ZJ, Hoffman BF. Effects of stretch on mechanical and electrical properties of cardiac muscle. *Am J Physiol* 1963;204:433.
7. Kaufmann R, Lab MJ, Hennekes R, et al. Feedback interaction of mechanical and electrical events in the isolated ventricular myocardium (cat papillary muscle). *Pflügers Arch* 1971;324:100-123.
8. Lab MJ. Mechanically dependent changes in action potentials recorded from the intact frog ventricle. *Circ Res* 1978;42:519-528.
9. Lerman BB, Burkhoff D, Yue DT, et al. Mechanoelectrical feedback: Independent role of preload and contractility in modulation of canine ventricular excitability [published erratum appears in *J Clin Invest* 1986;77:2053]. *J Clin Invest* 1985;76:1843-1850.
10. Levine JH, Guarnieri T, Kadish AH, et al. Changes in myocardial repolarization in patients undergoing balloon valvuloplasty for congenital pulmonary stenosis: Evidence for contraction-excitation feedback in humans. *Circulation* 1988;77:70-77.
11. Reiter MJ, Synhorst DP, Mann DE. Electrophysiological effects of acute ventricular dilatation in the isolated rabbit heart. *Circ Res* 1988;62:554-562.
12. Franz MR, Burkhoff D, Yue DT, et al. Mechanically induced action potential changes and arrhythmia in isolated and in situ canine hearts. *Cardiovasc Res* 1989;23:213-223.
13. Calkins H, Maughan WL, Kass DA, et al. Electrophysiological effect of volume load in isolated canine hearts. *Am J Physiol* 1989;256:H1697-H1706.
14. Calkins H, Maughan WL, Weisman HF, et al. Effect of acute volume load on refractoriness and arrhythmia development in isolated, chronically infarcted canine hearts. *Circulation* 1989;79:687-697.
15. Dean JW, Lab MJ. Effect of changes in load on monophasic action potential and segment length of pig heart in situ. *Cardiovasc Res* 1989;23:887-896.
16. Dean JW, Lab MJ. Regional changes in ventricular excitability during load manipulation of the in situ pig heart. *J Physiol (Lond)* 1990;429:387-400.

17. Hansen DE, Craig CS, Hondeghem LM. Stretch-induced arrhythmias in the isolated canine ventricle. Evidence for the importance of mechanoelectrical feedback. *Circulation* 1990;81:1094-1105.

18. Stacy GP Jr, Jobe RL, Taylor LK, et al. Stretch-induced depolarizations as a trigger of arrhythmias in isolated canine left ventricles. *Am J Physiol* 1992;263:H613-H621.

19. Hansen DE. Mechanoelectrical feedback effects of altering preload, afterload, and ventricular shortening. *Am J Physiol* 1993;264:H423-H432.

20. Coulshed DS, Cowan JC. Contraction-excitation feedback in an ejecting whole heart model—dependence of action potential duration on left ventricular diastolic and systolic pressures. *Cardiovasc Res* 1991;25:343-352.

21. Franz MR, Cima R, Wang D, et al. Electrophysiological effects of myocardial stretch and mechanical determinants of stretch-activated arrhythmias [published erratum appears in *Circulation* 1992;86:1663]. *Circulation* 1992; 86:968-978.

22. Hansen DE, Borganelli M, Stacy GP Jr, et al. Dose-dependent inhibition of stretch-induced arrhythmias by gadolinium in isolated canine ventricles. Evidence for a unique mode of antiarrhythmic action. *Circ Res* 1991;69:820-831.

23. Zabel M, Portnoy S, Franz MR. Effect of sustained load on dispersion of ventricular repolarization and conduction time in the isolated intact rabbit heart. *J Cardiovasc Electrophys* 1996;7:9-16.

24. Zabel M, Koller BS, Sachs F, et al. Stretch-induced voltage changes in the isolated beating heart: Importance of the timing of stretch and implications for stretch-activated ion channels. *Cardiovasc Res* 1996;32:120-130.

25. Reiter MJ, Zatelaki Z, Kirchhof CJ, et al. Interaction of acute ventricular dilatation and d-sotalol during sustained reentrant tachycardia around a fixed obstacle. *Circulation* 1994;89:423-431.

26. Lab MJ. Contraction-excitation feedback in myocardium. Physiological basis and clinical relevance. *Circ Res* 1982;50:757-766.

27. Craelius W, Chen V, El-Sherif N. Stretch activated ion channels in ventricular myocytes. *Biosci Rep* 1988;8:407-414.

28. Yang XC, Sachs F. Block of stretch-activated ion channels in Xenopus oocytes by gadolinium and calcium ions. *Science* 1989;243:1068-1071.

29. Yang XC, Sachs F. Characterization of stretch-activated ion channels in Xenopus oocytes. *J Physiol (Lond)* 1990;431:103-122.

30. Bustamante JO, Ruknudin A, Sachs F. Stretch-activated channels in heart cells: Relevance to cardiac hypertrophy. *J Cardiovasc Pharmacol* 1991;17(suppl 2):S110-S113.

31. Sigurdson W, Ruknudin A, Sachs F. Calcium imaging of mechanically induced fluxes in tissue-cultured chick heart: Role of stretch-activated ion channels. *Am J Physiol* 1992;262:H1110-H1115.

32. Ruknudin A, Sachs F, Bustamante JO. Stretch-activated ion channels in tissue-cultured chick heart. *Am J Physiol* 1993;264:H960-H972.

33. Sadoshima J, Takahashi T, Jahn L, et al. Roles of mechano-sensitive ion channels, cytoskeleton, and contractile activity in stretch-induced immediate-early gene expression and hypertrophy of cardiac myocytes. *Proc Natl Acad Sci U S A* 1992;89:9905-9909.

34. Davis MJ, Donovitz JA, Hood JD. Stretch-activated single-channel and whole cell currents in vascular smooth muscle cells. *Am J Physiol* 1992;262:C1083-C1088.

35. Popp R, Hoyer J, Meyer J, et al. Stretch-activated non-selective cation channels in the antiluminal membrane of porcine cerebral capillaries. *J Physiol (Lond)* 1992;454:435-449.

36. Sasaki N, Mitsuiwe T, Noma A. Effects of mechanical stretch on membrane currents of single ventricular myocytes of guinea-pig heart. *Jpn J Physiol* 1992;42:957-970.

37. Naruse K, Sokabe M. Involvement of stretch-activated ion channels in Ca2+ mobilization to mechanical stretch in endothelial cells. *Am J Physiol* 1993;264:C1037-C1044.

38. Hu H, Sachs F. Effects of mechanical stimulation on embryonic chick heart cells. *Biophys J* 1994;66:A170.

39. Franz MR, Burkhoff D, Spurgeon H, et al. In vitro validation of a new cardiac catheter technique for recording monophasic action potentials. *Eur Heart J* 1986;7:34-41.

40. Franz MR. Method and theory of monophasic action potential recording. *Prog Cardiovasc Dis* 1991;33:347-368.

41. Franz MR, Chin MC, Sharkey HR, et al. A new single catheter technique for simultaneous measurement of action potential duration and refractory period in vivo. *J Am Coll Cardiol* 1990;16:878-886.

42. Ino T, Karagueuzian HS, Hong K, et al. Relation of monophasic action potential recorded with contact electrode to underlying transmembrane action potential properties in isolated cardiac tissues: A systematic microelectrode validation study. *Cardiovasc Res* 1988;22:255-264.

43. Gillis AM, Wyse DG, Duff HJ, et al. Drug response at electropharmacologic study in patients with ventricular tachyarrhythmias: The importance of ventricular refractoriness. *J Am Coll Cardiol* 1991;17:914-920.

44. Han J, Moe GK. Nonuniform recovery of excitability in ventricular muscle. *Circ Res* 1964;14:44.

45. Merx W, Yoon MS, Han J. The role of local disparity in conduction and recovery time on ventricular vulnerability to fibrillation. *Am Heart J* 1977;94:603-610.

46. Kuo CS, Munakata K, Reddy CP, et al. Characteristics and possible mechanism of ventricular arrhythmia dependent on the dispersion of action potential durations. *Circulation* 1983;67:1356-1367.

47. Kuo CS, Reddy CP, Munakata K, et al. Mechanism of ventricular arrhythmias caused by increased dispersion of repolarization. *Eur Heart J* 1985;6(suppl D):63-70.

48. Fabritz CL, Kirchhof P, Behrens S, et al. Myocardial vulnerability to T wave shocks: Relation to shock strength, shock coupling interval, and dispersion of ventricular repolarization. *J Cardiovasc Electrophysiol* 1996;7:231-242.

Section VII

Ventricular Fibrillation and Defibrillation:
Introduction

Ventricular fibrillation is a complex and often fatal arrhythmia. However, since the advent of the implantable defibrillator there has been a dramatic decrease in mortality caused by this arrhythmia. This section summarizes novel research on the use of monophasic action potential (MAP) recordings to help us better understand the mechanisms that make the heart vulnerable to ventricular fibrillation, how antiarrhythmic drugs modulate the 'window of vulnerability," and how MAP recordings aid in our understanding of the mechanism of defibrillation. This section features the use of multiple simultaneous MAP recordings to gauge the effect of fibrillating and defibrillating shocks on the dispersion of ventricular repolarization.

42

Nonuniform Repolarization and the Wavelet Hypothesis of Cardiac Fibrillation

J. A. Abildskov, MD and Robert L. Lux, PhD

The wavelet hypothesis, which was formulated by Moe[1] more than 30 years ago, continues to explain the most likely mechanism of cardiac fibrillation. The existence of multiple, spatially discrete activation fronts, which was predicted by the hypothesis, has been experimentally demonstrated in atrial fibrillation and a variety of findings relating disparate recovery and vulnerability make it likely that the hypothesis is also applicable to ventricular fibrillation.[2-6] Nonuniform repolarization is an essential feature of the wavelet hypothesis and, since such repolarization can be measured with monophasic action potential (MAP) recordings, review of the hypothesis is appropriate in this volume. Review is also appropriate because there have been substantial additions to the original wavelet hypothesis.

Computer Model

The wavelet hypothesis is described in terms of a computer model of propagated excitation.[7] The model was originally developed to demonstrate

This work was supported by awards from the Nora Eccles Treadwell Foundation and the Richard A. and Nora Eccles Harrison Fund for Cardiovascular Research and grant HL42388 from the National Institutes of Health (Heart, Lung, and Blood Institute).
From Franz MR (ed): *Monophasic Action Potentials: Bridging Cell and Bedside.* ©Futura Publishing Company, Inc., Armonk, NY, 2000.

major features of the hypothesis and has continued to be useful for the definition of additional features. The model consists of individual units to which excitation can be propagated, and includes nonuniform cycle-length–dependent recovery of excitability and slow propagation during incomplete recovery. As implemented for studies of fibrillation, the model has included several hundred units arranged in a hexagonal structure such that each has 6 neighbors to which excitation can be propagated. Units were assigned intrinsic repolarization constants, K, which together with preceding cycle lengths determined the duration of refractoriness according to the relation $K\sqrt{CL}$. In that relation, CL represented the immediately preceding cycle length and the square root was an approximation of the cycle length-refractory period relation observed in cardiac muscle.

Time was represented in the model as discrete intervals, with one time step (TS) being the time required to transfer excitation from an excited unit to a fully excitable neighbor. Slow propagation during incomplete recovery was represented by additional time for the transfer of excitation to units in that condition. Specifically, 4, 3, and 2 TSs were necessary for transfer to units in successive stages of 2-TS duration, each following the absolute refractory period. Selected K values were randomly distributed in the matrix and simulated fibrillation was initiated by premature stimuli. Vulnerability was assessed as fibrillation threshold (FT), defined as the minimum duration of train stimulation at 1-TS intervals required to initiate self-sustained reentrant excitation persisting at least 200 TS following the stimuli. To minimize the effects of any particular distribution of K values, the average FT from 30 different random distributions of K values was determined.

In summary, the model simulated propagation, nonuniform cycle-length–dependent recovery of excitability, and slow propagation during incomplete recovery. These are all established factors in fibrillation as well as in other reentrant arrhythmias, and the merit of the model was that it allowed individual control of each, to identify its role in fibrillation and vulnerability.

Simulated Fibrillation

The essence of the wavelet hypothesis is nonuniform propagation of excitation expressed as the presence of multiple excitation fronts and by reentry occurring at changing locations. These features of fibrillation were evident in the behavior of the model in response to train stimulation as illustrated in Figure 1. Panel A illustrates uniform propagation of a response to stimulation when all units were fully excitable. Panel B, shows propagation of the first premature response to train stimulation in which the nonuniformity of propagation was due solely to nonuniform recovery related to the assigned K values. Panel C illustrates a second premature

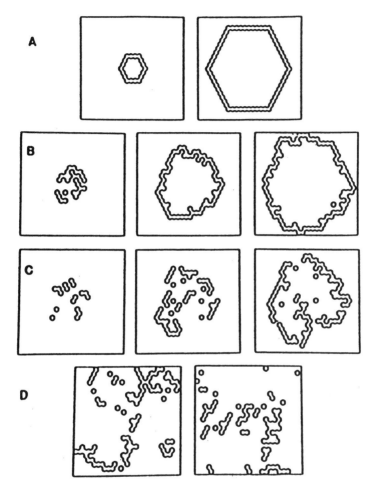

Figure 1. Matrix behavior during train stimulation from a single unit at the center of the matrix. Units scheduled for excitation at particular instants are shown. **A.** Propagation in fully recovered units. **B.** Propagation of the first premature response. **C.** Propagation of the second premature response. **D.** Spatially discrete wave fronts at two instants during simulated fibrillation. Reprinted from the *Japanese Journal of Electrocardiology*, with permission.

response having greater nonuniformity of propagation due to nonuniform cycle lengths of the previous response in addition to that of assigned K values. Additional premature responses result in further nonuniformity of propagation due to still more marked disparity of preceding cycle lengths. After a sufficient number of premature responses to stimulation, discrete wave fronts or wavelets occurred and excitation became self-sustained by means of reentry at changing locations. Panel D of Figure 1 shows wavelets at two instants during such simulated fibrillation.

Increasing nonuniformity of propagation with successive premature responses was an important factor in the initiation of simulated fibrillation. As noted above, this was the result of cycle length effects on recovery; the role of that factor is illustrated in Figure 2. A nonuniform activation index (NAI) was calculated as the sum of differences of activation time of each unit and its neighbors averaged over the entire matrix. As illustrated, the NAI increased during successive responses to the earliest stimuli that resulted in propagation.

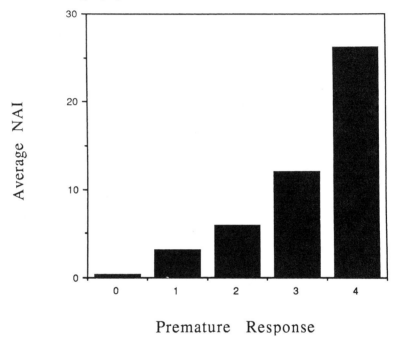

Figure 2. Nonuniform activation index (NAI) for successive responses. The response labeled 0 is in a fully excitable matrix, and 1 through 4 are responses to the earliest stimuli that resulted in propagated responses. Reprinted from the *Japanese Journal of Electrocardiology*, with permission.

Refractory Periods and Vulnerability

The duration and range of refractory periods are known to affect vulnerability to fibrillation in the heart. These effects were also evident in the model, and with the model it was possible to determine their individual mechanisms.[8] Figure 3 illustrates effects of varied K value mean and range on FT showing decreasing FT with increasing range and higher FT with

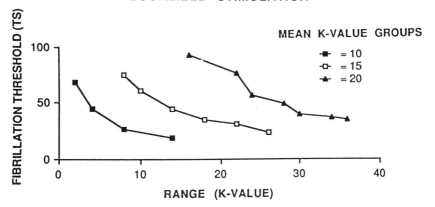

Figure 3. Relation of fibrillation threshold to range of K values for 3 mean K values. Fibrillation threshold values are the average of 30 determinations over different random distributions of each K value set. Reprinted from the *Japanese Journal of Electrocardiology*, with permission.

increasing mean. Increased range of K values resulted in greater disparity of refractory periods, which reduced FT by increasing the degree of nonuniform propagation per premature response. Fewer premature responses were therefore required to initiate fibrillation. Increased mean K value increased the average refractory period duration and increased FT by increasing the time required to initiate the number of responses necessary to induce fibrillation. These mechanisms could be documented by showing that the NAI following a premature response increased with increasing K value range but not with varied K value mean. The time required to initiate a particular number of premature responses, however, increased with increasing K value mean but did not change with varied range.

Nonuniform Propagation Required for Fibrillation

In addition to the degree of nonuniform propagation per premature response and the number of responses per unit time, the degree of nonuniformity itself that was required for fibrillation was affected by the range and mean of K values and resulting refractory periods.[9] Increasing K value and resulting refractory period range decreased FT by increasing the degree of nonuniform propagation with each premature response and also by decreasing the degree of nonuniformity necessary for fibrillation. Decreased mean K value and refractory period duration also reduced the degree of nonuniformity required for fibrillation, in addition to affecting the time necessary to initiate a particular number of responses. The degree of nonuniformity necessary for fibrillation was related to the minimum refractory period. Both increased refractory period range and decreased refractory period mean result in a decrease of the minimum refractory period. Evidence for these conclusions is illustrated in Figure 4. Panel B shows FT that decreased with increasing K value range and increased with increasing mean K value. The lower portion of the panel shows the degree of nonuniformity of propagation

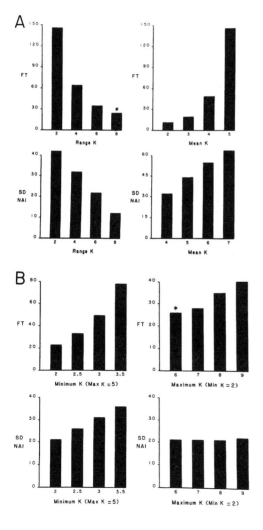

Figure 4. A. Fibrillation threshold (FT) to train stimulation with varied K value range and mean. In the lower portion of the panel, the degree of nonuniform excitation due to conduction defects that was required to initiate fibrillation is shown. The degree of nonuniformity required decreased with increasing range and increased with increasing mean K value. **B.** FT to train stimulation increasing with increasing minimum or increasing maximum K value. The lower portion of the panel shows standard deviation of the nonuniform activation index (NAI) produced by conduction defects that reflect the degree of nonuniform excitation required to initiate fibrillation in the presence of varied minimum and maximum K values. The degree of nonuniformity increased with increasing minimum K value but was not affected by maximum K value. Reprinted from the *Journal of Cardiovascular Electrophysiology*, with permission.

required to initiate fibrillation in the presence of the K values shown. That degree of nonuniformity was determined by observing simulations that had randomly distributed conduction defects in the model. Defects consisted of increased time for transfer of excitation, and severity was expressed as the range from 0 (no conduction defect) to the maximal additional time required for propagation. The range of conduction defects was increased in 1-TS increments until propagation of a single premature response was followed by simulated fibrillation. After the conduction defect range required to initiate fibrillation in a particular matrix was determined, K values were increased to prevent fibrillation, and the NAI of a propagated nonpremature response was measured. Propagation of that response was the same as that which preceded fibrillation, as both occurred when the matrix was fully excitable and the higher K value permitted measurement of the index without reentrant excitation. The average index from 5 different distributions of each set of K values was determined and represented the degree of nonuniformity of activation necessary to initiate fibrillation. As illustrated in Figure 4, both increased K value range and decreased mean K value resulted in reduction of the nonuniformity of excitation required to initiate fibrillation. As shown in panel B of Figure 4, increasing either minimum or maximum K value resulted in increased FT. Increasing minimum K value also increased the degree of nonuniformity necessary for fibrillation, but varying maximum K value did not alter the nonuniformity required. The mechanism of the different effects of minimum and maximum K values on the required degree of nonuniformity concerned the conditions necessary for reentry. It was necessary that excitation in some units be sufficiently delayed in order for neighboring units to become excitable. The minimum delay with that effect was therefore associated with the minimal refractory period, and was not affected by the refractory period maximum.

To summarize the effects of K values and resulting refractory periods on vulnerability: 1) increased range resulted in increased vulnerability due to increased nonuniformity of propagation per premature response and decreased nonuniformity necessary to initiate fibrillation; 2) decreased mean resulted in increased vulnerability due to decreased time necessary to initiate the required number of premature responses and decreased nonuniformity necessary to initiate fibrillation; 3) decreased minimum K value and resulting refractory period increased vulnerability by means of decreased average refractory period, increased refractory period range, and decreased degree of nonuniform excitation necessary for fibrillation; 4) decreased maximal K value and resulting refractory period increased vulnerability as the result of decreasing mean refractory period despite the opposing effect of decreased refractory period range and without an effect on the degree of nonuniformity necessary for fibrillation.

Vulnerable Period

It has been known since 1940 that fibrillation is most easily initiated during a limited portion of the cardiac cycle. That vulnerable period occurs during a window of incomplete recovery of excitability when propagation of premature responses is nonuniform. It does not begin, however, at the earliest time at which propagation is possible and at which maximal nonuniformity might be expected. The mechanism of that feature of the vulnerable period has been elucidated by means of the computer model, with use of distributions in which the K value range was sufficiently high and the K value mean sufficiently low that fibrillation could be induced by a single premature response.[10] In these simulations fibrillation occurred following stimuli at a time later than the earliest possible stimulus that resulted in propagation. The mechanism was slow propagation near the stimulus site during propagation of the earliest response. The time during that propagation allowed sufficient recovery in other regions so that further propagation occurred without reentry. Later stimulation resulted in more rapid propagation near the stimulus site and excitation of surrounding regions while recovery was markedly nonuniform. Nonuniformity of propagation was quantitated by means of the NAI and shown to increase with increasing premature cycle length before decreasing progressively.

Conduction Defects and Fibrillation

The wavelet hypothesis relates fibrillation to nonuniform propagation of premature responses secondary to disparate recovery of excitability. Similar but primary effects associated with nonuniform propagation due to conduction defects would be expected. It has been difficult to separate effects of disparate recovery and conduction defects experimentally, however, since interventions that result in such defects are also likely to affect recovery. In the model, conduction defects and repolarization could be independently varied and their individual effects determined.[9] Conduction defects consisting of increased time for transfer of excitation were randomly distributed in the matrix, together with units without defects. The severity of conduction defects was expressed as the range from 0 (no defect) to the maximal additional time required for activation.

The direct effect of randomly distributed conduction defects was nonuniform propagation of nonpremature as well as premature responses. Units that were excited at a particular time without a conduction defect were excited later when the defect was present. Hence, there was greater disparity of activation times between the unit and the one from which excitation was delivered. There were also secondary effects of these conduction defects on recovery that affected propagation of premature responses. With uniform K values, defects had the same effects on propagation of the initial response whether the response was premature or nonpremature. The defects resulted in nonuniform cycle lengths and the subsequent refractory periods became nonuniform even when K values were uniform. Premature responses were then affected by nonuniform refractoriness in addition to the continuing effect of the conduction defects, and propagation became increasingly nonuniform. When both conduction defects and nonuniform K values were present, propagation of the initial as well as subsequent premature responses was nonuniform due to both the defects and nonuniformity of refractory periods. In addition, propagation of each subsequent response was affected by nonuniform refractoriness due to both K values and conduction defects. Conduction defects reduced FT, and the magnitude of the decrease depended on the severity of the defects but also on the K values with which they were combined. The nonuniform propagation due to conduction defects increased with successive premature responses, and their effect on FT depended on the number of responses required to initiate fibrillation. As detailed previously, low mean K value or high K value range required a smaller number of responses to initiate fibrillation than higher mean or lower range. There was therefore less effect of conduction defects of a given severity on FT in the presence of high K range or low mean K value. In brief, conduction defects increased vulnerability but had less effect in the presence of marked disparity or low duration of refractoriness.

Premature Responses and Vulnerability

Effects (on vulnerability) of premature responses initiated at various times in the cardiac cycle and with various rates and conditions of refractoriness have been determined in the model.[11] FT was reduced by premature responses, and with decreasing prematurity there was an initial decrease followed by increasing FT. This is illustrated by the curve in panel A of Figure 5, which shows FT at intervals after premature responses with varied cycle lengths. The minimum FT was not associated with the earliest premature response, and the later occurrence of the minimum is an example of the vulnerable period described earlier. Following the minimum, there was an abrupt increase of FT associated with responses near the completion of refractory periods and having more uniform propagation as evidenced by decrease of the NAI shown with each FT. After propagation was uniform and the NAI was 0, FT continued to rise gradually due to effects of the longer premature cycle length on the subsequent refractory

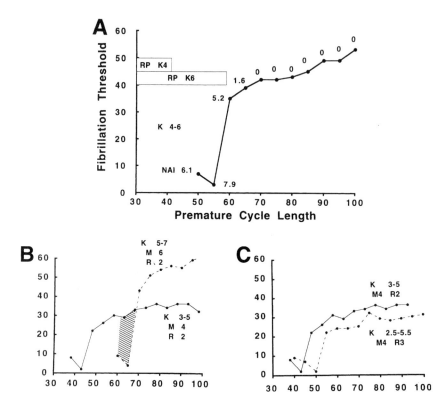

Figure 5. Curves of the fibrillation threshold (FT) in relation to the cycle length of premature responses. **A**. General features of such curves with the FT at the time of the earliest propagated response and at 5–time-step (TS) intervals. The earliest propagated response was not associated with the lowest FT, and following the minimum, the FT increased at first abruptly and then gradually. The nonuniform activation index (NAI) of a propagated response at each cycle length is shown and indicates an initial increase of nonuniformity followed by decreasing nonuniformity with increasing FT. The K values of the matrix from which the curve was obtained and the high and low refractory periods (RPs) following a basic cycle length of 100 TSs are shown. **B**. Effects of the varied mean K values: a high mean value shifted the curve upward and to the right and resulted in a lower FT during the period indicated by shading. **C**. Effects of the K value range on the FT, with a lower FT at most premature cycle lengths with the higher K range. Reprinted from the *Journal of Electrocardiology*, with permission.

period, which delayed the time at which reentry was possible. Altered mean or range of K values shifted the time phase of curves relating FT and premature cycle length. As illustrated in panel B of Figure 5, higher mean K value shifted the curve upward and to the right. The earliest response occurred later when the mean K value was higher so there was a range of premature cycle lengths associated with lower FTs, as indicated by the shaded area in the figure. This finding of lower FT with premature responses at some cycle lengths may be a factor in the proarrhythmia effects of drugs that prolong refractory periods. The compensatory pause following premature responses had a similar effect in that the earliest response following such a pause was later than the response before the pause and there was a range of premature cycle lengths associated with lower FTs after the pause. Similarly, a slower rate resulted in later occurrence of the earliest premature response and a range of premature cycle lengths associated with lower FT. Examples of the findings are shown by the calculated QRS complexes in Figure 6. Panel A shows a premature response at a cycle length of 50 TS that failed to initiate fibrillation when preceded by regular cycle lengths of 100 TS but did so after a compensatory pause. Panel B shows failure of a premature response at 49 TS to initiate

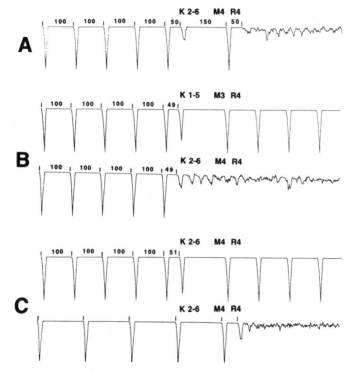

Figure 6. Calculated QRS complexes showing initiation of fibrillation by single premature responses. **A.** Five paced responses at a cycle length of 100 time steps (TSs) followed by a premature response at a cycle length of 50 TSs initiates fibrillation only after a compensatory pause. **B.** Five paced responses are followed by a premature response at a cycle length of 49 TSs, which fails to initiate fibrillation with a mean K value of 3 but does so with a mean K value of 4. **C.** Five paced responses are followed by a premature response at a cycle length of 51 TSs, which fails to initiate fibrillation with a pacing cycle length of 100 TSs but does so with a pacing cycle length of 150 TSs. Reprinted from the *Journal of Electrocardiology*, with permission.

fibrillation in the presence of K values with a mean of 3 but initiation of fibrillation in the presence of higher mean K values. Panel C shows failure of a premature response to initiate fibrillation when preceded by cycle lengths of 100 TS but initiation of fibrillation with a slower rate and cycle lengths of 150 TS.

Termination of Fibrillation

Conditions that terminated simulated fibrillation were the reverse of those that increased vulnerability to the initiation of fibrillation.[12] Sufficient increase of the mean K value dynamically terminated fibrillation by increasing refractory period duration and blocking propagation in reentry circuits. This occurred despite the fact that increased K values resulted in greater nonuniformity of propagation due to longer reentry circuits. These resulted in greater differences of activation times in initial and terminal limbs of the circuits. The magnitude of K value increase required to terminate fibrillation depended on K values present during fibrillation, and when these were high, a smaller increase was required to halt fibrillation then when they were low. The range of K values during fibrillation also affected the magnitude of K value increase needed to terminate fibrillation, a greater increase being necessary when K range was high.

Fibrillation could also be terminated by when the K value range was decreased; this resulted in less nonuniform propagation. With greater K value range during fibrillation, greater decrease of that range was required, and greater reduction was also required when the mean K value was low.

Summary

The original wavelet hypothesis related initiation of fibrillation to nonuniform propagation of premature responses and characterized fibrillation itself as multiple activation waves with reentry at changing locations. The most likely mechanism of fibrillation continues to be that proposed as the wavelet hypothesis, and a computer model based on the hypothesis continues to be useful for the further definition of fibrillation. Some additions to the wavelet hypothesis from studies using the model have been reviewed in this chapter.

Additions to the hypothesis include a more explicit description of the mechanisms by which refractory period range and duration affect vulnerability to fibrillation. Refractory period range affected the degree of nonuniform propagation per premature response while refractory period duration determined the time required to initiate the requisite number of responses to result in fibrillation. Evidence was also obtained that refractory period range and duration affected the degree of nonuniform propagation necessary to initiate fibrillation. For example, increased range of refractory periods increased vulnerability by increasing the degree of nonuniform propagation of each premature response and also by decreasing the degree of nonuniform propagation that resulted in fibrillation.

Another addition to the hypothesis was evidence that onset of the most vulnerable period occurred later than the earliest propagated response due to slower propagation of that response near the stimulus site. Conduction defects were found to increase vulnerability as expected, but the magnitude of that effect depended on the refractory periods with which they were associated. Nonuniformity of propagation due to conduction defects increased with successive premature responses so effects of the defects on vulnerability depended on the number of responses necessary to initiate fibrillation. High K value range, for example, required fewer responses, and the effect of conduction defects on vulnerability was therefore less than with lower K value range.

Vulnerability was found to increase following premature responses and, with increasing premature cycle length, there was an initial increase followed by progressive decrease of vulnerability. The time phase of curves relating vulnerability and premature cycle length was such that responses at some cycle lengths were associated with greater vulnerability in the presence of longer refractory periods, slower rates, or following a compensatory pause.

The main significance of findings reviewed in this chapter is their contribution to our understanding of the physiology of fibrillation and vulnerability to fibrillation. The medical significance depends on use of the findings in the prevention or management of fibrillation and reentrant arrhythmias in general. Those most likely to have such significance concern changes of vulnerability due to changing physiologic conditions or to drugs. For example, drugs that prolong refractoriness may have less effect on vulnerability when conduction defects are present, due to increasing effects of the defects when refractory periods are prolonged. As a further example, findings suggest that vulnerability following premature responses at certain cycle lengths may be increased by drugs that prolong refractoriness, and may be a factor in the proarrhythmia of such drugs. These and other possible medical applications of the findings with the model are speculative but may be useful for the design of experimental and clinical studies.

References

1. Moe GK. On the multiple wavelet hypothesis of atrial fibrillation. *Arch Int Pharmacodyn Ther* 1962;140:183-188.
2. Allessie MA, Lammers WJEP, Bonke FIM, et al. Experimental evaluation of Moe's multiple wavelet hypothesis of atrial fibrillation. In Zipes DP, Jalife J

(eds): *Cardiac Electrophysiology and Arrhythmias.* New York: Grune and Stratton, Inc.; 1985:265-275.

3. Han J, Moe GK. Nonuniform recovery of excitability in ventricular muscle. *Circ Res* 1964;14:44-60.

4. Han J, Garcia de Jalon PO, Moe GK. Fibrillation threshold of premature ventricular responses. *Circ Res* 1966;18:18-25.

5. Pogswizd SM, Carr PB. Mechanisms underlying the development of ventricular fibrillation during early myocardial ischemia. *Circ Res* 1990;66:672-695.

6. Janse MJ, Wilms-Schopman FJG, Coronel R. Ventricular fibrillation is not always due to multiple wavelet reentry. *J Cardiovasc Electrophysiol* 1995; 6:512-521.

7. Moe GK, Rheinboldt WC, Abildskov JA. A computer model of atrial fibrillation. *Am Heart J* 1964;67:200-220.

8. Abildskov JA. Vulnerability to fibrillation in a mathematical model. *Jpn J Electrocardiol* 1990;10:3-20.

9. Abildskov JA, Lux RL. Effects of nonuniform slowing of conduction on vulnerability to fibrillation in a computer model. *J Cardiovasc Electrophysiol* 1992;3:48-55.

10. Abildskov JA. Mechanism of the vulnerable period in a model of cardiac fibrillation. *J Cardiovasc Electrophysiol* 1990;1:303-308.

11. Abildskov JA, Lux RL. Effects of premature responses on vulnerability to fibrillation in a computer model. *J Electrocardiol* 1996;29:213-221.

12. Abildskov JA. Induced termination of fibrillation. *J Cardiovasc Electrophysiol* 1996;7:71-81.

43

Monophasic Action Potential Recordings During Ventricular Fibrillation Compared with Intracellular Recordings

C. Larissa Fabritz, MD, Paulus Kirchhof, MD, Ruben Coronel, MD, PhD, Tobias Opthof, PhD, Michael R. Franz, MD, PhD and Michiel Janse, MD

Monophasic action potentials (MAPs) are frequently used to record the time course of repolarization during ventricular fibrillation (VF) in vitro and in patients (Fig. 1, panel B).[1-7] Interpretation of MAPs during VF is based on the assumption that MAP recordings correspond to transmembrane action potential (TAP) recordings during VF as they do during regular rhythm (Fig. 1, panel A).[8] As the MAP records the summation potential of a large number of cells, microreentry and slow propagation of activation wave fronts might disturb the close correlation between MAP and transmembrane potential during VF (Fig. 1, panel B).[9,10] Specifically, superimposition of several asynchronous cellular action potentials could result in longer action potential durations (APDs) in the MAP during VF.

Reported capture of electrical stimuli during VF[11,12] is at variance with the hypothesis that local myocardial reactivation occurs at the earliest moment allowed by local refractoriness during VF.[2,13,14] Supernormal excit-

L. Fabritz and P. Kirchhof contributed equally to this chapter.

From Franz MR (ed): *Monophasic Action Potentials: Bridging Cell and Bedside.*
©Futura Publishing Company, Inc., Armonk, NY, 2000.

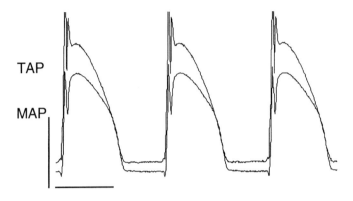

A.

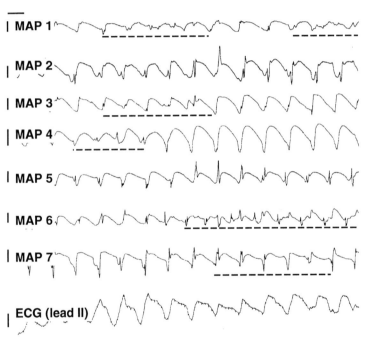

B.

Figure 1. A. Simultaneous recording of epicardial transmembrane action potential (TAP; top recording) and endocardial MAP (bottom recording) from the right ventricle during sinus rhythm. The vertical calibration bar indicates a 50-mV calibration for the TAP, and a 5-mV calibration for the MAP. The horizontal bar indicates a 100-millisecond period. **B.** Recording of 7 MAPs and a tissue bath electrocardiogram (ECG) (lead II) during sustained ventricular fibrillation. Recordings 1 and 2 are taken from the right ventricular epicardium, recordings 3 through 5 from the left ventricular epicardium, and recordings 6 and 7 from the left ventricular endocardium. The vertical calibration bars give a 5-mV reference for each MAP recording and a 1-mV reference for the ECG recording. The horizontal bar gives a 100-millisecond reference. Transient low-amplitude portions of MAP recordings are underlined by dashed lines.

ability of the myocardium or intermittent diastolic free intervals could explain these phenomena. Only few data exist on occurrence and duration of repolarized intervals during VF in patients,[2] partly due to difficulties in recording action potentials during tachyarrhythmias in vivo and in identifying recording artifacts in action potentials during VF.[15-17]

The study described in this chapter was therefore designed to compare MAPs and TAPs during VF, and to test whether fully repolarized, diastolic intervals can be observed during VF. For this purpose, activation and repolarization were measured simultaneously in closely spaced TAP and MAP recordings during VF in intact rabbit hearts.

Recordings

MAPs and TAPs were simultaneously recorded from 9 white male New Zealand rabbit hearts retrogradely perfused on a modified vertical Langendorff apparatus.[18] In 2 hearts, 2,3-butanedione monoxime was added at a concentration of 10 μM to impair movement of the ventricle. The hearts were positioned on a foam bed with the right ventricular free wall exposed, and fixed gently with use of a U-shaped fiber glass ring positioned on the right ventricle. MAP recordings were obtained by inserting a quadripolar MAP-pacing catheter into the right ventricular cavity.[18,19] The catheter tip was placed onto the apical endocardium or the free wall of the right ventricle. MAP recordings had an amplitude of greater than 6 mV during steady state rhythms.[18] They were preamplified with use of standard MAP preamplifiers for digitization and on-line display.

For recording of a TAP, a piece of right ventricular epicardium was removed. A standard glass microelectrode filled with 3 M KCl was inserted into a right ventricular subepicardial cell just opposite the endocardial MAP recording site (Fig. 2). The electrode was mounted on a silver spring wire connected to a micromanipulator. A silver-silver chloride wire was placed within the epicardium-free area as close as possible to the microelectrode tip, thereby providing a reference electrode for the TAP. TAPs were amplified by use of a custom designed differential direct current amplifier. Transmural distance between the microelectrode and the MAP catheter was ≤2 mm (Fig. 2). TAP amplitude was greater than 50 mV during VF.

Data Acquisition

MAP and TAP recordings were monitored with use of a 4-channel oscilloscope. After preamplification, both recordings were digitized at a sampling rate of 1000 Hz. Vertical resolution of the digitized data was less

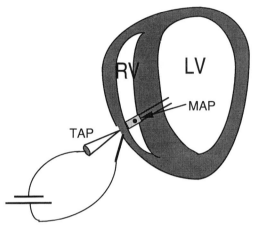

Figure 2. Vertical cross section of the isolated rabbit heart with the transmembrane action potential (TAP) and MAP electrodes in their recording positions. A standard MAP catheter was inserted into the right ventricular cavity. The catheter tip was placed onto the apical endocardium or the free wall of the right ventricle. For recording of a TAP, a standard glass microelectrode was inserted into the right ventricular subepicardium just opposite the endocardial MAP recording site. Transmural distance between the microelectrode and the MAP catheter was ≤2 mm.

than 0.5% of the maximal amplitude of the original signal per bit.[18] Data were recorded on digital storage media for off-line analysis.

Protocol

After verification of a stable MAP recording, VF was induced by application of 9 V of direct current to the left ventricular epicardium. The microelectrode was inserted into a subepicardial cell, and a maximum number of simultaneous recordings was obtained. In some recordings (n= 6), positioning of the microelectrode was performed prior to induction of VF. If VF did not terminate spontaneously after 5 minutes, a defibrillation shock was applied by an experimental defibrillator via two 5x3 cm opposing steel electrodes. After a rest period of 5 minutes and verification of MAP catheter position and signal stability, VF was induced again. Changes in MAP duration or morphology suggestive of ischemia during sinus rhythm[18] resulted in cessation of the experiment.

Data Analysis

MAP and TAP recordings were analyzed independently for cycle length and APD at 50% repolarization (APD_{50}) with use of modified custom interactive analysis software.[20] Only recordings showing maximal TAP amplitude greater than 50 mV and maximal MAP amplitude greater than 4 mV during VF were used for analysis. Activation was defined as the fastest upstroke during phase 0, cycle length as the interval between two activations, and APD_{50} as the interval from activation to the time point of repolarization to 50% of the action potential plateau.[7,20] Resting membrane potential was measured prior to induction of VF in both signals, and was controlled after each episode of VF. All parameters were visually controlled during analysis.[20] The same program was used to analyze both MAPs and TAPs. For statistical comparisons, a P value less than 0.05 was considered significant.

Simultaneous Recording of MAP and TAP During VF

Simultaneous recordings of MAPs and TAPs were obtained in 43 arrhythmia episodes, resulting in a total duration of 245 seconds of simultaneous arrhythmia recordings. Due to transient low-amplitude recordings in at least one of the signals, 42 seconds of simultaneous recordings were excluded from analysis. Transient low-amplitude potentials were recorded in both signals, MAP as well as TAP, during periods of less than 3 seconds' duration. They could be identified by a sudden increase in maximal diastolic potential and a sudden shortening of cycle length in the recording (Fig. 1, panel B), and occasionally showed 2:1 concordance of activation with the other recording.

APD and Cycle Length During VF

During VF, MAP and TAP recordings showed similar morphologies (Fig. 3). Cycle length was equal in the two recordings, averaging 89 ± 7

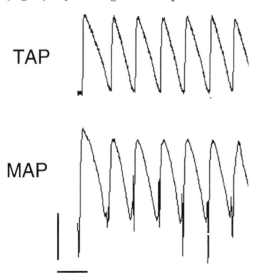

TAP

MAP

Figure 3. Simultaneous recording of transmembrane action potential (TAP) and MAP during ventricular fibrillation. The vertical calibration bar indicates 50 mV for the TAP and 5 mV for the MAP. The horizontal bar indicates 100 milliseconds. MAP and TAP recordings have almost identical activation times, cycle length, and action potential durations. Maximal repolarization levels change slightly from beat to beat, showing intermittent, completely repolarized intervals in both recordings.

milliseconds (TAP) and 89 ± 6 milliseconds (MAP; P=NS). APD was slightly longer in the MAP (63 ± 6 milliseconds) than in the transmembrane potential (57 ± 5 milliseconds; $P<0.001$; Fig. 4, panel A). Average activation time between the recordings was 2.8 ± 4 milliseconds. Activation times varied from -25 to $+25$ milliseconds. Usually, high activation times were transient and were preceded by a period of low-amplitude recordings in one of the two recordings.

In 9 of the 43 episodes, activation times between the two recordings did not change significantly over the entire recording. Based on the constant activation times between the two recording sites, these episodes were classified as ventricular tachycardia (VT). In these episodes, both APDs and cycle lengths were significantly longer than in the episodes of VF, showing average cycle lengths of 135 ± 7 milliseconds (MAP and TAP; P=NS), and APDs of 87 ± 11 milliseconds (TAP) and 94 ± 5 milliseconds (MAP). Again, there was no significant difference in cycle length between the two recordings, and APD was slightly longer in the MAP than in the TAP recording (difference = 7 milliseconds; $P<0.001$, Fig. 4, panel A). Both cycle lengths and APDs of MAPs correlated linearly with TAP durations. There was an almost perfect correlation for cycle length and a very close correlation for APD (Fig. 4, panel B).

Repolarized Intervals During VF

To quantify potentially excitable periods, the "repolarized interval" was analyzed as the time during which the action potential was repolarized to more than 50% of its plateau potential.[7,9] This repolarized interval averaged 26 ± 7 milliseconds per cycle in the MAP, and 32 ± 7 milliseconds per cycle in the TAP recording, corresponding to 36% of the total time for the transmembrane potential, and to 29% of the total time for the MAP. During VT, average repolarized intervals were significantly longer than in the VF episodes (48 ± 13 milliseconds [TAP], 41 ± 7 milliseconds [MAP]; $P<0.05$), and did at no point fall below 30 milliseconds. The duration of the repolarized interval correlated linearly with cycle length (Fig. 5), but not with APD ($r<0.2$).

Comparison of MAP and TAP Recordings During VF

MAP and TAP recordings were nearly indistinguishable in duration during sinus rhythm (Fig. 1, panel A), concordant with previous data.[8,9] During VF and VT, cycle length was equal in MAPs and TAPs (Fig. 4), while APD_{50} was slightly longer in the MAP than in the TAP, the 5-millisecond

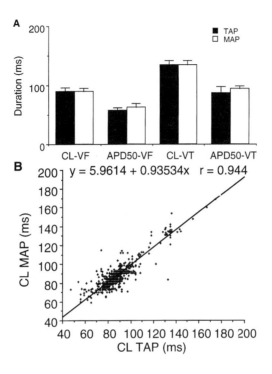

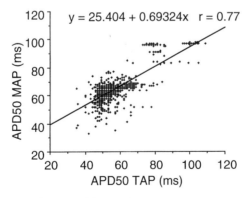

Figure 4. Comparison between MAP and transmembrane action potential (TAP) for action potential duration at 50% repolarization (APD50) and cycle length (CL). **A**. Comparison of mean values during ventricular fibrillation and ventricular tachycardia, expressed in milliseconds as mean ± standard deviation. **B**. Linear correlation between MAPs and TAPs for CL and APD.

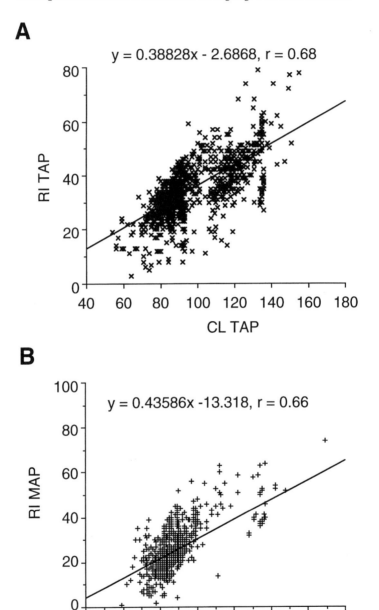

Figure 5. Linear correlation of repolarized intervals (RI) and cycle lengths (CL) in transmembrane action potential (TAP) and MAP data. **A**. Correlation in TAP recordings. **B**. Correlation in MAP recordings. All correlations were highly significant (r=0.66 to 0.69; $P<0.0005$).

difference being within the validity range of APDs.[20] Digital data processing contributed considerably to the accurate determination of the plateau potential during phase 2 of the action potential, and hence the exact time of 50% repolarization, especially in the more scattered MAP recordings.

Recording of multiple cellular potentials by the MAP can theoretically result in longer APDs than in the TAP by superimposing potentials of cells activated at slightly different moments, or of cells showing slightly dispersed repolarization.[9] Slow propagation of activation during VF[21-23] could enhance this effect. As the TAP was recorded close to the edge of the MAP's recording area in this study, estimation of MAP duration with twice the activation difference between MAP and TAP was performed according to the following formula:

$$MAPD_{est} = APD(TAP) + 2 \ \Delta AT_{TAP-MAP}$$

Estimated MAP duration ($MAPD_{est}$) was 63 ± 11 milliseconds during VF, and 93 ± 19 milliseconds during VT, which was not significantly different from measured MAP duration ($P > 0.2$). Superimposition of multiple cellular action potentials within the MAP's recording area can therefore explain the slight differences in APD between MAPs and TAPs observed in this study.

Cycle lengths were similar to cycle lengths measured by others in the fibrillating heart.[14,21] Fast changes in action potential morphology and activation time, and frequent observation of low-amplitude recordings, designate the arrhythmias recorded in this study as VF.[1,15-17] Slight differences in cycle length in comparison to other studies[7,24] can probably be explained by different experimental set ups and perfusion techniques.

Low-Amplitude Recordings

The transient nature of low-amplitude recordings in both MAPs and TAPs, and their occurrence in both recording types, makes a recording artifact unlikely. As low-amplitude recordings were concurrent with a decrease in cycle length, low-amplitude recordings might reflect simultaneous, superimposed recording of two or more asynchronous repolarization time courses, caused by electrotonic or direct addition of membrane potentials. Low-amplitude MAP recordings could result from recording over an area of conduction block or over the vortex of a reentrant wave.[23,25-27] The duration of low-amplitude recordings observed in this study (1 to 3 seconds) is comparable to the persistence time of activation wave fronts during VF as measured by epicardial activation mapping.[28] This observation supports a relation between low-amplitude MAP recordings and vortex rotors. The phenomena reflected by low-amplitude repolarization patterns during VF encourage further investigation involving other techniques of cardiac mapping.

Repolarization Levels During VF

In both recordings, maximal repolarization levels ranged from 50% to beyond 90% repolarization during VF (Fig. 3), a result that, from previous data, was not expected.[2,14-17,29] Correlation of repolarized intervals with cycle length, but not APD (Fig. 5), and large beat-to-beat variability of cycle lengths and maximal repolarization levels, support the assumption of intermittent excitable periods during repolarized intervals. Hence, in contrast to earlier hypotheses,[1,14,28] multiple activation wave fronts during VF do not always seem to result in reactivation at the earliest moment allowed by local refractoriness.

Repolarization beyond the level of relative refractoriness can explain regional capture of electrical stimuli during VF.[11,12] The 'random" response of fibrillating myocardium to electrical stimuli in experimental and clinical studies[10,30-32] could also be caused by different repolarization levels in regions of low shock field strength at the time of the shock. Analysis of repolarization during VF by MAP recordings in combination with other techniques of cardiac mapping[23,28,33-38] described in this book might result in characterization of repolarized intervals during VF. Understanding these phenomena and their spatial distribution in the heart at a given moment could eventually help us to understand the "random" character of the defibrillation threshold,[32] and may help us to develop finer techniques of electrical defibrillation.

Conclusions

Applying the quality criteria defined in this chapter, MAPs can be used to record repolarization during VF. This technique allows direct, continuous monitoring of repolarization during VF in experimental settings and in patients. We propose the following quality criteria for analysis of MAP recordings during VF:

1. MAP amplitude during VF greater than 60% of baseline MAP amplitude.
2. Exclusion of fractionated MAP recordings, recognized by loss of typical MAP morphology, sudden increase in maximal diastolic potential, and sudden shortening of cycle length.
3. Digital analysis of activation and plateau potential.

Regional capture of electrical stimuli during VF might be caused by intermittent repolarization to levels beyond refractoriness. Systematic investigation of repolarization levels during VF might help us to understand capture of electrical stimuli, and eventually might explain the random character of the defibrillation threshold.

References

1. Liem LB, Swerdlow CD, Franz MR. Distinctive features of ventricular fibrillation and ventricular tachycardia detected by monophasic action potential recording in human subjects. *J Electrophysiol* 1988;2:484-491.
2. Swartz JF, Jones JL, Fletcher RD. Characterization of ventricular fibrillation based on monophasic action potential morphology in the human heart. *Circulation* 1993;87:1907-1914.
3. Daubert JP, Frazier DW, Wolf PD, et al. Response of relatively refractory canine myocardium to monophasic and biphasic shocks. *Circulation* 1991;84:2522-2538.
4. Behrens S, Li C, Fabritz CL, et al. Shock-induced dispersion of ventricular repolarization: Implications for the induction of ventricular fibrillation and the upper limit of vulnerability. *J Cardiovasc Electrophysiol* 1997;8:998-1008.
5. Fabritz CL, Kirchhof PF, Moubarak J, et al. Mechanism of ventricular fibrillation induction by T wave shocks in patients. *J Am Coll Cardiol* 1996;27:402A. Abstract.
6. Fabritz CL, Kirchhof PF, Behrens S, et al. Myocardial vulnerability to T wave shocks: Relation to shock strength, shock coupling interval, and dispersion of ventricular repolarization. *J Cardiovasc Electrophysiol* 1996;7:231-242.
7. Kirchhof PF, Fabritz CL, Behrens S, Franz MR. Induction of ventricular fibrillation by T wave field-shocks in the isolated perfused rabbit heart: Role of nonuniform shock responses. *Basic Res Cardiol* 1997;92:35-44.
8. Franz MR, Burkhoff D, Spurgeon H, et al. In vitro validation of a new cardiac catheter technique for recording monophasic action potentials. *Eur Heart J* 1986;7:34-41.
9. Franz MR. Method and theory of monophasic action potential recording. *Prog Cardiovasc Dis* 1991;33:347-368.
10. Frazier DW, Wolf PD, Wharton JM, et al. Stimulus-induced critical point. Mechanism for electrical initiation of reentry in normal canine myocardium. *J Clin Invest* 1989;83:1039-1052.
11. Bonometti C, Hwang C, Hough D, et al. Interaction between strong electrical stimulation and reentrant wavefronts in canine ventricular fibrillation. *J Am Coll Cardiol* 1995;25(suppl):85A. Abstract.
12. KenKnight BH, Bayly PV, Gerstle RJ, et al. Regional capture of fibrillating ventricular myocardium. Evidence of an excitable gap. *Circ Res* 1995;77:849-855.
13. Ramdat-Misier A, Opthof T, van Hemel NM, et al. Dispersion of "refractoriness" in noninfarcted myocardium of patients with ventricular tachycardia or ventricular fibrillation after myocardial infarction. *Circulation* 1995;91:2566-2572.
14. Opthof T, Ramdat-Misier A, Coronel R, et al. Dispersion of refractoriness in canine ventricular myocardium. Effects of sympathetic stimulation. *Circ Res* 1991;68:1204-1215.
15. Akiyama T. Intracellular recording of in situ ventricular cells during ventricular fibrillation. *Am J Physiol* 1981;240:H465-H471.

16. Sano T, Tsuchihashi H, Shimamoto T. Ventricular fibrillation studied by the microelectrode method. *Circ Res* 1958;6:41-46.

17. Hogancamp CE, Kardesh M, Danforth WH, Bing RG. Transmembrane electrical potentials in ventricular tachycardia and fibrillation. *Am Heart J* 1959;57:214-222.

18. Kirchhof PF, Fabritz CL, Zabel M, Franz MR. The vulnerable period for low and high energy T wave shocks: Role of dispersion of repolarisation and effect of d-sotalol. *J Cardiovasc Res* 1996;31:953-962.

19. Franz MR. Long-term recording of monophasic action potentials from human endocardium. *Am J Cardiol* 1983;51:1629-1634.

20. Franz MR, Kirchhof PF, Fabritz CL, et al. Computer analysis of monophasic action potential recordings: Manual validation and clinically pertinent applications. *PACE* 1995;18:1666-1678.

21. Chen PS, Shibata N, Dixon EG, et al. Activation during ventricular defibrillation in open-chest dogs. Evidence of complete cessation and regeneration of ventricular fibrillation after unsuccessful shocks. *J Clin Invest* 1986;77:810-823.

22. Chen PS, Cha YM, Peters BB, Chen LS. Effects of myocardial fiber orientation on the electrical induction of ventricular fibrillation. *Am J Physiol* 1993;264:H1760-H1773.

23. Gray RA, Jalife J, Panfilov A, et al. Nonstationary vortexlike reentrant activity as a mechanism of polymorphic ventricular tachycardia in the isolated rabbit heart. *Circulation* 1995;91:2454-2469.

24. MacConaill M. Ventricular fibrillation thresholds in Langendorff perfused rabbit hearts: All or none effect of low potassium concentration. *Cardiovasc Res* 1987;21:463-468.

25. Restivo M, Gough WB, El-Sherif N. Ventricular arrhythmias in the subacute myocardial infarction period. High-resolution activation and refractory patterns of reentrant rhythms. *Circ Res* 1990;66:1310-1327.

26. Habbab MA, El-Sherif N. Recordings from the slow zone of reentry during burst pacing versus programmed premature stimulation for initiation of reentrant ventricular tachycardia in patients with coronary artery disease. *Am J Cardiol* 1992;70:211-217.

27. Ino T, Fishbein MC, Mandel WJ, et al. Cellular mechanisms of ventricular bipolar electrograms showing double and fractionated potentials. *J Am Coll Cardiol* 1995;26:1080-1089.

28. Cha YM, Birgersdotter-Green U, Wolf PL, et al. The mechanism of termination of reentrant activity in ventricular fibrillation. *Circ Res* 1994;74:495-506.

29. Zhou X, Wolf PD, Rollins DL, et al. Effects of monophasic and biphasic shocks on action potentials during ventricular fibrillation in dogs. *Circ Res* 1993;73:325-334.

30. Tang AS, Wolf PD, Afework Y, et al. Three-dimensional potential gradient fields generated by intracardiac catheter and cutaneous patch electrodes. *Circulation* 1992;85:1857-1864.

31. Souza JJ, Malkin RA, Ideker RE. Comparison of upper limit of vulnerability and defibrillation probability of success curves using a nonthoracotomy lead system. *Circulation* 1995;91:1247-1252.

32. Deale OC, Wesley R Jr, Morgan D, Lerman BB. Nature of defibrillation: Determinism versus probabilism. *Am J Physiol* 1990;259:H1544-H1550.

33. Millar C, Kralios F, Lux R. Correlation between refractory periods and ARIs from electrograms: Effect of rate and adrenergic interventions. *Circulation* 1985;72:1372.

34. Haws CW, Lux RL. Correlation between in vivo transmembrane action potential durations and activation-recovery intervals from electrograms. Effects of interventions that alter repolarization time. *Circulation* 1990;81:281-288.

35. Dillon SM. Synchronized repolarization after defibrillation shocks. A possible component of the defibrillation process demonstrated by optical recordings in rabbit heart. *Circulation* 1992;85:1865-1878.

36. El-Sherif N, Caref EB, Yin H, Restivo M. The electrophysiological mechanism of ventricular arrhythmias in the long QT syndrome. Tridimensional mapping of activation and recovery patterns. *Circ Res* 1996;79:474-492.

37. Laurita KR, Girouard SD, Rosenbaum DS. Modulation of ventricular repolarization by a premature stimulus. Role of epicardial dispersion of repolarization kinetics demonstrated by optical mapping of the intact guinea pig heart. *Circ Res* 1996;79:493-503.

38. Girouard SD, Pastore JM, Laurita KR, et al. Optical mapping in a new guinea pig model of ventricular tachycardia reveals mechanism for multiple wavelengths in a single reentrant circuit. *Circulation* 1996;93:603-613.

44

Extension of Refractoriness Mechanism for Ventricular Defibrillation

Oscar H. Tovar, MD and Janice L. Jones, PhD

Sudden cardiac death resulting from ventricular fibrillation is responsible for more than 350,000 fatalities per year in the United States alone.[1] Major advances in the treatment of this fatal arrhythmia have led to the development of transvenously implanted cardioverter defibrillators (ICDs) for patients who are susceptible to ventricular fibrillation, and automatic external defibrillators for patients who experience out-of-hospital ventricular fibrillation. However, mechanisms underlying fibrillation and electric defibrillation remain subjects of intense investigation. As our understanding of these fundamental mechanisms increases, we will be able to significantly improve the efficacy of defibrillation. In this chapter, we examine the research underlying the "extension of refractoriness" hypothesis for defibrillation with monophasic and biphasic defibrillator waveforms.

The "Extension of Refractoriness" Hypothesis for Defibrillation

During early ventricular fibrillation in dog and rabbit hearts, the individual myocytes are usually reexcited before they completely repolarize.[2,3]

This work was supported in part by NIH grants HL24606 and HL49089 and by a grant from the DVAMC.
From Franz MR (ed): *Monophasic Action Potentials: Bridging Cell and Bedside.* ©Futura Publishing Company, Inc., Armonk, NY, 2000.

The absence of diastolic intervals has been confirmed in humans by monophasic action potential (MAP) recordings acquired during induced fibrillation prior to nonthoracotomy defibrillator implantation.[4] This suggests that in both humans and in animals, the fibrillation cycle length is controlled primarily by the cellular refractory period. Therefore, in contrast to ventricular pacing where the shock is delivered during diastole, the defibrillating shock is usually delivered during the ventricular fibrillation action potential as shown in Figure 1. Since the action potential upstroke is very short compared with the total action potential duration, a defibrillating shock interacts primarily with cells during the absolute or relative refractory period. A defibrillating shock of sufficient intensity can alter the dynamics of fibrillation either by producing propagating action potentials, in which case fibrillation can continue,[5] or by producing graded responses from relatively refractory cells which can terminate fibrillation.[6,7] The extension of refractoriness hypothesis states that, if there is a sufficiently long postshock refractory period in all of or in a critical mass of the myocardium, this prolonged refractoriness will extinguish fibrillation because all fibrillation wave fronts will encounter refractory cells, as shown in Figure 1.

Probability of Successful Defibrillation and Extension of Refractoriness

A defibrillation shock creates a nonuniform electric field (ie, different local voltage gradients) throughout the heart.[8] Regions near the shock electrodes are exposed to relatively high shock intensities, while distant

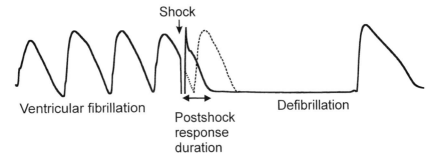

Figure 1. An episode of ventricular fibrillation in the isolated rabbit heart that is successfully terminated by an electric shock. The defibrillating shock, which was delivered during the relative refractory period of the fibrillation action potential, produced a graded response that extended refractoriness and terminated fibrillation. The dashed trace represents the likely course of fibrillation had the shock not been delivered. The extension of refractoriness produced by the shock caused the next fibrillation wave front to encounter refractory tissue. Therefore, the fibrillation wave front was blocked and fibrillation was terminated in that region.

regions are exposed to low intensities.[8-10] In most cases of failed defibrillation, the earliest postshock activations are recorded from the low potential gradient regions.[3,11,12] This suggests that the termination of fibrillation in these regions of the heart is a major determinant of the success or failure of the defibrillating shock. In dogs, successful defibrillation using monophasic shocks requires a minimum local voltage gradient of 5 to 7 V/cm in these low-gradient regions.[8,13]

During clinical and animal defibrillation, as well as in computer models,[3,5,9,14,15] the prolongation of refractoriness, especially in the low-gradient regions, appears to play a decisive role in the termination of fibrillation. MAP recordings from patients undergoing threshold determination prior to ICD implantation show that a successful defibrillating shock prolongs the fibrillation action potential (and presumably the refractory period).[15]

With use of MAP electrodes, similar recordings have been obtained from isolated rabbit hearts.[3] The degree of action potential prolongation in a low potential gradient region was measured as the postshock response duration and was correlated with the probability of successful defibrillation. Figure 2 illustrates the 3 possible defibrillation outcomes: immediate or type A defibrillation (ie, conversion of ventricular fibrillation to normal sinus rhythm [NSR] following diastole after the postshock response); pro-

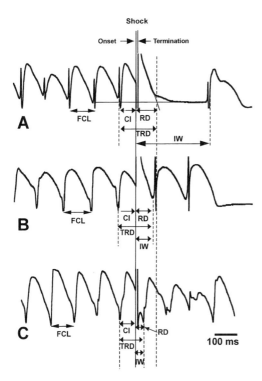

Figure 2. Three different outcomes of defibrillation attempts. **A.** Immediate defibrillation after a long postshock response. **B.** Progressive defibrillation after an intermediate postshock response. **C.** Failed defibrillation after a short postshock response. In these episodes the defibrillating shock was delivered at approximately the same coupling interval (marked as onset of the shock) to allow comparison of the different postshock responses. FCL = fibrillation cycle length; CI = coupling interval; RD = response duration; TRD = total response duration; IW = isoelectric window. Modified from Reference 3, with permission.

gressive or type B defibrillation (ie, defibrillation after 1 to 3 rapidly occurring action potentials without intermediate diastole following the shock)[11]; and failed defibrillation. The postshock response duration differed significantly with the success or failure of the shock to defibrillate. Overall response durations (mean ± SEM) associated with immediate successful defibrillation (97.7±3.4 milliseconds; n=23) were significantly longer than those associated with failed defibrillation (69.0±3.9 milliseconds; n=50). Immediate defibrillation did not occur when the response duration had a value less than 75 milliseconds. Response durations for progressive defibrillation (82.0±2.8 milliseconds; n=38) were intermediate between those for failed defibrillation and those for immediate successful defibrillation. The shortest response duration observed for successful progressive defibrillation was 47 milliseconds. The mean response duration in immediate defibrillation was 102% of the fibrillation cycle length, possibly due to complete repolarization of the cell membrane, which repolarizes only partially during fibrillation.

Shock Strength and Coupling Interval

The coupling interval and the shock intensity determine the duration of the postshock response.[9,16,17] Postshock response durations, obtained from a low shock intensity region at different coupling intervals, are shown in Figure 3. The data points in this figure can be considered as representing cells in various regions of the ventricle because, due to the continuously moving fibrillation wave fronts, cells in different regions of the heart are found at various stages of the fibrillation action potential at the time of the shock. Figure 3 shows that shocks delivered at long coupling intervals in a region of low potential gradient fail if the postshock response is short, even if the postshock response is long in other low potential gradient regions where the shock occurred at short coupling intervals. This is because the shock fails to defibrillate in the region with the short postshock response, as shown in panel C of Figure 2. In contrast, the shock is successful if it produces long responses at long coupling intervals and long responses at short coupling intervals, especially in the low potential gradient region (in other words, long responses throughout the ventricle). Consequently, it is at long coupling intervals—greater than 40% of the normalized coupling interval shown in Figures 3 and 4—that the degree of action potential prolongation correlates with the success or failure of defibrillation. A coupling interval of greater than 40% corresponds to 19% or greater repolarization of the action potential.[18] This implies that response durations from relatively refractory cells (those more than 19% repolarized) are critical for defibrillation success.

In the same study,[3] the probability of successful defibrillation increased with shock intensity and followed the classic shape, as shown in

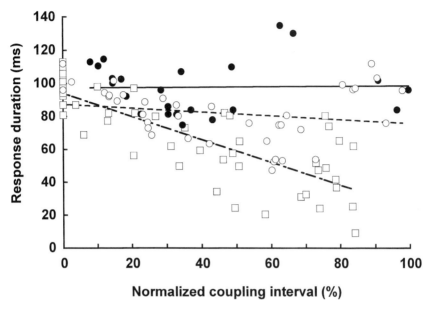

Figure 3. Response durations as a function of the normalized coupling interval. Normalized coupling interval was calculated as the percentage of the mean fibrillation cycle length. ● = immediate successful defibrillation; ○ = progressive successful defibrillation; □ = failed defibrillation. The corresponding regression lines are shown by solid, short-dashed, and long dashed lines. Modified from Reference 3, with permission.

Figure 4. The intensity of 2.4 A, which corresponded to 6 V/cm in the low potential gradient region, was associated with 90% probability of successful defibrillation. One hundred percent probability of successful defibrillation was reached at 2.8 A, which corresponded to a field strength of approximately 8.4 V/cm. However, at each intensity tested, successful defibrillation was associated with long response durations in the low potential gradient regions. Even at the low intensity of 1.2 A, corresponding to 3 V/cm, where the probability of successful defibrillation was only 43%, successful defibrillations were associated with long response durations, as shown in Figure 4. These findings suggest that, if a defibrillating shock produces long uniform response durations in a critical mass of the ventricle, then this shock will successfully defibrillate, even at low shock intensities.

Postshock Action Potentials After Progressive Defibrillation

Progressive defibrillation is less desirable than immediate successful defibrillation because when postshock activations occur, fibrillation may

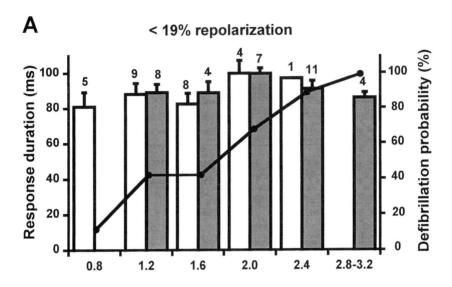

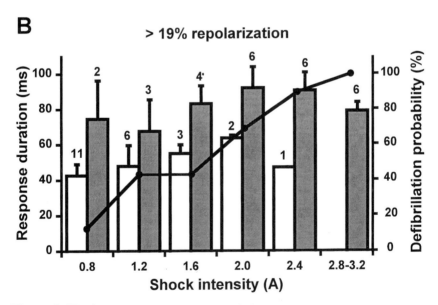

Figure 4. The bars represent the mean ± SEM of response durations obtained at each intensity tested for successful (gray bars) and failed defibrillation (white bars) obtained at (**A**) less than 19% repolarization, and (**B**) greater than 19% repolarization. Superimposed on both plots is the overall probability of successful defibrillation curve. The number of episodes is shown on top of each bar. Modified from Reference 3, with permission.

continue.[3,10] In the rabbit heart,[3] the probability of immediate defibrillation
(as a percentage of successful defibrillation) initially increased with shock
intensity, and reached its maximum probability (59%) at a shock intensity
of 2.4 A (corresponding to an electric field of 6.3 V/cm). At this intensity,
the overall probability of successful defibrillation was 90%, as shown in
Figure 5. The probability of immediate defibrillation then decreased with
increasing shock intensity so that it was only 10% at the higher current
intensities of 2.8 A to 3.2 A (8.4 V/cm), at which a 100% overall probability
of successful defibrillation was obtained.

Progressive Defibrillation at Low Shock Intensities

The high incidence of progressive defibrillation at low shock intensities is consistent with incomplete block of fibrillation action potentials by
intermediate duration postshock responses. Such a partial block, produced
in the low voltage gradient region, may be sufficient to alter fibrillation
dynamics by slowing reentry loops and to allow a gradual cessation of the
tachyarrhythmia.

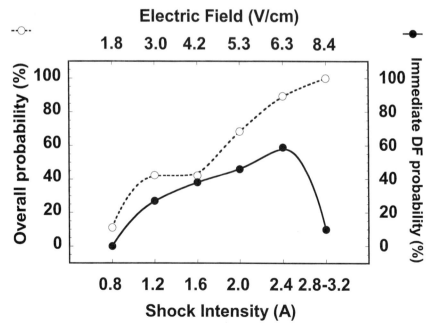

Figure 5. Overall probability of successful defibrillation (dashed curve) and probability of immediate successful defibrillation (solid curve) as a function of shock
intensity and the corresponding local electric field measurements from a low-
gradient region.

Progressive Defibrillation at High Shock Intensities

As discussed previously (Fig. 5), in the isolated rabbit heart, the probability of immediate defibrillation initially increased with shock intensity but then decreased as shock intensity continued to increase. Postshock activations in progressive defibrillation were present in 90% of successful defibrillations at a potential gradient of 8 V/cm or approximately 8 times diastolic threshold. At the cellular level, in myocardial cell aggregates during simulated NSR (pacing at cycle length of 600 milliseconds) and simulated fibrillation (pacing at cycle length of 180 milliseconds), similar postshock automatic activations were induced at shock intensities greater than 8 times diastolic threshold delivered in the relative refractory period, as shown in Figure 6.[19] Comparable dysfunction has been observed in chick myocytes[20] and in isolated guinea pig papillary muscle[21] when high-intensity shocks were delivered during diastole. Electroporation by high-intensity shocks is well known to cause calcium overload.[22,23] In a computer model, Ca^{++} release from the sarcoplasmic reticulum under conditions of calcium overload produced automaticity and triggered activity.[24]

In each of these cellular models, high shock intensities produced postshock automaticity. In the intact heart, similar postshock disturbances in the membrane potential produced by a defibrillation shock can cause focal ectopic activity and conduction dysfunction. These anomalies produce a few automatic activations before conversion to NSR (progressive defibrillation) if the cellular dysfunction is limited and recovery is sufficiently fast, or they allow refibrillation if recovery is slow or the injury is irreversible. Besides these immediate effects, there are delayed effects associated with high-intensity shocks. High-intensity shocks can be successful in defibrillating, but patients can have as a consequence depressed cardiac contractility[25] that has been associated with shock-induced decrease in Ca^{++} uptake by the sarcoplasmic reticulum, due to uncoupling of adenosine triphosphate (ATP) hydrolysis and Ca^{++} transport.[26] Even though the overall probability of successful defibrillation reaches 100% at higher shock intensities, as shown in Figure 5, the probability of immediate successful defibrillation is only 10%, suggesting that shocks at this intensity produce cellular injury. In the calf heart, the probability of success for transthoracic defibrillation initially increased with increasing shock intensity, but after reaching a peak value (not 100% for most waveforms), it decreased as intensity continued to increase.[27] At higher intensities where the probability of success was decreasing with increasing intensity, even successful defibrillations were followed by postshock arrhythmias. It may be that the progressive defibrillation seen at high intensities in the isolated rabbit heart model is the initial sign of postshock dysfunction, and that as intensity increased even further, actual defibrillation failure would have been observed similar to that seen in the calf model.

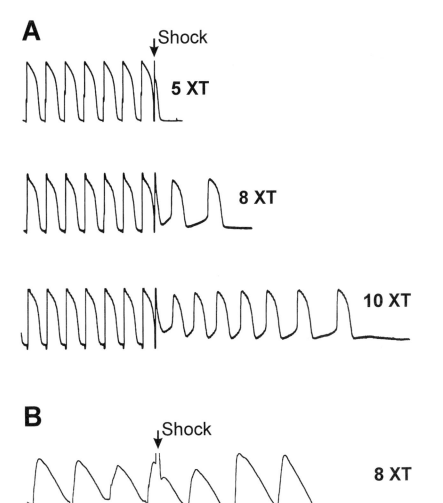

Figure 6. A. Myocardial cell aggregates paced with an electric field at a cycle length of 180 milliseconds to simulate fibrillation. The simulated defibrillation shock was an 8-millisecond monophasic waveform delivered at ≈80% repolarization. The panel shows 3 different shock intensities measured as multiples of diastolic threshold (XT). **B.** An episode of ventricular fibrillation in the isolated rabbit heart. The defibrillation shock, indicated by the arrow, was a monophasic waveform with an intensity of ≈8 times diastolic threshold recorded in a low shock intensity region of the heart.

Extension of Refractoriness with Biphasic Shocks

Selected biphasic waveforms have defibrillation energy thresholds 49% lower than monophasic waveforms of same total duration and tilt.[28] As mentioned previously, monophasic waveforms require a minimum voltage gradient in the heart of 5 to 7 V/cm,[8,13] or 3 to 6 times diastolic threshold[29] in those regions of lowest shock intensity far from the electrodes. In contrast, comparable biphasic waveforms require only about 2.7 V/cm[30] or about 1.5 times diastolic excitation threshold. An examination of the probability of successful defibrillation as a function of shock intensity curves for monophasic and biphasic waveforms can help to explain mechanisms through which biphasic waveforms reduce defibrillation threshold.[31,32] These curves show that the probability of successful defibrillation is similar for monophasic and biphasic waveforms for relatively high shock intensities at which both waveforms defibrillate in almost 100% of the cases, and for low shock intensities at which neither waveform defibrillates. There is, however, a "window" of intermediate shock intensities between these values for which the biphasic waveform has a higher probability of success than the monophasic waveform.

To determine the mechanism of the greater efficacy of biphasic waveforms at the intermediate "window" intensities, the effects of shock intensity and waveform on refractory period responses were studied in myocardial cell aggregates using an S1-S2 protocol, as shown in panel A of Figure 7. Fibrillation was simulated with 3 seconds of S1 pacing at a 180-millisecond cycle length.[17] Electric field shocks of 8 milliseconds' duration for monophasic waveforms and 4/4 milliseconds for biphasic waveforms were delivered at intensities of 1.5, 3, and 5 times diastolic threshold or approximately 2 to 7 V/cm. Monophasic shocks delivered in the last 10 milliseconds of the refractory period produced short responses (mean ± SEM; 8.8 ± 1.4 milliseconds) at 1.5 times diastolic threshold, and prolonged responses (53.0 ± 3.1 milliseconds) at 5 times diastolic threshold ($P < 0.01$). Biphasic shock response durations produced at the same coupling intervals (Fig. 7, panel B) were uniformly long and did not change significantly between 1.5 times diastolic threshold (35.1 ± 12.6 milliseconds) and 5 times diastolic threshold (46.2 ± 2.7 milliseconds). The window of intensities in which biphasic shocks had an advantage over monophasic shocks in extending the refractory period began at 1.5 times diastolic threshold (approximately 3 V/cm), and ended between 3 and 5 times diastolic threshold (approximately 5 to 7 V/cm).

Computer simulations confirmed these experimental findings, using similar S1-S2 protocols.[33,34] One model used the Drouhard-Roberge modification of the Beeler-Reuter model of the ventricular action potential to

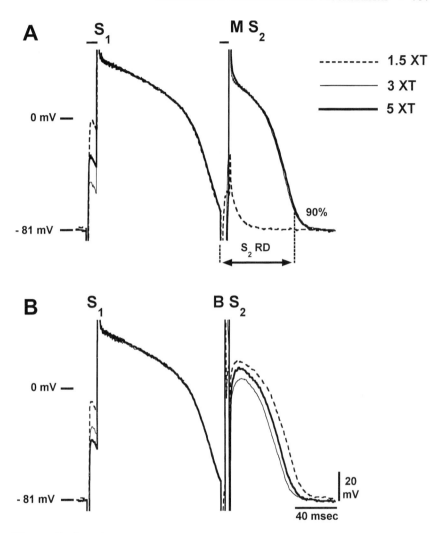

Figure 7. Superimposed recordings from isolated myocardial cells stimulated during the relative refractory period by an electric field at 1.5 times diastolic threshold (dashed line), 3 times diastolic threshold (thin solid line), and 5 times diastolic threshold (thick solid line). The small solid lines on top of the traces represent the duration of the S1 and S2 stimuli. **A**. Monophasic shocks. The arrow shows the response duration (RD) at 90% repolarization. **B**. Biphasic shocks. Modified from Reference 17, with permission.

determine postshock responses to monophasic and biphasic shocks.[34] Intensities of 1.5 and 3 times diastolic threshold were delivered at different coupling intervals with both waveforms. Within the relative refractory period, monophasic shocks produced markedly different responses between 1.5 and 3 times diastolic threshold while biphasic shocks produced uniformly long responses at the same intensities. In another study,[33] an 11-patch model of an isolated cardiac myocyte in a uniform electric field was used to determine postshock responses to monophasic and biphasic shocks between 1 and 4 times diastolic threshold at S1-S2 coupling intervals from 300 to 375 milliseconds (357 milliseconds was the normal time for repolarization). At the intermediate intensities of 1.5 to 3 times diastolic threshold, biphasic shocks produced longer and more uniform responses than did monophasic shocks.

These findings in computer models and in isolated cells predict that biphasic shocks lower defibrillation threshold by extending the refractory period at lower intensities than monophasic shocks. This prediction was directly tested in isolated rabbit hearts, with use of the Langendorff preparation.[35] Ventricular fibrillation and defibrillation were recorded with use of a MAP electrode placed in a low potential gradient region. Consistent with previous studies,[28] the E_{50} was 48% lower for biphasic shocks than for monophasic shocks. At the lowest and at the highest intensities tested, the probabilities of success were similar for monophasic and biphasic shocks. For the window intensities between 1.6 and 2.8 A, biphasic shocks produced longer responses than did monophasic shocks. The postshock response duration associated with successful defibrillation for a monophasic and biphasic shock was similarly long at all intensities. These results confirm the hypothesis that biphasic shocks reduce defibrillation threshold compared to monophasic shocks, by extending refractoriness at lower intensities and decreasing dispersion of refractoriness between low and high potential gradients.

Preconditioning Pulse

A mechanism through which specific biphasic waveforms effectively prolong refractory period responses at the window intensities was suggested by studies in which the previously described computer model of the ventricular action potential was used.[16] The S2 stimulus was either a 10-millisecond rectangular monophasic waveform or 10/10-millisecond symmetrical biphasic waveform. In order to examine the effect of the hyperpolarizing first phase ("conditioning prepulse") on the response produced by the subsequent depolarizing phase, the S1-S2 coupling interval for the biphasic waveform was defined as the start of the second phase, and was equal to the coupling interval for the monophasic waveform. At 1.5 times diastolic threshold, S2 monophasic shocks did not produce sodium current or prolonged postshock responses until the end of the refractory period. However, at the same coupling intervals, the biphasic waveform produced prolonged responses. The hyperpolarizing phase of the biphasic waveform allowed the subsequent depolarizing phase to produce significant sodium current in association with the prolonged responses. This study concluded that the hyperpolarizing prepulse induced recovery of the sodium channels from the inactivated state to the resting state, thereby setting the conditions for a larger, better defined response when the depolarizing pulse was delivered. Similar experiments performed on guinea pig papillary muscle that used an S1-S2 protocol and blocked sodium channels with 30 μM tetrodotoxin suggest that other mechanisms besides the reactivation of sodium channels may be involved in the prolongation of the action potential by biphasic waveforms.[36]

Relationship Between the Extension of Refractoriness and the Upper Limit of Vulnerability

The upper limit of vulnerability hypothesis proposes that, for hearts in normal rhythm, shocks with intensities below the upper limit of vulnerability can induce fibrillation[37,38] when delivered during the vulnerable period, whereas shocks above the upper limit of vulnerability do not induce fibrillation. This phenomenon can be explained by the fact that, during the vulnerable period, different regions of the heart are in various states of repolarization at the time of the shock. Therefore, a low-intensity shock below the upper limit of vulnerability creates dispersion of repolarization, which produces areas of slow or blocked conduction, and allows reentry leading to fibrillation. In contrast, a strong shock above the upper limit of vulnerability causes a uniform action potential extension that prevents reentry.

The "upper limit of vulnerability," as a hypothesis for defibrillation, states that shocks below the defibrillation threshold defibrillate, but that the nonuniform dispersion of refractoriness following the shock causes immediate refibrillation[11] leading to a failed defibrillation attempt. It can be deduced from this hypothesis that, in order to halt fibrillation without reinducing fibrillation, a successful shock must produce a relatively uniform refractoriness. Thus, the 'extension of refractoriness" hypothesis for defibrillation, which states that a successful shock must produce uniformly long postshock responses in all regions of the heart, can help to explain the upper limit of vulnerability. However, the extension of refractoriness hypothesis states that a low-intensity shock does not defibrillate if postshock responses are not long enough to block the fibrillation wave fronts. Thus, the fibrillation after the shock is a continuation of the fibrillation before the shock, not a conversion followed by a new episode of fibrillation.[10]

Correlation Between Postshock Response Duration and Activation Time Measured in Other Studies

Failed Defibrillation

When bipolar electrodes were used to examine activations in dogs,[11] an "isoelectric window" was measured from the time of the shock to the first postshock activation. This window was 64 milliseconds for failed defibrillation. In isolated rabbit hearts, MAP recordings, which allow analysis of the entire action potential,[3] revealed that this isoelectric window (see Fig. 2, panel C) was short because, for failed defibrillation attempts, the next postshock fibrillation activation occurred immediately following repolarization from the fibrillation action potential containing the shock. Therefore, the isoelectric window was similar to the postshock response duration (69 milliseconds).

Witkowski et al[10] used unipolar Ag/AgCl electrodes to show that, for failed defibrillation in dogs, the immediate postshock cycle length was similar (within 2 standard deviations) to the preshock fibrillation cycle length. Failed defibrillation was associated with at least one site on the ventricle where the first postshock activation was a continuation of the immediately previous fibrillation activity. Consistently, MAP recordings also showed that for failed defibrillation the total response duration, ie, the time measured from the upstroke of the last fibrillation action potential to the end of repolarization of the shock-induced response (mean 102.4 milliseconds; SD 20.1 milliseconds), was within 2 standard deviations of the preshock cycle length (mean 96.2 milliseconds; SD 13.2 milliseconds), suggesting the continuation of fibrillation.[3]

Successful Immediate Defibrillation

In the bipolar electrode study in dogs, the isoelectric window for successful defibrillation (339 milliseconds)[11] was similar to the time between the shock and the first postshock action potential upstroke (301.6 milliseconds) in the MAP study in which the isolated rabbit heart was used.[3] Additionally, the MAP study demonstrated that this long isoelectric window (Fig. 2, panel A) occurred because there was complete cessation of fibrillation leading to diastole until a new spontaneous activation was initiated and propagated.

The MAP recordings,[3] showing a postshock response duration of 97.6±3.4 milliseconds following successful immediate defibrillation, are similar to optical recordings of transmembrane potentials from isolated rabbit hearts (99.7±2.3 milliseconds).[39] For successful defibrillation, a uniformly long postshock response produced synchronization of repolarization throughout all phases of the fibrillation action potential in both studies, as shown in Figure 3.

Successful Progressive Defibrillation

Successful defibrillation following gradual termination of ventricular fibrillation in the Witkowski study was associated with at least one area of continued fibrillation, which self-extinguished within 3 activations. The MAP recordings in rabbits supported that finding and showed that with progressive successful defibrillation, there was no diastole between the postshock response and the action potential(s) before fibrillation termination (see Fig. 2, panel B).

In summary, according to the extension of refractoriness hypothesis, a successful defibrillating shock needs only to prolong refractoriness in regions of the myocardium where the shock is delivered to tissue late in fibrillation where the action potential is about to recover, but before a propagating action potential can be induced. In tissue where the shock is delivered early in the action potential, so that the postshock refractoriness would already be naturally long, there is no need for further prolongation.[40] This results in a uniformly long postshock refractoriness throughout the myocardium, including both the regions where postshock refractoriness was already long at the time of the shock and those regions where it needed to be prolonged, thereby terminating fibrillation.

References

1. Gillum RF. Sudden coronary death in the United States. *Circulation* 1989;79:756-765.
2. Akiyama T. Intracellular recording of in situ ventricular cells during ventricular fibrillation. *Am J Physiol* 1981;240:H465-H471.
3. Tovar OH, Jones JL. Relationship between "extension of refractoriness" and probability of successful defibrillation. *Am J Physiol* 1997;272:H1011-H1019.
4. Swartz JF, Jones JL, Fletcher RD. Characterization of ventricular fibrillation based on monophasic action potential morphology in the human heart. *Circulation* 1993;87:1907-1914.
5. Trayanova N, Bray MA. Membrane refractoriness and excitation induced in cardiac fibers by monophasic and biphasic shocks. *J Cardiovasc Electrophysiol* 1997;8:745-757.
6. Kao CY, Hoffman BF. Graded and decremental response in heart muscle fibers. *Am J Physiol* 1958;194(1):187-196.
7. Witkowski FX, Penkoske PA. Refractoriness prolongation by defibrillation shocks. *Circulation* 1990;82(3):1064-1066.

8. Wharton JM, Wolf PD, Smith WM, et al. Cardiac potential and potential gradient fields generated by single, combined, and sequential shocks during ventricular defibrillation. *Circulation* 1992;85:1510-1523.

9. Sweeney RJ, Gill RM, Steinberg MI, et al. Ventricular refractory period extension caused by defibrillation shocks. *Circulation* 1990;82:965-972.

10. Witkoswski FX, Penkoske PA, Plonsey R. Mechanism of cardiac defibrillation in open-chest dogs with unipolar DC-coupled simultaneous activation and shock potential recordings. *Circulation* 1990;82:244-260.

11. Chen PS, Shibata N, Dixon EG, et al. Activation during ventricular defibrillation in open-chest dogs. Evidence of complete cessation and regeneration of ventricular fibrillation after unsuccessful shocks. *J Clin Invest* 1986;77:810-823.

12. Chen PS, Wolf PD, Melnick SD, et al. Comparison of activation during ventricular fibrillation and following unsuccessful defibrillation shocks in open-chest dogs. *Circ Res* 1990;66:1544-1560.

13. Zhou X, Daubert JP, Wolf PD, et al. Epicardial mapping of ventricular defibrillation with monophasic and biphasic shocks in dogs. *Circ Res* 1993;72:145-160.

14. Dillon SM. Optical recordings in the rabbit heart show that defibrillation strength shocks prolong the duration of depolarization and the refractory period. *Circ Res* 1991;69:842-856.

15. Jones JL. Waveforms for implantable cardioverter defibrillators (ICDs) and transchest defibrillation. In Tacker WA Jr (ed): *Defibrillation of the Heart: ICDs, AEDs and Manual.* St. Louis: Mosby-Year Book; 1994:46-81.

16. Jones JL, Jones RE, Milne KB. Refractory period prolongation by biphasic defibrillator waveforms is associated with enhanced sodium current in a computer model of the ventricular action potential. *IEEE Trans Biomed Eng* 1994;41(1):60-68.

17. Tovar OH, Jones JL. Biphasic defibrillation waveforms reduce shock-induced response duration dispersion between low and high shock intensities. *Circ Res* 1995;77(2):430-438.

18. Tovar OH, Jones JL. Interaction of coupling interval and response duration in successful defibrillation. *Circulation* 1996;94(8):95. Abstract.

19. Tovar OH, Jones JL. Cellular basis of type B defibrillation occurring at high shock intensity. *Circulation* 1996;94(8):I100.

20. Jones JL, Lepeschkin E, Jones RE, et al. Response of cultured myocardial cells to countershock-type electric field stimulation. *Am J Physiol* 1978;235(2):H214-H222.

21. Kodama I, Shibata N, Sakuma I, et al. Aftereffects of high-intensity DC stimulation on the electromechanical performance of ventricular muscle. *Am J Physiol* 1994;267:H248-H258.

22. Jones JL, Jones RE, Balasky G. Microlesion formation in myocardial cells by high-intensity electric field stimulation. *Am J Physiol* 1987;253(22):H480-H486.

23. Tovar OH, Tung L. Electroporation and recovery of cardiac cell membrane with rectangular voltage pulses. *Am J Physiol* 1992;263:H1128-H1136.

24. Luo CH, Rudy Y. A dynamic model of the cardiac ventricular action potential. II. Afterdepolarizations, triggered activity, and potentiation. *Circ Res* 1994;74:1097-1113.

25. Jones DL. Response to a defibrillation shock: The good, the bad, and the ugly. *Am Heart J* 1992;124:834. Abstract.

26. Jones DL, Narayanan N. Defibrillation depresses heart sarcoplasmic reticulum calcium pump: A mechanism of postshock dysfunction. *Am J Physiol* 1998;274:H98-H105.

27. Gold JH, Schuder JC, Stoeckle H, et al. Transthoracic ventricular defibrillation in the 100 kg calf with unidirectional rectangular pulses. *Circulation* 1977;56(5):745-750.
28. Swartz JF, Fletcher RD, Karasik PE. Optimization of biphasic waveforms for human nonthoracotomy defibrillation. *Circulation* 1993;88(6):2646-2654.
29. Lepeschkin E, Jones JL, Rush S, et al. Local potential gradients as unifying measure for thresholds of stimulation, standstill, tachyarrhythmia and fibrillation appearing after strong capacitor discharges. *Adv Cardiol* 1977;21:268-278.
30. Zhou X, Wolf PD, Rollins DL, et al. Effects of monophasic and biphasic shocks on action potentials during ventricular fibrillation in dogs. *Circ Res* 1993;73:325-334.
31. Chapman PD, Vetter JW, Souza JJ, et al. Comparison of monophasic with single and dual capacitor biphasic waveforms for nonthoracotomy canine internal defibrillation. *J Am Coll Cardiol* 1989;14(1):242-245.
32. Jones JL, Swartz JF, Jones RE, et al. Increasing fibrillation duration enhances relative asymmetrical biphasic versus monophasic defibrillator waveform efficacy. *Circ Res* 1990;67:376-384.
33. Sobie EA, Tung L. Does the synchrony of repolarization after monophasic and biphasic field stimulation differ? A model study. *PACE* 1995;18(4):808. Abstract.
34. Jones JL, Tovar OH. Threshold reduction with biphasic defibrillator waveforms. Role of charge balance. *J Electrocardiol* 1995;28(suppl):25-30.
35. Tovar OH, Jones JL. Biphasic shocks improve defibrillation by extending refractoriness at lower intensities than monophasic shocks. *Circulation* 1997;96(8): I4035. Abstract.
36. Zhou X, Smith W, Justice R, et al. Mechanism of action potential prolongation by biphasic shocks. *Circulation* 1997;6(8):I635.
37. Behrens S, Li C, Fabritz CL, et al. Shock-induced dispersion of ventricular repolarization: Implications for the induction of ventricular fibrillation and the upper limit of vulnerability. *J Cardiovasc Electrophysiol* 1997;8:998-1008.
38. Watanabe Y, Dreifus LS. Ventricular arrhythmias. In *Cardiac Arrhythmias: Electrophysiologic Basis for Clinical Interpretation*. New York: Grune & Stratton Inc.; 1977:217-267.
39. Dillon SM. Synchronized repolarization after defibrillation shocks: A possible component of the defibrillation process demonstrated by optical recordings in rabbit heart. *Circulation* 1992;85:1865-1878.
40. Jones JL, Noe W, Tovar OH, et al. Can shocks timed to action potentials in low gradient regions improve both internal and out-of-hospital defibrillation? *J Electrocardiol* 1998;31(suppl):41-44. Review.

45

Mechanisms of Induction and Termination of Ventricular Fibrillation

Steffen Behrens, MD and
Michael R. Franz, MD, PhD

Introduction

Electrical field stimuli delivered during ventricular repolarization (T wave shock) can induce ventricular fibrillation (VF), and electrical field stimuli delivered during VF can defibrillate the heart.[1-3] Recently, a relationship between VF inducibility and defibrillation has been shown: the lowest shock strength that can successfully terminate VF, ie, the defibrillation threshold (DFT), closely correlates with the upper limit of vulnerability (ULV).[4-6] The ULV represents the highest strength of a T wave shock that is able to induce VF.[4,7,8] The observation of a close correlation between the ULV and DFT suggests a common mechanism for both VF induction and VF termination.[9,10] A better understanding of VF induction by field stimulation may thus increase our understanding of the mechanism that underlies defibrillation.

The mechanism of VF induction has been proposed to be due to the initiation of reentrant circuits within the ventricular myocardium.[9,11,12] Reentry may result if unidirectional block occurs, preventing activation wave fronts to travel in one direction but allowing propagation in another direction, only to excite the previously refractory zone after its recovery.[13]

From Franz MR (ed): *Monophasic Action Potentials: Bridging Cell and Bedside.* ©Futura Publishing Company, Inc., Armonk, NY, 2000.

Several years ago, Watanabe and Dreifus[14] postulated a direct relation between reentry initiation (VF induction) and dispersion of ventricular repolarization. They speculated that an electrical stimulus applied during repolarization would allow full excitation of cells of earlier repolarization, whereas cells of longer repolarization would become partially excited (graded response) or remain even unexcited (Fig. 1). The resulting dispersion of ventricular repolarization and its associated disparity in refractoriness would lead to slowing of impulse propagation or conduction block in unexcited or partially excited myocardium, thereby initiating reentry and VF. This hypothesis was based on focal electrical stimulation requiring propagation of activation wave fronts and exciting the ventricular myocardium sequentially. In contrast, electrical field stimuli alter the electrophysiologic condition of the myocardium simultaneously, allowing a more direct analysis of the relation between arrhythmia inducibility and the dispersion of ventricular repolarization. Data from mapping studies suggest that an electrical field stimulus of proper timing and strength may produce increased nonuniformity of refractoriness.[15-17] This is supported by studies that show that electrical field stimuli may affect the action potential duration (APD) (and thus the refractory period) by different degrees, depending

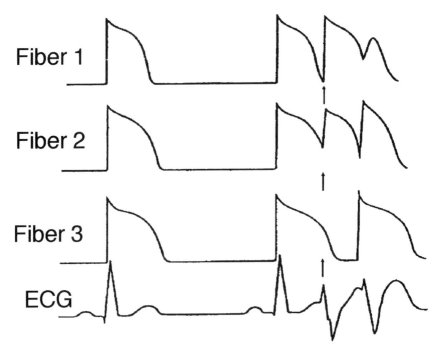

Figure 1. Hypothetical drawing of the effect of a premature stimulus (arrow) on the action potential response in 3 myocardial fibers with different action potential durations. Modified from Reference 14.

on the instantaneous repolarization state, the voltage gradient produced by the shock, and the myocardial fiber orientation at an individual ventricular site.[18-23] Thus, electrical field stimuli appear to modify ventricular repolarization, thereby creating the conditions for reentrant circuits to occur. These conditions that allow excitation wave fronts to form a reentry are discussed in this chapter. Data on the influence of the timing and strength of electrical field stimuli on the shock-induced dispersion of repolarization (SIDR)[24] are presented. This chapter further describes the relationship between SIDR and VF inducibility[24] and discusses the role of SIDR regarding the ULV. Additionally, the role of SIDR for defibrillation is discussed.

Experimental Set Up and Data Analysis

An isolated Langendorff-perfused rabbit heart model was used for the study. The heart was immersed in a tissue bath filled with warm Tyrode's solution as shown in Figure 2. Electrocardiogram (ECG) electrodes placed at the chamber's wall were used to record a volume-conducted ECG. Truncated exponential biphasic shocks were delivered for VF induction and defibrillation, using large stainless steel plate electrodes placed at opposite sides of the tissue bath. VF induction requires that shocks are delivered at coupling intervals within a specific time window during ventricular repolarization, known as the *vulnerable window*. A second requirement for VF induction by T wave shocks is that the shock strength must exceed the fibrillation threshold or lower limit of vulnerability (LLV), and must not be greater than the ULV. Thus, myocardial vulnerability to T wave shocks is defined 2-dimensionally as a function of shock coupling interval and shock strength.[8,25,26] VF inducibility and the corresponding SIDR were therefore determined as a function of both shock timing and shock strength. VF-inducing shocks were applied during paced rhythm (500-millisecond cycle length) over a wide range of coupling intervals and shock strengths, thereby exceeding the borders of the vulnerable window, the LLV, and ULV. Defibrillating shocks were applied 5 to 15 seconds after initiation of VF at shock strengths closely above or below the DFT. SIDR was measured from 10 monophasic action potentials (MAPs) recorded simultaneously from widely spaced sites of both ventricles. The precise location of MAP recordings is depicted in Figure 3. Eight MAPs were recorded from the epicardium, and 2 MAPs from the endocardium of the left and right ventricles. The analysis of MAP measures is shown in Figure 4. SIDR was defined as the range between the shortest and the longest postshock repolarization time (PSRT). PSRT was measured from the beginning of the shock artifact to the end of the repolarization phase in all 10 MAPs. In addition, the percentage of the shock-induced prolongation of

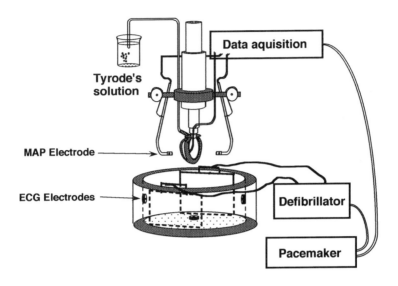

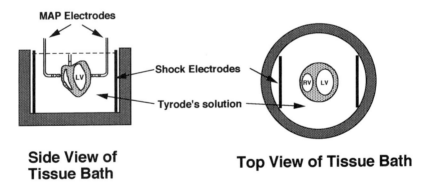

Side View of Tissue Bath   **Top View of Tissue Bath**

Figure 2. Experimental set up. The isolated rabbit heart was mounted on a vertical Langendorff apparatus. MAPs were recorded simultaneously from 8 epicardial and 2 endocardial sites of both ventricles (only 2 epicardial MAPs are shown). The heart was immersed in a tissue bath filled with warm Tyrode's solution. Two large shock plate electrodes were located on both sides of the tissue bath, to deliver electrical field stimuli to induce and terminate ventricular fibrillation. RV = right ventricle; LV = left ventricle.

ventricular repolarization during VF induction was estimated. This measure was defined as repolarization extension, and was calculated using the formula

$$(MAPD_S - MAPD_R) / MAPD_R \times 100\%$$

with $MAPD_S$ indicating the duration of the last regular beat before shock

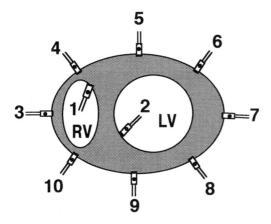

Figure 3. Cross section through the heart and arrangement of MAP recordings. MAP 1 was recorded from the endocardium of the right ventricular apex, MAP 2 from the left ventricular apex. MAPs 3, 4, and 10 were recorded from the right ventricular epicardium, MAP 5 through 9 from the left ventricular epicardium. RV = right ventricle; LV = left ventricle.

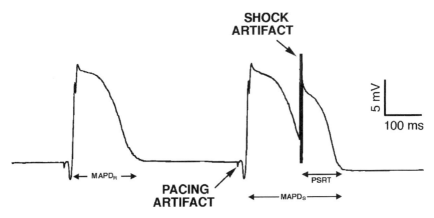

Figure 4. Analysis of MAP recordings during shock application. The pacing cycle length was 500 milliseconds. See text for details. $MAPD_R$ = MAP duration of the last regular beat before shock application; $MAPD_S$ = overall MAP duration of the beat during which the shock was applied; PSRT = postshock repolarization time.

application, and $MAPD_R$ the overall MAP duration of the beat during which the shock was applied.

Effects of Shock Timing and Strength on SIDR

Figure 5 illustrates an example of the repolarization response in 10 MAP recordings and the resulting SIDR produced by T wave shocks of various coupling intervals and strengths. The effects of shocks of different coupling intervals but the same strength (below the ULV) are shown in panels A through D of Figure 5. At short (panel A) and long (panel D)

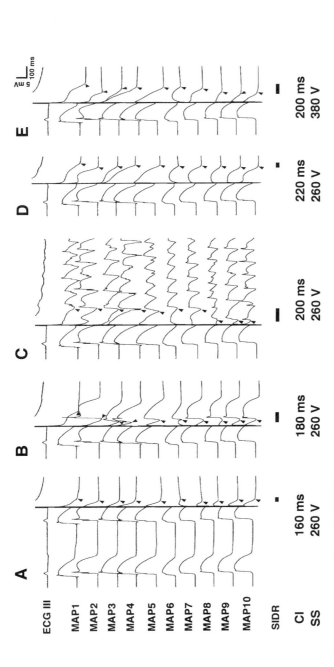

Figure 5. Original recording of 10 MAP recordings and lead III of a volume-conducted electrocardiogram, showing the effects of various shock coupling intervals (CI) and shock strengths (SS) on the repolarization response. In each tracing, the end of the postshock repolarization time is indicated by arrowheads. The shock-induced dispersion of repolarization (SIDR) is indicated by black bars below the tracings. In **A** through **D**, shocks of the same strength (below the upper limit of vulnerability) were delivered at 4 different coupling intervals, exceeding and comprising the vulnerable window. In **E**, the shock was delivered at the same coupling intervals as in C but at a strength above the upper limit of vulnerability. Ventricular fibrillation was induced in C where SIDR was large. See text for details. From Reference 24.

shock coupling intervals, the PSRT varies slightly in all tracings, resulting in small SIDR and no repetitive excitations. However, at intermediate shock coupling intervals, the PSRT varies substantially between different MAP recordings. In panel C of Figure 5, for example, new action potentials are directly excited by the shock in MAPs 1 through 7, whereas action potentials are only slightly prolonged in MAPs 8 through 10. This results in large SIDR and in the induction of VF. The effects of a shock of high strength (above the ULV) are shown in panel E of Figure 5. Although the shock coupling interval is the same as in panel C, the high-voltage shock produces a more uniform repolarization response resulting in less SIDR as compared to panel C and failure to induce VF.

Data from a single experiment are shown in Figure 6. The PSRT (upper panel) and the corresponding repolarization extension (lower panel) in each MAP recording are shown as functions of the shock coupling interval. The effects of weak shocks below the LLV (Fig. 6, panel A), of shocks of intermediate strength (Fig. 6, panel B), and of shocks above ULV strength (Fig. 6, panel C) are shown. VF induction occurs only at two shock coupling intervals (190 and 200 milliseconds) at the intermediate shock strength (indicated by "VF" in Fig. 6, panel B). At these two coupling intervals, PSRT among MAPs varies largely and is caused by a sudden increase of PSRT in some but not all MAPs (Fig. 6, panel B, upper image). In contrast, PSRT for shocks above ULV strength increases more continuously as shock coupling intervals are prolonged (Fig. 6, panel C, upper image). The large differences of PSRT among MAPs indicates large SIDR. Thus, at coupling intervals of 190 and 200 milliseconds, there is large SIDR for shock strengths below the ULV (Fig. 6, panels A and B) but not at high shock strengths above the ULV (Fig. 6, panel C). The lower image shows that repolarization extension is either ≈0% or ≥75% in the different MAP recordings if the shock strength is below the LLV (Fig. 6, panel A, lower image). This indicates that the shock causes either no MAP prolongation, or the excitation of new MAPs. This occurs at the same time at shock coupling intervals of 190 and 200 milliseconds (Fig. 6, panel A, lower image). In contrast, at shock strengths above the LLV and at the same two coupling intervals, the repolarization extension is ≈15% to 25% or greater than 65% in the different MAP recordings (Fig. 6, panel B, lower image), indicating that both MAP prolongation and excitation of new MAPs occurs at this higher shock strength.

Figure 7 shows, in a 3-dimensional graph, the average SIDR calculated over 8 experiments for each combination of shock coupling intervals and shock strengths. The graph shows that SIDR substantially changes as shock coupling intervals or shock strengths are altered. At coupling intervals less than 160 milliseconds and greater than 200 milliseconds, SIDR is small, regardless of the shock strength. At intermediate coupling intervals of 170

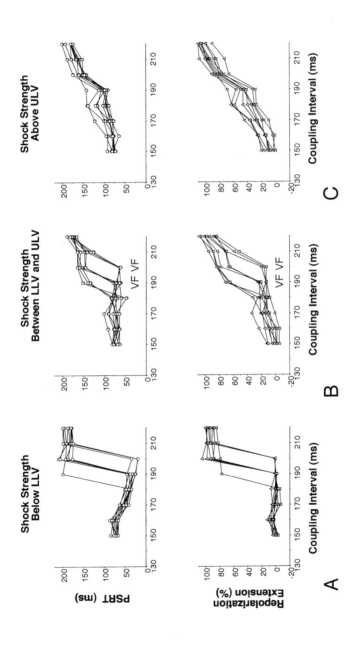

Figure 6. Effects of T wave shocks of different timing and 3 different shock strengths (A through C) on postshock repolarization time (PSRT) (upper panel) and repolarization extension (lower panel) in 9 MAP recordings, obtained from a single heart. Shock strengths were 140 V (A), 340 V (B), and 500 V (C). VF indicates the induction of ventricular fibrillation. See text for details. From Reference 24.

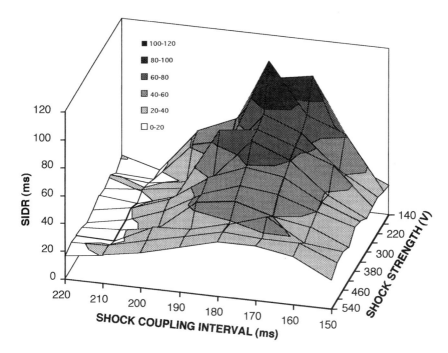

Figure 7. Three-dimensional graph of the average shock-induced dispersion of repolarization (SIDR) calculated over 8 experiments for several combinations of shock coupling intervals and shock strengths. From Reference 24.

to 190 milliseconds, however, SIDR is large at low shock strengths, and decreases progressively toward higher shock strengths.

These results derived from multiple MAP recordings of an intact beating heart are consistent with previous studies that analyzed the shock-induced response of action potentials on a cellular level by using transmembrane action potential recordings.[18-20] Kao and Hoffman[18] showed, in isolated myocardial tissue, that stimuli applied during the refractory period could extend the time course of repolarization, thereby creating prolongation of refractoriness. The duration of these so-called "graded responses" was dependent on the strength and timing of the stimuli. More recently, Knisley et al[19] showed that shocks delivered at different strengths and timings during the refractory period of rabbit papillary tissue caused either no change of the APD, an action potential prolongation, or a new action potential directly excited by the shock. Weak shocks (<4 V/cm) produced no or very small action potential prolongation at short coupling intervals but, with longer coupling intervals, APD increased suddenly, indicating a new action potential. In contrast, shocks delivered at high intensity and early during repolarization produced substantial action potential prolongation that prolonged progressively without a sudden increase, as shocks were applied at more complete repolarization levels. Zhou et al[20] studied the effect of timing of field shocks applied at an intermediate shock strength of 5 V/cm in canine hearts. They found that, as coupling intervals were prolonged, the APD prolonged slightly from 0% to ≈10% to 15%, until a sudden increase in the APD of approximately 80% occurred, indicating the excitation of a new action potential.

Thus, there is a sudden increase of the PSRT for shocks of low and intermediate strengths, and a more linear increase of the PSRT and the corresponding repolarization extension at high shock strengths above the ULV. At different MAP recording sites, the sudden increase of the PSRT for low and intermediate shock strengths occurs at different shock coupling intervals (Fig. 6, panels A and B), thereby causing spatial dispersion of ventricular repolarization. In summary, our data from the intact beating heart, and the results of the cellular studies mentioned above, demonstrate that SIDR is a function of both shock timing and strength. The relation between shock timing and SIDR reflects the role of the myocardial repolarization state at a given MAP recording site which is influenced by the activation time and the subsequent repolarization sequence.[25] The relation between the shock strength and SIDR reflects the role of the voltage-dependent repolarization extension of action potentials by field stimuli.[19]

VF Inducibility and SIDR

The previous paragraph described the various amounts of SIDR as a function of both shock timing and shock strength. However, what is the relation between VF inducibility and SIDR? To assess this, it is necessary to know the boundaries of VF vulnerability. These boundaries were measured in 8 experiments as follows: the ULV and LLV occurred at shock strengths of 390±48 V and 236±56 V, respectively, and the left and right borders of the vulnerable window at coupling intervals of 170±12 milliseconds and 195±5 milliseconds, respectively.

The relation between VF inducibility and SIDR is shown in Figures 8 and 9. In Figure 8, the relation between both parameters is depicted as a function of the shock timing. The graph shows that SIDR is large within the vulnerable window, but decreases as shock coupling intervals moves outside the borders of the vulnerable window where VF is no longer inducible. In Figure 9, the relation between SIDR and VF inducibility is depicted as a function of the shock strength. VF inducibility is indicated as the range between the LLV and ULV. With increasing shock strength, SIDR decreases progressively and reaches its lowest values above the ULV where VF is no longer inducible. At low shock strengths, however, SIDR further increases, reaching its largest values below the LLV.

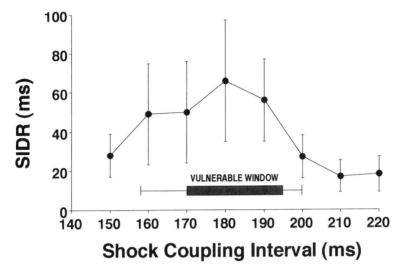

Figure 8. Relation between the shock-induced dispersion of repolarization (SIDR; mean ± SD) and ventricular fibrillation (VF) inducibility as a function of shock coupling interval. VF inducibility was expressed as the range between the left and right borders (mean ± SD) of the vulnerable window. From Reference 24.

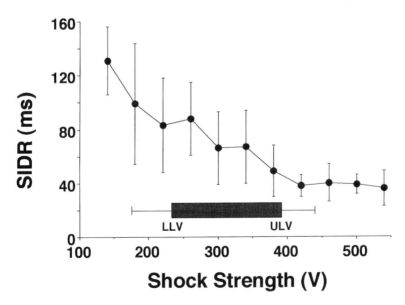

Figure 9. Relation between the shock-induced dispersion of repolarization (SIDR; mean ± SD) and ventricular fibrillation (VF) inducibility as a function of shock strength. VF inducibility was expressed as the range between the lower (LLV) and upper limit of vulnerability (ULV) (mean ± SD). From Reference 24.

Thus, SIDR is large during the vulnerable window (approximately 50 to 80 milliseconds) and decreases (<50 milliseconds) as shock coupling intervals move outside the borders of the vulnerable window. SIDR also decreases (<50 milliseconds) as shock strengths increase above the ULV. These findings suggest that VF inducibility and SIDR are related, and that a certain amount of SIDR is required for the induction of VF. However, this is only true for shocks above LLV strength. Below the LLV (ie, for shocks too weak to induce VF) SIDR is large (>80 milliseconds) due to the presence of both failure of repolarization extension and the excitation of new MAPs at the same time (Fig. 6, panel A). Although this condition causes large SIDR, VF is not inducible. This phenomenon appears to be related to the fact that a certain degree of shock-induced repolarization extension is required to create functional conduction block necessary to initiate reentry.[13] This repolarization extension for the weakest VF-inducing shocks was found to be $16.3 \pm 4.9\%$.[24] Thus, a repolarization extension in the range of 10% to 20 % appears to be critical for VF inducibility. This suggests that VF induction by T wave shocks occurs if both nonuniform repolarization and sufficient repolarization extension are present at the same time.

What is the mechanism of VF induction? A prerequisite for the induction of reentry and VF is the excitation of a propagating action potential and an area of functional block of conduction adjacent to the directly excited tissue.[8,12,13] Functional conduction block has been attributed to repolarization extension[27] and regional differences in refractoriness[15] caused by SIDR.[24] T wave shocks above the LLV strength cause VF if they produce large SIDR. Large SIDR occurs when both the excitation of new action potentials and a shock-induced MAP prolongation are present. New action potentials are directly excited in more repolarized myocardium. Shock-induced MAP prolongation produces extension of refractoriness and block of conduction[27] and occurs in regions less repolarized. VF will thus not be induced if a shock is delivered at a coupling interval too early to create new action potentials (to the left of the vulnerable window), or at a coupling interval too late to create action potential prolongation (to the right of the vulnerable window). However, if a shock is delivered at coupling intervals within the vulnerable window, it will create both new action potentials and action potential prolongation. This pattern is characterized by large SIDR, and VF will be induced.

VF is not inducible at shock strengths above the ULV and below the LLV.[6,28] However, the involved mechanisms are different. Decreasing SIDR at higher shock strength appears to be the mechanism underlying the ULV. Shocks at and above ULV strength produce small SIDR due to a high amount of shock-induced repolarization extension. This causes extension of refractoriness[29] and bidirectional block of conduction,[30] thereby not allowing the initiation of reentry and VF. For weak shocks below LLV strength, VF is not inducible despite large SIDR. In this case, repolarization is not sufficiently prolonged by these low-energy shocks to create unidirectional block of conduction thereby not allowing the initiation of reentry and VF. Thus, shocks of various strengths result in VF if both desynchronized ventricular repolarization and a critical magnitude of repolarization extension are produced by the shock.

Ventricular Defibrillation and SIDR

The close relation between the ULV and the DFT (the "ULV hypothesis of defibrillation"[31]) suggests that VF induction and VF termination by electrical field stimuli share a common mechanism. We therefore hypothesized that SIDR after successful defibrillation attempts is small (as was SIDR for shocks above the ULV), and that SIDR after unsuccessful defibrillation attempts is great (as was SIDR for shocks below the ULV). SIDR is measured after defibrillation attempts from 10 simultaneously recorded MAPs. Figure 10 depicts examples of both a successful (panel A) and an unsuccessful (panel B) defibrillation attempt. The bars below the figure indicate the SIDR in both examples. VF terminates (panel A) when SIDR is low, ie, ventricular repolarization has been synchronized as a consequence of the shock. Ineffective defibrillation, however, is characterized by great SIDR, indicating that the field shock was too weak to create uniformity of postshock repolarization. Figure 11 depicts SIDR at shock strengths

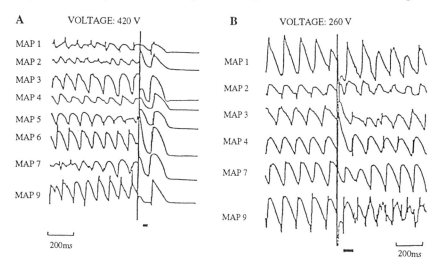

Figure 10. MAP recordings during a successful (**A**) and unsuccessful (**B**) defibrillation attempt. The shock-induced dispersion of repolarization is indicated by black bars below the tracings. See text for details.

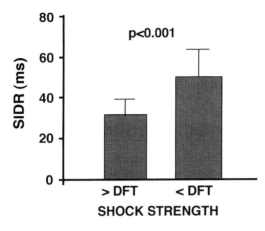

Figure 11. Shock-induced dispersion of repolarization (SIDR) for successful (shock strength > defibrillation threshold [DFT]; n=68) and unsuccessful (shock strength < DFT; n=75) defibrillation attempts.

slightly below and above the DFT. Shocks that were able to terminate VF were associated with smaller SIDR as compared to ineffective defibrillation shocks. These findings support the role of repolarization uniformity for successful defibrillation, and suggest that synchronized repolarization may be a mechanism not only for the ULV but also for the DFT.

Summary

T wave shocks influence the repolarization process and its global dispersion as a function of both shock timing and shock strength. SIDR for shocks above LLV strength and within the vulnerable window (where the shock induces VF) is large. SIDR decreases for shocks at and beyond the borders of the vulnerable window and the ULV. These findings suggest that shock-induced nonuniform repolarization is necessary for the induction of VF, and that uniform repolarization after a shock may explain why VF is not inducible above the ULV. An additional factor, however, is the amount of shock-induced MAP prolongation. Below LLV strength, shocks produce insufficient repolarization extension. This explains why low-energy shocks below the LLV do not induce VF despite large SIDR. Large SIDR after unsuccessful defibrillation attempts and small SIDR after successful defibrillation suggest that synchronized repolarization is a mechanism not only for the ULV but also for the DFT.

Acknowledgments The authors wish to thank Cuilan Li, PhD, Paulus Kirchhof, MD, and Larissa Fabritz, MD for their contribution in studying ventricular repolarization dispersion and its role for the induction and termination of VF.

References

1. Wiggers CJ, Wegren R. Ventricular fibrillation due to single localized induction in condenser shock supplied during the vulnerable phase of ventricular systole. *Am J Physiol* 1940;128:500-505.
2. Hoffman BF, Gorin EF, Wax FF, et al. Vulnerability to fibrillation and the ventricular excitability curve. *Am J Physiol* 1951;167:88-94.
3. Hoffman BF, Cranefield PF. *Electrophysiology of the Heart*. New York: McGraw-Hill; 1960.
4. Chen PS, Shibata N, Dixon EG, et al. Comparison of the defibrillation threshold and the upper limit of ventricular vulnerability. *Circulation* 1986;73:1022-1028.
5. Chen PS, Feld GK, Mower MM, Peters BB. Effects of pacing rate and timing of defibrillation shock on the relation between the defibrillation threshold and the upper limit of vulnerability in open chest dogs. *J Am Coll Cardiol* 1991;18:1555-1563.
6. Hwang C, Swerdlow C, Kass R, et al. Upper limit of vulnerability reliably predicts the defibrillation threshold in humans. *Circulation* 1994;90:2308-2314.
7. Lesigne C, Levy B, Saumont R, et al. An energy-time analysis of ventricular fibrillation and defibrillation thresholds with internal electrodes. *Med Biol Eng* 1976;14:617-622.
8. Shibata N, Chen PS, Dixon EG, et al. Influence of shock strength and timing on induction of ventricular arrhythmias in dogs. *Am J Physiol* 1988;255:H891-H901.
9. Shibata N, Chen PS, Dixon EG, et al. Epicardial activation after unsuccessful defibrillation shocks in dogs. *Am J Physiol* 1988;255:H902-H909.
10. Chen PS, Wolf PD, Ideker RE. Mechanism of cardiac defibrillation. A different point of view. *Circulation* 1991;84:913-919.
11. Chen PS, Wolf PD, Dixon EG, et al. Mechanism of ventricular vulnerability to single premature stimuli in open-chest dogs. *Circ Res* 1988;62:1191-1209.
12. Frazier DW, Wolf PD, Wharton JM, et al. Stimulus-induced critical point. Mechanism for electrical initiation of reentry in normal canine myocardium. *J Clin Invest* 1989;83:1039-1052.
13. El-Sherif N. Reentrant mechanisms in ventricular arrhythmias. In Zipes DP, Jalife J (eds): *Cardiac Electrophysiology: From Cell to Bedside*. Philadelphia: W. B. Saunders; 1995:567-582.
14. Watanabe Y, Dreifus LS. *Cardiac Arrhythmias: Electrophysiological Basis for Clinical Interpretation*. New York: Grune & Stratton, Inc; 1977.
15. Restivo M, Gough WB, El-Sherif N. Ventricular arrhythmias in the subacute myocardial infarction period. High-resolution activation and refractory patterns of reentrant rhythms. *Circ Res* 1990;66:1310-1327.
16. Knisley SB, Hill BC. Optical recordings of the effect of electrical stimulation on action potential repolarization and the induction of reentry in two-dimensional perfused rabbit epicardium. *Circulation* 1993;88:2402-2414.
17. Allessie MA, Bonke FI, Schopman FJ. Circus movement in rabbit atrial muscle as a mechanism of tachycardia. II. The role of nonuniform recovery of excitability in the occurrence of unidirectional block, as studied with multiple microelectrodes. *Circ Res* 1976;39:168-177.
18. Kao CY, Hoffman BF. Graded and decremental response in heart muscle fibers. *Am J Physiol* 1958;194:187-196.
19. Knisley SB, Smith WM, Ideker RE. Effect of field stimulation on cellular repolarization in rabbit myocardium. Implications for reentry induction. *Circ Res* 1992;70:707-715.

20. Zhou XH, Knisley SB, Wolf PD, et al. Prolongation of repolarization time by electric field stimulation with monophasic and biphasic shocks in open-chest dogs. *Circ Res* 1991;68:1761-1767.
21. Jones JL, Jones RE. Effects of monophasic defibrillator waveform intensity on graded response duration in a computer simulation of the action potential. *Proc Ann Int Conf IEEE Engl Med Biol Soc* 1991;13:598-599.
22. Jones JL, Jones RE, Milne KB. Refractory period prolongation by biphasic defibrillator waveforms is associated with enhanced sodium current in a computer model of the ventricular action potential. *IEEE Trans Biomed Eng* 1994;41:60-68.
23. Swartz JF, Jones JL, Jones RE, Fletcher R. Conditioning prepulse of biphasic defibrillator waveforms enhances refractoriness to fibrillation wavefronts. *Circ Res* 1991;68:438-449.
24. Behrens S, Li C, Fabritz CL, et al. Shock-induced dispersion of ventricular repolarization: Implications for the induction of ventricular fibrillation and the upper limit of vulnerability. *J Cardiovasc Electrophysiol* 1997;8:998-1008.
25. Fabritz CL, Kirchhof PF, Behrens S, et al. Myocardial vulnerability to T wave shocks. Relation to shock strength, shock coupling interval, and dispersion of ventricular repolarization. *J Cardiovasc Electrophysiol* 1996;7:231-242.
26. Behrens S, Li C, Kirchhof P, et al. Reduced arrhythmogenicity of biphasic versus monophasic T wave shocks. Implications for defibrillation efficacy. *Circulation* 1996;94:1974-1980.
27. Sweeney RJ, Gill RM, Steinberg MI, Reid PP. Ventricular refractory period extension caused by defibrillation shocks. *Circulation* 1990;82:965-972.
28. Chen PS, Feld GK, Kriett JM, et al. Relation between upper limit of vulnerability and defibrillation threshold in humans. *Circulation* 1993;88:186-192.
29. Sweeney RJ, Gill RM, Reid PR. Characterization of refractory period extension by transcardiac shock. *Circulation* 1991;83:2057-2066.
30. Gotoh M, Chen PS, Fishbein MC, et al. Cellular mechanism of the upper limit of vulnerability during electrical induction of reentry in vitro. *PACE* 1994;17:839. Abstract.
31. Chen PS, Shibata N, Dixon EG, et al. Activation during ventricular defibrillation in open-chest dogs. Evidence of complete cessation and regeneration of ventricular fibrillation after unsuccessful shocks. *J Clin Invest* 1986;77:810-823.

46

Effects of Monophasic and Biphasic Defibrillation Shocks on Dispersion of Ventricular Depolarization and Repolarization

Parwis C. Fotuhi, MD, Xiaohong Zhou, MD, Stephen B. Knisley, PhD and Raymond E. Ideker, MD, PhD

External and Internal Defibrillation with Monophasic and Biphasic Waveforms

In 1947 Beck et al[1] reported the termination of ventricular fibrillation by an electric shock during an open chest procedure. Nine years later, Zoll and coworkers[2] showed the feasibility of ventricular defibrillation in man by externally applied electric countershock. Over the past 5 decades, major changes and progress in defibrillation have been made, often achieved by driven individuals.[3] Today, transthoracic and intracardiac defibrillation are well accepted and widely used forms of therapy for life-threatening ventricular arrhythmias.[4,5]

From Franz MR (ed): *Monophasic Action Potentials: Bridging Cell and Bedside.*
©Futura Publishing Company, Inc., Armonk, NY, 2000.

One reason for the wide acceptance of internal defibrillation was the transition from an epicardial lead system, placed by an open chest procedure, to a less invasive, transvenously placed lead system. One factor that made this transition possible was the introduction of a new defibrillation waveform. Several animal and human studies have shown significant reduction in internal defibrillation energy requirements with use of biphasic instead of monophasic waveforms.[6-9] Based on the positive experience with biphasic waveforms in internal defibrillation, this type of waveform is now being investigated for use in improvement of transthoracic defibrillation.[10]

In spite of the wide use of defibrillators, the mechanisms by which an electrical shock halts fibrillation are still not completely understood. Wiggers[11] postulated that all activation fronts must be extinguished by the shock in order to terminate fibrillation. Mower and coworkers[12] and Zipes and coworkers[13] then proposed that all activations within a minimal volume or critical mass of myocardium must be eradicated by the shock in order for defibrillation to be successful. Mapping studies by Chen et al[14] suggested that a shock must not only halt the fibrillation wave fronts, but also must prevent the creation by the shock of new wave fronts that reinitiate fibrillation.

Many different monophasic and biphasic waveforms have been investigated in animal and clinical studies.[6-9,14-16] Those experimental studies that have focused on the mechanism of defibrillation have used animal preparations ranging from whole hearts in situ, to tissue sections, to single cardiac cells.[17-24] The recording systems used range from electrical mapping systems for whole hearts and tissue sections, to optical systems for isolated perfused hearts and single cells.[17-24]

The Effect of Electrical Stimuli on the Refractory Period

The prolongation of the action potential caused by electrical stimuli in combination with drugs such as quinidine, strophantine, and veratrine was shown many decades ago.[25-27] A graded and decremental response in heart muscle fibers[28] and a nonuniform recovery of excitability in ventricular muscle caused by electrical stimulation was later described.[29] It was found that sudden changes in activation rate,[30] premature depolarization, and the coupling interval to the preceding action potential all affected the amount of action potential prolongation caused by this graded response.[31] This work demonstrated a significant role of the action potential duration (APD) and of the duration of the refractory period on the initiation of ventricular arrhythmias. Tamargo and coworkers[32] and Prystowsky and Zipes[33] showed that a conditioning stimulus delivered during the relative refractory period could prolong ventricular refractoriness, and Windle and coworkers[34] showed that it could prevent electrical stimulation of a new action potential.

Based on these findings, it could be shown that the length and dispersion of the refractory periods play a crucial role in ventricular vulnerability.[35] Additionally, several groups[17-24,36-44] described prolongation of depolarization, extension of ventricular refractoriness, and reduction of dispersion of refractoriness by defibrillation shocks as possible underlying mechanisms for successful defibrillation. These studies are described briefly in the following section of this chapter.

Refractory Period Extension and Dispersion of Refractoriness Caused by Defibrillation Shocks

Studies by Chen et al[17] and Shibata et al[18] focused on the mechanism of myocardial vulnerability caused by premature stimuli, and the influence of shock strength and timing on the induction of arrhythmias, respectively. Based on their findings, these authors discussed the nonuniform dispersion of refractoriness as a possible factor for the reinitiation of reentry following defibrillation shocks.

This dispersion of refractoriness, caused by the prolongation of the refractory period by defibrillation strength shocks, was measured by Dillon and Wit.[21,39] These measurements were obtained by use of optical recordings during paced rhythm in perfused rabbit hearts. In a later study,[40] using the same animal model and recording technique, Dillon described the synchronization of repolarization by defibrillation shocks. He reported that defibrillation shocks applied during all phases of ventricular fibrillation caused the myocardium to repolarize at a constant time. This constant repolarization time was accompanied by a similar constancy in the return of myocardial excitability. The findings from other studies as well[41] show that shock-induced depolarization of refractory myocardium can prevent wave front propagation.

Similar results were obtained by Sweeney et al,[42] who showed an extension of the refractory period caused by shocks at defibrillation strengths. In the in situ dog heart preparation, S2 pacing stimuli and shocks of up to 30 J were delivered during the electrical systole of paced beats. An extension of the refractory period was caused by the shocks, but not by the pacing stimuli. Also, shocks delivered early during ventricular repolarization caused no refractory period extension, whereas shocks delivered midway or later into electrical systole caused a significant extension of the refractory period. In a second study, Sweeney et al[43] reported that changing the S1 pacing site, the pacing rate, or the pacing current did not significantly affect the amount of refractory period extension induced by S2 defibrillation strength shocks. These investigators also studied the effect of the local voltage gradient and the effect of ischemia on refractory period extension caused by the S2 defibrillation strength shocks. In this study, the major determinant for refractory period extension was the local voltage gradient caused by the S2 shock. A minimal voltage gradient was needed to produce refractory period extension, even with S1 pacing rates close to the activation rate of ventricular fibrillation. Acute ischemia, which occurs during ventricular fibrillation, had no significant effect on refractory period extension by S2 shocks.

In contrast to pacing site, pacing rate, pacing current, and ischemia, which had no significant effect on the prolongation of refractoriness, the number of phases of the shock waveform (ie, monophasic and biphasic) had a significant effect on the prolongation of refractoriness as first shown by Swartz and coworkers.[22] In this study, action potential recordings were made from cultured chicken embryo cells via capillary tubing. Eight intracellular monophasic S1 stimuli with a basic cycle length of 600 milliseconds were applied at 1.5 and 2 times the diastolic excitation threshold. A premature intracellular S2 stimulus of either monophasic or biphasic morphology was delivered at different coupling intervals. The monophasic S2 waveform was a 10-millisecond rectangular wave. The biphasic waveform consisted of two 10-millisecond rectangular phases of opposite polarity. The first phase was equal to the monophasic waveform in amplitude and duration, but was of opposite polarity. Equal duration square waves were used for the biphasic waveform so that the same amount of charge was delivered during both phases in these regions. The intent of this preconditioning phase was to hyperpolarize the tissue before the second phase of the biphasic waveform, which had the same polarity as and was thought to compare to the monophasic waveform, could depolarize the tissue. Figure 1 shows the total response duration for the two waveforms at 2 times diastolic threshold and how it changes with different S1-S2 coupling intervals. The total response duration is defined as the time from the upstroke of the action potential until the action potential is repolarized. It also includes the duration of the action potential prolongation caused by the shock. The greatest extension of the total repolarization time was achieved with the hyperpolarizing/depolarizing biphasic waveform at 2 times diastolic threshold. In the second part of the study, the stimulation protocol was repeated with waveforms of opposite polarities, and the result was compared to those in the first part of the study. The hyperpolarizing monophasic waveform had a total response duration of 190 milliseconds and the biphasic depolarizing/hyperpolarizing waveform had a total response duration of 210 milliseconds. Since these times are much shorter than the total repolarization time for the hyperpolarizing/depolarizing biphasic waveform, these results support the hypothesis that biphasic waveforms

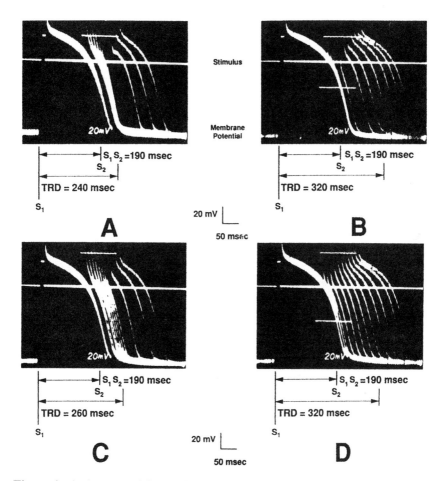

Figure 1. Action potential recordings from a single experiment showing superimposed membrane response to S2 stimuli at different S1-S2 coupling intervals scanning the S1 refractory period. The upper tracing in each panel shows the current stimulus waveform and amplitude as well as the 0 mV reference. The lower tracing shows the membrane potential response to 8 S1 and each S2 stimulus. TRD is the total response duration to an S2 stimulus given with an S1-S2 coupling interval of 190 milliseconds superimposed. The 20 mV label on the photographs is the voltage scaling placed on the screen by the oscilloscope. This vertical voltage scale, as well as the horizontal time scale, is shown by the length of the calibration lines between the panels. **A**. 1.5 times threshold monophasic S2 waveform; S1-S2 coupling intervals of 120 to 220 milliseconds are shown. **B**. 1.5 times threshold biphasic S2 waveform; S1-S2 coupling intervals of 130 to 230 milliseconds are shown. **C**. Two times threshold monophasic waveform; S1-S2 coupling intervals of 120 to 220 milliseconds are shown. **D**. Two times threshold biphasic S2 waveform; coupling intervals of 130 to 230 milliseconds are shown. Reproduced, with permission, from Reference 22: Conditioning prepulse of biphasic defibrillator waveforms enhances refractoriness to fibrillation wavefronts. Copyright 1991 American Heart Association.

are superior for defibrillation because hyperpolarization by the first phase has the preconditioning effect of restoring excitability, allowing the depolarizing second phase to cause greater extension of the refractory period. In the third part of the experiment, the authors showed that the biphasic S2 refractory period extension or graded response was indeed 60 milliseconds longer than the response following a monophasic S2 shock of the same strength and timing.

In a recent study by the same group, an 8-millisecond monophasic and a 4/4-millisecond biphasic truncated exponential waveform were delivered extracellularly and their effects compared.[44] These shocks were applied at strengths of 1.5, 3, and 5 times the diastolic threshold, resulting in a potential gradient ranging from 2 to 7 V/cm. For the monophasic waveform they found a significant increase in refractory period prolongation with an increase in the shock intensity from 1.5 to 5 times diastolic threshold. In contrast, changing the potential gradient for the biphasic waveform had no significant effect on refractory period prolongation. A similar refractory prolongation was seen for all 3 potential gradients caused by the biphasic shocks. Since the potential gradient varies widely across the ventricles during a defibrillation shock,[45] the similarity in the amount of refractory period extension indicates a smaller dispersion of refractoriness following the biphasic shock than following the monophasic shock (Fig. 2).

Tovar and Jones[44] suggest that biphasic shocks have a lower defibrillation threshold than monophasic shocks because of the effect on these regions of the myocardium where the first phase of the biphasic shock hyperpolarizes the cell membrane. This hyperpolarization could make the transmembrane potential sufficiently negative that the Na^+ channels will be reactivated, making it easier for the second phase to stimulate the cells in this region. These findings are discussed in greater detail in chapter 44.

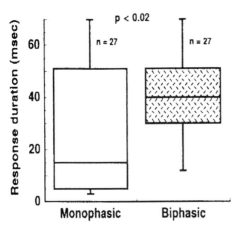

Figure 2. Box plot showing the median response duration for all measured S2 responses at functionally normalized coupling intervals ≤ 0 (-10, -5, and 0) milliseconds and intensities of 1.5 and 5 times. The line within the box represents the median value. The ends of the box represent the 25th (bottom line) and the 75th (top line) percentile, and the error bars represent the maximum and minimum values. Reproduced, with permission, from Reference 44: Biphasic defibrillation waveforms reduced shock-induced response duration dispersion between low and high shock intensities. Copyright 1995 American Heart Association.

Single capacitor truncated exponential biphasic waveforms, in which the leading edge voltage of the second phase equals the trailing edge of the first phase, were studied by Zhou et al.[36] Single capacitor biphasic waveforms deliver less current during the second phase than during the first phase, even when both phases are the same duration. In this open chest dog study, these investigators used a floating glass electrode to record monophasic action potentials (MAPs), in combination with 8 extracellular electrodes to measure the shock field. They investigated the amount of prolongation of the action potential caused by a 5-millisecond monophasic, a 2.5-millisecond monophasic, and a 2.5/2.5-millisecond biphasic truncated exponential waveform with a shock field of approximately 5 V/cm. The 5-millisecond monophasic shock had longer refractory period extension than the other two waveforms (Fig. 3). Interestingly, the S1-S2 interval induced not just refractory period extension but rather a new S2 stimulated action

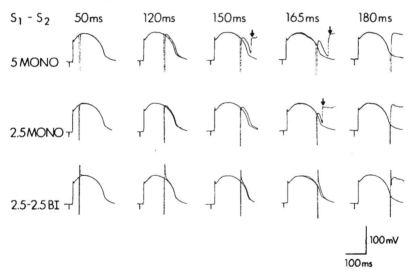

Figure 3. Prolongation of action potential duration following S2 shocks at different S1-S2 intervals in one animal. On the ordinate are the 3 different waveforms and on the abscissa are the S1-S2 coupling intervals of 50, 120, 150, 165, and 180 milliseconds. The action potential during which the S2 shock was given is superimposed on the preceding S1 action potential. As the S1-S2 action potential was lengthened, the action potential duration increased until an S2-induced new action potential was produced by all 3 waveforms at a 180-millisecond interval. At 150- and 165-millisecond S1-S2 intervals for the 5-millisecond monophasic shock (5MONO), and at the 165-millisecond interval for the 2.5-millisecond monophasic shock (2.5MONO), a new action potential (arrow) followed the prolongation of the last S1 action potential by the S2 shock. The voltage and time scales for the action potentials are shown in the lower right corner. 2.5-2.5BI = 2.5-2.5 millisecond biphasic shock. Reproduced, with permission, from Reference 36: Prolongation of repolarization time by electric field stimulation with monophasic and biphasic shocks in open chest dogs. Copyright 1991 American Heart Association.

potential that was significantly longer (179±11 milliseconds) for the 2.5/2.5-millisecond biphasic waveform and for the 2.5-millisecond monophasic waveform (175±11 milliseconds) when compared to the 5-millisecond monophasic waveform (171±13 milliseconds). Similar findings were obtained for the shortest S1-S2 interval that caused action potential prolongation. The 5-millisecond monophasic waveform had an S1-S2 interval of 143±11 milliseconds versus 166±13 milliseconds for the 2.5/2.5-millisecond biphasic waveform ($P \leq 0.05$), indicating a shorter effective refractory period for the monophasic than for the biphasic shock.

A limitation of the previously described studies by Tovar and Jones[44] and Zhou et al[36] was that they were performed during paced rhythm and not during ventricular fibrillation. It was not clear if the results obtained during paced rhythms held true during ventricular fibrillation, since Dillon[40] had reported that refractory period extension was not the same during fibrillation and paced rhythm.

The issue of refractory period extension caused by monophasic and biphasic shocks during ventricular fibrillation was addressed in a second study by Zhou et al.[37] The above-described study protocol and set up was modified and repeated with the use of a 5-millisecond and a 16-millisecond monophasic and a 2.5/2.5-millisecond and an 8/8-millisecond biphasic truncated exponential waveform to measure the effects of shocks on the APD during ventricular fibrillation. The investigators found a significant difference in the shortest coupling interval at which each waveform could capture the tissue. The shortest coupling interval for the 5-millisecond monophasic waveform, 61±5 milliseconds, was significantly shorter than that for the biphasic waveform, 66±6 milliseconds. Since the activation rate during ventricular fibrillation was 86±15 milliseconds, these coupling intervals imply that during ventricular fibrillation, cells were unexcitable during 71% of their ventricular fibrillation cycle length (61 milliseconds/86 milliseconds) for the 5-millisecond monophasic shock, and during 77% of their cycle length (66 milliseconds/86 milliseconds) for the 2.5/2.5-millisecond biphasic shock. Similar to their previous pacing study, Zhou et al[37] found that the APD during ventricular fibrillation was prolonged by all 4 waveforms. They found a greater ability of the longer waveforms (16-millisecond monophasic, 8/8-millisecond biphasic) to prolong the APD, especially at shorter coupling intervals when the cells were in an earlier portion of the action potential. The largest extension of refractoriness was seen with the 16-millisecond monophasic waveform (Fig. 4).

Initially, these results appeared to conflict with the finding of Swartz et al[22] and of Tovar and Jones.[44] These investigators found a greater extension of refractoriness by the biphasic than by the monophasic shock, while Zhou et al[36,37] reported a lesser extension of refractoriness by the biphasic than by the monophasic shock. The different waveforms used in the two studies (square wave and truncated exponential) may explain the different

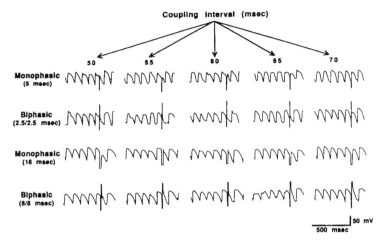

Figure 4. Examples of action potentials recorded before and after test shocks during ventricular fibrillation. On the y axis are the 4 different waveforms and on the x axis are the coupling intervals of 50 to 70 ms, timed from the upstroke of an action potential during fibrillation. The top two sets of tracings were recorded in one animal and the bottom two sets in another. The voltage and time scales are shown in the lower right corner. The action potential duration is increased 1) with an increase in coupling intervals for all shock waveforms; 2) for monophasic compared with biphasic waveforms of the same duration; and 3) for longer compared with shorter waveforms of the same number of phases. Reproduced, with permission, from Reference 37: Effects of monophasic and biphasic shocks on action potentials during ventricular fibrillation in dogs. Copyright 1993 American Heart Association.

results. Square wave biphasic waveforms with both phases equal in amplitude and duration used by the former investigators[22,44] do not defibrillate with a lower threshold than square wave monophasic shocks of the same duration.[46] Zhou et al[36,37] used the type of biphasic waveform that can be generated by a single capacitor resulting in waveforms in which the second phase is smaller in amplitude than the first phase. These waveforms have been shown to have lower defibrillation thresholds than the same duration monophasic shocks.[8,45]

The Potential Gradient and its Effect on Refractory Period Extension and Dispersion of Refractoriness

Similar to Chen et al[17] and Shibata et al,[18] whose studies focused on the reinitiation of reentry caused by the defibrillation shock, Frazier et al[19] investigated the hypothesis that the field of a premature S2 stimulus, interacting with relatively refractory tissue, can create unidirectional block and reentry in the absence of nonuniform dispersion of recovery. Recordings were made from the right ventricle using 117 to 120 transmural or epicardial electrodes. S1 pacing was done from a row of electrodes on one side of the mapped area, creating parallel activation isochrones and uniform parallel isorecovery lines (Fig. 5, panel A). S2 shocks ranging from 25 to 250 V were delivered through a mesh electrode along the bottom of the mapped area, scanning the refractory period. These shocks created isogradient electric field lines perpendicular to the isorecovery lines (Fig. 5, panel B).

Earliest activation following the S2 stimulus did not occur adjacent to the S2 electrode; rather it occurred where the S2 potential gradient was less than approximately 5 V/cm and where the tissue was just passing out of its refractory period (Fig. 5, panel C). It was assumed that the tissue closer to the S1 electrode, that had activated earlier following the S1 stimulus and hence had more time to recover, was directly excited by the S2 electric field (hatched region in Fig. 5, panel C). Where the electrode field generated by the S2 stimulus was weak, activation fronts after the S2 shock conducted away from the tissue that was directly excited by the shock toward tissue with greater refractoriness. Where the potential gradient of the shock potential field was above 5 V/cm, activations did not conduct away from the border of the region that was directly excited by the shock, leading to unidirectional conduction block.

Frazier et al[19] proposed that a possible mechanism for this unidirectional block was refractory period extension induced by the shock electric field. Based on their findings, they concluded that, since the amount of refractory period extension was directly related to the strength of the S2 electric field, the refractory period extension was sufficient to prevent conduction away from the directly excited region, where the potential gradient was greater than 5 V/cm, but that activation could occur where the refractory period extension was smaller and the shock potential gradient was less than 5 V/cm. The activation front that arose from the border of the directly excited region, where the shock field was less than 5 V/cm, propagated around and downward into the region where the shock field was greater than this value. This activation front slowed when it reached the region where the refractory period extension was assumed to have occurred (isochrones between 60 and 120 milliseconds in Fig. 5, panel C). It was assumed that during this time, the tissue directly excited by the S2 stimulus had sufficiently recovered so that it could again be excited. The activation front was then able to propagate into this region, initiating reentry that was present for several cycles until activation degenerated into ventricular fibrillation.

A

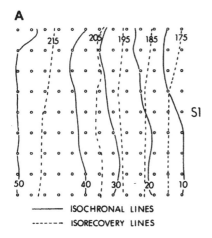

ISOCHRONAL LINES
ISORECOVERY LINES

B

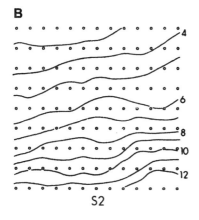

S2

C

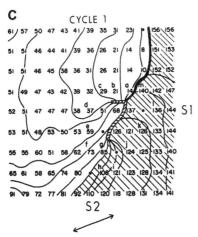

S2

Figure 5. Initiation of reentry and ventricular fibrillation following orthogonal interaction of myocardial refractoriness and potential gradient field created by a large stimulus. **A**. Distribution of activation time during the last S1 beat (solid lines) and recovery times to a local 2-mA stimulus (dashed lines) in milliseconds following this activation. **B**. Potential gradient field (V/cm) produced by an S2 stimulus of 150 V. **C**. Initial activation pattern following after the S2 stimulus delivered after a 191-millisecond S1-S2 interval. The hatched region is thought to be directly excited by the S2 stimulus field. Reproduced, with permission, from Reference 19: Stimulus induced critical point: Mechanism for electrical initiation of reentry in normal canine myocardium. Copyright 1989 *J Clin Invest.*

Frazier et al[19] showed that the location of the reentrant circuit could be altered by changing either the strength of the S2 premature stimulus or the S1/S2 coupling interval. The center of the reentrant pathway was always located where the tissue was just coming out of the refractory period at the time of the S2 stimulus and where the electric field of the S2 stimulus was approximately 5 V/cm. The existence of this critical point, where a critical value of the shock potential gradient (5 V/cm for the particular waveform used) and the critical level of refractoriness intersect, led to the "critical point" hypothesis for defibrillation. This hypothesis states that shocks slightly weaker than the defibrillation threshold fail to defibrillate because critical points are formed in the myocardium, where the critical potential gradient intersects tissue that is just evolving from its refractory period during fibrillation. Reentry occurs around these critical points, reinducing fibrillation. To defibrillate reliably, the shock strength must be increased until no critical points are formed throughout the myocardium. Thus, according to this hypothesis, the production of refractory period extension by the shock is crucial for the success or failure of defibrillation; by causing greater refractory period extension where the shock field is strong than where the shock field is weak, the shock can induce reentry that leads to the reinitiation of fibrillation. The fact that the minimum shock potential gradient that must be created throughout the ventricular muscle at the defibrillation threshold (4 to 6 V/cm, depending on the waveform) is similar to the critical potential gradient is consistent with the critical point hypothesis for defibrillation.

The hypothesis that greater refractory period extension in the regions of high potential gradients and less refractory period extension in the low potential gradient region is a cause for dispersion of refractoriness after the shock was also investigated in two studies by Knisley et al.[23,24] These studies focused not on the induction of fibrillation due to reentry, nor on the differences between monophasic and biphasic waveforms, but on the dispersion of repolarization induced by nonuniform shock fields that can occur during defibrillation. In one study, a glass microelectrode was used to record action potentials from frog ventricular strips in a tissue bath.[23] A high potential gradient was created on one side of the tissue bath. A low potential gradient was created on the other side of the tissue bath by shielding this section of the frog muscle from the current source. Table 1 shows changes in the APD produced by two shock field strengths. These changes induced a dispersion of repolarization between the low-gradient region and the adjacent high-gradient region.

In another study by Knisley et al,[24] the effect of 2.5, 8, and 14 V/cm shock potential gradients on the repolarization of perfused rabbit myocardium was investigated by use of the glass microelectrode technique. Despite different increases in APD caused by the different shock strengths, a decreased dispersion of repolarization was found to be caused by a

Table 1
Effect of Nonuniform Field Stimulation on Action Potential Duration

	Control	Paced	Shocked
APH	601±72	490±51	636±40*
APL	602±71	515±39	561±21†

Action potential duration (ms) for simultaneous intracellular impalements in regions of frog ventricular muscle having a high (APH) or low (APL) S2 potential gradient. The impalements were 1.4±0.4 mm apart (mean ± standard deviation; n = 6). Control values were obtained before beginning S2 shocks. Shocked values are for action potentials that received S2 during the plateau (S1-S2=300 ms). Paced values are for the last paced action potential preceding each shocked action potential. For the paced and shocked action potentials, the mean results for 13 to 20 S2 trials given over a period of 60 to 80 minutes in each experiment were averaged. The 5 ms S2 produced a potential gradient of 39±11 V/cm in the region of APH and 0.3±0.2 V/cm in the region of APL.

*$P<0.05$ APH compared with the simultaneously recorded APL. †$P<0.05$ compared with the preceding paced action potential. Reproduced from Reference 23, with permission.

shock that created a field strength of 8.4 V/cm (Fig. 6). A similar decrease in dispersion of repolarization was also found with shocks at the higher field strength. These shocks at the higher field strength induce action potential prolongation, which can also cause conduction block and reentry via the critical point mechanism, as hypothesized by Frazier et al[19] and shown by Knisley and Hill.[47]

These findings are also consistent with the critical point hypothesis for defibrillation (Fig. 7). In the region where the S2 electric field strength is 1.5 V/cm, an abrupt boundary (upper right) occurs between the tissue that is directly excited by the S2 and the tissue that is not directly excited. A large intracellular potential gradient at the boundary, 0.5 V/cm, can account for the initiation of propagation from the right to the left that has been reported in the region that has a low electric field strength. The large intracellular potential gradient at the boundary is comparable to that which occurs at a propagating wave front in myocardial tissue with normal inter-cellular connections.[24] In the region that has a high S2 electric field strength, there is no abrupt boundary between high and low intracellular potentials. Instead, on the line of an S2 strength of 15 V/cm, the largest intracellular potential gradient is only 0.017 V/cm, ignoring discontinuities of intracellular resistance. Also, the intracellular potentials on the 15 V/cm line are in the range in which sodium current is inactivated. The absence of a large intracellular potential gradient and the presence of intracellular potentials that inactivate sodium current, a current important for propagation, explain the absence of propagation after a shock where the electric field strength during the shock is high. In Figure 7 the spatial interactions between adjacent regions of myocardium are not taken into account because the response at each point is derived from a different shock episode in a

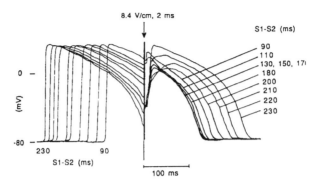

Figure 6. Action potential recordings illustrating the decrease in the dispersion of repolarization produced by an S2 having a strength of 8.4 V/cm oriented along the long axis of the myocardial fibers. The recordings, obtained from one cellular impalement, are aligned with the S2 time. An S1 stimulus was applied 3 milliseconds before the phase 0 depolarization of each of the recordings. The longest and shortest S1-S2 intervals tested, 230 and 90 milliseconds, are indicated beneath their respective phase 0 depolarization. In addition, the S1-S2 intervals for each of the responses after S2 are indicated to the right of the recordings. The dispersion of repolarization for cells that received S2 at these different times during the action potential is indicated by the variation of times of repolarization after S2. If S2 had no effect, the dispersion of repolarization for the various trials would be 140 milliseconds (the variation of times of phase 0 depolarization). The responses after S2 indicate that S2 decreased the dispersion of repolarization to 100 milliseconds (the variation of times of repolarization). A window of S1-S2 intervals occurred in which the dispersion of repolarization was negligible (S1-S2 = 130 to 170 milliseconds). For S2 given either earlier or later than this window, the repolarization time after S2 increased. Reproduced, with permission, from Reference 24: Effect of field stimulation on cellular repolarization in rabbit myocardium. Copyright 1992 American Heart Association.

myocardial fiber where there is neither a dispersion of shock strengths nor of refractory periods. As pointed out by Krassowska and Kumar[48] and by Gotoh et al,[49] consideration of the spatial interactions of the coupled myocardium with a dispersion of refractoriness and a dispersion of shock field strength may be necessary to fully understand the induction of reentry by the shock.

Defibrillation by Monophasic and Biphasic Waveforms Through Refractory Period Extension

The spatial effects of monophasic and biphasic shocks across a region of myocardium were compared by Daubert et al.[38] First they showed that the 2/1-millisecond biphasic waveform they were planning to study had a

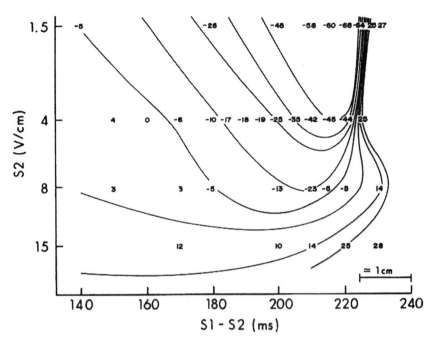

Figure 7. Intracellular potentials after S2 stimulation. The measurements were obtained from intracellular recordings with one cellular impalement for which various S2 electric field strengths oriented along the fibers and various S1-S2 stimulus intervals were tested. The intracellular potentials, given in millivolts within the graph, occurred 10 milliseconds after the S2 stimulus was applied. The intracellular potentials are graphed with the S2 field strength on the vertical axis and the state of refractoriness, or S1-S2 interval, on the horizontal axis to correspond with the spatially dispersed stimulus strength and states of refractoriness that induce reentry in the heart. The 1-cm calibration bar is approximate and is based on an assumed conduction velocity of 65 cm/s for the repolarization wave of the preceding S1 beat. The isopotential contours, determined by bivariate polynomial interpolation and smoothing by hand, represent intracellular potentials from −45 to 25 mV in 10-mV increments. Contours for intracellular potentials more negative than −45 mV are not shown because of uncertainty in the interpolation. Reproduced, with permission, from Reference 24: Effect of field stimulation on cellular repolarization in rabbit myocardium. Copyright 1992 American Heart Association.

lower defibrillation threshold than the 3-millisecond monophasic waveform they were planning to study. Similar to the study by Frazier et al,[19] they recorded epicardial shock potentials from 117 epicardial electrodes. Additionally, they recorded activation fronts of monophasic and biphasic shocks along with a single MAP signal in open chested dogs. They found that the 3-millisecond monophasic waveform excited refractory tissue more effectively than the 2/1-millisecond biphasic waveform. They also found that the biphasic shock caused less excitation of the tissue, and the conduction block at the border, where the potential gradient was approximately 4 V/cm, was closer to the defibrillation electrode than the conduction block caused by the monophasic shock (Fig. 8). Consequently, the strength-interval curve of the monophasic shock was shifted to the left in relation to the strength-interval curve of the biphasic waveform

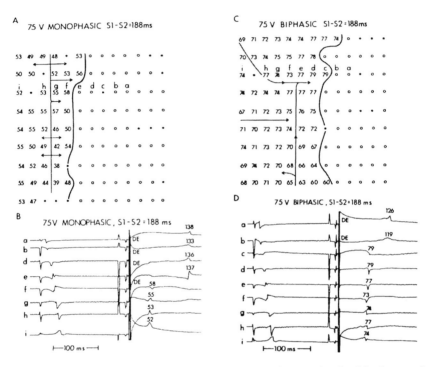

Figure 8. Activation maps and electrograms comparing conduction block caused by monophasic and biphasic shocks. Electrodes for delivering S1 and S2 stimuli were on the right. For monophasic shocks (**A**) conduction blocked at the directly excited border (solid line) where the potential gradient was ≈4 V/cm. An activation front then conducted through the mapped region beginning outside the mapped area (arrows). Open circles indicate electrodes recording over tissue directly excited by S2. Filled circles represent electrodes with technically poor recordings. S2 activation times in milliseconds are displayed at electrode sites for electrodes recording from tissue not directly activated by S2. **B.** Recordings for monophasic shocks from electrodes labeled a-i in A. The last S1 stimulus, S1 activation, S2 shock (with gain switch artifacts on either side), and post-S2 activations are shown. S2 activation times are shown above tracings. Electrodes recording from the directly excited (DE) zone activate during the S2 shock, and then again ≥90 milliseconds after S2. The directly excited activations occurred during the S2 stimulation and cannot be seen. **C.** A biphasic shock with the same setting as in A and B. Less tissue was directly excited than with the monophasic shock; conduction again blocked at the directly excited border. **D.** The electrogram labeled in C. Biphasic S2 stimulus can be seen between gain switch artifacts. Reproduced, with permission, from Reference 38: Response of relative refractory canine myocardium to monophasic and biphasic shocks. Copyright 1991 American Heart Association.

(Fig. 9). The simultaneous recording of the epicardial activation front and the MAP signal verified the existence of an area that was directly excited by the shock. A brief depolarization following the S2 shock was recorded with the MAP electrode when conduction was blocked at the border of the directly excited area. This brief depolarization caused a prolongation of the action potential. An explanation drawn from their findings for the greater defibrillation efficacy of biphasic waveforms is that the biphasic waveforms have a decreased tendency to initiate conduction block and reentry in areas with a shock gradient above 4 V/cm.

This decreased tendency of biphasic shocks compared to monophasic shocks to initiate block and reentry is supported by a computer model of cardiac field stimulation using these waveforms. This study by Fishler[50] investigated the spatial and temporal interactions of monophasic and biphasic field stimulation on the upstroke of a propagating wave front and on the other end of the wave front, the wave tail. Different monophasic and biphasic shock strengths were applied in this idealized computer model of a 1-dimensional cardiac strand. The suprathreshold monophasic and biphasic shocks depolarized the tissue in front of the wave front. This depolarized tissue led to conduction block and to termination of the wave front. A different effect was seen at the wave tail (Fig. 10). The low-strength monophasic shocks created a sharp spatial transmembrane potential by inducing an all-or-nothing response at the wave tail. This sharp spatial transmembrane potential initiated a new anterogradely propagating wave front (Fig. 10). The spatial response to the low-strength biphasic shock was not an all-or-nothing response. The cells underwent a graded response

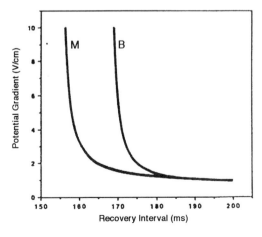

Figure 9. Monophasic (M) and biphasic (B) strength-interval curves for one animal superimposed. The biphasic curve is to the right of the monophasic curve, indicating that the biphasic waveform is less able to directly excite partially refractory myocardium. Absolute refractory period is the y asymptote of the strength-interval curve, whereas the diastolic threshold is the x asymptote. Absolute refractory periods are 155 milliseconds for the monophasic curve and 168 milliseconds for the biphasic curve. The diastolic threshold was 0.7 V/cm for the monophasic waveform and 0.6 V/cm for the biphasic waveform. Reproduced, with permission, from Reference 38: Response of relative refractory canine myocardium to monophasic and biphasic shocks. Copyright 1991 American Heart Association.

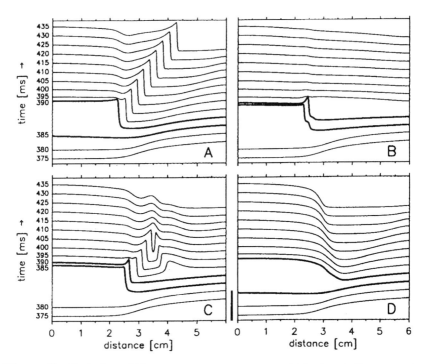

Figure 10. Evolution of fiber response to premature field stimuli. These panels present 4 series of snapshots of cellularly averaged transmembrane voltage profiles along the fiber in response to: **A**) monophasic S2 field stimulation at 1.10 times monophasic defibrillation threshold; **B**) monophasic S2 field stimulation at 2.50 times monophasic defibrillation threshold; **C**) monophasic S2 field stimulation at 1.75 times monophasic defibrillation threshold; and **D**) biphasic S2 field stimulation at 1.10 times monophasic defibrillation threshold. Emboldened profiles highlight the fiber response during the 10-millisecond S2 stimuli. Times in milliseconds indicated along the ordinate identify each profile and are specified relative to the time of the S1 stimulation (administered to the leftmost end of the fiber). Vertical calibration bar between panels C and D represents 100 mV. Reproduced from Reference 50, with permission.

with refractory period extension which was not sharp enough to initiate such a new wave front. A similar response was seen with the higher strength monophasic and biphasic shocks. These higher strength shocks had a "smoother" spatial transmembrane potential which did not initiate a new wave front (Fig. 10, panels C and D).

In agreement with this idea are the results of Behrens and coworkers,[20] who investigated the effect of monophasic and biphasic shocks on ventricular vulnerability. In a perfused rabbit heart model, shocks were timed to the T wave in paced rhythm and were delivered at different coupling intervals and shock strengths. These investigators found that the arrhythmogenicity of biphasic T wave shocks was significantly reduced compared to monophasic shocks. They also found that the zone where the shock induced ventricular fibrillation and the zone where the shock did not induce any arrhythmia were smaller for the biphasic waveform than for the monophasic waveform (Fig. 11). These findings are discussed in more detail in chapter 45.

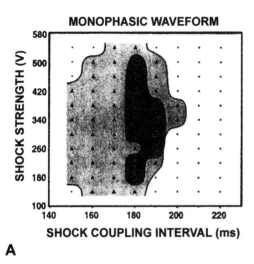

A

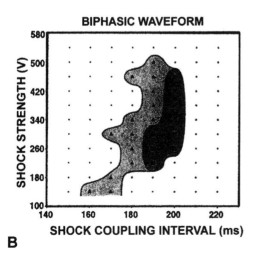

B

Figure 11. The area of vulnerability for monophasic (**A**) versus biphasic (**B**) shock waveforms. The shock-induced arrhythmic response is shown with a 2-dimensional grid of shock coupling intervals (x axis) and shock strengths (y axis). Squares represent the induction of ventricular fibrillation, triangles represent nonsustained arrhythmias, and small dots indicate no arrhythmia. The area of vulnerability (dark gray) and the area of nonsustained arrhythmias (light gray) are encircled by solid lines. Reproduced, with permission, from Reference 20: Reduced arrhythmogenicity of biphasic versus monophasic T-wave shocks. Copyright 1996 American Heart Association.

Implications of the Dispersion of Refractoriness on Defibrillation Efficacy of Monophasic and Biphasic Shocks

Previous work described above suggests two possible mechanisms by which refractory period extension induced by shocks can affect defibrillation. These two mechanisms are not mutually exclusive, and both may play a role in defibrillation. The first mechanism is induction of a critical point by the interaction of the shock field with refractory myocardium. Activation fronts arise after the shock and can be maintained for several cycles by reentry around a critical point. The second mechanism is the dispersion of refractoriness caused by refractory period extension following the shock, that will determine whether any activation fronts appearing after the shock will block, leading to the creation of new reentrant pathways during the postshock period. The different effects of monophasic and biphasic waveforms on refractory period extension may influence the defibrillation threshold through either or both of these two mechanisms.

The critical point has been shown to be different for biphasic and monophasic waveforms.[51] Since a biphasic waveform is less able to directly excite refractory tissue than a comparable monophasic waveform,[38] the critical point occurs in less refractory tissue. This effect depends on the waveform duration and waveform shape.[22,36,37,44] Daubert et al[38] showed that the biphasic strength-interval curve lay to the right of the monophasic curve. Based on this, the relative refractory tissue adjoining the directly excited area of biphasic shocks should be less refractory and should have less refractory period extension than the area of relative refractory tissue caused by monophasic shocks. This means that, after a biphasic shock, the activation front arising from the directly excited tissue would travel through more recovered tissue. Slow conduction is exhibited less or not at all in more recovered tissue. Without slow conduction, reinitiation of fibrillation and reentry is less likely.

Even though biphasic waveforms cause less refractory period extension than comparable monophasic waveforms, the dispersion of refractory periods following the shock has been shown by Tovar and Jones[44] and Behrens and coworkers[20] to be less for biphasic shocks than for comparable monophasic shocks. Since the dispersion of refractory periods is less, there is less likelihood that a propagating activation front will block, as block is thought to occur when an activation front encounters a region that is not yet recovered. Since block is thought to be less likely following biphasic shocks, the induction of reentry leading to the resumption of fibrillation should also be less likely.

Thus, possible explanations for the improved defibrillation efficacy of some biphasic waveforms compared to monophasic waveforms are that refractory period extension caused by biphasic waveforms 1) can better prevent the appearance of activation fronts after the shock, and 2) by decreasing the dispersion of refractoriness, can better prevent reentry of those activation fronts that do appear after a shock. It can be speculated that defibrillation efficacy might be increased by finding a waveform that further reduces the dispersion of refractoriness.

References

1. Beck P, Pritchard W, Veil H. Ventricular fibrillation of long duration abolished by electric shock. *JAMA* 1947;135:985-986.
2. Zoll P, Linenthal A, Gibson W. Termination of ventricular fibrillation in man by externally applied electric countershock. *N Engl J Med* 1956;254:727-732.
3. Mirowski M, Reid PR, Mower MM, et al. Termination of malignant ventricular arrhythmias with an implanted automatic defibrillator in human beings. *N Engl J Med* 1980;303:322-324.
4. Fogoros RN, Elson JJ, Bonnet CA, et al. Efficacy of the automatic implantable cardioverter-defibrillator in prolonging survival in patients with severe underlying cardiac disease. *J Am Coll Cardiol* 1990;16:381-386.
5. Fromer M, Brachmann J, Block M, et al. Efficacy of automatic multimodal device therapy for ventricular tachyarrhythmias as delivered by a new implantable pace-cardioverter-defibrillator. Results of a European multicenter study incorporating 102 implants. *Circulation* 1992;86:363-374.
6. Jones JL, Jones RE. Improved defibrillation waveform safety factor with biphasic waveforms. *Am J Physiol* 1983;245:60-65.
7. Schuder JC, Gold JH, Stoeckle H, et al. Defibrillation in the calf with bidirectional trapezoidal wave shocks applied via chronically implanted epicardial electrodes. *Trans Am Soc for Artif Int Org* 1981;27:467-470.
8. Dixon EG, Tang AS, Wolf PD, et al. Improved defibrillation thresholds with large contoured epicardial electrodes and biphasic waveforms. *Circulation* 1987;76:1176-1184.
9. Bardy GH, Ivey TD, Allen MD, et al. A prospective randomized evaluation of biphasic versus monophasic waveform pulses on defibrillation efficacy in humans. *J Am Coll Cardiol* 1989;14(3):728-733.
10. Bardy GH, Marchlinski FE, Sharma AD, et al. Multicenter comparison of truncated biphasic shocks and standard damped sine wave monophasic shocks for transthoracic ventricular defibrillation. *Circulation* 1996;94:2507-2514.
11. Wiggers CJ. The physiologic basis for cardiac resuscitation from ventricular fibrillation: Method for serial defibrillation. *Am Heart J* 1940;20:413-422.
12. Mower MM, Mirowski M, Spear JF, et al. Patterns of ventricular activity during catheter defibrillation. *Circulation* 1974;49:858-861.
13. Zipes DP, Fischer J, King RM, et al. Termination of ventricular fibrillation in dogs by depolarizing a critical amount of myocardium. *Am J Cardiol* 1975;36:37-44.
14. Chen PS, Shibata N, Dixon EG, et al. Activation during ventricular defibrillation in open chest dogs. Evidence for complete cessation and regeneration of ventricular fibrillation after unsuccessful shocks. *J Clin Invest* 1986;77:810-823.

15. Bardy GH, Hofer B, Johnson G, et al. Implantable transvenous cardioverter-defibrillators. *Circulation* 1993;87:1152-1168.
16. Winkle RA, Bach SM Jr, Mead RH, et al. Comparison of defibrillation efficacy in humans using a new catheter and superior vena cava spring-left ventricular patch electrodes. *J Am Coll Cardiol* 1988;11:365-370.
17. Chen PS, Wolf PD, Dixon EG, et al. Mechanism of ventricular vulnerability to single premature stimuli in open chest dogs. *Circ Res* 1988;62:1191-1209.
18. Shibata N, Chen PS, Dixon EG, et al. Influence of shock strength and timing on induction of ventricular arrhythmias in dogs. *Am Physiol Soc* 1988;255:H891-H901.
19. Frazier DW, Wolf PD, Wharton JM, et al. Stimulus induced critical point: Mechanism for electrical initiation of reentry in normal canine myocardium. *J Clin Invest* 1989;83:1039-1052.
20. Behrens S, Li C, Kirchhof P, et al. Reduced arrhythmogenicity of biphasic versus monophasic T-wave shocks. *Circulation* 1996;94:1974-1980.
21. Dillon SM. Optical recordings in the rabbit heart show that defibrillation strength shocks prolong the duration of depolarization and the refractory period. *Circ Res* 1991;69:846-856.
22. Swartz JF, Jones JL, Jones RE, et al. Conditioning prepulse of biphasic defibrillator waveforms enhances refractoriness to fibrillation wavefronts. *Circ Res* 1991;68:438-449.
23. Knisley SB, Afework J, Li J, et al. Dispersion of repolarization induced by a nonuniform shock field. *PACE* 1991;14:1148-1157.
24. Knisley SB, Smith WM, Ideker RE. Effect of field stimulation on cellular repolarization in rabbit myocardium. *Circ Res* 1992;70:707-715.
25. Drury AN, Love WS. The supposed lengthening of the absolute refractory period of frog's ventricular muscle by Veratrine. *Heart* 1926;13:77-85.
26. Love WS. The effect of quinidine and strophantine upon the refractory period and the tortoise ventricle. *Heart* 1926;13:87-93.
27. Lewis T, Drury AN. Revised views of the refractory period, in relation to drugs reputed to prolong it, and in relation to circus movement. *Heart* 1926;13:95-100.
28. Kao CY, Hoffmann BF. Graded and decremental response in heart muscle fibers. *Am J Physiol* 1958;194:187-196.
29. Han J, Moe GK. Nonuniform recovery of excitability in ventricular muscle. *Circ Res* 1964;14:44-60.
30. Janse MJ, Van der Steen ABM, Van Damm, et al. Refractory period of the dog's ventricular myocardium following sudden changes in frequency. *Circ Res* 1969;24:251-262.
31. Gettes LS, Morehouse N, Surawicz B. Effect of premature depolarization on the duration of action potentials in Purkinje and ventricular fibers of the moderator band of the pig heart. Role of proximity and the preceding action potential. *Circ Res* 1972;30:55-66.
32. Tamargo J, Moe B, Moe GK. Interaction of sequential stimuli applied during the relative refractory period in relation of ventricular fibrillation threshold in the canine ventricle. *Circ Res* 1975;37:534-541.
33. Prystowsky EN, Zipes DP. Inhibition in the human heart. *Circulation* 1983;68:707-713.
34. Windle JR, Miles WM, Zipes DP, et al. Subthreshold conditioning stimuli prolong human ventricular refractoriness. *Am J Cardiol* 1986;57:381-386.

35. Kuo CS, Munakata K, Reddy CP, et al. Characteristics and possible mechanism of ventricular arrhythmia dependent on the dispersion of action potential durations. *Circulation* 1983;67:1356-1367.
36. Zhou X, Knisley SB, Wolf PD, et al. Prolongation of repolarization time by electric field stimulation with monophasic and biphasic shocks in open chest dogs. *Circ Res* 1991;68:1761-1767.
37. Zhou X, Wolf PD, Rollins DL, et al. Effects of monophasic and biphasic shocks on action potentials during ventricular fibrillation in dogs. *Circ Res* 1993;73:325-334.
38. Daubert JP, Frazier DW, Wolf PD, et al. Response of relative refractory canine myocardium to monophasic and biphasic shocks. *Circulation* 1991;84:2522-2538.
39. Dillon SM, Wit AL. Transmembrane voltage changes recorded during countershock in normal rhythm. *Circulation* 1987;76:IV242. Abstract.
40. Dillon SM. Synchronized repolarization after defibrillation shocks. *Circulation* 1992;85:1865-1878.
41. Kwaku KF, Dillon SM. Shock-induced depolarization of refractory myocardium prevents wave-front propagation in defibrillation. *Circ Res* 1996;79:957-973.
42. Sweeney RJ, Gill RM, Steinberg MI, et al. Ventricular refractory extension caused by defibrillation shocks. *Circulation* 1990;82:965-972.
43. Sweeney RJ, Gill RM, Reid PR. Characterization of refractory period extension by transcardiac shock. *Circulation* 1991;83:2057-2066.
44. Tovar OH, Jones JL. Biphasic defibrillation waveforms reduced shock-induced response duration dispersion between low and high shock intensities. *Circ Res* 1995;77:430-438.
45. Tang AS, Wolf PD, Afework Y, et al. Three-dimensional potential gradient fields generated by intracardiac catheter and cutaneous patch electrodes. *Circulation* 1992;85:1857-1864.
46. Hillsley RE, Walker RG, Swanson DK, et al. Is the second phase of the biphasic defibrillation waveform the defibrillating phase? *PACE* 1993;16:1401-1411.
47. Knisley SB, Hill BC. Optical recordings of the effect of electrical stimulation on action potential repolarization and the induction of reentry in two-dimensional perfused rabbit epicardium. *Circulation* 1993;88:2402-2414.
48. Krassowska W, Kumar MS. The role of spatial interactions in creating the dispersion of transmembrane potential by premature electric shock. *Ann Biomed Eng* 1997;25:949-963.
49. Gotoh M, Uchida T, Mandel WJ, et al. Cellular graded response and ventricular vulnerability to reentry by a premature stimulus in isolated canine ventricle. *Circulation* 1997;95:2141-2154.
50. Fishler MG, Sobie EA, Tung L, et al. Modeling the interaction between propagating cardiac waves and monophasic and biphasic field stimuli: The importance of the induced spatial excitatory response. *J Cardiac Electrophysiol* 1996;7:1183-1196.
51. Ideker RI, Alferness C, Hagler J, et al. Rotor site correlates with defibrillation waveform efficacy. *Circulation* 1991;84:II499. Abstract.

Section VIII

Antiarrhythmic Device-Related Uses of Monophasic Action Potential Recording: Introduction

Nonpharmacologic, device-oriented interventions have taken center stage in the treatment of many types of cardiac arrhythmias. There are several ways in which monophasic action potential (MAP) recordings can be helpful in this field. By imbedding a MAP electrode in the tip of a radiofrequency electrode, investigators can obtain MAP recordings that can provide direct feedback on the progress of myocardial ablation. Atrial fibrillation is an arrhythmia that is difficult to overdrive-pace by focal electrical stimuli. MAP recordings provide continuous visualization of the repolarization phases, even during atrial fibrillation, and pinpoint the excitable gaps when they occur, thus improving the ability and recognition of local capture during pacing in atrial fibrillation. Multisite pacing during sinus rhythm has been proven to help prevent recurrence of atrial fibrillation, and it remains to be seen whether concomitant MAP recording can help to elucidate the mechanism and improve the success of this novel approach.

47

Real-Time Monitoring of Radiofrequency-Induced Myocardial Lesions by Simultaneous Recording of Monophasic Action Potentials

Michael R. Franz, MD, PhD, Hugh Sharkey, RN, Steward Edwards and Melvin M. Scheinman, MD

Radiofrequency (RF) catheter ablation of cardiac arrhythmias has become a widely used technique for curative treatment of supraventricular[1-4] and ventricular[5-9] tachyarrhythmias. RF produces thermal damage to myocardial tissue in close contact with the ablation electrode.[10-12] Newer ablation catheters have thermistors incorporated in the ablation electrode tip to monitor heat development at the RF application site.[12-16] Heat development at the electrode and the size of the lesion produced by it depend on a variety of factors including the strength and duration of the RF current,[11,12,16] the size and geometry of the electrode,[11,14,17] the electrical impedance at the interface between the electrode and the tissue or blood,[11,18] the firmness and stability of the electrode-tissue contact,[18] and the heat-sinking properties of the tissue or fluid surrounding the electrode surface.[19] When heat development is excessive, a protein coagulum may form at the elec-

Supported in part by a research grant R29-HL40483 from the NIHLB and an educational grant from EP Technologies, Inc., San Jose, CA.

From Franz MR (ed): *Monophasic Action Potentials: Bridging Cell and Bedside.* ©Futura Publishing Company, Inc., Armonk, NY, 2000.

trode surface, causing sudden impedance rise at the ablation electrode, and obstructing the transduction of heat into the targeted tissue.

Despite these recent advances, it may be desirable to have a direct *electrophysiologic* index that is capable of monitoring firm tissue contact and myocardial lesion formation *during* RF delivery. We developed a novel RF ablation catheter that is capable of recording monophasic action potentials (MAPs) simultaneously with RF delivery. The incorporation of a MAP electrode centrally into the tip of the ablation electrode was based on the following rationales: 1) MAPs can be recorded only when the tip electrode is seated firmly against myocardial tissue,[20,21] and 2) the tissue subjacent to the impinging tip electrode is viable and electrically coupled to the adjacent myocardium.[20,22] Thus, as RF creates an anatomic lesion at the recording site, the MAP signal should diminish in amplitude or even disappear completely. To validate this concept, the extent of loss of MAP amplitude at the end of RF delivery and 5 minutes later were correlated with postmortem anatomic lesion measurements.

Methods

Studies were performed in concordance with the guidelines of the American Heart Association and were approved by the University's Committee for experimental studies. Six adult mongrel dogs with weights from 20 to 25 kg were anesthetized with pentobarbital and subsequently respirated with room air through a cuffed endotracheal tube by a Harvard respirator. A femoral vein and artery were dissected free, and a 7F specially designed MAP-ablation catheter was inserted under fluoroscopic guidance via either route into the right or left ventricle. The design of this catheter is depicted in Figure 1. A platinum tip electrode, 4 mm in length, served as the RF ablation anode. Embedded centrally in the tip portion of the ablation electrode was the MAP recording electrode, which consisted of a nonpolarizable silver-silver chloride (Ag-AgCl) pellet of 1 mm^2 surface. The MAP electrode was insulated from the enclosing ablation electrode by a 0.1-mm spacing of non-conducting, heat-resistant epoxy material. Another Ag-AgCl electrode 5 mm proximal to the tip served as the reference electrode for the MAP recording circuit, and a platinum ring electrode (5 mm proximal to the ablation electrode) served as the bipolar electrogram reference. To stabilize endocardial contact of the MAP-ablation electrode, a 10 cm long elastic flat spring-steel member was imbedded in the distal portion of the catheter shaft. The MAP electrode configuration used in this ablation catheter is identical to the one described earlier, which has been demonstrated to accurately reproduce the time course of myocardial depolarization and repolarization as well as relative changes in the membrane resting and action potential magnitude, of the subjacent myocardium.[23]

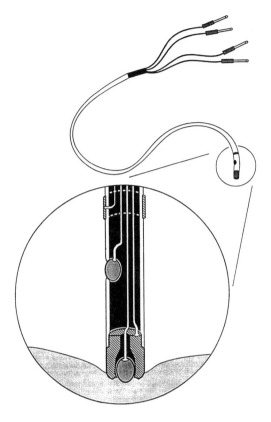

Figure 1. Illustration of MAP recording-ablation catheter that combines a 4-mm-long ablation and reference ring electrode with a silver-silver chloride MAP recording electrode pair. The exploring MAP electrode is centered within the ablation electrode tip and insulated from the latter by a 0.1-mm-thick layer of heat-resistant epoxy material, while the MAP reference is situated 5 mm proximal to the tip.

MAP signals were recorded with a high input-impedance, direct current (DC)-coupled, differential preamplifier with a frequency-response bandwidth of 0 to 5000 Hz. Surface electrocardiogram (ECG) recordings were obtained simultaneously with a conventional ECG amplifier. Both types of recordings were written out by a multichannel electrostatic recorder (Gould ES 1000, Gould Instruments, Cleveland, OH). RF energy was delivered between the platinum tip electrode and a back pad, with use of an EP Technologies (San Jose, CA) RF generator. A custom-designed narrow band-pass electronic filter (Stellartech, CA), introduced between the MAP electrode leads and the preamplifier, eliminated crosstalk between RF energy delivering electrodes and MAP recording electrodes so that MAPs free from RF noise and with only minimal DC offset could be recorded throughout the period of RF energy application (Fig. 2).

Protocols

RF energy delivery and simultaneous MAP recordings were performed at a total of 31 endocardial sites (Table 1). Of these, 4 were applied in the

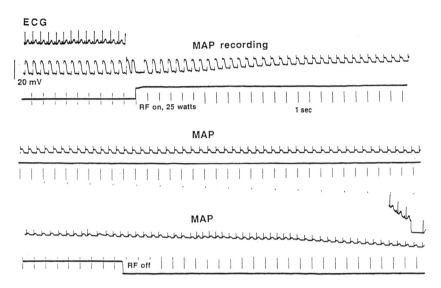

Figure 2. Original tracings of surface electrocardiogram (ECG) recordings and left ventricular endocardial MAP recordings during a 60-second radiofrequency (RF) delivery period and during 20 seconds after RF. Note that ECG recordings are offset from the screen during the RF delivery period and for some time thereafter, yet MAP recordings remain noise-free and show only minimal offset. See text for a more detailed description of MAP changes during RF application.

Table 1
Sites, Duration, and Power Levels of RF Delivery

Total number of applications	31
LV	27
RV	4
25 watts	23
60 seconds	13
7.1±2.0 seconds	7*
5 watts, 60 seconds	8

*Terminated due to early impedance rise. LV = left ventricle; RF = radiofrequency; RV = right ventricle.

right ventricle and 27 in the left ventricle. All catheter positions were documented by biplane cinematography. MAP recordings were monitored before and during RF delivery, and during a 5-minute post-RF observation period. RF was delivered at two energy levels. In group A (23 deliveries), RF of 25 W was delivered for a preset duration of 60 seconds. If sudden impedance rise (>130 Ω) occurred before the scheduled time (7 cases), RF energy was terminated immediately. In group B, 8 RF applications were delivered at 5 W for 60 seconds regardless of impedance changes. These different RF durations and power levels were chosen to produce a range of maximum, minimum, and intermediate lesion sizes that would serve as a basis for correlating the real-time MAP changes with the postmortem lesion sizes.

Data Analysis

The amplitude of the MAP was measured in millivolts as the distance from the diastolic baseline to the crest of the plateau of the MAP signal, as described earlier.[20] Because the baseline MAP amplitude varied between different endocardial sites, all MAP amplitude changes following the onset of RF are expressed in percentage of the baseline amplitude measured immediately before the start of RF.

At the end of the experiments, the dogs were sacrificed by intravenous infusion of concentrated potassium chloride, and the hearts were removed and fixed in formalin. The hearts were dissected and sliced, and the size of the ablative lesions was determined by planimetry for lesion depth (in mm) and volume (in mm³), as previously described.[17] Lesion volume was defined in mm^3 as the entire mass of denatured tissue in 3 dimensions, and lesion depth as the distance, in mm, extending from the endocardial contact site of the ablation electrode tip to the intramural lesion margin perpendicular to the electrode tip. The site of contact between the MAP-ablation electrode and the endocardium was identifiable by either myocardial indentations or burn marks at the endocardial surface. In vivo catheter positions and postmortem lesions could be matched for 27 of 31 sites. The remaining 4 sites could not be matched accurately between in vivo cinematographic data, and postmortem lesions and were excluded from analysis.

Statistical Analysis

The different energy levels and durations of RF delivery were expected to result in different degrees of MAP changes and anatomic lesion formation, and provided a basis for a statistical correlation between the decrease in MAP amplitude at the cessation and 5 minutes after RF, and the size of RF-induced anatomic lesions. Linear regression analysis was used to correlate the loss of MAP amplitude with either lesion depth or lesion volume. Statistical differences in MAP amplitude loss and lesion depth or volume between the different groups were determined by unpaired Student t test.

Qualitative Effects of RF Delivery on the Simultaneously Recorded MAP

Preceding each RF delivery, the MAP-ablation catheter was placed against the left ventricular or right ventricular endocardium so that stable MAP recordings (22±11 mV amplitude) were obtained from the Ag-AgCl electrode embedded in the tip of the ablation electrode. RF delivery to the ablation electrode produced rapid changes in the MAP recording. Due to the custom electronic filter in the MAP recording circuit, MAP changes could be observed *during* the period of RF delivery without noise or major DC offset. Figure 2 represents a typical example of the MAP changes seen during a 60-second period of RF energy delivery at 25 W. Within 3 to 5 seconds of RF initiation there was a marked decrease in the MAP amplitude, which subsequently decreased further to a fraction of the baseline value. Despite some DC offset, it can be appreciated that the decrease in MAP amplitude was due initially to a decrease in the MAP diastolic potential and subsequently to a combined decrease in diastolic and systolic MAP amplitude. At the end of the RF delivery period, the MAP amplitude (measured from the foot of the MAP to its plateau level) had decreased to approximately 10% of its value before RF delivery, rendering the MAP signal from its original monophasic appearance to a signal resembling a myocardial surface electrogram with an isoelectric ST segment followed by a T wave. Over the ensuing 5-minute postablation period, only minimal recovery of the MAP signal was seen.

RF Effects on MAP Amplitude During Abbreviated High-Energy or Continuous Low-Energy RF Deliveries

Of the 23 RF applications preset at 25 W, 7 were terminated prematurely (at 7.1±2.0 seconds) due to early impedance rise. An additional 8 RF deliveries, preset for an energy level of 5 W, could all be continued for 60 seconds without impedance rise (Table 1). The change in MAP amplitude during RF deliveries at 25 W, which were aborted early due to sudden impedance rise, is quantitatively shown in panel A of Figure 3. Despite the short duration of RF in these trials, the initial loss in MAP amplitude was marked (23.2±18.2% of pre-RF measured at 30 seconds after RF initiation) and sustained until 5 minutes after RF application, with only small recovery (25.6±15.0% of baseline; NS versus 30 seconds). During the 8 RF applica-

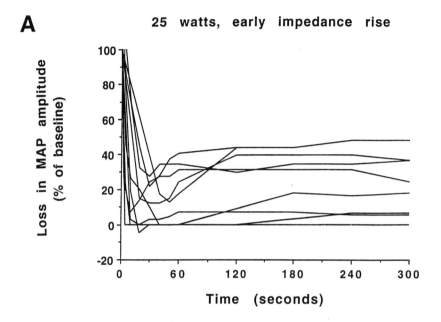

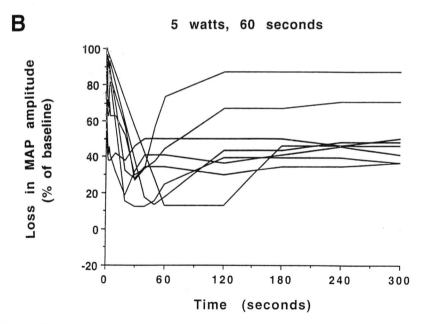

Figure 3. A. Individual time courses of MAP amplitude loss during and after 10 radiofrequency (RF) deliveries at 25 W that were terminated at 7.3±2.0 seconds due to early impedance rise. **B.** Individual time courses of MAP amplitude loss during and after 8 RF deliveries at 5 W for 60 seconds.

tions at 5 W, which were continued for 60 seconds without impedance rise, the relative loss in MAP amplitude developed with a slightly slower time course (29.8±8.2% of pre-RF at 30 seconds) were on average less pronounced at the termination of RF than the short-lasting and higher energy RF applications (35±12% of pre-RF; $P<0.05$), and showed a greater recovery at 5 minutes post RF (42.9±13% of pre-RF) (Fig. 3, panel B).

Effects of RF on MAP Amplitude During 60-Second High-Energy (25 W) RF Deliveries Uninterrupted by Early Impedance Rise

Thirteen of the 23 scheduled RF deliveries at 25 W (73% of all RF trials) could be administered for 60 seconds without significant impedance rise. These RF deliveries resulted in a decrease in the MAP amplitude that occurred with a negative exponential time course for the first 20 seconds of RF delivery. Thereafter, a slight (statistically nonsignificant) recovery of MAP amplitude was noted during the remaining 40 seconds of RF delivery and during the 5-minute period following cessation of RF (Fig. 4). The time course of the early reduction of MAP amplitude could be fitted by a single exponential, which reached half time within 3.6 seconds after onset of RF energy delivery and attained an amplitude of 13.8±12.3% of pre-RF baseline at 20 seconds. At 5 minutes post-RF, a small recovery to 20.6±15.0% of baseline was seen.

Relation Between Real-Time MAP Amplitude Decreases and Postmortem Lesion Size

RF delivery in the in situ hearts produced different degrees of relative loss in the MAP amplitude recorded at the RF ablation site, depending on the energy level and the duration of RF delivery. This diversity of in vivo outcomes at the end of different RF delivery times and at 5-minute recovery times provided the basis for a statistical correlation between the decrease in MAP amplitude during RF and the size of RF-induced anatomic lesions.

Postmortem analysis of RF delivery sites showed solid lesions of various sizes that extended from the tip electrode contact site concentrically into the myocardium. The lesions were contiguous with the endocardium at the RF electrode contact site; hence, there was no evidence that

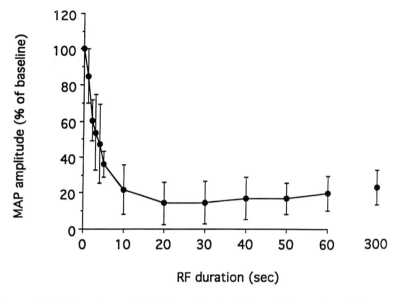

Figure 4. Relative change in MAP amplitude during a 60-second radiofrequency (RF) delivery period and at 5 minutes after RF delivery. Data represent the average ± standard deviation of 13 RF deliveries, which were applied for 60 seconds and which were not interrupted by significant impedance rise.

the MAP electrode embedded in the tip electrode had any shielding effect on the delivery of RF energy.

The loss in MAP amplitude at the end of RF delivery predicted postmortem lesion depth and lesion volume with linear correlation coefficients of 0.67 and 0.74, respectively, both significant at $P<0.0001$ (Fig. 5, panels A and B). The loss in MAP amplitude after a 5-minute post-RF recovery period showed a slightly greater linear correlation with postmortem lesion depth (r=0.72; $P<0.00001$) and lesion volume (r=0.80; $P<0.00001$) (Fig. 5, panels C and D). The loss of MAP amplitude predicted postmortem lesion formation even in those instances where early impedance rise curtailed the delivery of RF energy. On average, lesion volume tended to be slightly larger in cases of early impedance rise (118.4 ± 29.3 mm^3) than in those where RF energy was delivered for 60 seconds without impedance rise (94.2 ± 50.7 mm^3), but this difference was statistically not significant.

Discussion

This study demonstrates that MAP recordings obtained from a specially designed electrode imbedded centrally in the tip portion of an RF ablation electrode provides real-time monitoring of the electrophysiologic changes at the RF ablation site. Further, use of a custom designed RF

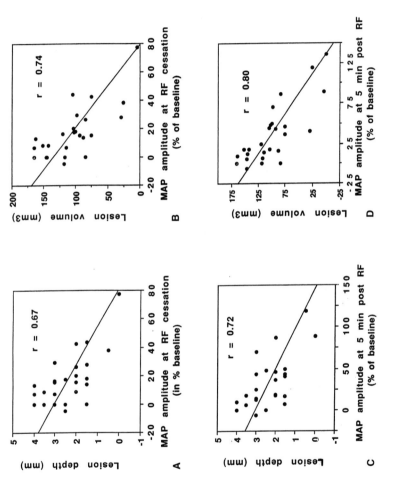

Figure 5. Correlations between loss of MAP amplitude and lesion depth and volume, respectively, at cessation of radiofrequency (RF) energy and after a 5-minute post-RF recovery period.

noise reduction filter allows MAP changes to be observed during RF, with minimal distortion. Most importantly, in this study, the relative loss in MAP amplitude reflected lesion formation as determined by postmortem analysis.

Time Course of MAP Amplitude Loss During RF

RF application caused a decrease in the MAP amplitude within seconds of RF initiation, often resulting in near complete abolition of the MAP signal within 10 to 30 seconds of RF energy application. In all experiments where RF was delivered at 25 W, the loss of MAP amplitude followed a (negative) exponential time course. This exponential decay of MAP amplitude bears a striking reciprocity with the rise in catheter tip temperature as reported by Haines and Watson,[10] in a thermistor-guided catheter ablation study. In that study, temperature rise followed a (positive) exponential time course, reaching stable levels at approximately 20 seconds. This supports the view that the relative loss in MAP amplitude during RF energy application reflects the effects of thermal injury on myocardial cells and that exceeding a critical temperature results in permanent tissue destruction.[10,11] However, temperature rise may occur also in the absence of effective tissue destruction (ie, when formation of denatured protein at the ablation electrode may produce temperature build-up in the absence of further tissue destruction). MAP recordings probe the electrophysiologic state of the myocardium itself,[20-23] and appear less subject to factors which may confound temperature measurements.[15-17]

Correlation of in Vivo MAP Amplitude Loss with Postmortem Lesion Size

As previously shown by us and others, MAPs can be recorded only from viable myocardium, while recordings from myocardial scars[20] or acutely infarcted myocardium[22,24] resemble electrograms with isoelectric ST segments. In this study, definitive tissue destruction by RF energy was verified post mortem and was found to correlate closely with the loss of MAP amplitude recorded during RF energy application. A decrease in MAP amplitude below 30% of baseline identified permanent tissue destruction of at least 50 mm^3 of lesion volume or 2 mm of lesion depth perpendicular to the ablation electrode tip. The rapid time course of MAP amplitude loss and its high correlation with postmortem lesion size, even with prematurely aborted RF energy deliveries, suggests that most of the tissue ablation was achieved within the first 10 to 20 seconds. Some recovery of MAP amplitude occurred during a 5-minute post-RF observation period, possibly indicating recovery of viability of myocardial cells injured only transiently. This may explain why anatomic lesion size correlated slightly better with MAP amplitude loss recorded at the end of the 5-minute recovery period than with MAP amplitude loss recorded immediately after cessation of RF energy.

Mechanism Underlying the Loss of MAP Amplitude During RF Ablation

According to current theory,[21] the MAP recorded by contact electrode provides information on the electrophysiology of subjacent myocardial cells by the following mechanism. Pressure of the MAP electrode against the myocardium causes depolarization of the *subjacent* tissue, rendering it unexcitable so it no longer participates in the periodic depolarizations and repolarizations of the *adjacent* myocardium. This creates an electrical gradient between the depolarized cells beneath the MAP electrode and the surrounding normal cells. This gradient causes current flow, which in turn creates a field potential, which mirrors the action potential time course of the cells outside the boundary. It follows that MAP signals can be recorded only if at least two conditions are fulfilled. The first is electrophysiologic viability of the myocardium underneath the exploring MAP tip electrode, and the second is firm contact between the MAP tip electrode and the myocardium.

Abolition of bypass tract conduction within only 1 to 2 seconds of RF energy delivery has led to speculation about whether RF energy exerts a direct electrical effect on myocardial tissue, causing interruption of impulse conduction even before thermal injury takes effect.[12] Our MAP recordings made during RF delivery serve as an argument that RF does not have a significant electrotonic effect on the underlying myocardial tissue. Following the onset of RF energy application, changes in MAP configuration and amplitude occurred gradually over several seconds and followed a monoexponential time course, reciprocal to the heat build-up reported by Haines and Watson.[10] Thus, it seems more likely that RF energy produces myocardial effects by thermal injury rather than by electrotonic effects, which would be expected to occur instantaneously.

Limitations

The MAP recording technique is likely to provide less reliable information on RF ablation effects when the tip electrode is not in direct contact with viable myocardium. For instance, catheter placement at the atrioventricular annulus may produce inadequate MAP recordings due to the fact that the MAP electrode is making contact predominantly with the collagenous tissue of the atrioventricular ring, which does not produce the electrical current flow required for MAP recordings.[21] Although it is conceivable that MAP signals may be recorded if the electrode were to ride directly on the bypass tract, the magnitude of these MAP potentials would be expected to be small because of the discrete myocardial tissue mass of an accessory atrioventricular connection. MAP recordings also may be less useful for guiding atrioventricular nodal ablation or modification procedures because of anticipated difficulties in placing the MAP catheter tip perpendicularly to the atrioventricular junction. This, however, might be overcome by new catheter designs.

Conclusions and Clinical Implications

MAPs recorded at the same site at which RF energy is delivered provide real-time physiologic feedback of the efficacy of RF energy in destructing myocardium subjacent to the ablation electrode. RF-induced loss of MAP amplitude predicts postmortem lesion formation, regardless of RF duration or whether impedance rise occurred. This may be helpful in limiting RF energy delivery to the shortest time necessary. Another advantage is that a stable MAP recording prior to application of RF energy helps to ascertain firm tissue contact. Finally, our data suggest that sudden impedance rise does not necessarily reflect inadequate tissue necrosis. If rapid MAP amplitude reduction occurs before and sustains after impedance rise, successful lesion formation might be assumed. If the arrhythmia persists despite abolition of the MAP signal, tissue necrosis most likely has occurred at a nontargeted site.

MAP recordings may be of particular interest in guiding ablation of ventricular tachyarrhythmias that originate from abnormal yet electrically active myocardium. The high precision of the MAP recording technique in identifying local myocardial activation,[21-23] and its unique ability to detect afterdepolarizations in vivo,[25-27] may be a useful adjunct in ablating ectopic or triggered ventricular tachycardias. Guidance of RF ablation by MAP and temperature monitoring are not mutually exclusive, and a combination of the two is probably of value. This study was confined to monitoring ablation of ventricular myocardium but MAP-guided ablation of *atrial* myocardium may also be of interest.[28,29]

References

1. Langberg JJ, Chin M, Schamp DJ, et al. Ablation of the atrioventricular junction with RF energy using a new electrode catheter. *Am J Cardiol* 1991;67:142-147.

2. Morady F, Scheinman MM, Kou WH, et al. Long-term results of catheter ablation of a posteroseptal accessory atrioventricular connection in 48 patients. *Circulation* 1989;79:1160-1170.

3. Jackman WM, Wang XZ, Friday KJ, et al. Catheter ablation of accessory atrioventricular pathways (Wolff-Parkinson-White syndrome) by radiofrequency current. *N Engl J Med* 1991;324:1605-1611.

4. Jackman WM, Beckman KJ, McClelland JH, et al. Treatment of supraventricular tachycardia due to atrioventricular nodal reentry, by radiofrequency catheter ablation of slow-pathway conduction. *N Engl J Med* 1992;327(5):313-318.

5. Langberg JJ, Desai J, Dullet N, et al. Treatment of macroreentrant ventricular tachycardia with RF ablation of the right bundle branch. *Am J Cardiol* 1989;63:1010-1013.

6. Cohen TJ, Chien WW, Lurie KG, et al. RF catheter ablation for treatment of bundle branch reentrant ventricular tachycardia: Results and long-term follow-up. *J Am Coll Cardiol* 1991;18:1767-1773.

7. Klein LS, Shih HT, Hackett K, et al. RF catheter ablation of ventricular tachycardia in patients without structural heart disease. *Circulation* 1992;85:1666-1674.

8. Morady F, Harvey M, Kalbfleisch SJ, et al. Radiofrequency catheter ablation of ventricular tachycardia in patients with coronary artery disease. *Circulation* 1993;87:363-372.

9. Gursoy S, Brugada J, Souza O, et al. RF ablation of symptomatic but benign ventricular arrhythmias. *PACE* 1992;15:738-741.

10. Haines DE, Watson DD. Tissue heating during RF catheter ablation: A thermodynamic model and observations in isolated perfused and superfused canine right ventricular free wall. *PACE* 1989;12:962-976.

11. Haines DE, Verow AF. Observations on electrode-tissue interface temperature and effect on electrical impedance during RF ablation of ventricular myocardium. *Circulation* 1990;82:1034-1038.

12. Nath S, DiMarco JP, Mounsey JP, et al. Correlation of temperature and pathophysiological effect during radiofrequency catheter ablation of the AV junction. *Circulation* 1995;92:1188-1192.

13. Pires LA, Huang SK, Wagshal AB, et al. Temperature-guided radiofrequency catheter ablation of closed-chest ventricular myocardium with a novel thermistor-tipped catheter. *Am Heart J* 1994;127:1614-1618.

14. Langberg JJ, Gallagher M, Strickberger SA, Amirana O. Temperature-guided radiofrequency catheter ablation with very large distal electrodes. *Circulation* 1993;88:245-249.

15. McRury ID, Whayne JG, Haines DE. Temperature measurement as a determinant of tissue heating during radiofrequency catheter ablation: An examination of electrode thermistor positioning for measurement accuracy. *J Cardiovasc Electrophysiol* 1995;6:268-278.

16. Tracy CM, Moore HJ, Solomon AJ, et al. Thermistor guided radiofrequency ablation of atrial insertion sites in patients with accessory pathways. *PACE* 1995;18:2001-2007.

17. Langberg JJ, Lee MA, Chin MC, et al. RF catheter ablation: The effect of electrode size on lesion volume in vivo. *PACE* 1990;13:1242-1248.

18. Strickberger SA, Vorperian VR, Man KC, et al. Relation between impedance and endocardial contact during radiofrequency catheter ablation. *Am Heart J* 1994;128:226-229.

19. Nakagawa H, Yamanashi WS, Pitha JV, et al. Comparison of in vivo tissue temperature profile and lesion geometry for radiofrequency ablation with a

saline-irrigated electrode versus temperature control in a canine thigh muscle preparation. *Circulation* 1995;91:2264-2273.

20. Franz MR. Long-term recording of monophasic action potentials from human endocardium. *Am J Cardiol* 1983;51:1629-1634.

21. Franz MR. Method and theory of monophasic action potential recording. *Prog Cardiovasc Dis* 1991;33:347-368.

22. Franz MR, Flaherty JT, Platia EV, et al. Localization of regional myocardial ischemia by recording of monophasic action potentials. *Circulation* 1984;69:593-604.

23. Franz MR, Burkhoff D, Spurgeon H, et al. In vitro validation of a new cardiac catheter technique for recording MAPs. *Eur Heart J* 1986;7:34-41.

24. Dilly SG, Lab MJ. Changes in monophasic action potential duration during the first hour of regional myocardial ischaemia in the anaesthetised pig. *Cardiovasc Res* 1987;21:908-915.

25. Ben-David J, Zipes DP. Differential response to right and left ansae subclaviae stimulation of early afterdepolarizations and ventricular tachycardia induced by cesium in dogs. *Circulation* 1988;78:1241-1250.

26. Zipes DP. Monophasic action potentials in the diagnosis of triggered arrhythmias. *Prog Cardiovasc Dis* 1991;33:385-396.

27. El-Sherif N, Bekheit SS, Henkin R. Quinidine-induced long QT interval and torsade de pointes: Role of bradycardia-dependent early afterdepolarizations. *J Am Coll Cardiol* 1989;14:252-257.

28. Elvan A, Pride HP, Eble JN, Zipes DP. Radiofrequency catheter ablation of the atria reduces inducibility and duration of atrial fibrillation in dogs. *Circulation* 1995;91:2235-2244.

29. Zipes DP. Radiofrequency ablation—what is left? *Eur Heart J* 1995;16(suppl G):24-27.

48

Electrophysiologic Basis for and Clinical Experience with Multisite Atrial Pacing for Prevention of Atrial Fibrillation

Sanjeev Saksena MD, FACC, Atul Prakash MD, MRCP and Ryszard B. Krol, MD

Introduction

The increasing use of multisite atrial pacing techniques for management of drug-refractory atrial fibrillation has spurred the investigation of the electrophysiologic mechanisms underlying its effectiveness.[1-3] Experimental and clinical investigation has been undertaken that bears on the mechanisms of atrial fibrillation and on their modification with multisite atrial pacing methods. Clinical studies have evaluated the electrophysiologic effects of these pacing methods and compared them with single-site pacing from traditional right atrial sites and novel pacing sites. While most clinical studies are acute evaluations, longer term clinical trial data have provided important insights into chronic effects of the therapy. It has become apparent that the electrophysiologic effects of the pacing techniques in question are diverse, as is the population of treated patients with atrial fibrillation. Thus, the discernible effects of the therapy, while categorized into specific actions, may be variable in extent for different

From Franz MR (ed): *Monophasic Action Potentials: Bridging Cell and Bedside.*
©Futura Publishing Company, Inc., Armonk, NY, 2000.

patient populations. These populations may be heterogeneous based on the associated conditions with atrial fibrillation including but not limited to the extent of coexisting bradyarrhythmia, atrial flutter, intra-atrial conduction defects, heart or lung disease, or prior cardiac surgery. There are, however, general abnormalities seen in diverse atrial fibrillation populations that appear to be associated with the arrhythmia. In this chapter, we summarize these abnormalities and examine the effects of atrial pacing that may have an antiarrhythmic role.

Electrophysiologic Abnormalities in Atrial Fibrillation

Since the original studies by Moe,[4] atrial fibrillation has been generally believed to be due to multiple wavelet reentry. The role of anatomic and functional abnormalities in the genesis and maintenance of the arrhythmia is now being vigorously investigated. A variety of experimental models have been used to study atrial flutter and atrial fibrillation. These models have included use of pharmacologic agents (aconitine, acetylcholine), inflammatory processes (talc-induced pericarditis), and, more recently, electrical pacing methods. These models have focused on the role of atrial premature beats and refractoriness in the genesis or maintenance of atrial fibrillation, and, to a lesser degree, have examined the effect of conduction abnormalities in the atria. The role of vagal stimulation in reducing atrial effective refractory periods and induction of atrial fibrillation has been long recognized. In experimental models of pacing-induced atrial fibrillation, the persistence of atrial fibrillation induces a rate-mediated reduction in atrial refractoriness.[5] This has been referred to as *atrial electrical remodeling*. The role of functional electrophysiologic abnormalities induced by long periods of rapid pacing in this model is particularly notable. Importantly, reverse remodeling with the elimination of atrial fibrillation has been suggested in this model. Regional atrial electrophysiology may vary at different atrial sites. Wood et al[6] have shown in another experimental model that there is a variability in action potential duration (APD) in the right atrium and left atrium. Prolongation of the APD in the left atrium relative to the right atrium was noted during pacing, regardless of the site of atrial pacing. This would result in dispersion of atrial refractoriness and, secondarily, repolarization. The role of conduction delays and block related to specific anatomic obstacles such as the crista terminalis has been emphasized in atrial flutter and now also in atrial fibrillation.[7,8] However, it has long been noted that atrial flutter and atrial fibrillation can coexist in the same individual and that atrial flutter can precede atrial fibrillation. Autonomic stimulation and atrial wall stress may also induce changes in the electrophysiologic properties of the atrium, leading to a propensity for an initiation or maintenance of atrial fibrillation.[9,10]

Early clinical studies demonstrated that delayed intra- and interatrial conduction was frequently observed in patients with atrial fibrillation. Cosio and coworkers[11] observed marked delays in intra-atrial conduction as measured by conduction intervals from the high right atrium to the right atrioventricular junction and coronary sinus in patients with atrial fibrillation as compared to those without this arrhythmia. Buxton et al[12] noted that such delays were seen in patients with both atrial fibrillation and atrial flutter. These delays were manifest as prolonged P wave durations, and later it was determined that the presence of a prolonged P wave duration could be an identifying marker for individuals with a propensity to atrial fibrillation, particularly after coronary bypass surgery.[13] Atrial effective refractory period is abbreviated in patients with atrial fibrillation, particularly in the right atrium. Rate adaptation of refractoriness is often absent.[14]

In addition to changes in the electrophysiologic substrate that may define the propensity to atrial fibrillation, the role of intercurrent influences on these factors has been emphasized. Increase in intra-atrial pressure can produce changes in refractoriness in the atria.[9] Nattel and Liu[10] have demonstrated that cholinergic stimulation can increase heterogeneity of atrial refractoriness and increase the propensity to sustenance of atrial fibrillation. A significant role for autonomic tone in the mediation of certain forms of atrial fibrillation has been recognized. Coumel and coworkers[15] have described forms of lone atrial fibrillation associated with conditions of high vagal tone such as bradycardia, during sleep, etc., as well as their prevention by pacing. Other clinical scenarios, such as atrial fibrillation after coronary bypass surgery, may involve heightened adrenergic tone. It can thus be readily appreciated that the effects of interventions to prevent atrial fibrillation must be directed at a multifactorial etiology for this arrhythmia.

Multisite Atrial Pacing Techniques

Two methods of multisite atrial pacing have been described. Daubert et al[16] have used stimulation at the high right atrium and the coronary sinus, with a triggered pacing algorithm. This allows for two electrical wave fronts to be initiated, with a small but quantifiable delay due to the triggered nature of the algorithm. This "biatrial" stimulation method has been employed, initially with distal coronary sinus stimulation, and more recently with proximal or mid coronary sinus locations.[16] We have described the method of dual-site right atrial stimulation, involving simultaneous stimulation at the high right atrium and at the ostium of the coronary sinus, wholly from the right atrium.[2] A continuous overdrive pacing approach has been developed. Initially due to the availability of technology, a high lower and upper rate limit were chosen to establish continuous pacing. More recently, other algorithms such as the continuous atrial pacing method using rate stabilization have become available in some devices and will be applied to achieve the same degree of atrial pacing.[17]

Potential Mechanisms of Efficacy

Table 1 enumerates the potential mechanisms of efficacy of atrial pacing methods in prevention of atrial fibrillation. There are a variety of potentially antiarrhythmic effects ranging from effects on triggering atrial premature beats, alteration of atrial electrophysiology, and prevention of conditions that promote initiation of atrial fibrillation such as bradycardia. Many of these mechanisms are equally applicable to single-site pacing and multisite pacing methods. However, effects on the atrial fibrillation substrate, impact on the dispersion of refractoriness, atrial fibrillation initiation, and mechanical, hormonal, and possibly autonomic effects may differ. The role of individual mechanisms can be considered, based on clinical studies.

Suppression of Triggering Premature Beats

The use of overdrive pacing for suppression of atrial premature beats is a long established concept. In a more formal study, Murgatroyd and colleagues[18] employed a crossover prospective study design to test a new overdrive pacing algorithm for atrial premature beat suppression in 70 patients. The pacing algorithm reduced atrial premature beats in 26% of patients and increased them in 11% (P=0.02). Atrial salvoes were reduced in 17% and increased in 11% (P=0.04). Overall, atrial fibrillation episodes were reduced in 16% and increased in 11% (P=NS). This was observed more often in patients with frequent atrial fibrillation. It can be concluded

---

Table 1
Prevention of AF by Dual RA Pacing

Electrophysiology

- Reduced RA and LA activation time
- Earlier recovery of excitability at sites of critical conduction delay
- Closely coupled APBs encounter less delayed conduction
- Window for AF initiation is decreased
- Biatrial pacing has similar effects

Clinical electrophysiologic effects of dual-site right atrial pacing inpatients with atrial fibrillation. AF = atrial fibrillation; APB = atrial premature beat; LA = left atrial; RA = right atrial.

that atrial overdrive pacing has favorable effects in selected patients and can reduce the density of atrial premature beats that trigger atrial fibrillation.

Prevention of Bradycardia

Bradycardia is associated with lengthening of atrial refractoriness and allows for the potential of long-short sequences with atrial premature beats. Sudden alterations in cycle length can unmask latent inhomogeneity in refractoriness in a substrate prone to reentrant arrhythmias. Importantly, bradycardia can allow the emergence of atrial premature beats with a variety of coupling intervals, further promoting the potential for initiating atrial fibrillation. As indicated earlier, suppression of atrial premature beats with continuous overdrive pacing can be achieved.

Direct Effects on Atrial Substrate

Atrial pacing alters the atrial activation sequence. Pacing from individual atrial sites can produce markedly different atrial activation patterns. Figure 1 illustrates the activation times for single- and dual-site pacing methods at specific atrial sites. Reduction in global atrial activation indicated by P wave duration is noted. Figure 2 summarizes the results of a recently reported series that examined atrial activation times at different right and left atrial regions in patients with atrial fibrillation.[19] Maximal conduction delay is present for high right atrial pacing at the proximal and distal coronary sinus. In contrast, coronary sinus ostial pacing encounters delayed activation at the crista terminalis and at interatrial septal sites. Multisite pacing using dual-site right atrial or biatrial pacing methods markedly alters the activation sequence of both atria. In addition, activation times are reduced at most right and left atrial sites to a similar extent by both methods. Note that single-site atrial pacing methods have variable effects in different atrial regions, advancing activation at some sites, causing no change at others, and occasionally even prolonging activation at other locations. More consistent reduction in activation time at multiple sites is seen with dual-site right atrial or biatrial pacing. These latter pacing modes achieve a reduction in P wave duration, unlike single-site pacing methods. Earlier activation at multiple atrial sites results in earlier recovery of excitability. These findings are of particular value in patients with advanced interatrial block, as well as those with relatively normal P wave duration. Daubert and coworkers[1] have described reduction and even normalization of P wave duration in patients with advanced interatrial block with biatrial

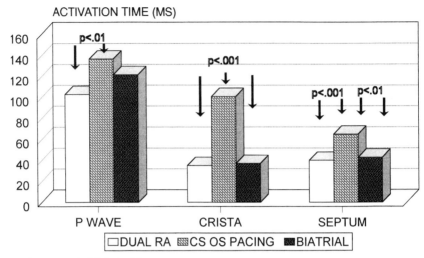

Delfaut et al: JACC Feb. 1977

Figure 1. Right atrial activation times at specific atrial sites and global atrial activation assessed by P wave duration in patients with atrial flutter or fibrillation during novel single- and dual-site pacing modes. Note that P wave duration is reduced by dual-site right atrial pacing, and atrial activation times are reduced at the measured right atrial sites with both dual-site pacing methods. BIATRIAL = dual-site pacing from high right atrium and distal coronary sinus; CS OS = coronary sinus ostial; DUAL RA = dual-site right atrial pacing from the high right atrium and ostium of the coronary sinus.

pacing, but could not achieve this with right atrial or left atrial pacing. Another potential mechanism that may be operative is pacing that is performed at a site contralateral to the site of origin of the triggering premature beat. In this scenario, the premature beat can fail to achieve a coupling interval of sufficient prematurity to initiate atrial tachyarrhythmias. This has been demonstrated acutely in the electrophysiology laboratory, with use of coronary sinus pacing with high right atrial extrastimuli.[19,20] For this method to be effective, it presupposes unifocal origin of atrial premature beats and usually a single arrhythmia substrate. Further evaluation of this method in long-term studies did not show any advantage over single-site atrial pacing from the high right atrium, but does not negate its value in a given patient.[21]

Reduction of Dispersion of Atrial Refractoriness

Dispersion of atrial refractoriness in different atrial regions has been described in patients with atrial fibrillation. In the study by Wood et al,[6] the basis for this may lie in APD variability in different atrial regions. Consistently, left atrial site had a longer APD. Multisite pacing methods synchronize atrial activation and reduce the dispersion in recovery of excitability. This reduction in dispersion may have significant antiarrhythmic benefit for preventing initiating reentrant rhythms. Mehra and Hill[22] have described a variety of circumstances including single-site pacing from within an abnormal region or dual-site pacing of normal and abnormal regions, which can result in reduction of conduction delay for subsequent premature beats by this mechanism.

Propagation of Atrial Premature Beats

The above-mentioned series of changes induced by atrial pacing, particularly multisite pacing, on the arrhythmia substrate translate into alteration of propagation and initiation of repetitive beats by atrial premature depolarizations. Multisite atrial pacing using both dual-site right atrial and biatrial pacing methods has resulted in reduction in incremental conduction delay for closely coupled (250 milliseconds) high right atrial extrastimuli.[19] The impact on moderately or late coupled extrastimuli (350 or 400 milliseconds) has not been discernible. This reduction in conduction delay has varied among different atrial regions and can range from 10% to 40% of the incremental delay.[19]

Prevention of Atrial Fibrillation Initiation

These electrophysiologic changes can acutely result in the suppression of inducible atrial fibrillation. Prakash et al[23] noted that reproducibly inducible atrial fibrillation and atrial flutter could be suppressed in 56% of patients with the spontaneous arrhythmia and coexisting heart disease. They used pretreatment with a dual-site right atrial pacing drive train of 8 paced beats, and showed arrhythmia suppression despite the application of the same premature extrastimuli at the identical site of application as well as after completion of a full stimulation protocol, using 3 premature beats and 2 or more right atrial pacing sites.[23] Experimental studies by Hill et al[24] and others have indicated that the window for initiation of atrial fibrillation is reduced by the application of this dual-site atrial pacing train, most probably due to the earlier recovery of excitability of the involved tissues in arrhythmogenesis. Yu et al[25] also noted that biatrial pacing suppressed reproducibly inducible atrial fibrillation in 67% of patients with lone atrial fibrillation.

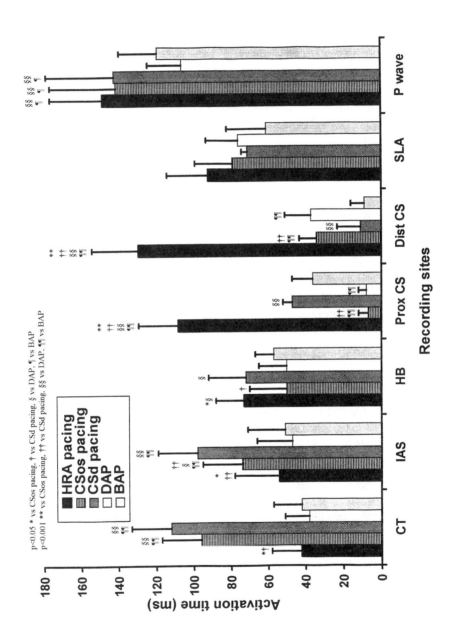

35693$48F2.TP

Clinical Experience

Dual-site atrial pacing methods have been applied chronically in a variety of arrhythmias and disease states. These include typical and atypical atrial flutter, paroxysmal, persistent, and chronic atrial fibrillation occurring in the setting of coronary disease, cardiomyopathies, valvular heart disease, hypertension, and congenital heart disease. Table 2 summarizes one series describing clinical application of biatrial pacing in patients with intra-atrial block and atypical atrial flutter.[1] Table 3 enumerates much of the clinical experience reported to date. Most clinical series report 75% to 80% or greater long-term efficacy when drug and pacing therapy is optimized. In contrast, lower success rates were obtained in some series, often related to lead problems or absence of concomitant drug therapy.

Clinical experience with dual-site pacing in patients with refractory symptomatic atrial fibrillation at our center now exceeds 65 patients. Clinical and arrhythmia characteristics in patients undergoing this procedure show a mean age of 67 years with a mean atrial fibrillation duration of 56 months. Paroxysmal atrial fibrillation was the presentation in 29 patients, persistent atrial fibrillation in 18 patients, and chronic atrial fibrillation in 13 patients. Figure 3 identifies the indication for pacemaker insertion in these patients. Fifty-one percent of all patients had no primary bradyarrhythmia with symptomatic refractory atrial fibrillation. Their mean left atrial diameter was 40 mm with a mean left ventricular ejection fraction

---

Table 2
Multisite Atrial Pacing for Arrhythmias in
Patients with Atrial Conduction Block

- 30 consecutive patients with IACB, mean age 68 yrs, 60% male
- Mean P wave duration 181 ms, IACT = 150 ms
- 83% had severe LA dilatation
- 63% had SND; 80% had AV block
- 80% had atrial flutter (type 2 in 1, atypical in 19 & both in 5); 43% had AF; 30% AT
- Failed an average of 2.5 drugs

Reported experience with patients with refractory atrial flutter and interatrial conduction block from Rennes, France. AF = atrial fibrillation; AT = atrial tachycardia; AV = atrioventricular; IACB = intra-atrial conduction block; IACT = intra-atrial conduction time; LA = left atrial; SND = sinus node dysfunction. From Reference 1.

Table 3
Pilot Observational Trials of Dual-Site Pacing
in Patients with Refractory Atrial Fibrillation

Author	Pts	Follow-up	Efficacy	Mode	Drug RX
Daubert	86	1–8 yrs	64%	Biatrial	Y
Saksena	85	1–6 yrs (n=30)	86% (n=30)	Dual RA	Y
Vardas	10	1.5 yrs	80%	Dual RA	Y
Hayes	10	0.5 yrs.	50%	Dual RA	N
Holt	14	1 yr	86%	Biatrial	?
Sopher	4	<2 yrs	25%	Biatrial	?
Boccadamo	19	2–12 mos	91%	Dual RA	Y
Total	155	2–60 mos	25%–87%		

Total and average values for each column are presented on the last line. Drug RX = concomitant antiarrhythmic drug therapy; Pts = patients; RA = right atrial.

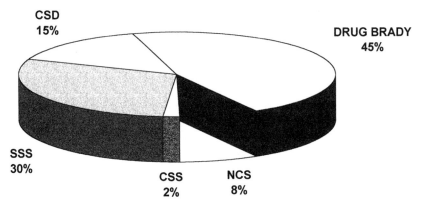

Figure 3. Indications for permanent pacemaker insertion in patients receiving dual-site right atrial pacing systems at the Atlantic Health System-Eastern Heart Institute during 1994 through 1997. CSD = conduction system disease; CSS = carotid sinus syndrome; DRUG BRADY = drug-induced bradycardia; NCS = neurocardiogenic syncope; SSS = sick sinus syndrome.

of 46%. They were refractory to an average of 3 antiarrhythmic drugs prior to insertion of the pacing system.

Clinical Results

The long-term results of the first 30 patients in the pilot study have been reported.[21] These patients had a mean arrhythmia-free interval of 8 days. Twenty-five of 30 patients maintained an atrial-based paced rhythm at last follow-up ranging from 3 to 43 months. One patient was censored due to heart transplant referral, and 4 patients continued in or progressed to chronic atrial fibrillation. During the initial crossover phase of the study, both single- and dual-site pacing were employed, but long-term patients have been maintained in the dual-site right atrial pacing mode alone. Patients were continued on previously ineffective antiarrhythmic drugs or drug therapy was discontinued.

During long-term follow-up, occasional atrial fibrillation recurrences were noted in the different pacing modes. Seven of 25 patients had a recurrence during single-site right atrial pacing. Four of these patients subsequently achieved control with dual-site right atrial pacing while 3 patients continued in or progressed to chronic atrial fibrillation. Three of 29 patients in dual-site right atrial pacing had recurrences of the arrhythmia that was subsequently controlled by change in antiarrhythmic drug therapy. There was a significant increase in arrhythmia-free intervals with all atrial pacing modes, and a significant incremental benefit of dual-site right atrial pacing during the initial crossover phase of the study (Fig. 4). On long-term follow-up, now up to 5 years, actuarial analysis shows freedom from symptomatic atrial fibrillation recurrences in 78% of patients at 1 year, 63% at 2 years, and 56% at 3 years with dual-site right atrial pacing. Long-term rhythm control was achieved in 86% of patients. The need for cardioversion therapy was 80%

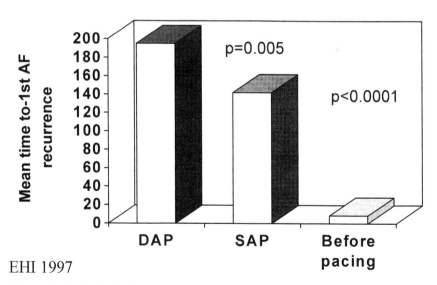

EHI 1997

Figure 4. Arrhythmia Suppression with Atrial Pacing: Arrhythmia-free intervals in days (Y axis) during preimplant pacing period (control), during single-site atrial pacing (SAP) and dual-site right atrial pacing (DAP) in the initial crossover period of the study. (Data derived from Reference 2.) Patients were continued on previously ineffective antiarrhythmic drugs. There is a significant improvement in this parameter with all atrial pacing modes with an incremental benefit of dual- over single-site atrial pacing. (See text for details.)

in the year prior to pacemaker insertion, declining to less than 20% of all patients during the follow-up period.[26] Recurrent cardioversion was rare, with no patient needing more than 3 shocks during the follow-up period. One patient who failed rhythm control had a system explant due to a pocket infection secondary to a surgical procedure at an adjacent site. There was a marked reduction in use of antiarrhythmic drugs and anticoagulation.[27]

Complications (Table 4)

Coronary sinus ostial lead dislodgment occurred intraoperatively in one patient, requiring immediate lead repositioning. There have been no late lead dislodgments or fractures. Other complications are similar to those noted during routine pacemaker insertion. These include high right atrial lead dislodgment (1 patient), right ventricular threshold rise (2 patients), pneumothorax requiring evacuation (1 patient), late pacemaker pocket infection (1 patient), and a local pocket twitch with the Y adapter (1 patient). One patient has come to generator replacement without evidence of lead or Y connector problems on pocket examination. Oversensing of ventricular activity by the wide bipole used in multisite atrial pacing has been noted by us and is often corrected by switching to unipolar sensing or shortening the atrioventricular conduction interval for the pacemaker.[28]

Clinical Trials of Dual-Site Right Atrial Pacing

Two prospective, randomized clinical trials have been initiated to compare the efficacy of dual-site atrial pacing, single-site atrial pacing, and support pacing. The Dual Site Atrial Pacing to Prevent Atrial Fibrillation (DAP-PAF) trial[29] has now been under way for approximately 1 year in North

---

Table 4
Safety Profile of Dual-Site Right Atrial Pacing from the
Atlantic Health System-Eastern Heart Institute Experience

- 65 implants (1994–1998)
- CS lead dislodgement
  - –Intraoperative = 1 (1.5%)
  - –Late = 0
- HRA lead dislodgement = 1 (1.5%)
- RV threshold rise = 2 (1.5%)
- Pneumothorax = 1 (1.5%)
- Lead pocket late infection = 1 (1.5%)
- Pocket complications = 2 (3%)

CS = coronary sinus; HRA = high right atrium; RV = right ventricular.

America. More than 85 patients have been enrolled, and the study has been expanded from the original 4 to 12 centers in North America. The study compares support pacing (DDI or VDI) with single-site atrial DDDR pacing and dual-site right atrial DDDR pacing in a randomized prospective study design. There is an initial 2-week optimization period for drug and device therapy. Combined pacing and drug therapy is encouraged to ensure a high degree of paced rhythm in the DDDR pacing modes in the trial. Six-month intervals are employed in each mode. The occurrence of two symptomatic atrial fibrillation recurrences prior to completion of each phase initiates a mode change. The primary endpoint is time to symptomatic atrial fibrillation recurrences with documented electrocardiogram or electrogram evidence. The details of the trial are described elsewhere.[28]

The SYNBIAPACE study compares 3 different modes of DDD pacing during 3-month periods in patients with atrial fibrillation and interatrial conduction delay.[1] The modes tested are conventional single-site atrial pacing, biatrial synchronous pacing, and no atrial pacing.

Conclusions

The electrophysiologic basis of dual-site atrial pacing methods and their impact on atrial fibrillation recurrences is now better understood due to experimental and clinical studies. Initial clinical experience is favorable, and randomized clinical trials will further evaluate and elucidate the patient population that benefits from atrial pacing, and select those suitable for dual-site atrial pacing methods.

References

1. Daubert C, Leclercq C, Pavin D, Mabo PH. Biatrial synchronous pacing: A new approach to prevent arrhythmias in patients with atrial conduction block. In Daubert JC, Prystowsky EN, Ripart A (eds): *Prevention of Tachyarrhythmias with Cardiac Pacing.* Armonk, NY: Futura Publishing Co., Inc.; 1997:99-119.
2. Saksena S, Prakash A, Hill M, et al. Prevention of recurrent atrial fibrillation with chronic dual site right atrial pacing. *J Am Coll Cardiol* 1996;28:687-694.
3. Saksena S, Prakash A, Madan N, et al. Prevention of atrial fibrillation by pacing. In Barold SS, Mugica J (eds): *Recent Advances in Cardiac Pacing: Goals for the 21st Century.* Armonk, NY: Futura Publishing Co., Inc.; 1998:101-114.
4. Moe GK. On the multiple wavelet hypothesis of atrial fibrillation. *Arch Int Pharmacodyn Ther* 1962;140:183-188.
5. Wijffels MCEF, Kirchhof CJHJ, Dorland RD, Allessie MA. Atrial fibrillation begets atrial fibrillation. A study in awake chronically instrumented goats. *Circulation* 1995;92:1954-1968.
6. Wood MA, Mangano RA, Schieken RM, et al. Modulation of atrial repolarization by site of pacing in the isolated rabbit heart. *Circulation* 1996;94:1465-1470.
7. Schoels W, Kubler W, Yang H, et al. A unified functional/anatomic substrate for circus movement atrial flutter: Activation and refractory patterns in the canine right atrial enlargement model. *J Am Coll Cardiol* 1993;21:73-84.

8. Cosio FG, Arribas F, Lopez-Gil M, Nunez A. Atrial flutter ablation: Electrophysiological landmarks. *J Intervent Cardiol* 1995;8:677-686.

9. Satoh T, Zipes D. Unequal atrial stretch in dogs increases dispersion of refractoriness conducive to developing atrial fibrillation. *J Cardiac Electrophysiol* 1996;7:833-842.

10. Nattel S, Liu L. Differing sympathetic and vagal effects on atrial fibrillation in dogs: Role of refractoriness heterogeneity. *Am J Physiol* 1997;273:H805-H816.

11. Cosio FG, Palacios J, Vidal JM, et al. Electrophysiologic studies in atrial fibrillation. Slow conduction of premature impulses: A possible manifestation of the background for reentry. *Am J Cardiol* 1983;51:122-130.

12. Buxton AE, Waxman HL, Marchlinski FE, et al. Atrial conduction: Effects of atrial extrastimuli with and without atrial dysarrhythmias. *Am J Cardiol* 1984;54:755-761.

13. Buxton AE, Josephson ME. The role of the P wave duration as a predictor of postoperative atrial arrhythmias. *Chest* 1981;80:68-73.

14. Luck JC, Engel T. Dispersion of atrial refractoriness in patients with sinus node dysfunction. *Circulation* 1979;60:404-411.

15. Coumel P, Friocourt P, Mugica J, et al. Long-term prevention of vagal atrial arrhythmias by atrial pacing at 90/minute: Experience with 6 cases. *PACE* 1983;6:552-560.

16. Daubert C, Mabo PH, Berder V, et al. Atrial tachyarrhythmias associated with high degree interatrial conduction block: Prevention by permanent atrial resynchronisation. *Eur J C P E* 1994;1:35-44.

17. Ricci R, Puglisi A, Azzolini P, et al. Consistent atrial pacing algorithm to suppress recurrent paroxysmal atrial fibrillation: A randomized prospective cross over study. *PACE* 1998;35(II):798.

18. Murgatroyd FD, Nitzsche R, Slade AKB, et al. A new pacing algorithm for overdrive suppression of atrial fibrillation. *PACE* 1994;17:1966-1973.

19. Prakash A, Delfaut P, Krol RB, Saksena S. Regional right and left atrial activation patterns during single- and dual-site atrial pacing in patients with atrial fibrillation. *Am J Cardiol* 1998;82:1197-1204.

20. Papageorgiou P, Anselme F, Kirchhof CJ, et al. Coronary sinus pacing prevents induction of atrial fibrillation. *Circulation* 1997;96:1893-1898.

21. Delfaut P, Saksena S, Prakash A, Krol RB. Long-term outcome of patients with drug-refractory atrial flutter and fibrillation after single- and dual-site right atrial pacing for arrhythmia prevention. *J Am Coll Cardiol* 1998;32:1900-1908.

22. Mehra R, Hill MRS. Prevention of atrial fibrillation/flutter by pacing techniques. In Saksena S, Luderitz B (eds): *Interventional Electrophysiology.* 2nd ed. Armonk, NY: Futura Publishing Co., Inc.; 1996:521-540.

23. Prakash A, Saksena S, Hill M, et al. Acute effects of dual-site right atrial pacing in patients with spontaneous and inducible atrial flutter and fibrillation. *J Am Coll Cardiol* 1997;29:1007-1014.

24. Hill M, Mongeon L, Mehra R. Prevention of atrial fibrillation: Dual site atrial pacing reduces the coupling window of induction of atrial fibrillation. *PACE* 1996;19(II):630. Abstract.

25. Yu W-C, Chen S-A, Tai C-T, et al. Effects of different atrial pacing modes on atrial electrophysiology. *Circulation* 1997;96:2992-2996.

26. Prakash A, Saksena S, Krol R, et al. Necessity for atrial defibrillation shocks during and after implantation of a dual site right atrial pacing system. *PACE* 1997;20(II):1128. Abstract.

27. Prakash A, Delfaut P, Giorgberidze I, et al. Long-term outcome of dual site right atrial pacing and drug therapy in atrial fibrillation: Is elimination of anticoagulant and antiarrhythmic therapy feasible? *Circulation* 1997;96(I):I208. Abstract.
28. Delfaut P, Prakash A, Lewis A, et al. Novel pacing modes interfere with pacemaker diagnostic for atrial fibrillation detection. *J Am Coll Cardiol* 1997;29(2):149A. Abstract.
29. Fitts SM, Hill MRS, Mehra R, et al. Design and implementation of the Dual Site Atrial Pacing to Prevent Atrial Fibrillation (DAPPAF) clinical trial. *J Interven Cardiac Electrophysiol* 1998;2:139-144.

49

Local Capture by Atrial Pacing in Chronic Atrial Fibrillation Monitored by Monophasic Action Potential Recordings

Claudio Pandozi, MD, Mauro Villani, MD and Massimo Santini, MD, FACC, FESC

Introduction

Atrial fibrillation is maintained by multiple wandering wavelets that are continuously reentering themselves.[1-3] The number of wavelets is related to the atrial mass and to the wavelength (product of refractoriness and conduction velocity) of the reentrant circuits.[4,5] Short wavelengths allow the simultaneous presence of a greater number of wavelets, while long wavelengths reduce their number, increasing the probability of their simultaneous extinction and the termination of the arrhythmia.[6]

The types of circuits that have been identified in atrial fibrillation models include leading circle reentry,[7] random reentry,[7] and spiral wave reentry.[8] Each of these mechanisms has typical electrophysiologic features, so that the actual importance of a given model of reentry in human atrial fibrillation can be established.

From Franz MR (ed): *Monophasic Action Potentials: Bridging Cell and Bedside.* ©Futura Publishing Company, Inc., Armonk, NY, 2000.

Local Capture and Local Capture Extension in Human Chronic Atrial Fibrillation

Local atrial pacing capture has been demonstrated in dogs with induced atrial fibrillation[9] and in humans with chronic atrial fibrillation[10] (types I and II according to the Wells classification [Figs. 1 and 2])[11] The possibility of local pacing capture in humans has important implications regarding the electrophysiologic mechanisms underlying the maintenance of chronic atrial fibrillation. In fact, because local capture implies the presence of an excitable gap in at least some phases, it is clear that leading circle reentry (in which there is no excitable gap) is not the only electrophysiologic mechanism maintaining atrial fibrillation in humans.[12] Although the presence of random reentry[13] cannot be excluded, it is unlikely that the very short excitable gap associated with this pattern can account for the frequency of pacing capture observed during chronic atrial fibrillation in humans.[10] Therefore, local pacing capture suggests the presence, at least in some moments, of reentrant circuits with large excitable gaps.[7] An alternative explanation has been proposed in the spiral wave hypothesis,[8] which states that the core of the reentrant wave fronts remains excitable but is not excited during reentry.

In our study[10] of the possibility of local pacing capture during chronic atrial fibrillation, we used a Franz catheter for pacing and monophasic action potential (MAP) recordings, and a quadripolar standard lead with 2-mm spacing, which allowed contemporary recording of bipolar electrograms from the distal and proximal pairs, as well as unipolar recording from the distal electrode. To improve the specificity of our results, local atrial capture was assumed to have occurred only when all of the following criteria were met: 1) MAP, unipolar, and bipolar electrograms phase-locked to the stimulus artifact; 2) local atrial cycle length equal to the pacing cycle length; 3) constant morphology of the unipolar and bipolar atrial electrograms and MAPs; 4) constant activation sequence in electrograms from the distal and proximal pairs of the atrial catheter; and, finally, 5) the appearance of endocavitary recordings typical of atrial fibrillation (variable morphology, amplitude, cycle length, and activation sequence of local atrial electrograms and MAPs) at loss of capture or cessation of pacing. Although the use of these strict criteria undoubtedly increased the specificity of our findings, sensitivity was also reduced, since episodes of transient capture or capture limited to the MAP catheter were not considered (see below).

In another study,[14] we evaluated the extension of atrial capture in the lateral wall of the right atrium. An octopolar lead (5-mm interelectrode distance; 6 mm between pairs) was positioned, in the 30° left anterior

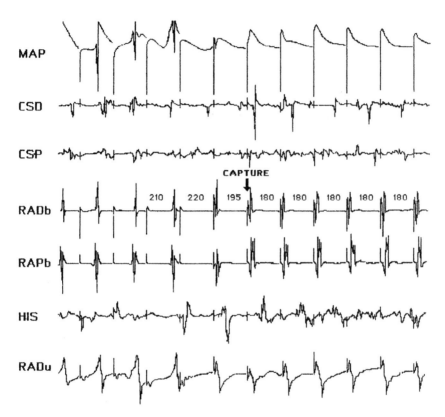

Figure 1. Endocavitary recording showing local capture during type I atrial fibrillation. During pacing at the midlateral right atrial wall level (cycle: 180 milliseconds), the spikes initially fall in the absolute atrial refractory period, as clearly shown by the MAP, and are evidently out of phase with respect to the MAP and to the local unipolar and bipolar electrograms. At the moment indicated by the arrow, the MAP, the unipolar, and both the proximal and distal bipolar electrograms from the lateral right atrial wall become constantly phase-locked to the stimulus artifact. The configuration of the electrograms becomes uniform, as does the local activation sequence, indicating that capture has occurred. Capture does not extend to the septal right atrium and to the coronary sinus, which show autonomous electrical activity. CSD = coronary sinus distal; CSP = coronary sinus proximal; RAD = lateral right atrium distal; RAP = lateral right atrium proximal; His = septal right atrium; b = bipolar recording; u = unipolar recording.

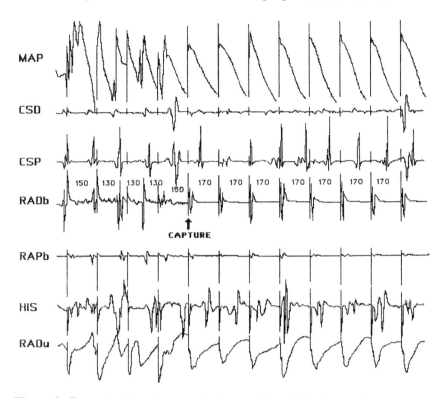

Figure 2. Example of local capture during type II atrial fibrillation. During pacing at the low-lateral right atrial wall level (cycle: 170 milliseconds), at the moment indicated by the arrow, the MAP, the unipolar, and the bipolar atrial electrogram of the lateral atrial wall become phase-locked to the stimulus artifacts and the configuration of the electrograms becomes constant, as does the local activation sequence, suggesting that local atrial capture has occurred. Septal right atrium and coronary sinus show autonomous electrical activity. CSD = coronary sinus distal; CSP = coronary sinus proximal; RAD = lateral right atrium distal; RAP = lateral right atrium proximal; His = septal right atrium; b = bipolar recording; u = unipolar recording.

oblique view, in the lateral right atrium and simultaneous recording of bipolar electrograms were obtained from the 4 pairs. A Franz catheter was used for MAP recording and pacing. The octopolar and MAP catheters were positioned approximately 10 mm apart in the midlateral atrial wall. Capture extended radially up to 40 mm from the pacing site in roughly half of the capture episodes, and up to 30 mm in the other half (Figs. 3 and 4). In only 2 of the 48 episodes, more limited capture extension (≤20 and ≤10 mm) was observed. Pacing termination of atrial fibrillation was never observed, and the mean capture extension in patients treated with antiarrhythmic drugs was significantly greater than that seen in untreated patients.

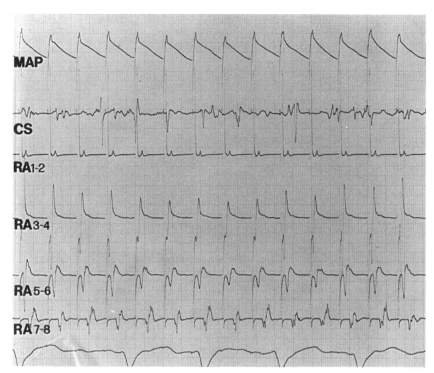

Figure 3. Endocavitary recording showing local capture of all 4 bipolar pairs implying capture extension of approximately 4 cm. During pacing at the midlateral right atrial wall site (cycle: 160 milliseconds), the MAP and all 4 bipolar electrograms are constantly phase-locked to the stimulus artifact. The configuration of the electrograms is uniform, as is the local activation sequence, indicating that capture has occurred. No capture is observed from the coronary sinus pair. CS = coronary sinus; RA1-2, RA3-4, RA5-6, RA7-8 = electrograms from the 4 bipolar pairs of the octopolar at 1-cm distance from the pacing Franz catheter. RA1-2 is the electrogram recorded by the pair nearest, and RA7-8 is the electrogram recorded by the most distant pair from the Franz catheter tip. (Paper speed: 100 mm/s.)

Extensive local capture during atrial fibrillation has important theoretical implications for treatment of this arrhythmia. It suggests that atrial fibrillation might be terminated by reducing the fibrillating tissue mass below the critical value necessary for perpetuation of the arrhythmia[2]—a goal that could theoretically be achieved by simultaneous multisite pacing. Pacing capture might produce a more organized form of atrial fibrillation, thus reducing the defibrillation threshold.[15] The latter phenomenon might have important implications regarding the diffusion of low-energy intracardiac cardioversion of atrial fibrillation using temporary leads or automatic atrial defibrillator.

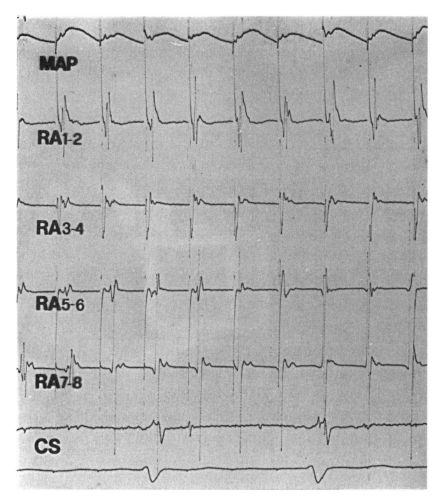

Figure 4. Endocavitary recording showing local capture at only 2 of the 4 bipolar pairs implying capture extension of approximately 2 cm. During pacing at the midlateral right atrial wall site (cycle: 180 milliseconds), the MAP and the two bipolar electrograms nearest to the pacing site (RA1-2, RA3-4) are constantly phase-locked to the stimulus artifact, while the 3rd and the 4th bipolar electrogram and the coronary sinus (RA5-6, RA7-8, and CS) are clearly out of phase with respect to the spikes. Moreover, the configuration of the two electrograms nearest to the pacing site is uniform, as is the local activation sequence, confirming that capture has occurred. CS = coronary sinus; RA1-2, RA3-4, RA5-6, RA7-8 = electrograms from the 4 bipolar pairs of the octopolar at 1-cm distance from the pacing Franz catheter. RA1-2 is the electrogram recorded by the pair nearest, and RA7-8 is the elecrogram recorded by the most distant pair from the Franz catheter tip. (Paper speed: 100 mm/s.)

MAP Characteristics During Atrial Fibrillation

MAP recordings during atrial fibrillation are generally very irregular, and the depolarization phase is slowed and distorted.[16] The severity of these alterations is related to the degree of synchronization of the arrhythmia at a specific site and to the recording site itself. In fact, local atrial fibrillation in the right lateral wall anteriorly to the crista terminalis appears to be more organized than that occurring in the septum. We have demonstrated that the degree and the changes in the severity of MAP alterations occurring during atrial fibrillation are not artifacts but are related to the organization and variation in the degree of organization of the arrhythmia, respectively.[17] Bipolar electrograms were recorded simultaneously from the distal and proximal pairs of a quadripolar lead, and MAPs were obtained from a Franz catheter positioned 10 mm from the latter. Using the Wells method,[11] we classified the atrial fibrillation as: type I (discrete electrograms separated by an isoelectric baseline free of perturbations), type II atrial fibrillation (discrete electrograms, with perturbation of the baseline), or type III (absence of discrete complexes and isoelectric intervals). MAPs were arbitrarily classified, based on their morphology, as: type I (almost normal, similar to that recorded during atrial flutter), type II (partially altered, with depolarization and repolarization phases that were markedly slowed, distorted, and of variable amplitude), and type III (totally altered, in which the normal phases were no longer discernible). In basal recordings we found a perfect correspondence (100%) between type I and type III atrial fibrillation and type I and type III MAP, respectively; type II MAPs were recorded in approximately 70% of the sites showing type II atrial fibrillation. Morphologic changes in bipolar electrograms occurred during recording at 23 sites. Again, perfect correspondence (100%) was found between type I and III atrial fibrillation and type I and III MAPs, respectively, while type II MAPs were observed in approximately 70% of the situations in which type I or III atrial fibrillation changed to type II. We have concluded that MAP morphology and MAP modifications are not related to recording artifacts but to the complexity of local atrial fibrillation and to changes in local activation. Therefore, MAP recording allows validation of the Wells classification[11] of local atrial fibrillation.

Another aspect of the MAP during chronic atrial fibrillation is its triangular shape, which is the result of a shorter phase 2 and the decreased slope of phase 3.[18] It is very interesting to note how these MAP features, which were described many years ago, are in total agreement with more recent findings regarding atrial electrical remodeling and the changes in membrane ion flux underlying the latter phenomenon.[18-21] The ionic remodeling responsible for action potential changes in a canine model of atrial fibrillation is predominantly due to a reduction in I_{ca}, although I_{to} decreases have also been reported.[22] The reduction in I_{ca} accounts for the shortening of the MAP and the refractory period, and for the loss of the plateau that gives the MAP its specific triangular shape. In fact, the same effects on MAP morphology are produced by nifedipine, while exposure of fibrillating atrial cells to Bay K 8644, a drug that enhances I_{ca}, restores the plateau and MAP duration.[18]

Advantages of MAP Recording During Atrial Fibrillation Local Capture Attempts

The use of MAP recording during local capture attempts also has some practical advantages. First, calculation of the FF interval, and consequently the occurrence of capture, can sometimes be evaluated using only the distance between two consecutive MAP upstrokes.[23] Our experience confirms that, at least for type I or type II MAPs, the upstroke and its notch, which correspond to the intrinsic deflection of the unipolar recording, are always well defined. In contrast, the FF interval cannot always be evaluated using the intrinsic deflection on the unipolar recording because of the low amplitude of the signal and/or contamination by electrical activity in the neighboring area. Sometimes the FF interval and the occurrence of capture are difficult to determine in the bipolar recording. This can occur when capture extension is limited and there is fusion between the spontaneous activation of atrial fibrillation and pacing activation at the bipolar recording site. Second, episodes of very local capture, missed by both unipolar and bipolar recordings, can be detected only by MAP recordings, due to the particular configuration of the Franz catheter, in which the pacing and recording sites are almost identical (Fig. 5). The presence of transient or very local capture in our study is demonstrated by shortening of the local FF interval that occurs before the achievement of "true" capture, ie, that defined by our strict study criteria.[2] In these cases, if we look very carefully at the tracing, we often find that transient capture limited to the MAP recordings actually occurs before the achievement of stable capture of the unipolar and bipolar recordings, which explains the acceleration of the local atrial fibrillation observed during pacing "before capture." A third advantage of MAP recording is that it can be useful for clarifying the mechanism of capture failure or delay of capture after the initiation of pacing. For example, in Figure 1, it is clear from the MAP recording that initially capture is not achieved, because the spikes fall during the atrial repolarization phase. Capture actually begins when the spike falls outside of the phase of atrial refractoriness. Finally, the use of the Franz catheter not only provides MAP recordings, it is also associated with

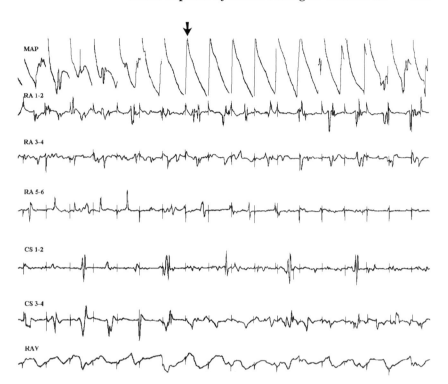

Figure 5. Episode of possible very local capture limited to the MAP recordings. During pacing at the midlateral right atrial wall site (cycle: 170 milliseconds), initially the spikes are clearly out of phase with respect to the MAP and to the local unipolar and bipolar electrograms. At the moment indicated by the arrow, the MAP becomes phase-locked to the stimulus artifact for 4 beats, while the unipolar and bipolar electrograms from the lateral right atrial wall remain out of phase, suggesting that local capture limited to the MAP catheter has occurred. CS 1-2 = distal coronary sinus; CS 3-4 = proximal coronary sinus; RA 1-2, RA 3-4, RA 5-6 = electrograms from 3 bipolar pairs of the octopolar lead at 1-cm distance from the pacing Franz catheter. (Paper speed: 100 mm/s.)

a very low pacing threshold.[16] This is important, because it is obviously not possible to test the pacing threshold during local capture attempts. Moreover, low-energy stimulation may reduce the amplitude of the spike and the distortion of the electrogram by the spike itself, facilitating interpretation of the tracings.

Future Research on Local Atrial Capture Using MAP Recordings

MAP recording with use of the Franz catheter has other advantages that have not yet been fully utilized. We have demonstrated atrial capture only in type I and type II atrial fibrillation, but capture of type III atrial fibrillation cannot be excluded, because our criteria are applicable only to capture episodes involving at least 15 mm of atrial tissue. Local capture might also be possible in type III atrial fibrillation, but its extension would probably be more limited than in type I and type II atrial fibrillation. In fact, type III atrial fibrillation is a very complex arrhythmia in terms of the number of reentrant circuits, the presence of lines of conduction block, and the frequency of activation of atrial cells. Capture extension is therefore limited by the activation of atrial cells near the pacing site by fibrillation wavelets with an interval shorter than that of the pacing interval, that therefore collide with the paced wave fronts. Moreover, intra-atrial conduction block of the paced wave front may occur. Our criteria would not detect transient capture extending only few millimeters. It can be detected only by a careful analysis of MAP recordings from the Franz catheter, because the stimulation and recording sites are almost identical. In fact, in Figure 6, during type III atrial fibrillation, at a certain moment

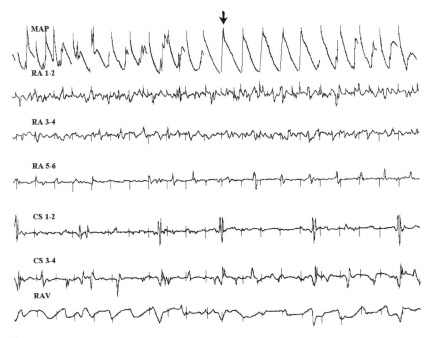

Figure 6. Episode of possible capture limited to the MAP recordings during type III atrial fibrillation. At a certain moment and only for few beats (arrow) MAPs seem to be in phase with the stimulus artifact, and the local atrial cycle length is equal to the pacing cycle length (150 milliseconds). In contrast, type III atrial fibrillation is still being recorded by the bipolar pairs of the quadripolar lead 1 cm away from the Franz catheter. This behavior strongly suggests that capture of type III atrial fibrillation limited to the MAP catheter could have occurred. (Paper speed: 100 mm/s.)

and only for few beats, MAPs seem to be in phase with the stimulus artifact, and the local atrial cycle length is equal to the pacing cycle length. In contrast, type III atrial fibrillation is still being recorded by the bipolar pairs of the quadripolar lead 1 cm away from the Franz catheter. This behavior strongly suggests that capture of type III atrial fibrillation limited to the MAP catheter has occurred. With the same method, the window of capture during type III atrial fibrillation could also be determined. Although further studies are necessary to confirm these preliminary observations, the careful analysis of the MAP recordings seems to suggest that local pacing capture is also possible in some phases of type III atrial fibrillation, but its extension is more limited than in type I and type II atrial fibrillation. This means that, in type III atrial fibrillation as well, leading circle reentry is not the only mechanism, and that an excitable gap is present at least at some moments during this complex and disorganized arrhythmia. These findings are consistent with the results of Konings et al[7] in induced atrial fibrillation in humans. They found a shifting leading circle in only 3% of the fibrillation cycles in the more organized forms of the arrhythmia (corresponding to type I of the Wells classification) and in 66% of those in the more complex forms (corresponding to Wells type III atrial fibrillation).

Conclusions

Experimental atrial fibrillation and atrial fibrillation induced in human beings have been shown to be maintained by mechanisms other than leading circle reentry or random reentry. The achievement of local pacing capture during spontaneous chronic atrial fibrillation in humans indicates that leading circle reentry is not the unique mechanism maintaining the arrhythmia. Atrial MAP recordings present particular features during atrial fibrillation, and the MAP characteristics reflect the effects of electrical remodeling induced by the arrhythmia. Moreover, the MAP morphology and its changes are not secondary to recording artifacts, but are truly related to the degree of synchronization of the arrhythmia and to changes in its complexity. During local pacing capture attempts, MAP recordings facilitate calculation of the FF interval and clarify the reason for capture failure or delay. They allow detection of episodes of local pacing capture with limited temporal and spatial extension. Finally, MAP recordings with the Franz catheter may disclose episodes of transient and spatially limited capture during type III atrial fibrillation.

References

1. Moe GK. On the multiple wavelet hypothesis of atrial fibrillation. *Arch Int Pharmacodyn Ther* 1962;140:183-188.

2. Allessie MA, Lammers WJEP, Bonke FIM, Hollen J. Experimental evaluation of Moe's multiple wavelet hypothesis of atrial fibrillation. In Zipes DP, Jalife J (eds): *Cardiac Electrophysiology and Arrhythmias.* Orlando: Grune & Stratton; 1985:265-275.

3. Allessie MA, Lammers WJEP, Rensma PL, Bonke FIM. Flutter and fibrillation in experimental modes: What has been learned that can be applied to humans. In Brugada P, Wellens HJJ (eds): *Cardiac Arrhythmias: Where to Go from Here.* Mount Kisco, NY: Futura Publishing Co., Inc.; 1987:67-82.

4. Smeets JL, Allessie MA, Lammers WJEP, et al. The wavelength of the cardiac impulse and reentrant arrhythmias in isolated rabbit atrium. *Circ Res* 1986;58:96-108.

5. Rensma PL, Allessie MA, Lammers WJEP, et al. Length of excitation wave and susceptibility to reentrant atrial arrhythmias in normal conscious dogs. *Circ Res* 1988;62:395-410.

6. Allessie MA, Wijffels MCEF, Kirchhof CJ. Experimental models of arrhythmias: Toys or truth? *Eur Heart J* 1994;15(suppl A):2-8.

7. Konings KTS, Kirchhof CJ, Smeets JRLM, et al. High-density mapping of electrically induced atrial fibrillation in humans. *Circulation* 1994;89:1665-1680.

8. Ikeda T, Uchida T, Hough D, et al. Mechanism of spontaneous termination of functional reentry in isolated canine right atrium. Evidence for the presence of an excitable but nonexcited core. *Circulation* 1996;94:1962-1973.

9. Kirchhof C, Chorro F, Scheffer GJ, et al. Regional entrainment of atrial fibrillation studied by high-resolution mapping in open-chest dogs. *Circulation* 1993;88:736-749.

10. Pandozi C, Bianconi L, Villani M, et al. Local capture by atrial pacing in spontaneous chronic atrial fibrillation. *Circulation* 1997;95:2416-2422.

11. Wells JL Jr, Karp RB, Kouchoukos NT, et al. Characterisation of atrial fibrillation in man: Studies following open heart surgery. *PACE* 1978;1:426-438.

12. Allessie MA, Bonke FIM, Schopman JG. Circus movement in rabbit atrial muscle as a mechanism of tachycardia. III. The "Leading Circle" Concept: A new model of circus movement in cardiac tissue without the involvement of an anatomical obstacle. *Circ Res* 1977;41:9-18.

13. Allessie MA, Konings, Kirchhof C. Mapping of atrial fibrillation. In Olsson SB, Allessie MA, Campbell RW (eds): *Atrial Fibrillation: Mechanisms and Therapeutic Strategies.* Armonk, NY: Futura Publishing Co., Inc.; 1994:37-49.

14. Pandozi C, Villani M, Castro C, et al. Spatial extension of local pacing capture in the lateral wall of the right atrium during clinical chronic atrial fibrillation. *G Ital Cardiol* 1999;29:107-114.

15. Kalman JM, Olgin JE, Karch MR, Lesh MD. Regional entrainment of atrial fibrillation in man. *J Cardiovasc Electrophysiol* 1996;7:867-876.

16. Franz MR. The role of monophasic action potential recording in atrial fibrillation. In Olsson SB, Allessie MA, Campbell RW (eds): *Atrial Fibrillation: Mechanisms and Therapeutic Strategies.* Armonk, NY; Futura Publishing Co., Inc.; 1994;109-125.

17. Pandozi C, Villani M, Toscano S, et al. Electrophysiologic characteristics of chronic atrial fibrillation: Results obtained by recording both bipolar electrograms and monophasic action potential. *Eur Heart J* 1996;17(suppl):523. Abstract.

18. Yue L, Feng J, Gaspo R, et al. Ionic remodeling underlying action potential changes in a canine model of atrial fibrillation. *Circ Res* 1997;81:512-525.

19. Wijffels M, Kirchhof C, Dorland R, Allessie M. Atrial fibrillation begets atrial fibrillation. A study in awake chronically instrumented goats. *Circulation* 1995;92:1954-1968.
20. Tieleman RG, De Langen CDJ, Van Gelder IC, et al. Verapamil reduces tachycardia-induced electrical remodeling of the atria. *Circulation* 1997;95:1945-1953.
21. Daoud EG, Knight BP, Weiss R, et al. Effect of verapamil and procainamide on atrial fibrillation-induced electrical remodeling in humans. *Circulation* 1997;96:1542-1550.
22. Van Wagoner DR, Pond AL, McCarthy PM, et al. Outward K+ current densities and Kv1.5 expression are reduced in chronic human atrial fibrillation. *Circ Res* 1997;80:772-781.
23. Hedin E, Yuan S, Pripp CM, et al. Evaluation of the atrial refractoriness during atrial fibrillation using the monophasic action potential recordings. *Eur Heart J* 1997;18(suppl):317. Abstract.

50

A Novel Automated Method to Detect FF Intervals During Atrial Fibrillation Using the Monophasic Action Potential Technique

Michèle Adam, MD, Vincenzo Barbaro, PhD,
Pietro Bartolini, PhD, Giovanni Calcagnini, PhD,
Sandra Morelli, PhD, Fulvio Bellocci, MD,
Paolo Zecchi, MD and
Annibale Sandro Montenero, MD

Introduction

Despite the latest advances in therapies, atrial fibrillation is a common arrhythmia that remains difficult to treat with drugs or with interventional techniques. Even though the mechanism that maintains atrial fibrillation was well described by Moe[1] and by Allessie et al,[2] part of the problem still lies in the poor understanding of the mechanisms that initiate it.

Moe and Allessie et al have shown that atrial fibrillation is based on the continuous propagation of various individual wavelets in the atria that reenter themselves or one another (multiple wavelet reentry). Later studies, performed during cardiac surgery with high-density atrial mapping, docu-

From Franz MR (ed): *Monophasic Action Potentials: Bridging Cell and Bedside.*
©Futura Publishing Company, Inc., Armonk, NY, 2000.

mented that multiple wavelets wander around both anatomic and functional obstacles during recently induced atrial fibrillation.[3,4]

The recording of the monophasic action potentials (MAPs) with a contact electrode catheter provides a panel of data on the morphology of the repolarization and the diastolic interval, and better information on local atrial activation time. The measurement of the duration of the diastolic interval is of utmost importance in clinical electrophysiology, in order to determine, with appropriate sensing, when pacing should be delivered. Without a reliable measurement of the electrophysiologic intervals, synchronized pacing cannot be done and the effect of capture of the arrhythmia (entrainment) cannot be evaluated. The MAP recording technique, first introduced by Franz in the 1980s,[5] permits both recording and pacing at the same site, making possible the simultaneous measurement of effective refractory period and action potential duration.

As the analysis of MAP recordings may remain long and tedious, we developed an automated analysis of FF intervals that allows, with the same accuracy as the electrophysiologist's, to measure FF intervals. This gave us a better understanding of local capture, and might open new pathways in the treatment of atrial fibrillation.

Atrial Fibrillation Types as Seen from MAP Recordings

In general, atrial fibrillation is defined as a rapid atrial rhythm (cycle length <200 milliseconds) with a variable beat-to-beat cycle length (>20 milliseconds), variable morphology, and variable amplitude of recorded electrograms.

With a MAP recording, we were able to define the 3 classic types of atrial fibrillation in a new way:

Type I atrial fibrillation corresponds to irregular atrial complexes of consistent morphology that follow each other with no obvious diastolic interval in between successive depolarizations.

Type II atrial fibrillation would be an intermediate between type I and type III.

Type III is characterized by fragmented atrial complexes. The depolarization is markedly slowed, distorted, and of variable amplitude because the potential does not return to its normal diastolic level but is frequently interrupted by the subsequent depolarization at various degrees of incomplete repolarization (fractionated MAP).

As proposed by Franz,[6] these irregularities in the MAP pattern may reflect the interdigitation of multiple wavelets and the variability of local refractoriness in the area where the MAP is recorded. This supports the multiple wandering wavelets theory.

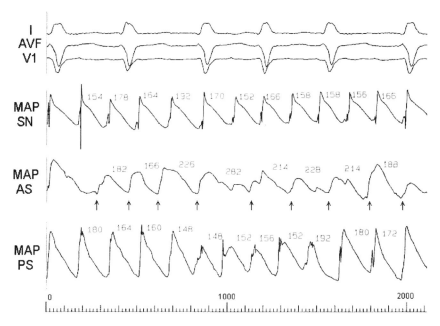

Figure 1. Surface electrocardiogram leads I, aVF, V1, MAP SN, MAP AS, and MAP PS. Arrows indicate the onset of MAP signal. Numbers identify the duration of FF intervals in milliseconds. MAP recordings show 3 different patterns of local atrial activation. At the MAP sinus node (MAP SN) site, the activity recorded is regular and organized (type I atrial fibrillation). The MAP signal at the anterior septum (AS) site is the most fractionated and disorganized (type III atrial fibrillation). At the posterior septum (PS) site, the activity is intermediate between types I and III (type II atrial fibrillation). Fractioning of electrograms might represent different wavelets that collide with each other.

Figure 1 was recorded in a patient in which all 3 types can be simultaneously identified. Type I is recorded by a MAP catheter placed close to the sinus node, type II with one placed on the posterior septum of right atrium, and type III with a MAP catheter placed on the anterior septum of right atrium.

Definition and Measurement of FF Intervals

During atrial fibrillation, the FF interval is defined as the distance between two apexes or nadir of atrial fibrillation waves. It can be measured manually or on paper, or, better, with an on-screen caliper (Fig. 1). As this procedure is long and tedious when a great number of FF intervals must be analyzed, we used a computerized method. This adjustable threshold-crossing algorithm permitted us to identify, with very good accuracy, the FF intervals, even when the electrograms were very fractionated such as in type III atrial fibrillation. It was developed by the engineers of the Italian National Health Institute,[7] and validated by use of the method described by Bland and Altman.[8]

Figure 2 shows an example of the automated FF interval recognition that allowed us to analyze 100 FF intervals and determine the mean FF (MFF) and the shortest FF (SFF) local interval at each site studied.

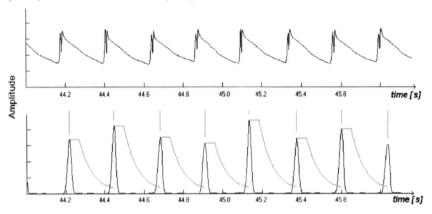

Figure 2. Example of the automated FF interval recognition. Top trace shows the original signal (MAP). Bottom trace shows the filtered signal used for the automated recognition procedure (black line) and the markers of the detected peaks (red lines). The exponential threshold is also depicted (blue lines). See color plate.

Electrophysiology of Atrial Fibrillation

After Moe[1] and Allessie et al[2] provided the experimental evidence that atrial fibrillation is based on multiple wavelet reentry, high-density mapping studies of the electrical excitation of the atria, performed during surgery in humans, showed a variable spectrum of atrial activation due to the complexity of the arcs of conduction block and areas of slow conduction.[3,4] The direction, size, and shape of each wavelet evolves with time, determined by the complex interaction of activation wave fronts with spatially and temporally varying tissue excitability and refractoriness. It has been hypothesized[9] that sustained atrial fibrillation can be determined by the magnitude of the tissue wavelength, defined as the product of refractoriness and conduction velocity. The atrium is activated at a very high rate, and local atrial activation varies continuously in cycle length and morphology.

A relation between local atrial activation during atrial fibrillation and atrial refractoriness has been demonstrated,[10,11] with the assumption that the SFF interval reflects local refractoriness because cardiac cells can be reexcited soon after the refractory period (leading circle reentry).

However, the variation of cycle length during atrial fibrillation might be also caused by the fact that, once their excitability has been recovered, the fibers are reentered after a slight delay by one of the wandering wavelets. This might result in a small gap of excitability because the atrial fibers are not activated at their maximal rate (random reentry). However, the electrophysiologic mechanism of atrial fibrillation still remains poorly understood in clinical electrophysiology, mainly because of the limited capacity of conventional catheters to record local activation time.[12,13]

Atrial Pacing and Local Capture During Atrial Fibrillation

Local capture has been defined as follows: 1) phase-lock of stimulus artifact with the local atrial activation; 2) local atrial cycle length identical to the set pacing cycle length; or 3) local shortening of the atrial fibrillation cycle length.

Several recent studies[14-17] have reported local capture. The presence of an excitable gap during atrial fibrillation has been reported by Kirchhof et al,[14] in a dog model of pacing-induced atrial fibrillation where the area of local capture had a mean diameter from ≤4 cm to ≈6 cm.

In our study, we measured MFF and SFF in each site, before and after pacing, in patients with idiopathic paroxysmal atrial fibrillation in whom the atrial fibrillation was either spontaneous or induced by pacing.

To evaluate the effects of pacing on atrial fibrillation, atrial pacing with a cycle length 10% shorter than SFF was delivered. The choice of the site was based on catheter stability, MAP amplitude, and local FF cycle length. Pacing stimuli were delivered according to the method described by Capucci et al.[15]

Pacing during atrial fibrillation with a cycle length slightly shorter than the mean fibrillation intervals resulted in penetration of the paced wave fronts into an excitable gap between the wandering fibrillation wavelets. The shortening of the pacing cycle length resulted in acceleration of atrial fibrillation and loss of capture. This pacing-induced acceleration of atrial fibrillation was thought to be due to the induction of small leading circle reentry circuits near the site of pacing, maybe determined by a rate-dependent shortening of the refractory period, which is a facilitating mechanism for the induction of this small leading circle reentry. Capucci et al[15] confirmed the existence of an excitable gap during atrial fibrillation in patients suffering from drug refractory paroxysmal atrial fibrillation by using atrial pacing to accelerate the MFF interval at the stimulation site. This acceleration was short-lived and followed by resumption of the original atrial fibrillation rate.

Capture of the right atrium during induced atrial fibrillation was also obtained by Daoud et al[16] in patients referred for supraventricular or ventricular tachycardia catheter ablation. This overdrive pacing during atrial fibrillation resulted, at times, in transient disorganization of the right atrial electrograms, consistent with the hypothesis of the induction of transient small circle leading reentry circuits.

In patients with chronic atrial fibrillation, local atrial capture was obtained in 87% of the sites considered for pacing by Pandozi et al,[17] showing that an excitable gap might also exist in this condition, at least in some phases.

On the basis of the previously reported studies, our experience confirms that atrial pacing shorter than the MFF can locally entrain the recorded wavelets, as demonstrated by the phenomena of capture and acceleration.

Atrial Pacing of Atrial Fibrillation and Loss of Capture

In some patients, capture was lost before the pacing was stopped, and "local capture" lasted from 15 to 30 seconds of stimulation, which, as demonstrated by Janse et al[18] in the canine ventricular myocardium, may be the time required by the atrial fibers to reach a new steady state value of refractoriness at given pacing cycle lengths. This further shortening of refractoriness led to penetration of the local recorded area by new wandering wavelets, which resulted in both acceleration of the FF intervals and loss of capture. An example is shown in Figure 3.

The loss of capture before pacing interruption was also demonstrated by Pandozi et al,[17] but no atrial fibrillation acceleration was detected for the first 20 FF intervals. In their study, the presence of a short interval between the last captured beat and the first noncaptured beat was explained by spontaneous variation in the FF interval. The difference between our observations and those of Pandozi et al might be explained by the fact that during chronic atrial fibrillation the atrial fibers are already activated at their maximal rate and no further shortening of refractoriness can be achieved.

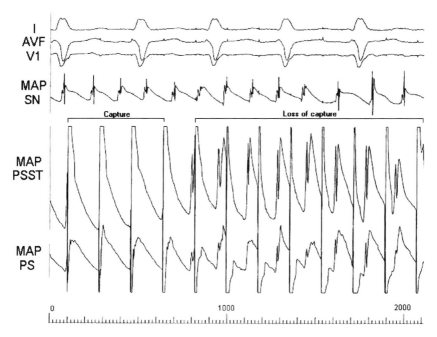

Figure 3. Surface electrocardiogram leads I, aVF, V1, MAP SN, MAP PSST, and MAP PS. This figure shows pacing of atrial fibrillation followed by loss of capture due to the shortening of FF interval.

Atrial Pacing of Atrial Fibrillation Without Loss of Capture

In a few patients, local capture lasted until the interruption of pacing and resulted in a long postpacing interval, perhaps because the capture of a single wandering wavelet was achieved. It is worth noting that, in these 3 patients, the mFF local cycle length before pacing was slightly but not significantly longer than the MFF of the overall population, perhaps reflecting wider and more stable wavelets. An example is shown in Figure 4.

Utility of Multisite MAP Recording During Atrial Fibrillation

In the first part of our study, we simultaneously recorded 3 MAPs in the right atrium during sinus rhythm and during atrial fibrillation. The first MAP catheter was placed close to the sinus node (SN), the second was placed on the anterior septum (AS), and the third on the posterior septum (PS), close to the orifice of the coronary sinus.

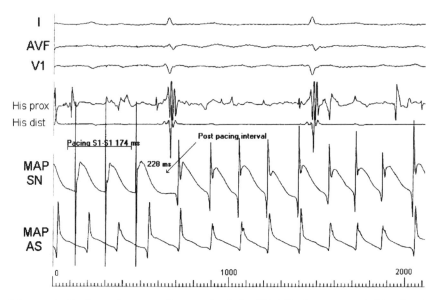

Figure 4. Surface electrocardiogram leads I, aVF, V1, His proximal, His distal, MAP SN, and MAP AS. In this patient, capture was maintained as long as the site was paced. No shortening of MFF interval is visible when pacing is interrupted. The postpacing interval observed confirms the effectiveness of capture. Also note the regular pattern and the more reliable morphology of MAPs recorded at any site compared with atrial electrograms recorded at the His site.

Before pacing, there was no significant statistical difference in MFF or SFF between the 3 sites. We did, however, observe morphologic differences between the sites. In most cases, the atrial fibrillation was more organized on the free wall of the right atrium, with a type I atrial fibrillation, whereas it was least organized on the septum, with a type III atrial fibrillation.

The Effects of Pacing: Interest of Radar Graph Representation and Clinical Implications

In the second part of the study, pacing was delivered in 1 of the 3 atrial sites, either at SN or at PS site, which was then considered as a proximal site. Simultaneous recording was obtained at the two other atrial sites, which were defined as distal sites. For each patient, MFFs at every site were plotted before and after pacing.

We observed that atrial pacing significantly shortened the MFF intervals at the proximal sites, whereas no modification was observed at the distal sites. An example is shown in Figure 5, in which atrial pacing at the AS site does not influence the two other sites.

For each patient, we plotted the FF intervals measured before pacing against those after pacing in a radar graph representation. The intent of this representation is to show, in a very immediate way, the effect of pacing or its absence (Fig. 6).

This technique is helpful in order to understand atrial activation during atrial fibrillation, supporting, at least in part, the multiple wandering wavelets theory described by Moe[1] and Allessie et al,[2] and may improve the algorithms for the detection of atrial fibrillation in new dual-chamber implantable cardioverter defibrillators.

Even if there has been no evidence that multiple-site pacing converts atrial fibrillation to sinus rhythm, it has been shown to reduce recurrences in patients with paroxysmal atrial fibrillation. Thus, MAP recordings might increase atrial sensing during atrial fibrillation in order to deliver an appropriate pacing.

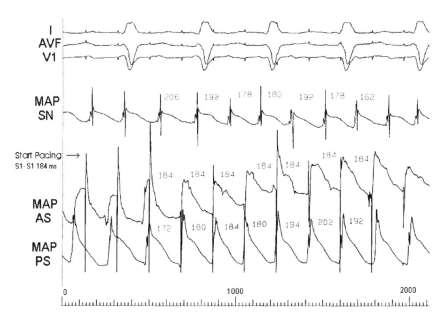

Figure 5. Surface electrocardiogram leads I, aVF, V1, MAP SN, MAP AS, and MAP PS. Arrows indicate the onset of the MAP signal. Numbers identify the duration of FF intervals in milliseconds. This figure shows that pacing with a cycle length of 184 milliseconds captures atrial fibrillation at the anterior septum (AS) site but does not influence sinus node (SN) or posterior septum (PS) sites.

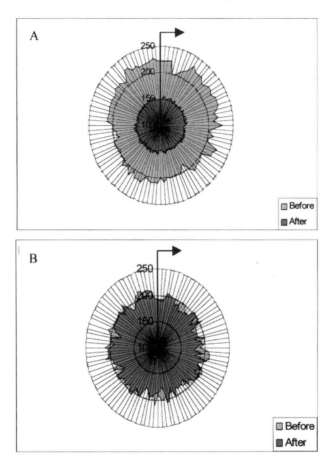

Figure 6. This figure shows 100 FF intervals plotted in radar graph representation. Mean FF intervals are depicted in blue before pacing and in red after pacing. The scale from center to top of figure indicates the FF intervals in milliseconds. Left: marked shortening of FF intervals after pacing (patient A). Right: absence of modification of FF intervals before and after pacing (patient B). See color plate.

Conclusions

MAP recordings are feasible and reliable for use during a standard electrophysiology procedure. This technique improves the detection of atrial activity and helps to differentiate the different types of atrial fibrillation. The automated FF interval recognition allows an efficient and time-saving analysis of atrial fibrillation patterns. The radar graph representation gives immediate feedback of beat-to-beat FF interval modifications provocated either by drugs or pacing.

Our study demonstrates that atrial pacing does not influence other than locally the atrial activation pattern during atrial fibrillation, even when delivered with the most appropriate sensing represented by MAP recording. Although we cannot conclude whether pacing results in a true capture of the local wavelets or in a simple variation of the local refractoriness, it has become evident the local pacing can affect local activation during atrial fibrillation.

References

1. Moe GK. On the multiple wavelet hypothesis of atrial fibrillation. *Arch Int Pharmacodyn Ther* 1962;140:183-188.
2. Allessie MA, Lammers WJEP, Bonke FIM, Hollen J. Experimental evaluation of Moe's multiple wavelet hypothesis of atrial fibrillation. In Zipes DP, Jalife J (eds): *Cardiac Arrhythmias*. New York: Grune & Stratton; 1985:265-276.
3. Cox JL, Canavan TE, Schuessler RB, et al. The surgical treatment of atrial fibrillation. II. Intraoperative electrophysiological mapping and description of the electrophysiological basis of atrial flutter and atrial fibrillation. *J Thorac Cardiovasc Surg* 1991;101:406-426.
4. Konings KTS, Kirchhof CJHJ, Smeets JRLM, et al. High density mapping of electrically induced atrial fibrillation in man. *Circulation* 1994;89:1665-1680.
5. Franz MR. Long term recording of monophasic action potential from human endocardium. *Am J Cardiol* 1983;51:1629-1633.
6. Franz MR. The role of monophasic action potential recording in atrial fibrillation. In Olsson SB, Allessie MA, Campbell RWF (eds): *Atrial Fibrillation: Mechanism and Therapeutic Strategies*. Armonk, NY: Futura Publishing Co., Inc.; 1996:109-125.
7. Barbaro V, Bartolini P, Bernarducci R, et al. An algorithm for the detection and the classification of atrial fibrillation from intra-atrial electrograms. *Proceedings of the VIII Mediterranean on Medical and Biological Engineering and Computing* (MEDICON "98), 1998; acts on CD Rom.
8. Bland JM, Altman DG. Statistical methods for assessing agreement between two methods of clinical measurement. *Lancet* 1986;1:307-310.
9. Allessie MA, Rensma PL, Lammers WJEP, Kirchhof CJHJ. The role of refractoriness conduction velocity and wavelength in initiation of atrial fibrillation in normal conscious dogs. In Attuel P, Coumel P, Janse MJ (eds): *The Atrium in Health and Disease*. Mount Kisco, NY: Futura Publishing Co., Inc.; 1989:27-41.
10. Ramdat Misier AR, Opthof T, Van Hemel NM, et al. Increased dispersion of refractoriness in patients with idiopathic paroxysmal atrial fibrillation. *J Am Coll Cardiol* 1992;19:1531-1535.
11. Lammers WJEP, Allessie MA, Rensma PL, Schalij MJ. The use of fibrillation cycle length to determine spatial dispersion in electrophysiological properties and to characterize the underlying mechanism of fibrillation. *New Trends Arrhythmias* 1986;2:109-112.
12. Wells JL, Karp RB, Kouchoukos NT, et al. Characterization of atrial fibrillation in man: Studies following open heart surgery. *PACE* 1978;1:426-438.
13. Waldo AL. Atrial fibrillation following open heart surgery. In Olsson SB, Allessie MA, Campbell RWF (eds): *Atrial Fibrillation: Mechanism and Therapeutic Strategies*. Armonk, NY: Futura Publishing Co., Inc.; 1996:211-223.
14. Kirchhof C, Chorro F, Jan Scheffer G, et al. Regional entrainment of atrial fibrillation by high-resolution mapping in open-chest dogs. *Circulation* 1993;88:736-749.

15. Capucci A, Biffi M, Boriani G, et al. Dynamic electrophysiological behaviour of human atria during paroxysmal atrial fibrillation. *Circulation* 1995;92:1193-1202.
16. Daoud E, Pariseau B, Niebauer M, et al. Response of type I atrial fibrillation to atrial pacing in humans. *Circulation* 1996;94:1036-1040.
17. Pandozi G, Bianconi L, Villani M, et al. Local capture by atrial pacing in spontaneous chronic atrial fibrillation. *Circulation* 1997;95:2416-2422.
18. Janse MJ, van der Steen ABM, van Dam RH, Durrer D. Refractory period of the dog's ventricular myocardium following sudden changes in frequency. *Circ Res* 1969;24:251-262.

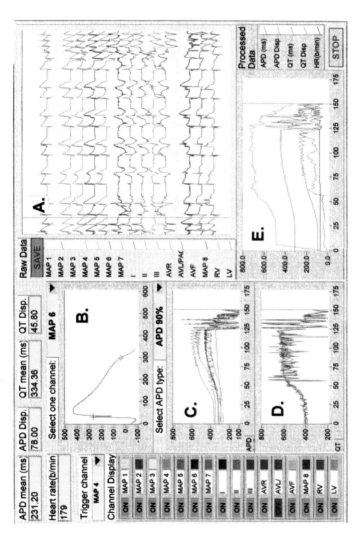

Figure 8-4. Front panel display of a real-time MAP analysis program during the induction of torsades de pointes with d-sotalol and low potassium. **A.** Original recordings from 10 MAP (top) and 6 electrocardiographic (ECG) leads. **B.** Enlarged MAP lead 6 with marks for the beginning and end of the action potential duration at 90% repolarization (APD$_{90}$) interval, measured for each beat. **C.** Beat-to-beat changes in APD$_{90}$ measurements from 10 MAP leads. Note the marked APD prolongation after approximately 25 beats and the progressively increasing APD alternans after 75 beats. **D.** QT measurements from 5 ECG leads (AVL display turned off). **E.** Display of mean APD$_{90}$, APD dispersion, mean QT duration, QT dispersion, and heart rate versus beat number.

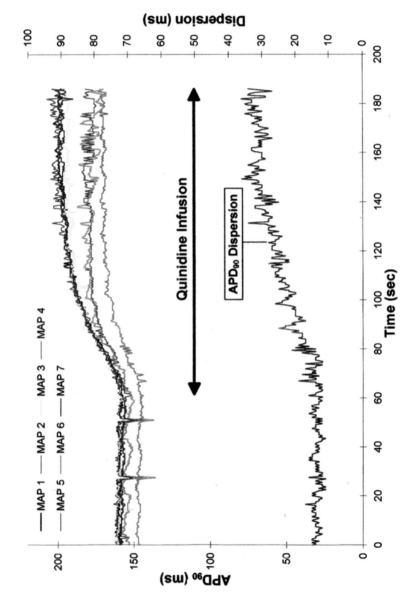

Figure 8-5. Real-time analysis of changes in APD$_{90}$ and dispersion of repolarization in response to perfusion with 20 µM quinidine in an isolated, perfused rabbit heart.

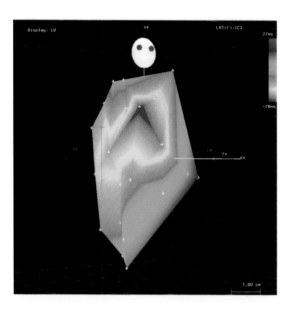

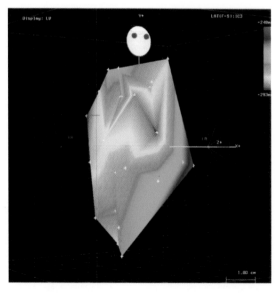

Figure 22-1. Right anterior oblique view of a 3-dimensional electroanatomic map of the swine left ventricle (LV). **A.** Activation map of the LV during sinus rhythm. The earliest activation site, represented by the red area is located at the anterosuperior septum. The activation then spread to the rest of the endocardium, with the postero-basal area activated last (blue and purple areas). Yellow and green represent areas with intermediate local activation times (LATs). Total activation time of this ventricle was 47 milliseconds. **B.** Activation-recovery interval (ARI) map of the same ventricle. Colors represent ARI values recorded at each site, with red corresponding to sites with the longest ARIs, blue and purple indicating short ARIs, and yellow and green representing areas with intermediate values. Note the homogenous gradient of ARI resembling the activation sequence, with the longest ARIs (red) located along the septum (earliest activation). *Continues.*

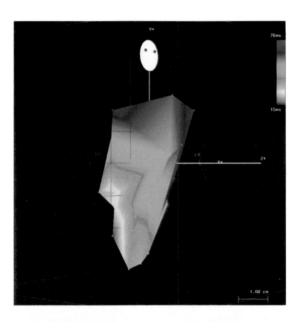

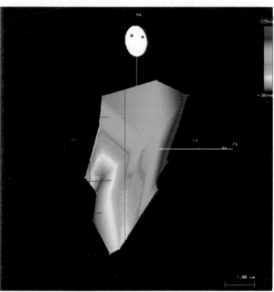

Figure 22-1 (*continued*). **C**. Activation map of the LV during pacing from the RV inferior septum (cycle length = 350 milliseconds). Total activation time was 61 milliseconds. **D**. ARI map of the same ventricle during pacing. Note again the inverse spatial correlation between ARIs and activation times, with the longest ARIs (red) located at the sites of earliest activation and than shortens gradually as activation proceeds.

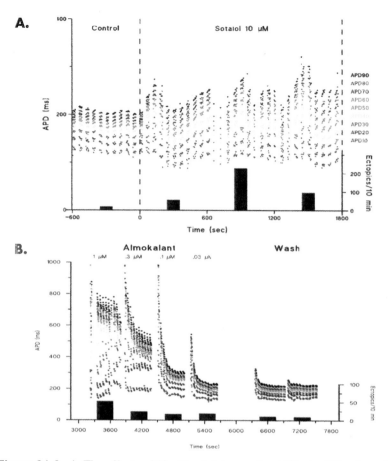

Figure 24-6. A. The effects of 10-μM sotalol upon the APD_{10} to APD_{90} (exp. 8321). Every minute, a train of 30 action potentials was applied at 1 Hz and the durations of every fourth nonectopic action potential are plotted (when there are many ectopics, fewer points are plotted, eg, from 660 to 780 seconds). Note that sotalol not only lengthens the APD, it also markedly slows repolarization especially between APD_{30} and ADP_{90}. In addition, the stability of the action potential is greatly reduced, especially between 40% and 80% repolarization: scatter of points is much increased, sometimes so markedly that the colors representing different APDs start mixing. **B.** The effects of almokalant (exp. 8537) on APD_{10} to APD_{90}. At 1 μM, the drug elicits numerous arrhythmias while the APD exhibits very marked variability. At 0.3 μM, the arrhythmias decline markedly but the variability remains extensive. Due to overlap of the points, the magnitude is somewhat underestimated. But note example APD_{10} and APD_{20}, and, although more difficult to see, the variability is even more marked as repolarization proceeds (see APD_{90}). At 0.1 μM there is only variability left at APD_{90}. At 0.03 μM the only remaining effect is the reverse use dependence (seen as a marked increase in APD following a long rest period). However, during wash also, this latter effect declines as the APDs approach the control values. Permission for publication of these data kindly provided by Dr. G. Duker from Astra-Hassle.

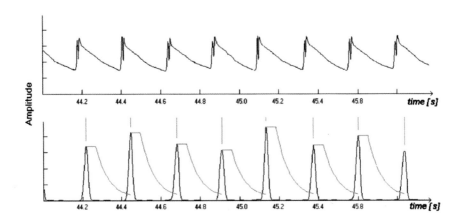

Figure 50-2. Example of the automated FF interval recognition. Top trace shows the original signal (MAP). Bottom trace shows the filtered signal used for the automated recognition procedure (black line) and the markers of the detected peaks (red lines). The exponential threshold is also depicted (blue lines).

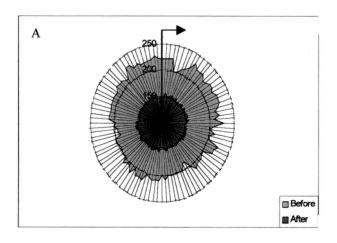

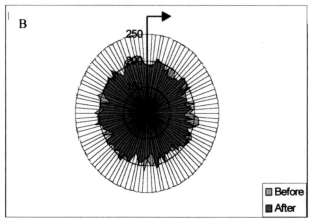

Figure 50-6. This figure shows 100 FF intervals plotted in radar graph representation. Mean FF intervals are depicted in blue before pacing and in red after pacing. The scale from center to top of figure indicates the FF intervals in milliseconds. Left: marked shortening of FF intervals after pacing (patient A). Right: absence of modification of FF intervals before and after pacing (patient B).

Index

878 • *Monophasic Action Potentials: Bridging Cell and Bedside*

QT dispersion
  M cell in, 596-597
  measurement of, 322-323
  ventricular recovery and, 327-328
  ventricular repolarization and, 337-338, 341-347
QT interval, 319-321
  antiarrhythmic drugs and, 307-308
  clinical correlates of, 330-334
  discussion of, 328-329
  electrolytes and, 258
  epicardial ventricular recovery and, 323-329
  exercise and, 258-259
  findings of, 327-328
  MAP recordings of, 323-324
  measurement of, 322-323
  potassium channel blockers and, 664
  real-time MAP analysis and, 139
  signals of, 324-327
  sympathetic stimulation and, 256-257
  temperature and, 257
  T wave and, 254-260
  ventricular arrhythmias and, 160, 163
  ventricular effective refractory period and, 166, 167
Quality criteria for monophasic action potential recordings, 135-136
Quinidine
  action potential duration and, 310, 311
  in atrial flutter, 426, 523-524
  in combination therapy, 479, 480
  ERP/APD modulation and, 96, 97
  M cells and, 585
  QT interval and, 664
  refractoriness and, 473-474
  reverse use dependence and, 476
  safety of, 432
  in sodium channel blockade, 387
  suction electrode method and, 10
  ventricular repolarization and, 307-308, 312, 313

Rabbit heart, isolated
  activation-repolarization sequence memory in, 149-156
  myocardial ischemia in, 195-207; *See also* Myocardial ischemia
  torsades de pointes and, 665-667, 668
  ventricular dilatation in, 679-692; *See also* Ventricular dilatation
  vulnerable window of fibrillation and, 396-397
Radar graph representation in atrial pacing, 860-861, 862
Radiofrequency-induced myocardial lesions, 807-821
  clinical implications of, 819
  data analysis of, 811
  discussion of, 815-818
  limitations of, 818-819
  MAP amplitude and, 812-815, 816
  methods for, 808-809, 810
  protocols for, 809-811
  simultaneously recorded MAP and, 812
  statistical analysis of, 811
Rapid pacing, 160-165
Rate adaptation of monophasic action potential duration, 11-13
Rate dependence, inverse, 433-438
Rate-dependent modulation of action potential duration, 147-288
  activation-repolarization sequence memory and, 149-156
  atrial memory and, 171-182; *See also* Atrial memory
  bradycardia and, 157-169; *See also* Bradycardia
  cardiac memory and, 183-193; *See also* Cardiac memory
  myocardial ischemia and, 195-225; *See also* Myocardial ischemia
  regional ischemia and reperfusion and, 271-288; *See also* Regional ischemia and reperfusion
  T wave alternans and vulnerability and, 253-269; *See also* T wave alternans
  ventricular vulnerability to reentry and fibrillation and, 227-251; *See also* Ventricular vulnerability to reentry and fibrillation
RBBB; *See* Right bundle branch block
Recovery in T wave alternans, 258-259
Reentry
  atrial flutter and, 512-513
  initiation of, 241, 242
  ventricular vulnerability to; *See* Ventricular vulnerability to reentry and fibrillation
Refractoriness
  altered loading conditions and, 695-702
  atrial fibrillation and, 828-829
  class Ia antiarrhythmic drugs and, 473-474